Health Literacy:

Breakthroughs in Research and Practice

Information Resources Management Association
USA

IGI GLOBAL
DISSEMINATOR OF KNOWLEDGE

www.igi-global.com

Published in the United States of America by
IGI Global
Medical Information Science Reference (an imprint of IGI Global)
701 E. Chocolate Avenue
Hershey PA, USA 17033
Tel: 717-533-8845
Fax: 717-533-8661
E-mail: cust@igi-global.com
Web site: http://www.igi-global.com

Library of Congress Cataloging-in-Publication Data

Names: Information Resources Management Association, editor.
Title: Health literacy : breakthroughs in research and practice / Information Resources Management Association, editor.
Other titles: Health literacy (Information Resources Management Association)
Description: Hershey, PA : Medical Information Science Reference, [2017] | Includes bibliographical references.
Identifiers: LCCN 2016049645| ISBN 9781522519287 (hardcover) | ISBN 9781522519294 (ebook)
Subjects: | MESH: Health Literacy--trends | Health Communication--trends
Classification: LCC RA418 | NLM WA 590 | DDC 362.1--dc23 LC record available at https://lccn.loc.gov/2016049645

British Cataloguing in Publication Data
A Cataloguing in Publication record for this book is available from the British Library.

For electronic access to this publication, please contact: eresources@igi-global.com.

List of Contributors

Table of Contents

Preface

The constantly changing landscape surrounding health literacy makes it challenging for experts and practitioners to stay informed of the field's most up-to-date research. That is why IGI Global is pleased to offer this one-volume comprehensive reference collection that will empower students, researchers, and academicians with a strong understanding of these critical issues by providing both broad and detailed perspectives on cutting-edge theories and developments. This compilation is designed to act as a single reference source on conceptual, methodological, and technical aspects, as well as to provide insight into emerging trends and future opportunities within the discipline.

Health Literacy: Breakthroughs in Research and Practice is organized into four sections that provide comprehensive coverage of important topics. The sections are:

1. Health Technology
2. Medical Practice and Treatment
3. Patient Care
4. Patient Education

The following paragraphs provide a summary of what to expect from this invaluable reference source:

Section 1, "Health Technology," opens this extensive reference source by highlighting the latest computational tools in the medical industry. Through perspectives on web-based communication, electronic health records, and gamification, this section demonstrates the benefits and importance of e-health initiatives. The presented research facilitates a better understanding of how emerging technologies are transforming healthcare delivery and medical practices.

Section 2, "Medical Practice and Treatment," includes chapters on emerging strategies for optimized procedures and processes in medical treatment. Including discussions on medical errors, chronic disease, and healthcare service delivery, this section presents research on the latest trends and practices in medical institutions. This inclusive information assists in advancing current practices in medical treatment.

Section 3, "Patient Care," presents coverage on the improvement of patient care strategies. Through innovative discussions on multimedia, social networking, and the aging population, this section highlights the changing scope of patient engagement. These inclusive perspectives contribute to the available knowledge on optimizing patient care in contemporary healthcare settings.

Section 4, "Patient Education," discusses coverage and research perspectives on the promote health education initiatives in contemporary society. Through analyses on decision making, women's health, and technological tools, this section contains pivotal information on the latest developments in patient education. The presented research facilitates a comprehensive understanding of how medical information and knowledge transforms the landscape of patient care.

Although the primary organization of the contents in this work is based on its four sections, offering a progression of coverage of the important concepts, methodologies, technologies, applications, social issues, and emerging trends, the reader can also identify specific contents by utilizing the extensive indexing system listed at the end.

As a comprehensive collection of research on the latest findings related to Health Literacy. *Health Literacy: Breakthroughs in Research and Practice* provides researchers, practitioners, and all audiences with a complete understanding of the development of applications and concepts surrounding these critical issues.

Section 1
Health Technology

Chapter 1
Health, Digitalization, and Individual Empowerment

Alena Lagumdzija
Karolinska University Hospital, Sweden

Velmarie King Swing
Southern Nazarene University, USA

ABSTRACT

Internet, eHealth and digitalization have opened information access for patients and medical health users. Digitalization provides an opportunity for telemedicine, storage of Electronic Patient Records (EPRs) and net communication for both medical staff and patients with access. Digitalization and technical improvement have increased the usage of Internet based technologies and telephones for positive health coaching and digital-learning applications for all medical users, school staff, and students. The effect of Information Technology on healthcare and medical services can be described as revolutionary. Increasingly, the utilization of digital equipment and medical technology are employed in patients' homes.

INTRODUCTION

The term 'information society', which encapsulates globalization and Information Technology (IT) phenomena, is often used to describe a society in which data production and consumption becomes increasingly vital in society functions. Many individuals are connected to different networks of one form or another in an information society. Such networks include cable and satellite television, telephone, computer-to-computer, person to computer communications and online information services (Webster, 2014). There are many benefits of IT in healthcare including the utilization of computer software application programs to enhance safety, efficiency, and real-time decision support to medical and healthcare practitioners (Blumenthal & Tavenner, 2010). IT presents solutions to current complex healthcare challenges. Progress from IT comes with higher medical expenses (Callahan, 2008; Deloitte Centre for health solutions, 2015; Wang et al., 2003). Also, long-term care of individuals and the cost of hospitalization are increasing significantly in different countries for different reasons (Callahan, 2008).

DOI: 10.4018/978-1-5225-1928-7.ch001

Several complementary investments are required for the integration of successful techniques in organizational, business, and educational developments. In other words, Information Technology does not simply mean the implementation of new technology. The need to adapt and integrate existing systems with care work operations and processes is essential. Equally essential is the education of clinical personnel, nurses, and physicians. Finally, an integrative approach to the resolution of legal issues and responsibilities associated with home and ambulatory care is essential.

The first objective of the chapter, from a Swedish perspective, is to explore the above issues and highlight the importance and difficulties involved in using information technology in globalized healthcare and medical services. These measures are concerns of politicians, policy-makers, healthcare authorities, schools, and private participants. The second objective is to explore how the information society has dealt with the challenge of integrating IT in healthcare in response to citizens' expectations and requirements.

Cost of Healthcare

Rapid development in medical science can offer new medical solutions, however, with potential high costs. Future development and improvement of medical techniques should relieve the currently overloaded primary healthcare system. Ethical concerns include justification of cost constrained solutions to the increasing complexity of individuals' health requirements. Technical progress is more than a prerequisite for the integration of information technology in healthcare and medicine.

Many countries are facing an aging population, which requires increased budgetary allocations for the elderly segment of the population due to disproportionate healthcare costs. For example, Sweden and Japan are countries known for low mortality. According to the World Health organization (WHO, 2014), Life expectancy for women in Japan is 87, the longest in the world. This is followed by Spain, Switzerland and Singapore. Men in Japan have a life expectancy of 80 years. life expectancy in Sweden it is 81.1 years (OECD, 2013). However, individuals with increased longevity can experience poor health from diseases such as dementia, mental health disorders, cancer, diabetes or other ailments. Possible chronic diseases or mental health illnesses may require multiple points of care by primary and specialist health care providers. Increased life expectancy drives the need for treatment capabilities in terms of long-term treatments and planning across complex care provider chains (Gröne, & Garcia-Barbero, 2001; Kodner, & Spreeuwenberg, 2002; Mur-Veeman, Raak van, & Paulus, 2008). Chronic diseases can require more than one point of care. The multiple care points can cause potential risks of errors that can cause additional health complications.

Information Technology

Documentation and regulatory compliance activities detract from actual face-to-face meeting between patient and medical staff. In the past years, technology push has been increasing. The term 'technology push' refers to new technology research and development that drives the production and sales of new products onto the market without market research or proper consideration of whether or not such products satisfy individual needs (Martin, 1994). Examples of technology push in medical care include wearable technologies such as bio-sensing wearables, digital hearing aids, blood pressure monitors and so on. Technology-Enabled Care (TEC), and collecting telemedicine, telecare, digital and mobile health are also examples of eHealth. Cultural and regulatory barriers to the adoption of TEC in different countries, the record keeping, digitalization, physician consultation problems as well as the national care agreements and guarantors are hot topics in the globalized world (Deloitte Centre for health solutions, 2015).

The effect of Information Technology on healthcare and medical services can be described as revolutionary. Increasingly, the utilization of digital equipment and medical technology are employed in patients' homes. The home environment would relieve nursing care, reduce transportation costs and the eventual medical intervention can occur at an earlier stage of the disease process. A study by Lindberg, Nilsson, Zotterman, Söderberg, and Skär, (2013) found that patients who utilized telecare at home preferred a combination of telecare and traditional healthcare delivery. Moreover, healthcare professionals could use Information and Communication Technology (ICT) applications in homecare as a tool to support people living with chronic illnesses (Lindberg et al. 2013). This brings up questions on how individuals can take advantage of technologies to improve their life and how digitalization of healthcare can help individuals become healthier?

The first indication of improvements is in the use of technology such as synchronized IT systems and centralized patients´ medical records to make the medical and healthcare system more efficient. Centralized medical records are necessary because many countries in the world, European and Japan are facing challenges of an aging society. A report by the Organization for Economic Cooperation and Development (OECD) showed that in 2011 the average life expectancy exceeded 80 years across OECD countries. Individual Swiss, Japanese, and Italians are expected to live longest among OECD countries (OECD, 2013).

Advancements in technology have caused greater availability of data for medical professionals and made data driven analysis possible for a variety of clinical methods. Data can be collected, processed into information, and accessed across the healthcare provider chain to effectively advance a patient´s status and treatment. However, digitalization of medical records has been developed using a top-down approach that affects the push of technology solutions in the medical industry.

A second response has been to engage people and help them take active and preventive care of their own health and to deal with current medical problems (OECD, 2013). With increased general welfare and rapid technology development, the Internet is currently considered as a basic standard service in everyday life. To facilitate communication between patients and clinicians, many health care providers have developed digital guides for those who need orientation in how to manage personal medical problem. The digital guides also connect patients with similar medical problems to collaborate in collecting relevant information. Swedish residents, for example, can study digitally available information about the medical treatment and results obtained by health providers in different areas (Sveriges Riksdag, 2012).

When prepared patients succeed in establishing a good dialog with the medical staff, increased understanding of the diagnosis can further motivated the patients to participate in the recommended treatment. As understanding of individual diagnosis increases, patients will more likely seek second and third opinions about treatment options. A third response is to develop technical and institutional solutions. Given the fact that many countries have aging societies, improved knowledge of IT and healthcare providers is essential in the development of technical and institutional solutions that connect providers and patients.

When considering the use of distance medical services, the legality of who is responsible should problems arise, need to be addressed. Additionally, retention of experienced personnel with technology and service provider activities may assist in the cost effectiveness of resolving issues.

In 2012 there were over 40,000 medical and health related apps, available for smartphones (Pelletier, 2012). This provides the opportunity for learning, but is also very important that everyone can share benefits regardless of the age and status. However, validation of information may become difficult and contextualizing within a particular situation. Enhanced individualized learning opportunities and searching in the 'overflow of information' is essential in discovering how to utilize available options and effectively evaluate information.

An example is the use of digital systems by a specialist while leading a surgery team at a distance. Teleconsultations are now widespread in almost all developed and developing countries (Jennett, et al., 2004) and empowers patients and facilitates disease management by allowing physicians and patients to confer on specific plans of care, specifically in cases where a control of a given disease, such as diabetes, depends on patients' self-care endeavour. Telemedicine technology is also useful in the identification of disaster victims and the administration of triage, which is typically the first step in pre-hospital medical treatment and transportation of casualties. As underdeveloped countries catch up with the digital requirements, i.e., the Internet and the World Wide Web, teleconsultations are certain to spread to such countries.

Individual Empowerment

As one of the world's most computer mature nations, Sweden is far ahead in terms of technology for the creation and implementation of e-courses at universities, secondary schools and companies. The Swedish schools are increasing applications of ICT as teaching tools needed to achieve their aims. The program, ICT for Everyone, which is a Digital Agenda for Sweden, proposed that Swedish school-children and teachers should have access to modern learning tools that are required for contemporary education and that every student, on completing primary and lower secondary school, should be able to use modern technology as a tool for knowledge-seeking, communication, creation and learning (Swedish Ministry of Enterprise, Energy and Communications [SMEEC], 2011). To apply knowledge, teachers need to be competent in usage of digital equipment and have a clear vision of how and why digital tools are used. Every individual learns in a different way. By using digital programs, teachers can customize pedagogical methods at different levels of school education and give students the tools, knowledge and digital skills required to understand the Internet and the digital environment (MEEC, 2011).

Moreover, present generations are accustomed to searching for new information and communicating with each other through computers, mobiles and digital games. Essary (2011) reported that 75% of millennials are connected to the Internet through Facebook. However, despite e-learning advantages, personal student-teacher contact can be lacking the relationships one develops with classmates in a classroom and school in the online setting. University students create social networks that are both personality stimulating and a place to make friends for life. It can also be difficult to replace the daily discussions with classmates, teachers or friends at campus.

The rapid IT and ICT progress that have so far been achieved could make traditional universities leery of e-learning. Sweden and other developed countries are facing revolutionary changes in high education. Although a large majority has not succumbed to it, many US universities currently provide courses online. Allen and Seaman (2013) have reported that by the fall of 2002, 1.6 million higher education students were taking courses online. Allen and Seaman also reported that 62.4% of higher education institutions began offering complete online programs in 2012 compared to 34.5% who did in 2002.

Unlike the United States, Japan, UK, Ireland, Australia (OECD, 2012), Swedes view higher education as a non-commercial product. Education in Sweden is a public practice with 40% of the population of 8.3 million enrolled (Boucher, 2014). For example, there are over a million 7-17 year-olds in compulsory basic education (*Grundskola*), 16-19 year-olds enrolled in integrated upper secondary school (*Gymnasieskola*), and 270,000 adults taking school level courses administered by local governments

(Swedish National Agency for Education, 2016). If the Swedish students in the future choose MOOC trainings it is likely that it will negatively affect the municipalities with higher education institutions. However, the use of online courses could have greater implications for developing countries when the cost of technology is calculated.

Distance learning and e-learning became popular concepts in the discussions on IT and educational issues. This concept in Sweden has been replaced by 'flexible learning'. A common international term, 'blended education' is a combination of e-learning and traditional learning, which address the different forms of teaching and learning. Perhaps the IT-health sector could learn from the education system so that the 'e-Health' is regarded as an integrated part of 'health' and not something outside or alternative to 'health'

Globalization

Globalization has allowed the transfer of patients, capital, knowledge, technology, and other services across borders. In recent years globalization has increased rapidly. Globalization has provided the ability for establishing stronger relationships between developed and developing nations. However, globalization can have positive and negative outcomes. A positive affect is increased accessibility to medical services, which promises to be one of the defining attributes of the 21st century. Apart from ethical considerations, the transmigration of medical personnel, from advanced economies to impoverished countries, is one of the benefits accruing to individuals the world over. Advancements in science have contributed to preventive healthcare by reducing the prospect of an individual acquiring severe and life-threatening illnesses. It is important to note that global communication technologies facilitate increases in scientific communications, information, knowledge sharing and the development of new techniques, methods, medicines, and vaccines. Tracking and monitoring outbreaks of particular diseases has been enhanced by IT.

Migration of highly trained medical specialists from thinly populated countries, e.g., Island (Solberg, et al., 2013) to other countries and cultures in reaction to economic conditions is one of the disadvantages of globalization. Another example of the disadvantages of globalization is the growing migration, tourism, and increased spread of infectious diseases such as, for instance, SARS and EBOLA, that can potentially exert a negative influence on both poor and rich countries (Pang & Guindon, 2004). Globalization can lead to increased exchange and influence of different cultures, customs, attitudes and philosophies of life. Regarding migration, a previous study explored the effects of poor working conditions and a desire for greater access to enhanced equipment and technology in medical care can be important (Astor, et al., 2005).

While longevity can reflect good health, ageing societies such as Japan, Germany, and Sweden are experiencing falling fertility rates, declining workforce, and increasing medical costs (Harper, 2013). Sweden's ageing society has increasing needs and associated costs for the medical services and emergency transportation (The Swedish Association of Local Authorities and Regions, 2014). For example, in 2014, the Swedish elderly care and nursing costs were approximately 25% of total costs (The Swedish Association of Local Authorities and Regions, 2014). In addition, most hospitals are overburdened and there is shortage of doctors, particularly in rural areas and in home care for elderly. However, elderly individuals prefer, as much as possible, to receive medical services at home (Burholt, & Naylor, 2005; Linhart, 2010; Dale, et al., 2008). In Sweden, the demographic aspect of an increasing aging population is only a partial portion of the burden on society. Providing an increased quality of life is becoming a higher priority.

Since the early 1990's, EU implemented a high-quality eHealth to facilitate obtaining healthcare in other European member states. The program´s goal was to secure infrastructure and coordinate communication between cross-border regions, healthcare stakeholders, the system and the citizen (European Commission, 2007).

An example of implemented projects is the European Health Insurance Card (EHIC) introduced across the European Union in 2004. The EHIC allows EU citizens to access healthcare while traveling and instantaneously assured participating hospitals accept the insurance of travellers and guaranteed fast reimbursement via electronic transfer of administrative data (European Commission, 2007, 2015). Additionally, the European eHealth initiated a commitment by all EU member states to develop eHealth schemes providing a transparent view of the eHealth national landscapes. The vision of EU was that European eHealth space should be able to deliver high quality healthcare to all European citizens independent of the location when in need of acute or medical care (European Commission, 2007).

The implementation of eHealth across Europe has progressed and an example is the EU project known as epSOS (Smart Open Services for European Patients). The epSOS was a European large-scale project financed and guaranteed by the EU and the 23 Member States. The project´s goal was to implement cross-border exchanges of electronic medical information and connect EU member countries by eHealth. The connection can improve patient care by using the electronic patient record system when citizens traveling abroad are in need of help (Linden, 2009). The epSOS program will allow health professionals to access patient records and eHealth information in doctors' original languages with an original copy.

Currently, epSOS consists of patient summary and ePrescriptions. The patient summary contains information from the patients' home countries, i.e., patient´s name, gender, birth, a list of the current medication. Crucial clinical patient data – current medical issues, allergies, major surgical procedures are also included in the epSOS. For security and protocol purposes, a recording of the information about whom and when treatment occurred is generated and updated. The epSOS and ePrescriptions contain the current prescriptions in patients' home countries and are transmitted electronically to pharmacies in countries using the epSOS system.

Primary Care vs. National Systems Computing

Sweden has provided digitalization and boosted personal empowerment through the common use of computers in Swedish homes. The rapid progress of digitalization occurred in the middle of the 1990s across diverse sectors of the society, including the medical segment. In 2010 Internet access in Sweden was 88.3% of all households, compared with Japan's 78% household Internet access in the same period (OECD, 2015).

Scandinavian countries (Denmark, Sweden, and Norway) are among the most advanced in terms of operational telecommunication infrastructure, broadband connection and fully operational national Information and Communication Technology infrastructures for communications support in the health sector (European Commission, 2007). In primary healthcare, providers are required to deliver preventive and acute care, thus facing the challenge of integrating and managing an enormous amount of information.

For enhanced coordination of patient care, Swedish healthcare providers have utilized Electronic Health Records (EHR) for prescriptions since 1997. In 2012, the EHR was fully implemented in Swedish primary care, hospitals, and psychiatry. EHR contain information from all providers involved in patient´s care. EHR allows a patient´s health record to move to other health care providers, hospitals, nursing homes and even across national borders. EHR allows instant access to information about patients' medical history, and became a valuable tool in crisis, enabling providers to reduce time in making treatment decisions.

Three factors that have contributed to the accessibility of information for both patients and medical professionals are: the Internet, eHealth, and digitalization. Digitalization provides an opportunity for many things including telemedicine, storage, retrieval of electronic patient records (EPRs), and communication among medical staff and patients. Digitalization and technical improvement have increased the usage of Internet based technologies and telephones for positive health coaching and digital-learning applications for all medical users, school staff, and students.

Beside advancements in Information and Communication technology (ICT) infrastructure, Sweden is unique in terms of citizens´ registration by personal identity number, utilizing the Modulus-10-system that is considered a very secure system and organized identification of citizens with very low or no risk for mixing people up (Ludvigsson, Otterblad-Olausson, Pettersson, & Ekbom, 2009). However, there is no single centralized national database for patients' medical records to date. An interesting note about Sweden is the ability to have centralized ePrescriptions, however, it lacks the centralized national patient records. A council of 21 counties, 290 municipalities, private organizations, and the central government share the centralization of records. There are no hierarchical relationships. Each county, council, and municipality can have individual self-governing local authorities and budgets for medical services with responsibility for different activities. The exception is the Swedish island of Gotland, where the municipality has the responsibilities and tasks normally associated with a county council.

The fractured structure can make communication and decision-making difficult. Part of the reason is that the system was constructed by IT specialists in the medical sector, who designed and developed a top-down system with inadequate knowledge or experience in business operations. Very few have a complete command over both information technologies and the business operations. Consequently, multiple IT medical record systems in use are difficult to connect to one common system.

There are advantages with an organizational structure such as the Swedish system, however, reaching a national or European level of connecting systems may be difficult. Undoubtedly, Swedish citizens are open-minded, however cautious. The government is focused on efforts to deploy various departments and authorities that would provide and control the future security of personal information access and transfer. This added complex hierarchy of authority renders the decision-making and implementation process more complicated. Examples of the supervisory authorities within the health sector are the Swedish Government Agency Health and Social Care Inspectorate and the Swedish eHealth Agency. The newly created authorities are aiming to increase the development of the national eHealth infrastructure, e.g. individuals' access to individual medical health records by personal health account and e-prescriptions.

Another authority that the Swedish government initiated was the National Patient Summary (*Nationell Patientöversikt, NPÖ*). The aim of NPÖ is to increase cooperation by making it possible for all health care providers, including private ones, to directly access a patient's medical records that are stored by other health care providers, provided all legal requirements are fulfilled (Jerlvall, & Pehrsson, 2012).

In contrast to Sweden, Norway and Denmark use national eHealth infrastructures that support electronic exchange of various healthcare related messaging and other services. Meanwhile, Finland's regional networks are allowing the exchange of various types of patient records (European Commission, 2007). However, there are many differences and common challenges between regions and countries in the delivery and founding of medical care (Hall & Walton, 2004; Haux, Ammenwerth, Herzog, & Knaup, 2002; Nytrø & Faxvaag, 2004). One example of a common challenge for both Sweden and Denmark is that hospitals are mainly public and are a part of the regional healthcare structure. Hospital departments and healthcare canters are responsible for individual facility budgetary control (Glenngård et al., 2005; Kjellberg et al., 2007). Facility budgets may create a limited initiative for increased activities in the healthcare centres or hospital departments.

The current payment system fails to reward cross-sectoral activities, which contributes to a lack of collaboration between hospital departments and healthcare centres (Glenngård et al., 2005; Vrangbaek & Christiansen, 2005). In turn, the lack of collaboration results in IT systems with different development levels and functional scopes.

Future points for consideration are the IT systems synchronizations and solutions. In order to respond effectively, the government has to find a balance between bottom-up and top-down dialog to identify common system requirements and goals. An essential aspect of the system development either in public, private, or medical sectors, is the application of preliminary solution plan known as 'Architectural principle' (Lindström, 2005). The architectural principle describes how to synchronize information content systems with each other. Systems that should communicate with other systems are also described, along with the person in charge of managing all systems. There is also the guidance required for specifications and evaluation of different alternatives that can affect decision making for IT product purchase and technique choices (Lindström, 2005).

Challenges of Digitalization

Addressing differences in healthcare between patients that have Internet access and those that lack connection is imperative to ensure that healthcare is provided for all. Sweden was identified as a world leader in the use of Information and Communication Technology (ICT), which contributed to the country's productivity growth. Since 2002, Sweden's 80 public hospitals, 800 primary care centres, 950 pharmacies and large number of private healthcare centres have been connected via *Sjunet*, a federated fibre-optical eHealth network (SMHSA, 2006; Stroetmann, Dobrev, Lilischkis, & Stroetmann, 2014). The Sjunet, which was developed as a regional project separated from the Internet, allows a secure exchange of confidential data, e.g., patient`s personal data, pictures and medical applications, images, e-prescription system and video conferencing. Additionally, Sjunet links regional administrations, pharmacies, health care, and county councils.

eHealth and the national social services efforts are focused on practical improvements in Swedish industries, healthcare, medical and social services. According to SMEEC (2011), the correct use of technology could allow physicians to receive all relevant information from the electronic patient medical record regarding severely ill patients that are admitted to the emergency or hospital wards.

On the other hand, beside positive Internet effects, privacy and identity security issues are some of problems that are often associated with being a member of a social network. There is also a new trend for bulling in schools or at working places thru mobile messages, social networking, or mails. Computers allow people to become victims of the so-called cyber-bullying (Hiduja, & Patchin, 2010). Internet access opens many ways for harassment and bullying that invade the lives of victims. Cyber-bullying can lead to more depression, discouragement, loneliness, and in the worst-case scenario, suicide (Hiduja, & Patchin, 2010).

Visiting social media Web sites are common activities of many technology savvy learners. However, dangers persist for those vulnerable children. Whereas many millennials are conversant with the Internet, some are exposed to cyber crimes, including bullying, extortion, and the like (Tokunaga, 2010). Children, 30 percent of whom use the Internet without parental supervision (ChildrenOnline, 2015), are exposed to the dangers of being dragged from home because they click with cyber tormenters. The number of children and teens that are exposed to crime on the Internet from home is rapidly growing. According to ChildrenOnline, one in every 25 teenagers has received online sexual solicitation and more than 70 percent between the ages of 12 and 17 have social media profile.

Cyber crime demands the attention of everyone, including patients, parents, school and medical administrators (Keith, & Martin, 2005). To prevent Internet harassment, it is crucial to teach users and creators of all ages early. Given that online education and telemedicine are here to stay as aspect of the 21st-Century culture, it is important to offer education that will help learners become aware of the pros and cons of online learning, including the ethics, safely, and legal issues at the early stages of schooling (*Digitaliseringskommissionen*, 2014).

The Wealth of Health (Medical Tourism)

The use of digital health across Europe has become increasingly globalized. Digital health has progressed from public discussions to applied eHealth and medical services. More patients, often from high-income EU countries, cross borders to developing countries in order to seek treatment and different types of medical services. The reasons are either shorter waiting time or lower cost of health service in developing countries. The trend has become known as medical tourism.

The definition of medical tourism takes into account the territorially bounded nature of health systems, where access to healthcare is often but not always limited to national boundaries (Carrera, & Bridges, 2006). Medical tourism constitutes an individual solution to what is traditionally considered a government concern in Sweden. Individuals, mostly from richer countries, basically try to solve their health problems by seeking cheaper and efficient treatment, mostly from relatively poorer countries in Asian and Latin America. In 2003, it is reported that nearly 350,000 patient travelled from developed countries as medical tourists to developing countries (Horowitz, Rosensweig, & Jones, 2007).

Notably, the health sector in Southeast Asia is expanding rapidly, attributable to rapid growth of the private sector and, medical tourism, which is emerging as a lucrative business opportunity (Pocock, & Phua, 2011). These countries combine high quality medical services and competitive pricing with tourist packages in capitalizing on the popularity of medical patients as tourist. Thailand, for example, has established cosmetic surgery and sex change operations, while Singapore is attracting patients at the high end of the market for advanced treatments such as cardiovascular and neurological surgeries and stem cell therapy (Pocock, & Phua, 2011; UNESCAP, 2007). In addition, Singapore, Malaysia and Thailand alone, had an estimated 2 million medical travellers visiting in 2006-2007 with earning of over US $ 3 billion in treatment costs (Pocock, & Phua, 2011). Many poor countries find it difficult to retain medical staff attracted by higher pay in rich countries.

Indeed, medical tourism can bring economic benefits to countries, including additional resources for investment in healthcare. However, unless properly managed and regulated on the policy side, the financial benefits of medical tourism for health systems may come at the expense of access and use of health services by local consumers. Pocock and Phua (2011) argued that governments and industry players would do well to remember that health is wealth for both foreign and local populations.

Generally speaking, the relationship among globalization, the medical sector, and education development is complex. Increased globalization makes it easier for medical workers to migrate to other countries (Mahroum, 2001). It can as well provide opportunities for high-income countries to increase economic investment and enhanced technology for developing countries. There is also potential to learn from countries that may be ahead in planning and development.

While it is important to observe recent improvements in telemedicine (Jennett, et al., 2004), especially in the treatment of prisoners, military personnel, and victims of natural disaster, at the same time it is necessary to be aware that more training is needed in order to extend the trend to more peoples of the world, including people in poorer countries. Although various studies suggest that telemedicine through teleconsultation is acceptable to a great number of patients, Perednia, and Allen (1995) found that further studies are needed to derive its precise health benefits.

Health, Linguistic and Cultural Divide

The progress in medical science and development of new therapies significantly reduced the need for hospital care. Nonetheless, it is predicted that there will not be enough resources for the healthcare sector due to rapid demographic changes (Anell, Glenngård, & Merkur, 2012). To accommodate the increased demand on healthcare, higher technical knowledge and further progress in development and usage of medical digital equipment are needed. For example, robots are being developed to assist family members or medical staff involved in homecare.

Patients do not always use the Emergency Department (ED) to conform to the original design and for the intended purpose. The ED is a specialized service equipped with specialized resources and personnel for the treatment of urgent and emergency life-threatening problems. However, research shows that Emergency Department personnel are routinely assigned to patients that do not meet the criteria of life-threatening emergency needs. According to Göransson, Ehrenberg, and Ehnfors (2005), 81% ED staff were assigned to patients who did not arrive at the hospital by ambulance.

Inequality happens to show a certain degree of pervasiveness in the Swedish health and medical system. While life expectancy for both men and women has improved, such improvement does not extend to people employed in menial jobs (Whitehead, Evandrou, Haglund, & Diderichsen, 1997). Apart from individual health conditions and wellbeing, attributes that determine the quality of a good health care system, from a European perspective, includes but not limited to, (a) the comfort of the physical environment, (b) availability of information, (c) adequate communication, (d), interpersonal relations between health care personnel–nurses, physicians, technicians, and the like (Johansson, Oleni, & Fridlund, 2002). If an individual were able to establish a dialogue with medical staff, she/he would be able to acquire a better understanding of his diagnosis, which in turn would help, to a large degree, his prognosis communication with a physician. It might help the patient become more motivated toward recommended treatment.

Individual empowerment is possible in health care due to the current Digital Age of the World Wide Web of Internet connections. The Internet allows the proliferation of apps that can collect and dispense medial information to promote and maintain healthy lifestyles as well as to treat various illnesses. Given the rampant nature of Internet provided information, it is important that patients are able to distinguish valuable and valueless information (Metzger, & Flanagin, 2013). As Cassel and Guest (2012) have suggested, the quantity of care and information is not necessarily equivalent to quality care and information. Nonetheless, well-informed patients should be capable of preventing or diagnosing disease by themselves.

Electronic health records enable the transfer and analysis of patient data among healthcare professionals. Despite the progress that have been made in Information and Communication Technology (ICT), there is still planet of room for growth (Aarts, & Berg, 2006; Aarts, Doorewaard & Berg 2004;

Littlejohns, Wyatt, & Garvican, 2003; Wears, & Berg 2005). In addition, ICT adoption by healthcare organizations is a slow process and Sweden is not the only country facing slow progression of ICT utilization. Professor emeritus K. Lundgren (2007) from Swedish Royal Institute of Technology claimed that approximately 70% of IT projects worldwide are unsuccessful. Electronic Health Record (EHR) systems are rarely successfully implemented in countries other than where they were developed (Kajbjer, Nordberg, & Klein, 2010).

What began as a series of pilot projects, computerized health support system has been available in Swedish hospitals as early as the mid-1960. The Karolinska Hospital in the Stockholm region gained notoriety due to the implementation of batch processing of medical records, limited in volume and scope nonetheless (Kajbjer et al, 2010). In the 1970s and early 1980s a system known as PAX was developed locally, in Gothenburg. A central mainframe computer with dumb terminals was developed to help manage patient invoicing and the allocation of hospital beds. Computerized in primary care medial records system was implemented in the mid-1980s. Among many commercialized computerized systems imported from Norway, Denmark, or Iceland in the 1990s, Journal III, Melior, and VAS were in use in Sweden. By 2009, approximately 85% of hospital wards were using Electronic Health Record (EHRs).

Kajbjer et al. (2010) explained that the popularity of these system is based on the fact that the clinical staff, nurses, and physicians were allowed to influence many of the details regarding how the system functions, although it took more than twenty years after the initial trials before EHR system was installed in the Swedish primary care. It is important that eHealth is based on a solid foundational structural where information processes are analyzed and management has established clear operational procedures. However, efforts to establish national information structures, standardizations, and the like, have either been delayed or failed to take hold. Many information systems have failed to communicate with each other because of technical, organizational, institutional, or frequent problems with security and reliability (Lundgren, 2007).

In many areas, including the home care environment, digitalization has neither contributed to improvements in working conditions, nor ensured better relationships with elderly patients. Digitalization in the home care environment has diminished individual autonomy and exerted increased external control over patients. In other words, rather than dialogues with the patient, digitalization has guaranteed bureaucratic demands. This is often the case in the medical sector. The organization is divided in autonomous island structures rather than a synchronized whole with clear goals and strategies.

The lack of dialog is partly one reason for many IT-projects to fail. According to previously published reports, large public sector IT-projects may experience failure because of inadequate dialog and knowledge transfer between management and IT-professionals, and because of unclear formulation of operational strategy development (Swedish National Audit Office, 2002). The famous American innovation researcher, von Hippel, stated that technical knowledge was more general, i.e., it was easier to communicate with a counterpart than it is for organizations to communicate its knowledge to suppliers (von Hippel, 1994, 1998). Knowledge of an organization´s goal, together with its customers, suppliers, as well as the knowledge and relationship among co-workers, are often based on specific company experience. For von Hippel (1994, 1998), the rational process is to make users solve problems and generate technical knowledge within an organization than to hire technicians from outside, who are not familiar with the organisation´s goal, to take that responsibility. von Hippel also pointed out that it would be more rational if more IT-technicians were hired by IT consuming organizations rather than within the IT producing companies, wich could allow the development of competence of the IT users' information solutions (von Hippel, 1994, 1998).

eHealth can enhance individual wellbeing by making important information available to healthcare professionals, independent of their location. However, eHealth requires developmental demands, which include educating people and finding ways to reach those that are not so easy to reach. Because of the digital nature of data, which is transmitted over the Internet, monitoring patients involves issues relating to security and privacy (Atkinson & Gold, 2002). The balance between security and efficiency constitutes a challenging risk factor.

The current healthcare system in Sweden has long been known to suffer many problems (Hjern, Grindefjord, Sundberg, & Rosén, 2001; Wahlberg, Cedersund, & Wredling, 2003). There are problems of communication among government institutions, IT-professionals, patients and professional care providers. Effective and enduring solutions in healthcare are connected to leadership as an all-complex organization.

FUTURE RESEARCH DIRECTIONS

The role of patients in the healthcare sector is essential for a fully functional medical and healthcare system. Future challenges include a determination of the means by which citizens can effectively use Information Technology as a tool for managing their own health. Possible innovation processes in IT within the medical and healthcare sectors have been characterized by too much technology push and too little demand-pull. Clinical systems that have been developed in close cooperation with doctors and nurses have been more successful than systems developed with a top-down approach. Unfortunately, such systems are less prevalent.

It is important to be aware of the fact that the most essential user of any system is an individual. All future systems that do not include user input as part of the solution will likely fail. Hence, the success of any patient related healthcare system is probably measured in terms of the extent to which it facilitates the empowerment of patients. A necessary ingredient of a successful system is the development of the soft infrastructure, i.e., the structuring of information and tools that make it possible for people to understand and evaluate information and available services.

Early use of ICT and digital education can assist school students to increase knowledge transfer by using computers and technology. This could also promote students to increase self-discipline and select a preferred path towards learning. The best way of teaching ethics should be by combining knowledge and collaboration between schoolteachers and different area specialists such as medicine, computer scientists and engineers.

CONCLUSION

The lives of 21st Century individuals are expected to be vastly different from those of progenitors. It is in the 21st Century that life expectancy is expected to improve due to the development of newer effective drugs and the globalization of healthcare. The Information Age is also responsible for the digitization of healthcare documents to the advantage of patients, physicians, and researchers. The rapid development of technology needs to be matched with a rapid training and development of human resources that will be able to use the new technology in more areas that extend beyond medicine and healthcare.

Both developed and developing countries are faced with similar problems in terms of understanding the organization activities. Moreover, countries face problems with the establishment and implementation of Information Technology in healthcare. Organizational development and knowledge are strongly dependent on customer voices, which are the reference points in healthcare delivery. No consumer-oriented system can be constructed without such reference points. Sometimes decision-making is achieved more efficiently with top-down solutions and technology push. Other means of creating successful systems includes the ability to anticipate problems and to be ready to provide solutions as they develop. Solutions are more appropriate with input by consumers or end-users.

In order to successfully implement digitalization of the medical sector internationally both absorptive and sender capacities are needed. Evidently, building up and implementing new systems is a long-term project. For successful implementation of eHealth, governments should first consider and create new policies and strengthen laws for medical sector digitalization to better dialog on trade, education and health. An approach to match the patient with identifying data developed can assist in the follow up data in long-term, eHealth implementation to be institutionalised with clear contracts and trust in patients´ confidentiality.

REFERENCES

Aarts, J., & Berg, M. (2006). Same systems, different outcomes comparing the implementation of computerized physician order entry in two Dutch hospitals. *Methods of Information in Medicine*, *45*(1), 53–61. PMID:16482371

Aarts, J., Doorewaard, H., & Berg, M. (2004). Understanding implementation: The case of a computerized physician order entry system in a large Dutch university medical center. *Journal of the American Medical Informatics Association*, *11*(3), 207–216. doi:10.1197/jamia.M1372 PMID:14764612

Allen, I. E., & Seaman, J. (2013). Changing course: Ten years of tracking online education in the United States. Newburyport, MA: Sloan. Available from http://onlinelearningsurvey.com/reports/changing-course.pdf

Ammenwerth, E., Talmon, J., Ash, J. S., Bates, D. W., Beuscart-Zephir, M. C., Duhamel, A., & Geissbuhler, A. et al. (2006). Impact of CPOE on mortality rates-contradictory findings, important messages. *Methods of Information in Medicine*, *45*(6), 586–593. Available from http://www.lina-schwab.de/Publikationen/z42.pdf PMID:17149499

Andersson, G., & Karlberg, I. (2000). Integrated care for the elderly: The background and effects of the reform of Swedish care of the elderly. *International Journal of Integrated Care*, *1*(1), 1–10. Available from http://citeseerx.ist.psu.edu/viewdoc/download?doi=10.1.1.276.9726&rep=rep1&type=pdf PMID:16902694

Anell, A., Glenngård, A. H., & Merkur, S. (2012). Sweden: Health system review. Health systems in transition. *European Observatory on Health Systems and Policies, 14*(5), 1-159. Retrieved from http://www.euro.who.int/__data/assets/pdf_file/0008/164096/e96455.pdf

Astor, A., Akhtar, T., Matallana, M. A., Muthuswamy, V., Olowu, F. A., Tallo, V., & Lie, R. K. (2005). Physician migration: Views from professionals in Colombia, Nigeria, India, Pakistan and the Philippines. *Social Science & Medicine*, *61*(12), 2492–2500. doi:10.1016/j.socscimed.2005.05.003 PMID:15953667

Atkinson, N. L., & Gold, R. S. (2002). The promise and challenge of eHealth interventions. *American Journal of Health Behavior*, *26*(6), 494–503. doi:10.5993/AJHB.26.6.10 PMID:12437024

Bates, D. W., & Gawande, A. A. (2003). Improving safety with information technology. *The New England Journal of Medicine*, *348*(25), 2526–2534. doi:10.1056/NEJMsa020847 PMID:12815139

Blumenthal, D., & Tavenner, M. (2010). The "meaningful use" regulation for electronic health records. *The New England Journal of Medicine*, *363*(6), 501–504. doi:10.1056/NEJMp1006114 PMID:20647183

Boucher, L. (2014). *Tradition and change in Swedish education*. Oxford, UK: Elsevier.

Burholt, V., & Naylor, D. (2005). The relationship between rural community type and attachment to place for older people living in North Wales, UK. *European Journal of Ageing*, *2*(2), 109–119. doi:10.1007/s10433-005-0028-3

Burström, K., Johannesson, M., & Diderichsen, F. (2001). Health-related quality of life by disease and socio-economic group in the general population in Sweden. *Health Policy (Amsterdam)*, *55*(1), 51–69. doi:10.1016/S0168-8510(00)00111-1 PMID:11137188

Callahan, D. (2008). *Health care costs and medical technology*. The Hastings Center. Available from http://healthcarecost-monitor.thehastingscenter.org/uploadedFiles/Publications/Briefing_Book/health%20care%20costs%20chapter.pdf

Carrasquillo, O., Orav, E. J., Brennan, T. A., & Burstin, H. R. (1999). Impact of language barriers on patient satisfaction in an emergency Department. *Journal of General Internal Medicine*, *14*(2), 82–87. doi:10.1046/j.1525-1497.1999.00293.x PMID:10051778

Carrera, P. M., & Bridges, J. F. (2006). Health and medical tourism: What they mean and imply for health care systems. *Health and Ageing, 15*. Retrieved from https://www.genevaassociation.org/media/75240/ga2006-health15-carrerabridges.pdf

Cassel, C. K., & Guest, J. A. (2012). Choosing wisely: Helping physicians and patients make smart decisions about their care. *Journal of the American Medical Association*, *307*(17), 1801–1802. doi:10.1001/jama.2012.476 PMID:22492759

ChildrenOnline. (2015). *Internet safety newsletter: Children online research 2007– 2008*. Retrieved from http://www.childrenonline.org

Coiera, E. (1996). Clinical communication: a new informatics paradigm. In Proceedings of the AMIA Annual Fall Symposium (pp. 17–21). American Medical Informatics Association. Available from http://www.ncbi.nlm.nih.gov/pmc/articles/PMC2233204/

Coiera, E. (2000). When conversation is better than computation. *Journal of the American Medical Informatics Association*, *7*(3), 277–286. doi:10.1136/jamia.2000.0070277 PMID:10833164

Coiera, E. (2004). *Handbook of health information management: Integrating information and communication technology in health care work*. London, UK: Routledge.

Coiera, E., & Tombs, V. (1998). Communication behaviours in a hospital setting: An observational study. *British Medical Journal*, *316*(7132), 673–676. doi:10.1136/bmj.316.7132.673 PMID:9522794

Crane, J. A. (1997). Patient comprehension of doctor-patient communication on discharge from the emergency department. *The Journal of Emergency Medicine, 15*(1), 1–7. doi:10.1016/S0736-4679(96)00261-2 PMID:9017479

Dale, B., Sævareid, H. I., Kirkevold, M., & Söderhamn, O. (2008). Formal and informal care in relation to activities of daily living and self-perceived health among older care-dependent individuals in Norway. *International Journal of Older People Nursing, 3*(3), 194–203. Doi:.10.1111/j.1748-3743.2008.00122.x

Deloitte Centre for health solutions. (2015). *Connected health. How digital technology is transforming health and social care*. London, UK: The creative studio at Deloitte. Retrieved from http://www2.deloitte.com/content/dam/Deloitte/uk/Documents/life-sciences-health-care/deloitte-uk-connected-health.pdf

Donchin, Y., Gopher, D., Olin, M., Badihi, Y., Biesky, M. R., Sprung, C. L., & Cotev, S. et al. (1995). A look into the nature and causes of human errors in the intensive care unit. *Critical Care Medicine, 23*(2), 294–300. doi:10.1097/00003246-199502000-00015 PMID:7867355

Essary, A. C. (2011). The impact of social media and technology on professionalism in medical education. *The Journal of Physician Assistant Education, 22*(4), 50–53. doi:10.1097/01367895-201122040-00009 PMID:22308935

European Commission. (2007). *eHealth ERA report. eHealth-priorities and strategies in European countries. Toward the establishment of a European eHealth research arena*. Retrieved from http://www.ehealth-era.org/documents/2007ehealth-era-countries.pdf

European-Commission. (2015). *European health insurance card*. Retrieved June 10, 2015 from http://ec.europa.eu/social/main.jsp?langId=en&catId=559&newsId=2281&furtherNews=yes

Glenngård, A. H., Hjalte, F., Svensson, M., Anell, A., & Bankauskaite, V. (2005). *Health systems in transition*. Retrieved from http://old.hpi.sk/cdata/Documents/HIT/Sweden_2005.pdf

Göransson, K. E., Ehrenberg, A., & Ehnfors, M. (2005). Triage in emergency departments: National survey. *Journal of Clinical Nursing, 14*(9), 1067–1074. doi:10.1111/j.1365-2702.2005.01191.x PMID:16164524

Gosden, T., Forland, F., Kristiansen, I. S., Sutton, M., Leese, B., Giuffrida, A., & Pedersen, L. et al. (2001). Impact of payment method on behaviour of primary care physicians: A systematic review. *Journal of Health Services Research & Policy, 6*(1), 44–55. doi:10.1258/1355819011927198 PMID:11219360

Gröne, O., & Garcia-Barbero, M. (2001). Integrated care: A position paper of the WHO European office for integrated health care services. *International Journal of Integrated Care, 1*(2), e21. doi:10.5334/ijic.28 PMID:16896400

Hall, A., & Walton, G. (2004). Information overload within the health care system: A literature review. *Health Information and Libraries Journal, 21*(2), 102–108. doi:10.1111/j.1471-1842.2004.00506.x PMID:15191601

Harper, S. (2013). *Ageing societies: Myths, challenges and opportunities*. New York, NY: Routledge.

Haux, R., Ammenwerth, E., Herzog, W., & Knaup, P. (2002). Health care in the information society. A prognosis for the year 2013. *International Journal of Medical Informatics, 66*(1-3), 3–21. doi:10.1016/S1386-5056(02)00030-8 PMID:12453552

Hiduja, S., & Patchin, J. W. (2010). Bullying, Cyberbullying, and Suicide. *Archives of Suicide Research, 14*(3), 206–221. doi:10.1080/13811118.2010.494133 PMID:20658375

Hjern, A., Grindefjord, M., Sundberg, H., & Rosén, M. (2001). Social inequality in oral health and use of dental care in Sweden. *Community Dentistry and Oral Epidemiology, 29*(3), 167–174. doi:10.1034/j.1600-0528.2001.290302.x PMID:11409675

Horowitz, M. D., Rosensweig, J. A., & Jones, C. A. (2007). Medical Tourism: Globalization of the healthcare marketplace. Medscape General Medicine. *The Medscape Journal of Medicine, 9*(4), 24–30. Available from http://www.ncbi.nlm.nih.gov/pmc/articles/PMC2234298/

Jennett, P. A., Scott, R. E., Affleck, H. L., Hailey, D., Ohinmaa, A., Anderson, C., & Lorenzetti, D. et al. (2004). Policy implications associated with the socioeconomic and health system impact of telehealth: A case study from Canada. *Telemedicine Journal and e-Health, 10*(1), 77–83. doi:10.1089/153056204773644616 PMID:15104919

Jerlvall, L., & Pehrsson, T. (2012). *eHealth in Swedish county councils*. Inventory comissioned by the SLIT group, CEHIS (swe: Center för eHälsa i Sverige/Eng: Center for eHealth in Sweden).

Johansson, P., Oleni, M., & Fridlund, B. (2002). Patient satisfaction with nursing care in the context of health care: A literature study. *Scandinavian Journal of Caring Sciences, 16*(4), 337–344. doi:10.1046/j.1471-6712.2002.00094.x PMID:12445102

Kajbjer, K., Nordberg, R., & Klein, G. O. (2010). Electronic health records in Sweden: from administrative management to clinical decision support. In History of Nordic Computing 3 (pp. 74–82). Springer Berlin Heidelberg. Available from http://dl.ifip.org/db/conf/hinc/hinc2010/KajbjerNK10.pdf

Keith, S., & Martin, M. E. (2005). Cyber-bullying: Creating a culture of respect in a cyber world. *Reclaiming Children and Youth, 13*(4), 224. Available from http://bienestaryproteccioninfantil.es/imagenes/tablaContenidos03SubSec/13_4_Keith_Martin.pdf

Kjellberg, J., Sørensen, J., Hansen, J., Andersen, S., Avnstrøm, L., & Borgstrøm, L. (2007). Almen praksis som koordinator—en international belysning. [General practice as coordinator—an international review]. *Copenhagen: Danish Institute for Health Services Research (DSI),* Report No. 02. [in Danish].

Klevens, R. M., Edwards, J. R., Richards, C. L., Horan, T. C. Jr, Gaynes, R. P., Pollock, D. A., & Cardo, D. M. (2007). Estimating health care-associated infections and deaths in US hospitals, 2002. *Public Health Reports, 122*(2), 160–166. PMID:17357358

Kodner, D. L., & Spreeuwenberg, C. (2002). Integrated care: Meaning, logic, applications, and implications–a discussion paper. *International Journal of Integrated Care, 2*(4), 1–6. doi:10.5334/ijic.67 PMID:16896389

Lindberg, B., Nilsson, C., Zotterman, D., Söderberg, S., & Skär, L. (2013). Using Information and Communication Technology in Home Care for Communication between Patients, Family Members, and Healthcare Professionals: A Systematic Review. *International Journal of Telemedicine and Applications*. doi:.10.1155/2013/461829

Linden, F. (2009). epSOS local data providers. *Acta Informatica Medica, 17*(3), 142. Retrieved from http://www.ejmanager.com/mnstemps/6/6-1299792486.pdf?t=1457826043

Lindström, Å. (2005). *On the Syntax, Semantics, and Pragmatics of Architectural Principles.* Working paper. Retrieved from http://www.ics.kth.se/Publikationer/Working%20Papers/EARP-WP-2005-03.pdf

Lindström, Å. (2006). *Using architectural principles to make the it-strategy come true* (Doctoral dissertation, KTH, Royal Institute of Technology Stockholm, Sweden). Retrieved from http://citeseerx.ist.psu.edu/viewdoc/download?doi=10.1.1.64.8686&rep=rep1&type=pdf

Linhart, M. (2010). *Independence in old age: Older German women living alone.* Saarbrücken: Lambert.

Littlejohns, P., Wyatt, J. C., & Garvican, L. (2003). Evaluating computerised health information systems: Hard lessons still to be learnt. *British Medical Journal, 326*(7394), 860–863. doi:10.1136/bmj.326.7394.860 PMID:12702622

Ludvigsson, J. F., Otterblad-Olausson, P., Pettersson, B. U., & Ekbom, A. (2009). The Swedish personal identity number: Possibilities and pitfalls in healthcare and medical research. *European Journal of Epidemiology, 24*(11), 659–667. doi:10.1007/s10654-009-9350-y PMID:19504049

Lundgren, K. (2007). *Draken i tiden: IT-nationen Sverige* [Dragon in time: IT-nation of Sweden]. Stockholm: Studieförbundet näringsliv och samhälle (SNS). [in Swedish]

Mahroum, S. (2001). Europe and the immigration of highly skilled labour. *International Migration (Geneva, Switzerland), 39*(1), 27–43. doi:10.1111/1468-2435.00170

Maier, C. B., Glinos, I. A., Wismar, M., Bremner, J., Dussault, G., & Figueras, J. (2011). Cross-country analysis of health professional mobility in Europe: the results. *Health professional mobility and health systems. Evidence from, 17*, 23-66. Available from http://apps.who.int/iris/bitstream/10665/170421/1/Health-Professional-Mobility-Health-Systems.pdf#page=36

Martin, M. J. C. (1994). Managing innovation and entrepreneurship in technology-based firms. New York: Wiley IEEE. Retrieved from https://books.google.se/books?id=fnE7R732COMC&printsec=frontcover&redir_esc=y#v=onepage&q&f=false

Metzger, M. J., & Flanagin, A. J. (2013). Credibility and trust of information in online environments: The use of cognitive heuristics. *Journal of Pragmatics, 59*, 210–220. doi:10.1016/j.pragma.2013.07.012

Mur-Veeman, I., van Raak, A., & Paulus, A. (2008). Comparing integrated care policy in Europe: Does policy matter? *Health Policy (Amsterdam), 85*(2), 172–183. doi:10.1016/j.healthpol.2007.07.008 PMID:17767975

Nytrø, Ø., & Faxvaag, A. (2004). *Healthcare informatics towards 2020. In Infosam 2020, Information Society of 2020* (pp. 127–133). Trondheim, Norway: NTNU.

OECD. (2012). *Education Indicators in focus.* Retrieved from http://www.oecd.org/education/skills-beyond-school/49729932.pdf

OECD. (2013). Health at a Glance 2013: OECD Indicators, OECD, Paris. OECD Publishing.

OECD (2015). *Internet access (indicator).* doi: 10.1787/69c2b997-en

Pang, T., & Guindon, G. E. (2004). Globalization and risks for health. *EMBRO Rep*, *5*(Supplement 1), S11–S16. doi:10.1038/sj.embor.7400226 PMID:15459728

Pelletier, S. G. (2012). *Explosive growth in health care apps raises oversight questions.* Association of American Medical Colleges. Retrieved from; https://www.aamc.org/newsroom/reporter/ october2012/308516/health-care-apps.html

Perednia, D. A., & Allen, A. (1995). Telemedicine technology and clinical applications. *Journal of the American Medical Association*, *273*(6), 483–488. doi:10.1001/jama.1995.03520300057037 PMID:7837367

Pocock, N. S., & Phua, K. H. (2011). Medical tourism and policy implications for health systems: A conceptual framework from a comparative study of Thailand, Singapore and Malaysia. *Globalization and Health*, *7*(12). doi:10.1186/1744-8603-7-12 PMID:21539751

Sarver, J., & Baker, D. W. (2000). Effect of language barriers on follow-up appointments after an emergency department visit. *Journal of General Internal Medicine, 15*(4), 256-264. Doi:.10.1111/j.1525-1497.2000.06469.x

Schoen, C., Osborn, R., Huynh, P. T., Doty, M., Peugh, J., & Zapert, K. (2006). On the front lines of care: Primary care doctors' office systems, experiences, and views in seven countries. *Health Affairs*, *25*(6), w555–w571. doi:10.1377/hlthaff.25.w555 PMID:17102164

Shapiro, J., & Saltzer, E. (1981). Cross-cultural aspects of physician-patient communication patterns. *Urban Health*, *10*, 10–15. Available from http://europepmc.org/abstract/med/10254342 PMID:10254342

Silverstein, M., & Parker, M. G. (2002). Leisure activities and quality of life among the oldest old in Sweden. *Research on Aging*, *24*(5), 528–547. doi:10.1177/0164027502245003

Singleton, K., & Krause, E. (2009). Understanding cultural and linguistic barriers to health literacy. *OJIN: The Online Journal of Issues in Nursing*, *14*(3). doi:10.3912/OJIN.Vol14No03Man04

SMEEC. (2011). *Swedish Ministry of Enterprise, Energy and Communications. ICT for everyone - A Digital Agenda for Sweden* (Reference No. N2011.19). Stockholm: Sweden. Åtta.45. Retrieved from http://www.government.se/reports/2011/12/ict-for-everyone---a-digital-agenda-for-sweden/

SNBHW. (2003). *Årsrapport NPS—En analys av barnmorskors, sjuksköterskors, läkares, tandhygienisters och tandläkares arbetsmarknad.* [Annual report NPS—an analysis of midwifes', nurses', doctors', dental hygienists' and dentists' labor market]. Stockholm, Sweden: Socialstyrelsen [Swedish National Board of Health and Welfare]]. Retrieved from http://www.socialstyrelsen.se

Solberg, I. B., Tómasson, K., Aasland, O., & Tyssen, R. (2013). The impact of economic factors on migration considerations among Icelandic specialist doctors: A cross-sectional study. *BMC Health Services Research*, *13*(524), 7. PMID:24350577

Stetson, P. D., McKnight, L. K., Bakken, S., Curran, C., Kubose, T. T., & Cimino, J. J. (2002). Development of an ontology to model medical errors, information needs, and the clinical communication space. *Journal of the American Medical Informatics Association*, *9*(Supplement 6), S86–S91. doi:10.1197/jamia.M1235

Stroetmann, K. A., Dobrev, A., Lilischkis, S., & Stroetmann, V. (2014). eHealth is worth it. *The economic benefits of implemented eHealth solutions at ten European sites. eHealth Impact*. Retrieved from http://www.ehealth-impact.org

Stroetmann, K. A., Jones, T., Dobrev, A., & Stroetmann, V. N. (2006). eHealth is Worth it. *The economic benefits of implemented eHealth solutions at ten European sites*. Available from http://www.ehealth-impact.org/download/documents/ehealthimpactsept2006.pdf

Suetens, C., Hopkins, S., Kolman, J., & Diaz Högberg, L. (2013). Point prevalence survey of healthcare associated infections and antimicrobial use in European acute care hospitals: 2011-2012. Stockholm, Sweden: European Centre for Disease Prevention and Control (ECDC). doi:10.2900/86011

Sveriges Riksdag. (2012). *Rapport från riksdagen 2011/12:RFR5. eHälsa-nytta och näring* [eHealth-advantage and industry]. Retrieved from https://www.riksdagen.se/sv/Dokument-Lagar/Utredningar/Rapporter-fran-riksdagen/eHalsa---nytta-och-naring_GZ0WRFR5/

Swedish Institute. (2013-2015). Retrieved from https://sweden.se/migration/#2013

Swedish Ministry of Health and Social Affairs. (2006). *National strategy for eHealth-Sweden*. Stockholm, Sweden: Socialdepartementet. Retrieved from http://sweden.gov.se/content/1/c6/06/43/24/f6405a1c.pdf

Swedish National Audit Office [Riksrevisionsverket]. (2002). *IT i verksamhetsutvecklingen-Bättre styrning av myndigheternas IT investeringar I IT-baserad verksamhetsutveckling*. Stockholm, Sweden: Riksrevisionens publikationsservice. Retrieved from http://www.riksrevisionen.se

Swedish National Agency for Education. (2016). Retrieved from http://www.skolverket.se/statistik-och-utvardering

The Swedish Association of Local Authorities and Regions. (2014). *Vägval för framtiden. Våra territoriella och kulturella gränser*. Retrieved from http://skl.se/download/18.547ffc53146c75fdec079e4b/1404478740292/skl-15-trender-vagval-for-framtiden-2025.pdf

Tokunaga, R. S. (2010). Following you home from school: A critical review and synthesis of research on cyberbullying victimization. *Computers in Human Behavior*, *26*(3), 277–287. doi:10.1016/j.chb.2009.11.014

UNESCAP. (2007). *Medical travel in Asia and the Pacific: challenges and opportunities. Thailand.* Retrieved from http://www.unescap.org/ESID/hds/lastestadd/MedicalTourismReport09.pdf

von Hippel, E. (1994). Sticky information and the locus of problem solving: Implications for innovation. *Management Science*, *40*(4), 429–439. doi:10.1287/mnsc.40.4.429

von Hippel, E. (1998). Economics of product development by users: The impact of "sticky" local information. *Management Science*, *44*(5), 629–644. doi:10.1287/mnsc.44.5.629

Vrangbæk, K., & Christiansen, T. (2005). Health policy in Denmark: Leaving the decentralized welfare path? *Journal of Health Politics, Policy and Law*, *30*(1-2), 29–52. doi:10.1215/03616878-30-1-2-29 PMID:15943386

Wahlberg, A. C., Cedersund, E., & Wredling, R. (2003). Telephone nurses' experience of problems with telephone advice in Sweden. *Journal of Clinical Nursing*, *12*(1), 37–45. doi:10.1046/j.1365-2702.2003.00702.x PMID:12519248

Wang, S. J., Middleton, B., Prosser, L. A., Bardon, C. G., Spurr, C. D., Carchidi, P. J., & Bates, D. W. et al. (2003). A cost benefit analysis of electronic medical records in primary care. *The American Journal of Medicine*, *114*(5), 397–403. doi:10.1016/S0002-9343(03)00057-3 PMID:12714130

Wears, R. L., & Berg, M. (2005). Computer technology and clinical work: Still waiting for Godot. *Journal of the American Medical Association*, *293*(10), 1261–1263. doi:10.1001/jama.293.10.1261 PMID:15755949

Webster, F. (2014). *Theories of the Information Society*. New York: Routledge.

Whitehead, M., Evandrou, M., Haglund, B., & Diderichsen, F. (1997). As the health divide widens in Sweden and Britain, what's happening to access to care? *British Medical Journal*, *315*(7114), 1006–1009. Retrieved from http://www.ncbi.nlm.nih.gov/pmc/articles/PMC2127673/pdf/9365303.pdf

WHO. (2014). *Large gains in life expectancy. World Health Statistics 2014*. Available from http://www.who.int/mediacentre/news/releases/2014/world-health-statistics-2014/en/

World Health Organization. (2010). *The burden of health care-associated infection worldwide: A summary*. Retrieved from http://www.who.int/gpsc/country_work/summary_20100430_en.pdf

ADDITIONAL READING

Anderson, C. L., & Agarwal, R. (2011). The digitization of healthcare: Boundary risks, emotion, and consumer willingness to disclose personal health information. *Information Systems Research*, *22*(3), 469–490. doi:10.1287/isre.1100.0335

Angst, C. M., & Agarwal, R. (2009). Adoption of electronic health records in the presence of privacy concerns: The elaboration likelihood model and individual persuasion. *Management Information Systems Quarterly*, *33*(2), 339–370. Available at http://www.jstor.org/stable/20650295

Baum, F. (2003). The new public health (No. Ed. 2). Oxford University Press.

Eysenbach, G. (2000). Consumer health informatics. *British Medical Journal*, *320*(7251), 1713–1716. doi:10.1136/bmj.320.7251.1713 PMID:10864552

Tang, P. C., Ash, J. S., Bates, D. W., Overhage, J. M., & Sands, D. Z. (2006). Personal health records: Definitions, benefits, and strategies for overcoming barriers to adoption. *Journal of the American Medical Informatics Association*, *13*(2), 121–126. doi:10.1197/jamia.M2025 PMID:16357345

KEY TERMS AND DEFINITIONS

E-Health: The use of ICT (Information and Communications Technologies). It is used in support of health related fields.

EHIC: The European Health Insurance Card.

EHR: Electronic Health Records. A real-time longitudinal electronic record of patient's health information.

EPRs: Electronic patient records.

***EpSOS*:** Smart Open Services for European Patients.

EU: European Union.

Globalization: The worldwide movement toward economic, financial, trade, and communications integration.

HAIs: Healthcare-associated infections.

ICT: Information and Communication Technology.

IT: Information Technology.

OECD: The Organization for Economic Co-operation and Development.

TEC: Technology-Enabled Care.

This work was previously published in the Handbook of Research on Individualism and Identity in the Globalized Digital Age edited by F. Sigmund Topor, pages 380-402, copyright year 2017 by Information Science Reference (an imprint of IGI Global).

Chapter 2
Using the Communication AssessmenT Checklist in Health to Assess the Communication Quality of Web Based Resources for Prostate Cancer

Juliana Genova
University of Ottawa, Canada

Curtis A. Olson
Geisel School of Medicine at Dartmouth, USA

Jackie Bender
University Health Network, Canada

ABSTRACT

Introduction: The communication quality of web resources for patients is unknown. The purpose of this study was to assess prostate cancer websites using the Communication AssessmenT Checklist in Health (CATCH). Methods: CATCH is a theory-based tool consisting of 50 elements nested in 12 concepts. Two raters independently applied it to 35 HON certified websites containing information on prostate cancer treatment. Results: Websites contained a mean 24.1 (SD= 3.6) CATCH items. The concepts Language, Readability, Layout, Typography and Appearance were present in over 80% of sites. Content, Risk Communication, Usefulness, and Scientific Value were present in 50% or less. Discussion: The prostate cancer websites evaluated in this study did not present treatment information in a useful, informative or credible way for patients. The communication quality of these resources could be improved with a clear strategic intent focused on decision-making, using CATCH as a guiding framework.

DOI: 10.4018/978-1-5225-1928-7.ch002

INTRODUCTION

There is a growing emphasis on shared decision-making (Makoul & Clayman, 2006; Wong et al., 2000) as a means to enhance patient care. Partnerships with patients can improve the planning and carrying out of therapies (Brett et al., 2014; Brown, Brown, & Sharma, 2000), facilitate adaptation of new knowledge to specific patient communities (Brett et al., 2014; Collier, 2011; Fagerlin, Zikmund-Fisher, & Ubel (2011); Frank, Basch, & Selby, 2014) and make information more accessible to patients by making it more user-friendly (Brett et al., 2014).

There is, however, a gap in our understanding of the process that occurs between the creation of knowledge and its use (Bero et al., 1998; Dopson, Locock, Gabbay, Ferlie, & Fitzgerald, 2003; Lang, Wyer, & Haynes, 2007). In fact, academic researchers have often studied knowledge dissemination and implementation as a two-step process, the first step of which is distilling and packaging the evidence (Cohen et al., 2008; Grimshaw et al., 2006), and the second step is studying the adoption of evidence, taking into consideration behaviour-change factors (Ajzen & Albarracen, 2007; Ajzen, Czasch, & Flood, 2009; Michie, Johnston, Abraham, & Walker, 2005; Michie, van Stralen, & West, 2011). Those steps overlap and are well documented. But the factors affecting the effectiveness of the resources used to communicate new health knowledge and influence behaviour remains largely unexplored.

There are several instruments designed to help streamline health information, filter it and make it more usable. Four instruments evaluate the implementability of clinical guidelines and incorporate a communication dimension. The Guideline Implementability Appraisal tool (GLIA) (Shiffman et al., 2005) proposes a "Presentation and Formatting" dimension comprising two items, while ADAPTE (T. A. Collaboration, 2009) highlights the importance of Context of Use", "Strength of Evidence" and " Risks and Benefits". Two others– Appraisal of Guidelines for Research & Evaluation (AGREE) (Brouwers et al., 2010; A. Collaboration, 2001; Klazinga, 2003) and GRADE (Guyatt et al., 2011; Guyatt et al., 2012; Oxman & GRADE Working Group, 2004) assess the scientific value of the evidence, its scope and purpose, rigor of development, clarity and presentation. Another set of instruments analyses the quality of information provided in web resources for prostate cancer. LIDA (Borgmann et al., 2015; Soobrah & Clark, 2012) and DISCERN (Charnock, Shepperd, Needham, & Gann, 1999) measure the accessibility, usability and reliability of the information; the Information Comprehensiveness Tool (Warren, Footman, Tinelli, McKee, & Knai, 2014) assesses its comprehensiveness; and a framework developed by Ferreira, Carreira, Silva and Lunet (2013) evaluates its relevance.

The first instrument to address the overall suitability of materials for patients, is Suitability Assessment of Materials (SAM), developed by Doak, Doak and Root (1994). Although SAM was developed for use with print materials, it has also been used to assess video- and audio-taped instructions to patients.

However, the existing tools give little or no attention to the communication characteristics of the resource and the message it contains. To the best of our knowledge, there is no instrument for evaluating the communication qualities of online health-related materials and the concepts that could trigger behaviour change and to ensure that patients have accurate, spin-free information.

In this chapter, we present a version of CATCH (Communication AssessmenT Checklist in Health), a new instrument based on communication theories for assessing health messages. We modified the original CATCH tool for application to web-based resources. We will demonstrate its use by applying it to web-based resources for prostate cancer patients. Our aim is to show how the modified CATCH tool can be used to identify the communication concepts exemplified on prostate cancer treatment websites designed for patients and suggest ways to further tailor those online messages to make them more effective.

BACKGROUND

Prostate cancer is the most common cancer among men in Canada (Society, Records, & Registries, 1987), and the fourth most common cancer worldwide, after lung, breast and bowel cancer (Collin et al., 2008). In Canada, every year 23,600 men are diagnosed with prostate cancer (Carter, Miller, Murphy, Payne, & Bryant-Lukosius, 2014). Prostate cancer is also one of the more difficult cancers for patients to comprehend because of the variety of treatment options available (Clark, Wray, & Ashton, 2001; Stamey, McNeal, Yemoto, Sigal, & Johnstone, 1999) including: watchful-waiting, active surveillance, surgery, external beam radiation, brachytherapy, hormone therapy, cryotherapy, chemotherapy and high frequency ultrasound therapy (Loblaw et al., 2007). Each option has its pros and cons, which vary according to the patient's age, genetics and overall health.

It is important that prostate cancer patients educate themselves on the treatment options available to them, because treatment options are numerous, decisions are largely patient driven and the side effects can be distressing, and in some cases, long term.

Nowadays the most popular source for health information is the Internet. It may have the greatest potential for health related behaviour change and decision-making (Chua et al., 2011). Data from the World Bank (2015) indicates that at least 85.6% of people in Canada and 84.2% in US use the Internet. According to the Pew Internet and American Life Project Health Fact Sheet (2012), 72% of adults in the US use the Internet to obtain health information.

Not surprisingly, the Internet is a popular source for prostate cancer information for patients. A 2014 multi-province, population-based survey of Canadian men with prostate cancer found that 79% reported using the Internet and 68% reported using the Internet for information on prostate cancer treatment during the diagnosis and treatment period (Wong et al., 2000).

There are, however, significant challenges, the first of which is the low eHealth literacy of much of the population (Jacobs, Lou, Ownby, & Caballero, 2014; Sullivan, 2011; Tennant et al., 2015). eHealth literacy is defined as "the ability to seek, find, understand, and appraise health information from electronic sources and apply the knowledge gained to addressing or solving a health problem" (Norman & Skinner, 2006a; Norman & Skinner, 2006b). 50% of Canadian men with prostate cancer reported not knowing how to judge the quality of information on the Internet and whether it was personally applicable, and 25 to 30% reported poor search skills and difficulty finding information that they could understand (Norman & Skinner, 2006a; Norman & Skinner, 2006b). As evidence suggests, low levels of eHealth literacy are associated with inferior health outcomes, increased hospitalization and morbidity (Van der Vaart et al., 2011). One approach to address the issue is to tailor online messages to individuals' needs, preferences and circumstances and make them easy to understand, acceptable, easily deployed, accessible and cost-effective (Chua et al., 2011), (Aakhus, Granlund, Oxman, & Flottorp, 2015; Davison, Szafron, Gutwin, & Visvanathan, 2014; Falk et al., 2014; Salonen, Ryhänen, & Leino-Kilpi, 2014). Tailored interventions, consistently proven to be more effective in inducing behavior change (Hoffman et al., 2013; Norman & Skinner, 2006), can help consumers find and evaluate information, monitoring their health status, and understand financial constraints (Kobayashi, Wardle, & von Wagner, 2014; Smith et al., 2015)

Numerous studies have assessed the quality of prostate cancer information on the Internet (Black & Penson, 2006; Pruthi, Belsante, Kurpad, Nielsen, & Wallen, 2011; Routh, Gong, Cannon, & Nelson, 2011) (Hellawell, Turner, Le Monnier, & Brewster, 2000). When systematically reviewed by Black and Penson (2006), websites containing information on prostate cancer were found to be of sufficient quality to aid in decision making but lacked currency, attribution, balance of evidence and comprehensiveness.

Prostate cancer websites have also been assessed for readability – the ease with which information is read and understood. Using Flesch Kindcaid Grade Level and Flesch Reading Ease Level tools, Ellimoottil, Polcari, Kadlec and Gupta (2012) analysed 62 eligible websites containing information on prostate cancer treatment options and only found 3 that were written below a high school reading level. Concerning findings given that one third of the US population reads below a high school reading level (Ellimoottil et al., 2012). To our knowledge, the communication quality of prostate cancer websites has not been studied.

The CATCH Instrument

CATCH (Table 1), whose development and preliminary validation is described in a prior publication, (Genova et al., 2014) is based on SAM (Doak et al., 1994), fundamental communication concepts from the theories of risk communication (Fischhoff, Brewer, & Downs, 2011), Tarde's theory of social values (Tarde, 1890; Tarde, 1902a; Tarde, 1902b), and concepts related to user-centred design (Neuhauser, 2011; Nielsen, 2004). The original CATCH is composed of 55 elements nested in 12 concepts ranging from appearance, form and content to fundamental communication concepts such as numeracy, objectivity, credibility, effectiveness, scientific value and usefulness. CATCH was initially applied to a set of PEMs with proven effectiveness (Giguère et al., 2012) distributed to clinicians and demonstrated good ability to discriminate between resources that are different based on the quality of communication concepts, suggesting good construct validity (Genova et al., 2014). As a theory-based instrument, CATCH can, in our view, be applied to print or online content, using different medias and targeting different audiences.

Because we modified CATCH specifically for web-based resources for prostate-cancer patients, its validity and reliability must be re-assessed. The present study is a pilot designed to show how CATCH can be applied to online resources; further studies are needed to formally assess its performance.

Tailoring of CATCH for Web Resources

The concepts underlying CATCH (Table 1) for patients and CATCH for physicians are the same. Both versions contain the same 12 concepts, but the CATCH for patients contains 5 fewer elements. Table 1 presents each concept and element.

Table 1. Concepts and elements for the Communication AssessmenT Checklist in Health (CATCH)

Concept	Element: Description
Appearance	1. Pictures, special fonts and colors 2. Length: the material is no more than a page long.
Layout and typography	3. Clear layout: the text and graphics attract the reader's attention and create a visual path. 4. Short to-the-point paragraphs: the resource uses short sentences of no more than 12 words, paragraphs of no more than 10 sentences with a single idea, and short and simple words. 5. Subtitles: subtitles or subheadings are used to clearly group the information. 6. Font size: the text is easy to read because the font size is not excessively small or large, at least 12 point, serif. 7. Text clearly laid out and delimited by spaces: the text is well organized and easy to follow. 8. Italics and capitals are used appropriately for references and subtitles or to enhance the layout.

continued on following page

Table 1. Continued

Concept	Element: Description
Content	9. Purpose of the text is clearly stated in the title, illustration, or introduction. 10. Limited scope: the scope of the resource is relevant to the stated purpose and is limited to defining the problem and the rationale, and providing a solution. 11. Summary: the resource provides a summary or a review that reiterates and explains the central information. 12. Information limited to key messages: the resource covers only a few key messages, ideally no more than three or four. 13. Desired behaviours explained or modeled: best practices or recommended therapy procedures are clearly described.
Language and readability	14. Active voice: Sentences are written in the active voice whenever possible. 15. Context given first: the situation is explained to the reader at the beginning of the message. 16. Organizers (sometimes called "road signs") such as headers, captions, or transition words or statements briefly inform the reader of what is coming next.
Graphics	17. Graphics to facilitate understanding: the graphics are self-explanatory and facilitate understanding of the text. 18. Relevance of graphics: graphics match and enhance the content; they should be simple in their meaning, without additional details that distract the reader. Moreover, they depict the recommended behaviour. 19. Captions: captions and/or legends are used for each figure, list, table, or other display supporting the text.
Risk communication	20. Risk clarity: the risk is clearly presented and defined. There is no ambiguity. 21. Likelihood of the event: there is a greater than 50% likelihood that the event described in the message will happen. 22. Risks presented in order of priority: risks are presented starting with the most important, to clarify all the issues at stake at each level of risk. 23. Objective presentation of both harms and benefits: the resource provides complete information on harms and benefits. For example, reporting survival rates for 1 year is incomplete compared to 5 years. 24. Standardized presentation of harms and benefits: for all the outcomes, harms are defined the same way and use the same variable as benefits. 25. Absolute risk difference used 26. Consistent denominators and whole numbers: the resource uses the same denominators to present harms and benefits to ensure consistency, as well as whole numbers, which are easier to understand than fractions or decimals. 27. Consistent time frames for harms and benefits: the resource expresses harms and benefits in the same temporal patterns. 28. Clear difference between the risks at baseline and the risks at follow-up: Risks at baseline and following treatment are clearly presented so that the reader can evaluate the degree of change between the two time periods. 29. Use of positive and negative frames: the message highlights not only the harms, but also the benefits of the recommended action, and uses positive framing that is more productive than negative framing (e.g., survival versus mortality). 30. Symbols (numbers, graphs, statistics, etc.): symbols are used to clearly convey the meaning of the probabilities presented.
Scientific value	31. Effectiveness of the recommendations: it is stated in the resources that adherence to the recommendations yields concrete and specific results. 32. Robustness of the evidence: it is stated in the resource that the message is supported by sufficient, high quality data. It is convincing for professionals.
Emotional appeal	33. Communication of urgency: the message raises concerns that should be answered immediately to reduce the morbidity or mortality of patients. 34. Timeliness and visibility of the topic: the resource addresses a topic covered by popular media because of a public debate, a scientific controversy, or because it features a celebrity with a disease. 35. Vibrancy or intensity: a fast pace and the choice of words show that the author is invested in the subject or driven by the urgency to convey something. The resource, through its appearance and language, conveys a sense of urgency. 36. Threat of the event: the message depicts a serious threat that cannot be ignored. 37. Newness of the message: the document provides a new perspective or represents an innovation. 38. Highlighting of danger: the message highlights a potential threat or danger relative to the topic presented.
Relevance	39. Consistency with experience, logic, and language of reader: the message's language, format, and structure correspond to the reader's level of education, language, and/or professional background. 40. Cultural match: the resource is adapted to the culture of readers and takes into account their background, customs, beliefs, and expectations. 41. Narrative included: contains personal testimonies or real life-examples to drive the message home.

continued on following page

Table 1. Continued

Concept	Element: Description
Social value/ Source credibility	42. Endorsement by renowned individuals or organizations: the document is "validated" by renowned clinicians, research scientists, professional organizations, or the government. 43. Background of the author: the resource clearly states that its author has relevant experience. 44. Disclaimer of conflict of interests: an official statement attests to the absence of any conflict of interest.
Social value/ Usefulness for the patient	45. Time saving the resource states that the recommended behaviour saves time. 46. Money saving: the resource states that the recommended behaviour helps save money. 47. Non-threatening: the message does not highlight deficiencies or lack of training in the medical staff or the health system. 48. Building of self-efficacy: the resource describes a technology or innovation that will give more self-confidence to the clinician and allow them to make an informed decision or trust his or her own judgment. 49. Increased ease: the resource offers an easier and better way to do things. 50. Better quality of life: the resource states that adherence to the targeted behaviour will facilitate healthcare processes and improve organization of the environment.

The concepts of Layout, Typography, and Clarity of Content (elements 2 to 11) which relate to information design, as well as the elements of risk communication (elements 20 to 30) were appropriate for PEMs and for web resources, as well as for physicians and patients.

We adjusted the concepts "Source Credibility" and "Usefulness" from Tarde's Theory of Social Value (Katz, 1999; Lazzarato, 2002; Tarde, 1890; Tarde, 1902). The adjustment was simple: we removed all elements pertaining to usefulness for the physician or the health system. The rest (elements 42 to 50) remain the same.

Also, we did not include the element of Increased Ease, as it related to the ease of operation for the physician, or the elements Incentive and Promotion of Health, because they seemed irrelevant for patients as written.

THEORETICAL FRAMEWORK FOR CATCH

CATCH is a new evaluation framework based on several theories.

Risk Communication

The first theory is risk communication, and one of its most important dimensions is objectivity. We operationalized objectivity and included the elements numeracy, standard definitions, constant denominators and timeframes. If risks and benefits are in numerical expressions, they are easier to use and more comprehensible for patients in distress with a decreased ability to process information (Fagerlin et al., 2011). In decision-making, patients with better numeracy skills rely more on abstract information, such as numbers and graphs, while less numerated patients use emotion-based information, such as narratives (Salmon & Atkin, 2003), and whole numbers (e.g., 1 in 10,000) (Peters, 2012b; Sheridan et al., 2011).

Objectivity is better conveyed with standard definitions, constant denominators and timeframes about risks, costs and benefits, especially if they are enumerated in order of importance (Fischhoff, 2012; Fischhoff et al., 2011; Fischhoff, Watson, & Hope, 1984; Peters, 2012b). While enumerating choices, less is more: research shows that less cognitive effort results in better decision quality choices for patients

(Peters, Dieckmann, Dixon, Hibbard, & Mertz, 2007) - less messages and fewer options for patients have bigger impact (Zikmund-Fisher, Windschitl, Exe, & Ubel, 2011).

Novelty, urgency and visibility of the danger are three elements that are usually intertwined. Novelty and urgency increase the perception of risk (Bandura, 2001) and this has more impact on arguments (Ajzen, 1971) and opinion change (Murphy et al., 1998). The relationship between stronger fear-arousing conditions and greater message acceptance is a linear one (Berkowitz & Cottingham, 1960; Sutton & Eiser, 1984). Witte and Allen (2000) conclude in their meta-analysis of over hundred fear appeal articles "the stronger the fear aroused by a fear appeal, the more persuasive it is" (p. 601). Visibility increases the impact of those elements.

There is also a subjective dimension to risk communication. A patient with high self-efficacy (Witte & Allen, 2000) is more likely to perform the recommended action. Michie and Abraham (2008) and Woolf, Grol, Hutchinson, Eccles and Grimshaw (1999) define self-efficacy as control of material and social environment, perceived behavioural control, self-esteem and self-confidence. Also, Ruiter and Kok (2011) show that people are more likely to act if the response will lead to a quick, sure and efficient change (Witte & Allen, 2000). The effectiveness of the recommended response may lead to behaviour change.

The message has to be relevant to the public. People relate to a message that is consistent with their experience, logic and language and they are more likely to adopt it. Patients tend to make sense of their environment through narrative, they think with stories (Morris, 2001) and are influenced by their own history and memories. Cultural match, as the expression " on-going negotiation within societal groups and conflicts of cultures" (Harter, Japp, & Beck, 2005), allows them to identify with the information and ultimately, to adopt it.

Conveying risks and benefits depend also on the formulation of the message. Effective messages highlight the positive outcomes of a treatment or behaviour (gain frames), especially when the outcome is clear (Ruiter & Kok, 2011; Salmon & Atkin, 2003). When the tone of the message is vibrant, commanding or intense, the conviction of the author is perceived by people and they use better the information (Peters, 2012a).

Tarde's Theory of Social Value

Gabriel Tarde based his theory on societal change on innovation and imitation, both triggered by value-credit (Tarde, 1902). Value-credit is composed of value-usefulness, value-beauty and value-truth. We operationalized value-truth, related to credibility of the source (Atkin, 1994), as endorsement by experts and disclaimer of interests. Value-usefulness is operationalized as time-saving, money-saving (Brownson, Fielding, & Maylahn, 2009) and non-threatening for the patient. Value-beauty is operationalized as "healthy environment" that promotes healing, or a treatment that avoids unnecessary surgical interventions or undesirable side effects.

Plain Language, Graphics and Content

CATCH incorporates also some elements of SAM (Doak et al., 1994) and comprises notions related to the plain language, such as active voice, use of short sentences and words which break the information into easier-to-process words (US Federal Plain Language Guidelines, 2010) and clean layout that facilitates reading (US Department of Health and Human Services, 2010) and creates a visual path (Doak, Doak,

& Root, 1996) (Neuhauser, 2011). As for graphics, they should be culturally appropriate (Doak et al., 1996; Potomac & Doak, 2002), simple (Wright, 2001) and show only the behaviours to be encouraged (US Federal Plain Language Guidelines, 2010).

METHODS

Conceptualization and Operationalization

CATCH was created based on a literature review of commonly accepted communication theories. We defined some concepts that could be applied to evidence-based material, operationalized them and applied them, using a mapping approach, first to PEMs and then to web-based resources for prostate-cancer patients.

Sample of Web-Based Resources for Prostate-Cancer Patients

We conducted a search using the HON code search engine and the key words "prostate cancer treatment'. The Health on the Net Code (HON Code) is the oldest and most common quality standard for health related online information (Health On the Net Foundation, 2014). To achieve the HON code seal of approval, websites must conform to a number principles: have authoritative, reliable and accessible information, support patient-physician relation and confidentiality, and mention funding sources (Health On the Net Foundation, 2014) We hypothesized that the HON code certification guarantees, at least to some degree, the credibility of health information or the fact that it is reviewed by medical professionals. In addition, the results from the HON code search engine correspond well with the top ten web sites obtained using Google. More than 75% of patients begin their search with one of these three search engines (Pew Internet and American Life Project Health Fact Sheet, 2012), and visit only the top 10 web sites listed in the results [16]. To assess a diverse sample of content, we included the first four search results from each organization that pointed to different content, and selected the first 35 search results.

Application of CATCH

A conceptual mapping approach was used to apply CATCH to the selected sample of web pages. Two raters (JB, JG) independently applied the 50 elements of the CATCH instrument to each web-based resources for prostate-cancer patients.

Each web resource was rated along each CATCH element using a dichotomous scale indicating the presence/absence of the element. We wanted to find the presence or absence of each CATCH element and to compute the total occurrences. Once all the elements computed, this would give a comprehensive picture of the strategies used, their advantages and also disadvantages.

Analysis and Scoring

We used Excel and SPSS Version 21 to calculate the sum and sum percentage for each CATCH item and the total summary score for each web resource. We computed the scores for CATCH concepts by calculating the mean value of the items pertaining to each concept.

Rating Procedure

The raters compared their ratings and resolved any disagreements through discussion, which in some cases resulted in rewording of an element. Most disagreements among raters resulted from an unclear description of the elements or misunderstandings as to the degree of specificity required when coding for the presence or absence of an element.

RESULTS

Frequent Concepts

Table 2 and Figure 1 show that the most commonly addressed CATCH concepts. In order of frequency, they were Language and Readability, Layout & Typography, and Appearance. These elements were present in 80% to 93% of the web resources. As shown in Figure 2, the majority of the web resources evaluated contained less than 50% of the CATCH items. The mean CATCH summary score of the web-resources was 24.1 (SD= 3.6). The scores ranged from 15 to 33, out of a possible 50.

Table 2. Summary scores for CATCH concepts and elements (N=35)

CATCH Concepts and Items		Summary Score Sub-scale: X, SD (%), Item: n (%)
Appearance		28, 7.1 (80)
	1. Pictures, special fonts and colours	33 (94)
	2. Length: the material is no more than a page long.	23 (66)
Layout and Typography		31.3, 1.6 (86)
	3. Clear layout	31 (89)
	4. Short to-the-point paragraphs	30 (86)
	5. Subtitles	33 (94)
	6. Font size	29 (83)
	7. Text clearly laid out and delimited by space	32 (91)
	8. Italics and capitals	33 (94)
Content		19, 11.7, (54)
	9. Purpose of the text	27 (77)
	10. Limited scope	32 (91)
	11. Summary	4 (11)
	12. Information limited to key messages	10 (29)
	13. Desired behaviours explained or modelled	22 (63)
Language and Readability		32.7, 2.1 (93)
	14. Active voice	32 (91)
	15. Context given first	35 (100)
	16. Organizers	31 (89)

continued on following page

Table 1. Continued

CATCH Concepts and Items		Summary Score Sub-scale: X, SD (%), Item: n (%)
Graphics		13, 1.7 (37)
	17. Graphics to facilitate understanding	14 (40)
	18. Relevance of graphics.	14 (40)
	19. Captions	11 (31)
Risk Communication		11.6, 12.2 (33)
	20. Risk clarity	27 (77)
	21. Likelihood of the event	33 (94)
	22. Risks presented in order of priority	15 (43)
	23. Objective presentation of both harms and benefits	7 (20)
	24. Standardized presentation of harms and benefits	1 (3)
	25. Absolute risk difference used	0 (0)
	26. Consistent denominators and whole numbers	0 (0)
	27. Consistent time frames for harms and benefits	0 (0)
	28. Clear difference between the risks at baseline and the risks at follow-up	2 (6)
	29. Use of positive and negative frames	20 (57)
	30. Symbols (numbers, graphs, statistics, etc.)	0 (0)
	Scientific Value	16, 7.1 (51)
	31. Effectiveness of the recommendations	23 (66)
	32. Robustness of the evidence	13 (37)
Emotional Appeal		19.2, 11.8 (55)
	33. Communication of urgency	7 (20)
	34. Timeliness and visibility of the topic	34 (97)
	35. Vibrancy or intensity	7 (20)
	36. Threat of the event	32 (91)
	37. Newness of the message	15 (43)
	38. Highlighting of danger	20 (57)
Relevance		12.7, 16.3 (36)
	39. Consistency with experience, logic, and language of reader	31 (89)
	40. Cultural match	7 (20)
	41. Narrative included	0 (0)
Social Value/ Source Credibility		8.0, 8.0 (23)
	42. Endorsement by renowned individuals or organizations	16 (46)
	43. Background of the author	8 (23)
	44. Disclaimer of conflict of interests	0 (0)
Social Value/Usefulness for the Patient		8.3, 11.8 (24)
	45. Time saving	1 (3)
	46. Money saving	2 (6)

continued on following page

Table 1. Continued

CATCH Concepts and Items		Summary Score Sub-scale: X, SD (%), Item: n (%)
	47. Non-threatening	31 (89)
	48. Building of self-efficacy	2 (6)
	49. Increased ease	12 (34)
	50. Better quality of life	2 (6)

Figure 1. CATCH element scores

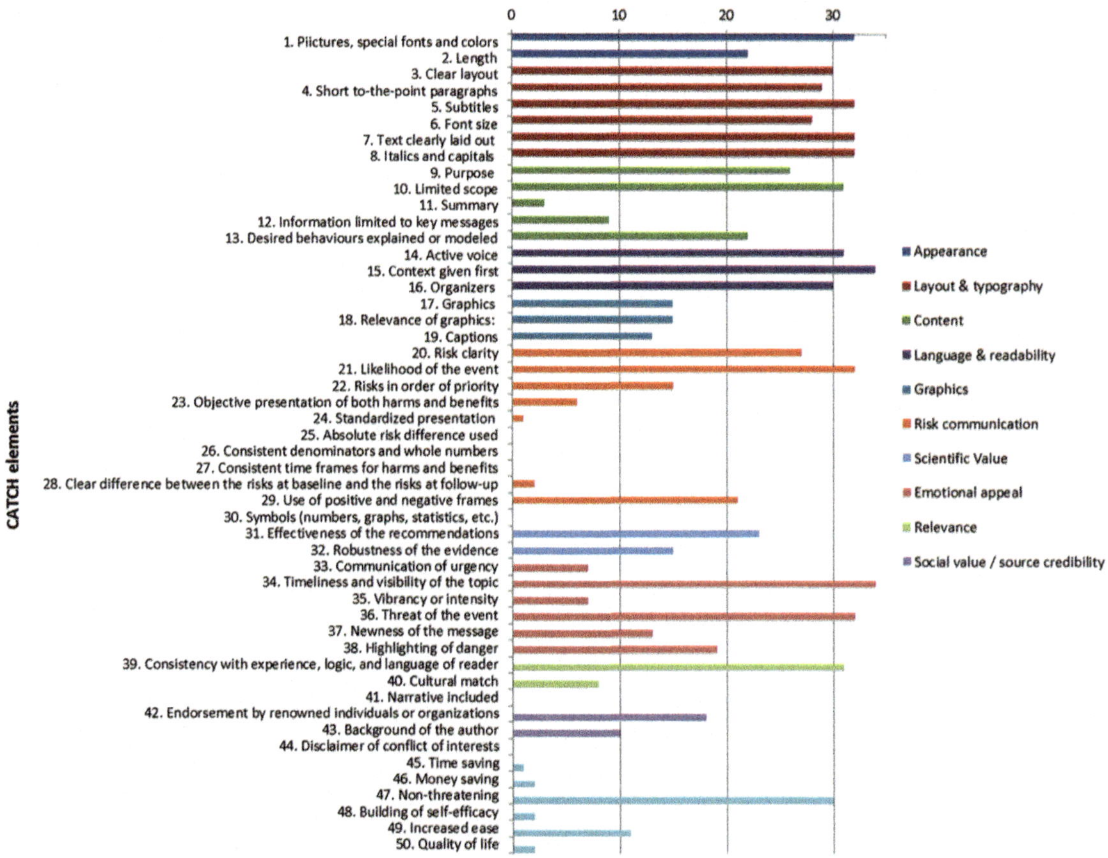

Nearly all the web resources appropriately used italics and capitals, had clearly laid out text, sub-titles and easy to read fonts. Although Appearance came in a close second, only 66% of the resources were the appropriate length for the web, about a screen long, and while many had graphics, most graphics were a simple stock image of the prostate gland. A handful of web resources contained embedded videos. In most cases, these were relevant to and facilitated understanding of the text.

Figure 2. CATCH instrument score

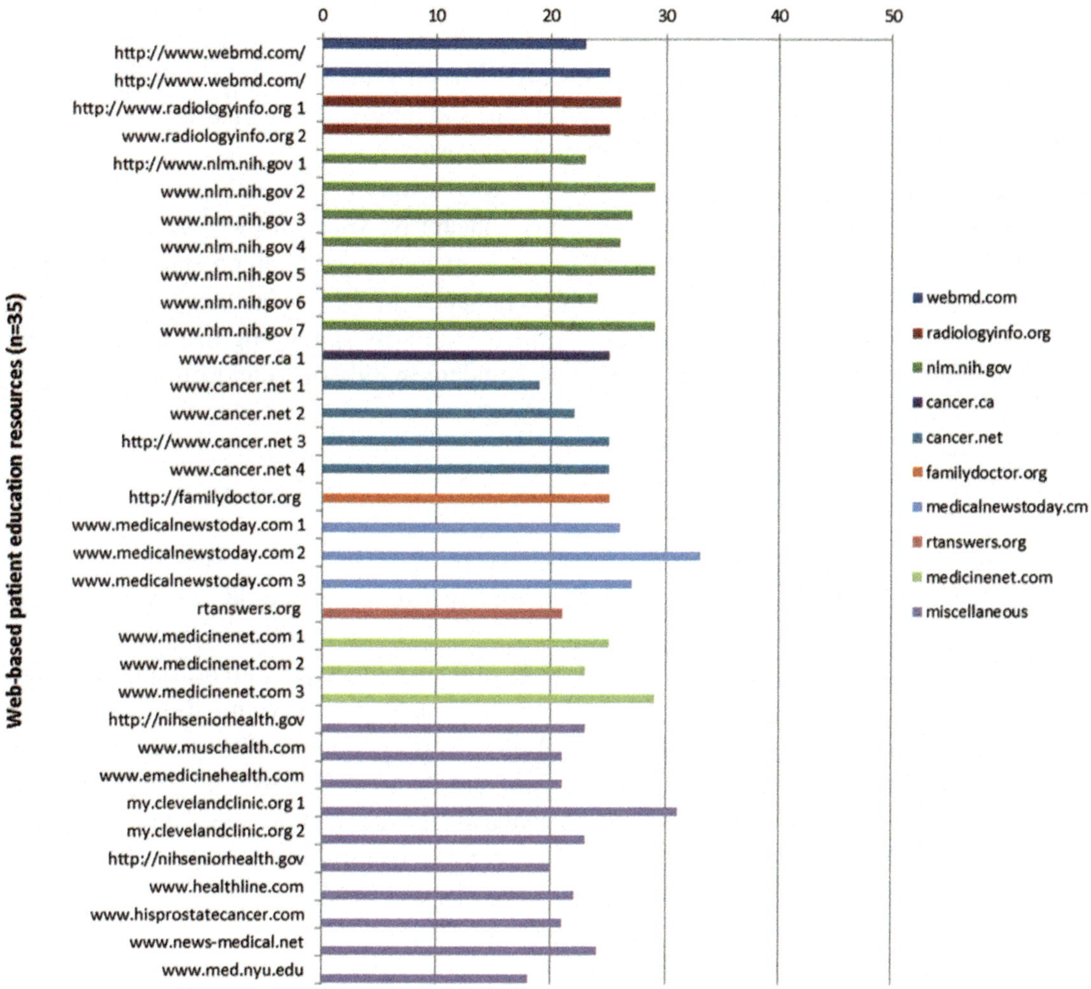

Poorly Represented Concepts

The concept Content was unequally distributed. Almost all of the resources had limited scope, clearly stated the context and were written in active voice. But only 4 had summaries and 29% contained key messages or recommended a particular behaviour or course of action. Web-based resources that did provide a recommendation, advised their readers to consult their physician.

Risk communication was poorly covered, beyond Risk Clarity and Likelihood of the Event, which were present in 94% and 77% of web resources respectively. Only 20% of resources contained a clear and objective presentation of the risks and benefits associated with each treatment option. Few web resources contained numeric presentation of the information, such as in a chart, graph or table, and none reported absolute risks or used consistent denominators or timeframes to describe the likelihood of harms and benefits. Positive and negative (gain and loss) frames, to invite patients to adopt a recommended behaviour, were not used.

The Scientific Value of the web resources for prostate-cancer patients was also poorly addressed. Two-thirds conveyed the effectiveness of the treatment options, but only 37% indicated that the message was supported by high quality evidence. This finding goes hand-in-hand with the results for the concept Credibility. Less than 50% of the web resources for prostate-cancer patients reported that they were reviewed by a medical professional or organisation, and only 23% reported the background of the author. We did not find any disclaimers of conflict of interests.

As for the concept Emotional Appeal, only two elements were consistently covered: Threat of the Event, Timeliness and Visibility. With regards to the concept Newness of the Message, less than half of the web resources provided a new perspective or reported an innovation in prostate cancer treatment, and only about 20% of web resources conveyed the concepts Vibrancy or Intensity, or Urgency.

The concept Usefulness for the patient was also poorly addressed, ranging from 6 to 34%, with the exception of the element Non-Threatening which was evident in 89% of web resources.

DISCUSSION

In this section we discuss the communication concepts exemplified on Web sites for prostate cancer patients. We will also highlight concepts and features that are missing or could be given more attention to improve the communication of the evidence.

CATCH was used to assess the Appearance, Layout and Typography, Content, Language and Readability, Graphics, Communication of Risks, Emotional Appeal, Scientific Value, Relevance, Usefulness for the patient and Source Credibility of HON certified sites for prostate cancer patients.

In general, only the concepts of Appearance, Layout and Typography and Language and Readability were well represented in the web resources on prostate cancer treatment options. This result can be explained with the fact that there are established user-centered design standards and guidelines to present content on websites (Nielsen, 1999, 2004; User-Centered Design Basics, 2015).

However, essential concepts were frequently missing. We found only 14 graphics, mostly similar stock images of the prostate gland. Pictures speak volumes, especially to an audience with lower literacy levels, like the general public (Ellimoottil et al., 2012). Similarly, Bender, Yue, To, Deacken and Jadad (2013) found that a significant proportion of smartphone apps for cancer (at least 30%) used basic and repetitive images. Genova et al. (2014) also found poor use of graphics in printed education materials for clinicians; the pictures were only remotely connected to the content and overly complicated.

As far as the concept of Content is concerned, the most revealing finding is that there was no explicit statement of the purpose of the web-based resources for prostate-cancer patients, except in the fact that the title of the page corresponded to the content. In that sense, these resources lacked a clear *strategic intent.* The purpose of the web resources for prostate cancer patients had to be inferred from the content and the organization of the materials. The purpose was not well defined and this ambiguity translated into poor communication of risks and incomplete information. If we suppose that patient education materials are supposed to inform and guide patient action, our evaluation shows these materials were not well-designed to achieve that purpose. In terms of guidance, only a few web resources took what might be called a minimalist approach to patient empowerment (e.g., recommending that patients ask their doctor about participation in a clinical trial).

This lack of strategic intent may in fact explain why many prostate cancer websites lack sufficient detail about treatment options (Ogah & Wassersug, 2013). It may also account for why risk factors were not presented objectively or consistently. We did not find any numerical representations of risks and advantages, such as charts, graphs, or numbers, aiming to facilitate decision-making and give them clear understanding of the situation. Timeframes, symbols and risk difference were not at all used. As for the organization of risks, most web materials did not present the serious side effects of prostate cancer treatments, the risks associated, and the eventual benefits. All those factors are important for informed shared decision making.

Also, the web resources did not use the strength of Emotional Appeal elements to encourage or empower patients: positive frames were barely used; the tone was neutral, without patient narratives or a mention of cultural match.

The lack of strategic intent of the web-based materials evaluated is further illustrated by the low summary scores for credibility and scientific value. The names, credentials and background of the authors or reviewers were rarely present, and none of the sites provided disclaimers of conflict of interests - results that are quite curious for medical web sites. This finding is consistent with studies of the quality or credibility of information on prostate cancer websites, which has been reported to be lacking in currency, attribution, balance of evidence and disclosure (Black & Penson, 2006).

Web resources are not ends in themselves but rather a means to an end. Evaluating web resources entails assessing the fit between the content and the intended purpose. If a health information material is designed with a strategy in mind - whether it is to inform, change perceptions or even attract visitors - it should be useful for the intended purpose. The prostate cancer websites in our sample did not score well in terms of Usefulness for patients - they did not adequately address the concerns that motivate patients to seek out this information: quality of life (except for impotency); reducing physical and emotional discomfort; saving time and money; or inconvenience. Warren et al. (2014) found that many prostate cancer websites do not adequately address topics identified as important to patients, particularly related to treatment, recovery and quality of life issues (Warren et al., 2014). To improve the usefulness of websites containing information on prostate cancer treatment options, Ogah and Wassersug (2013) advise website developers to: (1) present all evidence-based treatment options, (2) regularly update and time stamp information, (3) acknowledge that treatment recommendations may become out of date quickly, and (4) direct viewers to information on relevant, active clinical trials (Rot, Ogah, & Wassersug, 2012).

CONCLUSION

CATCH is a theoretically based framework that can be used to evaluate the quality of various materials, whether they are patient or physician oriented, print or web-based.

The present study reveals that frequently consulted websites for prostate-cancer patients are not optimally designed to present health information in a way that is useful, informative and credible for patients. If the strategic intent is what guides content developers to create meaningful and valuable resources, with attention to detail, this was not the case here.

Communicating risks can be improved with more objective presentations of risks and benefits, numerical presentation of facts and consistent timeframes. The purpose of the information on the web sites must be clearer. The information should be more credible and geared towards informed decision-making, not just gaining knowledge about diseases and treatments. The web resources did not show any innovative approach or new treatment, the danger was downplayed and the risks and benefits were organized just by gravity of the treatment. If the web resources are to change attitudes and behaviour and more effectively support patients' active involvement in decisions related to their own care, communication elements such as vibrant tone and empathy with patients should become more common features of Web-based patient resources.

REFERENCES

Aakhus, E., Granlund, I., Oxman, A., & Flottorp, S. (2015). Tailoring interventions to implement recommendations for the treatment of elderly patients with depression: a qualitative study. *International journal of mental health systems, 9*(1), 1-24.

Ajzen, I. (1971). Attitudinal vs. normative messages: An investigation of the differential effects of persuasive communications on behavior. *Sociometry, 34*(2), 263–280. doi:10.2307/2786416

Ajzen, I., & Albarracen, D. (2007). *Predicting and changing behavior: A reasoned action approach.* Mahwah, NJ: Lawrence Erlbaum Associates Publishers.

Ajzen, I., Czasch, C., & Flood, M. G. (2009). From Intentions to Behavior: Implementation Intention, Commitment, and Conscientiousness1. *Journal of Applied Social Psychology, 39*(6), 1356–1372. doi:10.1111/j.1559-1816.2009.00485.x

Atkin, C. (1994). Designing persuasive health messages. *Effective dissemination of clinical health information*, 95-0015.

Bandura, A. (2001). Social cognitive theory: An agentic perspective. *Annual Review of Psychology, 52*(1), 1–26. doi:10.1146/annurev.psych.52.1.1 PMID:11148297

Bender, J., Yue, R., To, M., Deacken, L., & Jadad, A. (2013). A lot of action, but not in the right direction: Systematic review and content analysis of smartphone applications for the prevention, detection, and management of cancer. *Journal of Medical Internet Research, 15*(12), e287. doi:10.2196/jmir.2661 PMID:24366061

Berkowitz, L., & Cottingham, D. R. (1960). The interest value and relevance of fear arousing communications. *Journal of Abnormal and Social Psychology, 60*(1), 37–43. doi:10.1037/h0045247 PMID:13799520

Bero, L. A., Grilli, R., Grimshaw, J. M., Harvey, E., Oxman, A. D., & Thomson, M. A. (1998). Closing the gap between research and practice: An overview of systematic reviews of interventions to promote the implementation of research findings. *BMJ (Clinical Research Ed.), 317*(7156), 465–468. doi:10.1136/bmj.317.7156.465 PMID:9703533

Black, P., & Penson, D. (2006). Prostate cancer on the Internet-information or misinformation? *The Journal of Urology, 175*(5), 1836–1842. doi:10.1016/S0022-5347(05)00996-1 PMID:16600774

Borgmann, H., Wölm, J., Vallo, S., Mager, R., Huber, J., Breyer, J., & Tsaur, I. et al. (2015). Prostate Cancer on the Web-Expedient Tool for Patients' Decision-Making? *Journal of Cancer Education.* PMID:26234650

Brett, J., Staniszewska, S., Mockford, C., Herron-Marx, S., Hughes, J. R., Tysall, C., & Suleman, R. (2014). Mapping the impact of patient and public involvement on health and social care research: A systematic review. *Health Expectations*, *17*(5), 637–650. doi:10.1111/j.1369-7625.2012.00795.x PMID:22809132

Brouwers, M., Kho, M., Browman, G., Burgers, J., Cluzeau, F., Feder, G., & Hanna, S. et al. (2010). AGREE II: Advancing guideline development, reporting and evaluation in health care. *Canadian Medical Association Journal*, *182*(18), E839–E842. doi:10.1503/cmaj.090449 PMID:20603348

Brown, G., Brown, M., & Sharma, S. (2000). Health care in the 21st century: Evidence-based medicine, patient preference-based quality, and cost effectiveness. *Quality Management in Health Care*, *9*(1), 23–31. doi:10.1097/00019514-200009010-00004 PMID:11185879

Brownson, R. C., Fielding, J. E., & Maylahn, C. M. (2009). Evidence-based public health: A fundamental concept for public health practice. *Annual Review of Public Health*, *30*(1), 175–201. doi:10.1146/annurev.publhealth.031308.100134 PMID:19296775

Canadian Cancer Society, National Cancer Institute of Canada. Advisory Committee on Records, & Registries. (1987). Canadian cancer statistics. Canadian Cancer Society.

Carter, N., Miller, P., Murphy, B., Payne, V., & Bryant-Lukosius, D. (2014). Healthcare providers' perspectives of the supportive care needs of men with advanced prostate Cancer. *Paper presented at the Oncology nursing forum*. doi:10.1188/14.ONF.421-430

Charnock, D., Shepperd, S., Needham, G., & Gann, R. (1999). DISCERN: An instrument for judging the quality of written consumer health information on treatment choices. *Journal of Epidemiology and Community Health*, *53*(2), 105–111. doi:10.1136/jech.53.2.105 PMID:10396471

Chua, H. F., Ho, S. S., Jasinska, A. J., Polk, T. A., Welsh, R. C., Liberzon, I., & Strecher, V. J. (2011). Self-related neural response to tailored smoking-cessation messages predicts quitting. *Nature*, *20*(1), 1. PMID:21358641

Clark, J., Wray, N., & Ashton, C. (2001). Living with treatment decisions: Regrets and quality of life among men treated for metastatic prostate cancer. *Journal of Clinical Oncology*, *19*(1), 72–80. PMID:11134197

Cohen, D. J., Crabtree, B. F., Etz, R. S., Balasubramanian, B. A., Donahue, K. E., Leviton, L. C., & Green, L. W. et al. (2008). Fidelity versus flexibility. *American Journal of Preventive Medicine*, *35*(5), 381–389. doi:10.1016/j.amepre.2008.08.005 PMID:18929985

Agree Collaboration. (2001). Appraisal of guidelines for research & evaluation (AGREE) instrument.

Collaboration, The ADAPTE. (2009). *The ADAPTE Process: Resource Toolkit for Guideline Adaptation. Version 2.0.* Retrieved from http://www.adapte.org

Collier, R. (2011). Federal government unveils patient-oriented research strategy. *Canadian Medical Association Journal*, *183*(13), E993–E994. doi:10.1503/cmaj.109-3978 PMID:21876023

Collin, S. M., Martin, R. M., Metcalfe, C., Gunnell, D., Albertsen, P. C., Neal, D., & Donovan, J. et al. (2008). Prostate-cancer mortality in the USA and UK in 1975-2004: An ecological study. *The Lancet Oncology*, *9*(5), 445–452. doi:10.1016/S1470-2045(08)70104-9 PMID:18424233

Davison, B., Szafron, M., Gutwin, C., & Visvanathan, K. (2014). Using a web-based decision support intervention to facilitate patient-physician communication at prostate cancer treatment discussions. *Revue canadienne de soins infirmiers en oncologie [Canadian Oncology Nursing Journal]*, 24(4), 241-247.

Doak, C. C., Doak, L. G., & Root, J. H. (1994). Suitability assessment of materials (SAM). *Paper presented at the American Public Health Association Annual Meeting*, Washington, DC.

Doak, C. C., Doak, L. G., & Root, J. H. (1996). Teaching patients with low literacy skills. *AJN The American Journal of Nursing*, *96*(12), 16M. doi:10.1097/00000446-199612000-00022

Dopson, S., Locock, L., Gabbay, J., Ferlie, E., & Fitzgerald, L. (2003). Evidence-based medicine and the implementation gap. *Health*, *7*(3), 311–330. doi:10.1177/1363459303007003004

Ellimoottil, C., Polcari, A., Kadlec, A., & Gupta, G. (2012). Readability of websites containing information about prostate cancer treatment options. *The Journal of Urology*, *188*(6), 2171–2176. doi:10.1016/j.juro.2012.07.105 PMID:23083852

Fagerlin, A., Zikmund-Fisher, B. J., & Ubel, P. A. (2011). Helping patients decide: Ten steps to better risk communication. *Journal of the National Cancer Institute*, *103*(19), 1436–1443. doi:10.1093/jnci/djr318 PMID:21931068

Falk, E. B., O'Donnell, M. B., Tompson, S., Gonzales, R., Chin, S. D., Strecher, V., & An, L. (2014). *Neural systems associated with self-related processing predict population success of health messages.* Mass Commun Health.

Ferreira, D., Carreira, H., Silva, S., & Lunet, N. (2013). Assessment of the contents related to screening on Portuguese language websites providing information on breast and prostate cancer. *Cadernos de Saude Publica*, *29*(11), 2163–2176. doi:10.1590/0102-311x00150312 PMID:24233032

Fischhoff, B. (2012). *Communicating Risks and Benefits: An Evidence Based User's Guide*. Government Printing Office.

Fischhoff, B., Brewer, N. T., & Downs, J. S. (2011). *Communicating risks and benefits: an evidence-based user's guide*. Food and Drug Administration.

Fischhoff, B., Watson, S. R., & Hope, C. (1984). Defining risk. *Policy Sciences*, *17*(2), 123–139. doi:10.1007/BF00146924

Frank, L., Basch, E., & Selby, J. (2014). The PCORI Perspective on Patient-Centered Outcomes Research. *Journal of the American Medical Association*, *312*(15), 1513–1514. doi:10.1001/jama.2014.11100 PMID:25167382

Genova, J., Nahon-Serfaty, I., Dansokho, S. C., Gagnon, M. P., Renaud, J. S., & Giguère, A. (2014). The Communication AssessmenT Checklist in Health (CATCH): A Tool for Assessing the Quality of Printed Educational Materials for Clinicians. *The Journal of Continuing Education in the Health Professions*, *34*(4), 232–242. doi:10.1002/chp.21257 PMID:25530293

Giguière, A., Légaré, F., Grad, R., Pluye, R., Haynes, B., Cauchon, M., & Labrecque, M. et al. (2012). Decision boxes for clinicians to support evidence-based practice and shared decision making: The user experience. *Implementation Science; IS*, *7*(72). PMID:22862935

Grimshaw, J., Eccles, M., Thomas, R., MacLennan, G., Ramsay, C., Fraser, C., & Vale, L. (2006). Toward Evidence-based Quality Improvement. *Journal of General Internal Medicine*, *21*(Suppl. 2), S14–S20. PMID:16637955

Guyatt, G., Oxman, A., Akl, E., Kunz, R., Vist, G., Brozek, J., & deBeer, H. et al. (2011). GRADE guidelines: 1. Introduction-GRADE evidence profiles and summary of findings tables. *Journal of Clinical Epidemiology*, *64*(4), 383–394. doi:10.1016/j.jclinepi.2010.04.026 PMID:21195583

Guyatt, G., Oxman, A. D., Sultan, S., Brozek, J., Glasziou, P., Alonso-Coello, P.,... & Jaeschke, R. (2012). GRADE guidelines: 11. Making an overall rating of confidence in effect estimates for a single outcome and for all outcomes. *Journal of clinical epidemiology*.

Harter, L. M., Japp, P. M., & Beck, C. S. (2005). *Narratives, health, and healing: Communication theory, research, and practice*. Mahwah, NJ: Lawrence Erlbaum.

Health On the Net Foundation. (2014). Retrieved from http://www.healthonnet.org/HONcode/Conduct.html

Hellawell, G., Turner, K., Le Monnier, K., & Brewster, S. (2000). Urology and the Internet: An evaluation of Internet use by urology patients and of information available on urological topics. *BJU International*, *86*(3), 191–194. doi:10.1046/j.1464-410x.2000.00831.x PMID:10930912

Hoffman, A., Volk, R., Saarimaki, A., Stirling, C., Li, L., Härter, M., & Llewellyn-Thomas, H. et al. (2013). Delivering patient decision aids on the Internet: Definitions, theories, current evidence, and emerging research areas. *BMC Medical Informatics and Decision Making*, *13*(Suppl. 2), S13. doi:10.1186/1472-6947-13-S2-S13 PMID:24625064

Jacobs, R., Lou, J., Ownby, R., & Caballero, J. (2014). A systematic review of eHealth interventions to improve health literacy. *Health Informatics Journal*. PMID:24916567

Katz, E. (1999). Theorizing diffusion: Tarde and Sorokin revisited. *The Annals of the American Academy of Political and Social Science*, *566*(1), 144–155. doi:10.1177/0002716299566001012

Klazinga, N. (2003). Development and validation of an international appraisal instrument for assessing the quality of clinical practice guidelines: The AGREE project. *Quality & Safety in Health Care*, *12*(1), 18–23. doi:10.1136/qhc.12.1.18 PMID:12571340

Kobayashi, L. C., Wardle, J., & von Wagner, C. (2014). Limited health literacy is a barrier to colorectal cancer screening in England: Evidence from the English Longitudinal Study of Ageing. *Preventive Medicine*, *61*, 100–105. doi:10.1016/j.ypmed.2013.11.012 PMID:24287122

Lang, E., Wyer, P., & Haynes, R. (2007). Knowledge translation: Closing the evidence-to-practice gap. *Annals of Emergency Medicine*, *49*(3), 355–363. doi:10.1016/j.annemergmed.2006.08.022 PMID:17084943

Lazzarato, M. (2002). *Puissances de l'invention: la psychologie Économique de Gabriel Tarde contre l'Économie politique*. Paris: Empêcheurs de penser en rond.

Loblaw, D., Virgo, K., Nam, R., Somerfield, M., Ben-Josef, E., Mendelson, D., & Talcott, J. et al. (2007). Initial hormonal management of androgen-sensitive metastatic, recurrent, or progressive prostate cancer: 2007 update of an American Society of Clinical Oncology practice guideline. *Journal of Clinical Oncology*, *25*(12), 1596–1605. doi:10.1200/JCO.2006.10.1949 PMID:17404365

Makoul, G., & Clayman, M. L. (2006). An integrative model of shared decision making in medical encounters. *Patient Education and Counseling*, *60*(3), 301–312. doi:10.1016/j.pec.2005.06.010 PMID:16051459

Michie, S., & Abraham, C. (2008). Advancing the science of behaviour change: A plea for scientific reporting. *Addiction (Abingdon, England)*, *103*(9), 1409–1410. doi:10.1111/j.1360-0443.2008.02291.x PMID:18783495

Michie, S., Johnston, M., Abraham, C., & Walker, A. (2005). Making psychological theory useful for implementing evidence based practice: A consensus approach. *Quality & Safety in Health Care*, *14*(1), 26–33. doi:10.1136/qshc.2004.011155 PMID:15692000

Michie, S., van Stralen, M. M., & West, R. (2011). The behaviour change wheel: A new method for characterising and designing behaviour change interventions. *Implementation Science; IS*, *6*(1), 42. doi:10.1186/1748-5908-6-42 PMID:21513547

Morris, D. B. (2001). Narrative, ethics, and pain: Thinking with stories. *Narrative*, 55-77.

Murphy, M., Black, N., Lamping, D., McKee, C., Sanderson, C., Askham, J., & Marteau, T. (1998). Consensus development methods, and their use in clinical guideline development. *Health Technology Assessment (Winchester, England)*, *2*(3), i. PMID:9561895

Neuhauser, L. (2011). Readability, Comprehension and Usability. In B. Fischhoff, N. Brewer, & J. S. Downs (Eds.), *Communicating Risks and Benefits: An Evidence-Based User's Guide. US Department of Health and Human Services Food and Drug Administration. Risk Communication Advisory Committee and consultants.*

Nielsen, J. (1999). *Designing web usability: The practice of simplicity*. New Riders Publishing.

Nielsen, J. (2004). *Designing web usability*. Pearson Deutschland GmbH.

Norman, C. D., & Skinner, H. A. (2006a). eHEALS: The eHealth literacy scale. *Journal of Medical Internet Research*, *8*(4), e27. doi:10.2196/jmir.8.4.e27 PMID:17213046

Norman, C. D., & Skinner, H. A. (2006b). eHealth literacy: Essential skills for consumer health in a networked world. *Journal of Medical Internet Research*, *8*(2), e9. doi:10.2196/jmir.8.2.e9 PMID:16867972

Ogah, I., & Wassersug, R. (2013). How reliable are "reputable sources" for medical information on the Internet? The case of hormonal therapy to treat prostate cancer. *Paper presented at the Urologic Oncology: Seminars and Original Investigations.*

Oxman, A.GRADE Working Group. (2004). Grading quality of evidence and strength of recommendations. *BMJ (Clinical Research Ed.)*, *328*(19), 1490–1494. PMID:15205295

Peters, E. (2012a). Affect and emotion. Communicating Risks and Benefits: An Evidence Based User's Guide, 89.

Peters, E. (2012b). Quantitative information. In B. B Fischhoff, N. Brewer, & J. S. Downs (Ed.), Communicating Risks and Benefits: An Evidence Based User's Guide: An Evidence Based User's Guide (pp. 53). US Department of Health and Human Services Food and Drug Administration. Risk Communication Advisory Committee and consultants.

Peters, E., Dieckmann, N., Dixon, A., Hibbard, J. H., & Mertz, C. K. (2007). Less is more in presenting quality information to consumers. *Medical Care Research and Review*, *64*(2), 169–190. doi:10.1177/1077558707064002030l PMID:17406019

Pew Internet and American Life Project Health Fact Sheet. (2012). *Pew Internet*. Retrieved from http://www.pewinternet.org/fact-sheets/health-fact-sheet/

Potomac, M., & Doak, C. C. (2002). Pfizer Principles for Clear Health Communication.

Pruthi, R., Belsante, J., Kurpad, R., Nielsen, M., & Wallen, E. (2011). Robotic cystectomy and the Internet: Separating fact from fiction. *Paper presented at the Urologic Oncology: Seminars and Original Investigations*. doi:10.1016/j.urolonc.2009.04.010

Rot, I., Ogah, I., & Wassersug, R. (2012). The language of prostate cancer treatments and implications for informed decision making by patients. *European Journal of Cancer Care*, *21*(6), 766–775. doi:10.1111/j.1365-2354.2012.01359.x PMID:22574619

Routh, J. C., Gong, E. M., Cannon, G. M. Jr, & Nelson, C. P. (2011). Does a controversial topic affect the quality of urologic information on the Internet? *Urology*, *78*(5), 1051–1056. doi:10.1016/j.urology.2011.06.050 PMID:21945281

Ruiter, R. A. C., & Kok, G. (2011). Planning to frighten people? Think again! In *Writing Health Communication: An Evidence-Based Guide for professionals*.

Salmon, C. T., & Atkin, C. (2003). Using media campaigns for health promotion. Handbook of health communication, 285-313.

Salonen, A., Ryhänen, A., & Leino-Kilpi, H. (2014). Educational benefits of Internet and computer-based programmes for prostate cancer patients: A systematic review. *Patient Education and Counseling*, *94*(1), 10–19. PMID:24021418

Sheridan, S. L., Draeger, L. B., Pignone, M. P., Keyserling, T. C., Simpson, R. J., Rimer, B., & Gizlice, Z. et al. (2011). A randomized trial of an intervention to improve use and adherence to effective coronary heart disease prevention strategies. *BMC Health Services Research*, *11*(1), 331. doi:10.1186/1472-6963-11-331 PMID:22141447

Shiffman, R., Dixon, J., Brandt, C., Essalhi, A., Hsiao, A., Michel, G., & O'Connell, R. (2005). The GuideLine Implementability Appraisal (GLIA): Development of an instrument to identify obstacles to guideline implementation. *BMC Medical Informatics and Decision Making*, *5*(23). doi:10.1186/1472-6947-5-23 PMID:16048653

Smith, S. C., O'Conor, R., Curtis, L., Waite, K., Deary, I., Paasche-Orlow, M., & Wolf, M. S. (2015). Low health literacy predicts decline in physical function among older adults: findings from the LitCog cohort study. *Journal of epidemiology and community health*, jech-2014-204915.

Soobrah, R., & Clark, S. K. (2012). Your patient information website: How good is it? *Colorectal Disease*, *14*(3), e90–e94. doi:10.1111/j.1463-1318.2011.02792.x PMID:21883807

Stamey, T. A., McNeal, J. E., Yemoto, C. M., Sigal, B. M., & Johnstone, I. M. (1999). Biological determinants of cancer progression in men with prostate cancer. *Journal of the American Medical Association, 281*(15), 1395–1400. doi:10.1001/jama.281.15.1395 PMID:10217055

Sullivan, G. M. (2011). A primer on the validity of assessment instruments. *Journal of graduate medical education, 3*(2), 119-120.

Sutton, S. R., & Eiser, J. R. (1984). The effect of fear-arousing communications on cigarette smoking: An expectancy-value approach. *Journal of Behavioral Medicine, 7*(1), 13–33. doi:10.1007/BF00845345 PMID:6716470

Tarde, G. (1890). *Les lois de l'imitation*. Paris: Kimé éditeur.

Tarde, G. (1902). *Pstchologie économique. Tome second.* Paris.

Tarde, G. (1902). *Psychologie économique. Tome premier.* Paris.

Tennant, B., Stellefson, M., Dodd, V., Chaney, B., Chaney, D., Paige, S., & Alber, J. (2015). eHealth Literacy and Web 2.0 Health Information Seeking Behaviors Among Baby Boomers and Older Adults. *Journal of Medical Internet Research, 17*(3), e70. doi:10.2196/jmir.3992 PMID:25783036

The World Bank Group. (2015). Retrieved from http://Worldbank.org

US Department of Health and Human Services. (2010). *CfMMS*. Toolkit for Making Written Material Clear and Effective.

US Federal Plain Language Guidelines. (2010). Retrieved from http://www.plainlanguage.gov/howto/guidelines/bigdoc/fullbigdoc.pdf

User-Centered Design Basics. (2015). Retrieved from http://www.usability.gov/what-and-why/user-centered-design.html

Van der Vaart, R., van Deursen, A., Drossaert, C., Taal, E., van Dijk, J., & van de Laar, M. (2011). Does the eHealth Literacy Scale (eHEALS) measure what it intends to measure? Validation of a Dutch version of the eHEALS in two adult populations. *Journal of Medical Internet Research, 13*(4), e86. doi:10.2196/jmir.1840 PMID:22071338

Warren, E., Footman, K., Tinelli, M., McKee, M., & Knai, C. (2014). Do cancer-specific websites meet patient's information needs? *Patient Education and Counseling, 95*(1), 126–136. doi:10.1016/j.pec.2013.12.013 PMID:24447523

Witte, K., & Allen, M. (2000). A meta-analysis of fear appeals: Implications for effective public health campaigns. *Health Education & Behavior, 27*(5), 591–615. doi:10.1177/109019810002700506 PMID:11009129

Wong, F., Stewart, D., Dancey, J., Meana, M., McAndrews, M., Bunston, T., & Cheung, A. (2000). Men with prostate cancer: Influence of psychological factors on informational needs and decision making. *Journal of Psychosomatic Research, 49*(1), 13–19. doi:10.1016/S0022-3999(99)00109-9 PMID:11053599

Woolf, S. H., Grol, R., Hutchinson, A., Eccles, M., & Grimshaw, J. (1999). Clinical guidelines: Potential benefits, limitations, and harms of clinical guidelines. *BMJ: British Medical Journal, 318*(7182), 527–530. doi:10.1136/bmj.318.7182.527 PMID:10024268

Wright, S. M. (2001). Contribution of a lecturer-practitioner in implementing evidence-based health care. *Clinical Effectiveness in Nursing, 5*(1), 30–34. doi:10.1054/cein.2000.0170 PMID:11761876

Zikmund-Fisher, B. J., Windschitl, P. D., Exe, N., & Ubel, P. A. (2011). 'I'll do what they did": Social norm information and cancer treatment decisions. *Patient Education and Counseling, 85*(2), 225–229. doi:10.1016/j.pec.2011.01.031 PMID:21367557

KEY TERMS AND DEFINITIONS

Better Quality of Life or Better Organization of the Environment: In some cases, treating the disease requires a full reorganization of the patient environment, daily routine or practices (e.g. cases of depression). Better quality of life refers also to a treatment that is not intrusive and respects the person – for instance, a breast cancer operation may be life-saving, but is very invasive for the patient and does not enhance her quality of life.

Effectiveness of the Recommended Response: The recommended response (in evidence-based practice) will be efficient and quick, promoting the user to adopt it.

Narrative: Quite often, diseases are personified and different social groups color the description of the disease. Cancer is a typical example – patients describe it as "a silent killer" and they often see themselves as "warriors", a narrative that will appeal to readers who are cancer patients.

Negative Frame: The message is negative, p.ex. "If you smoke, you will die a painful death."

Objective Presentation of Harms and Benefits: Evidence-based practice aims to provide complete information on risks and advantages for the patient, based on standardized presentation of harms and benefits, outcomes, dosages and periods of evaluation, and using consistent denominators and whole numbers. The difference between the risks at baseline and the risks at follow-up should be clearly explained. Risks are presented in order of priority.

Positive Frame: The message is expressed in positive terms, p.ex. "If you stop smoking, you will see your grandchildren grow".

Purpose of the Text: The main messages of the text are clearly stated in the title, the illustration are relevant and the introduction and conclusion sum up clearly the content. The content is limited in scope and relevant – it defines the problem, the rationale and suggests a solution.

Risk Clarity: The risk is clearly presented and defined. There is no ambiguity. Presenting the risks. Absolute risk reduction is more objective than relative risk reduction.

Self-Efficacy: Feeling of confidence in one's abilities. Self-confidence is considered a game changer when it comes to behavior-change and adoption of new practices.

Urgency, Vibrancy or Intensity of the Tone: The reader can feel, in the tone of the message, in the choice of words, active voice and dynamic verbs, that the author is sincere and communicates his or her emotions on the topic. This feeling is usually communicated to the reader and it has a bigger impact.

This work was previously published in Transformative Healthcare Practice through Patient Engagement edited by Guendalina Graffigna, pages 163-191, copyright year 2017 by Medical Information Science Reference (an imprint of IGI Global).

Chapter 3
E-Health:
Modern Communication Technology Platforms for Accessing Health Information

Wayne Usher
Griffith University, Australia

ABSTRACT

This chapter will identify how Australian university students access and use various forms of technology (Web 1.0 – Internet, Web 2.0 – social media - SM) to retrieve personal health information. This chapter will move beyond Web 1.0, to present a theoretical basis of claim, concerning the extent to which other forms of technology (e.g. Web 2.0 and wireless monitoring devices) have impacted on youth. What is more, attention will be directed towards outlining to what degree this has shaped their patterns of health information retrieval. Importantly, this chapter aligns with contemporary literature that suggests a need for further studies into the area of human - technology interactions, which promotes sustainable action plans and strategies that will create and encourage reform throughout e-health programs and interactive communication platforms. Given that Australian university students are prolific users of modern forms of communication technology and that youth, in general, characteristically undertake relatively high levels of risky health behaviours and unhealthy lifestyle choices, such a chapter would seem warranted.

INTRODUCTION

There is limited rigorous cross sectional research, investigating and comparing Australian university students' and their technology usage to access health information. What is more, research outlining contrasting patterns of Web 1.0, Web 2.0 and wireless monitoring device adoption by university students to address chronic disease (CD) is narrow. Therefore, this chapter builds on past and presents contemporary research that outlines how modern forms of communication technologies are impacting on individuals' health information access, implementation and health care delivery into the early 21st century. Hence, a broad objective of this chapter is to address how emerging health technologies have the potential to manage CD and heighten health information access and dissemination. A more specific objective is to

DOI: 10.4018/978-1-5225-1928-7.ch003

demonstrate how technologies, such as the Internet/World Wide Web (Web 1.0), social media (SM - Web 2.0), and various wireless mobile monitoring devices / platforms, are being collectively harnessed and have the potential to address Australia's CD epidemic, especially amongst youth.

The chapter is organized as follows. First, a synopsis of the current university students and Australia's CD epidemic is presented. Within this section it will be highlighted as to what are the major contributing risk factors and CD conditions represented both globally and nationally. Second, a summary of major technology (Web 1.0) innovations and university students' will be presented with further attention given to user trends. This section will draw on research by Usher et al., (2015) which goes to provide evidential baseline data concerning the current landscape as it stands. Such approaches are legitimised by drawing on past and contemporary research. Third, the remaining body of this section describes and discusses past research in the area of Web 1.0 and university students' usage trends and access to technology for the purpose of health information retrieval.

The fourth section gives reference to potential future research directions, with specific attention given to outlining how Web 2.0 technologies have created a new healthcare ecosystem. Emphasis is directed towards outlining how new communication technologies have heightened an active pre-eminence of health content creation, accessibility, delivery and adoption over passive content consumption. This section concludes by presenting how that enabling technologies, such as Web 2.0, offer for the first time the potential for individuals to be connected into a healthcare ecosystem that can deliver actionable information in a timely manner, overcoming the barriers of multiple data silos across many platforms.

Lastly, the chapter concludes by offering a glimpse into future possibilities surrounding emerging strategies, technologies and potential recommendations to heighten the uptake as to the sustainability of e-health and how they could potentially provide a framework that legitimizes university students' participation in discourses around health information access and implementation.

BACKGROUND

University Students and Australia's Chronic Disease Epidemic

University students typically enter a dynamic transitional period of new independence from their parents that is characterised by rapid, interrelated changes in body, mind, and social relationships (Pullman et al., 2009). Arnett (2000) has distinguished the period between ages 18 and 25 as a phase of "emerging adulthood," a liminal period between adolescence and adulthood. Although the university years are often viewed as a key phase for personal growth and development, they also represent a period of increased risk for injury, morbidity, and mortality associated with multiple health behaviours (Binkowska-Bury & Januszewicz, 2010). More precisely, many university students fail to meet recommended nutritional guidelines, have decreased physical-activity (Lowery et al., 2000; Hendricks et al., 2006; Reddy et al.,. 2011) and many first-year boarding university female students are significantly more likely to start binge eating (Barker, 2007).

Australian university students are becoming less physically active and have increasingly adopted a sedentary lifestyle centered on computer use and television viewing (Alricsson et al., 2008), leading to increased health risks. Correspondingly, chronic diseases are currently contributing to around 70% of the total burden of illness and injury experienced by the Australian population, with the expected proportion to increase to 80% by 2020 (Department of Health and Ageing, 2008). There are 8 identified health areas which contribute significantly to the burden of illness and injury in Australia, identified as National Health Priority Areas, these being:

1. Arthritis,
2. Musculoskeletal conditions,
3. Asthma,
4. Cardiovascular health,
5. Diabetes mellitus,
6. Injury,
7. Obesity, and
8. Mental health.

With a chronic disease epidemic emerging throughout the Australian population, Yee et al., (2008) argued that current health care delivery, management and education models pertaining to chronic disease and addressing health inequalities will not meet future demands, and that productivity and efficiency of future healthcare and education will be sustainable only if organisations leverage advances in technology (i.e. the Internet). As health provision moves into the early 21st century, it is important for health care providers to adopt new initiatives in an attempt to cater to modern health problems, chronic diseases, and escalating health care costs (Towards a National PHC Strategy, 2008; World Health Organisation, 2010). Such ideologies are underpinned by the perception that healthy lifestyles depend on the early adoption of healthy living habits and readily accessible information; unhealthy lifestyles among youths are strongly linked to unhealthy habits in adulthood (Lowery et al. 2000; Landsberg et al. 2010).

As young people are seen to be in a unique stage of knowledge absorption and personality shaping and are prolific in their technology usage (Anderson, 2001; Bernhardt & Hubley, 2001), it would seem appropriate that early intervention programs should be aimed at combining young peoples' health awareness and communication networks as a strategy for combating Australia's growing illness epidemic. Thus, the understanding and evaluation of healthy lifestyles and knowledge management via modern communication networks (i.e. the Internet) among university students are essential for the promotion of their healthy growth and for guiding early preventative programs. Furthermore, Landsberg et al. (2010) identifies that the university environment is an ideal and cost-effective means of developing healthy lifestyles.

MAIN FOCUS OF THE CHAPTER

Internet (Web 1.0) and University Students

With the advent of the Internet (Web 1.0), has come an increase in information retrieval. From its earliest conception and implementation, Web1.0 technology has become the information *ether* to which has permeated every aspect of society, with an unprecedented impact on the Australian healthcare industry. Kamel Boulos & Wheeler (2007) identified that the Internet has been presented as an enabler in health information retrieval and health care, for patients, organizations, clinicians and lay persons. What is more, such an invention as Web 1.0 has provided the necessary e-platform for creating and sustaining positive behavioural changes in patients suffering from CD (Ritterband, Thorndike, Cox, Kovatchev, & Gonder-Frederick, 2009). They go on to comment that:

Website use leads to behaviour change via different mechanisms of change (e.g., knowledge and motivation). Behaviour change impacts physiology and target behaviours to bring about symptom improvement, and treatment maintenance helps users maintain these gains. (p.20).

Usher (2009) supports such claims by identifying that individuals who access, understand and use health websites that possess a high degree of reliability, interactivity and are user-friendly, demonstrate a higher degree of self-efficacy when it comes to their individual health literacy levels.

Web 1.0 Usage Trends Amongst University Students

It is a given that university students use the Internet (Anderson, 2001). University students continue to be early adopters of new Internet tools and applications in comparison to general Internet-using populations (Johnson-Yale *et al.,* 2009). A recent report indicated that American college students were heavy users of the Internet, with 74% of the students surveyed reportedly using the Internet for "four or more hours per week" (Pew Internet & American Life Project, 2009). The Internet is increasingly becoming part of our lives, its use being centered on the younger age-group of citizens between 15 and 24 (90.3%) and between 25 and 34 years of age (78.3%) are Internet users. Correspondingly, as access improves into the early 21st century, people will increasingly use the Internet to find health information (Fox & Jones, 2009; Uden-Kraan, 2009). Research has indicated that between the years 1998–2005, the number of Australian households, with access to the Internet, rose from 1,098,000 to 4,039,000, a rise of 268% (ABS, 2005). Similarly, a recent Nielsen's Internet & Technology Report (2010) indicates that the average Australian Internet user spent 17.6 hours per week online throughout 2009, up from 16.1 hours in 2008. Consequently, with such exponential growth and access to the Internet, it is expected that online health information access and use will steadily grow throughout all Australian demographics; especially with university students. Furthermore, numerous publications (Nöthlings et al., 2010; Hu et al., 2011; Reddy et al., 2011) have shown that healthy lifestyle practices and readily accessible information / education do reduce disease occurrence and mortality rates.

Cain et al., (2009) posit that the transformation of health information dissemination is mirrored in the steady increase in access and usage demonstrated by individuals when concerned with the Internet. Commonly cited estimates over the years have suggested that more than half (Brodie et al., 2000; Fox et al., 2000) and as much as 80% of young adults with Internet access have used it for health care purposes. In a similar study, it was found that more than 60% reported that they frequently searched the Internet for information and that they used various search engines and multiple websites to find health information (Escoffery et al., 2005). For the past 20 years we have been immersed in what has been termed the 'information age', during which the availability of information of all types, including health information, has been greatly improved by the advent of computers and the Internet (Fox & Jones, 2009; Hitlin & Rainie, 2005).

Global and US health website traffic rankings reveal that individuals are increasingly accessing the Internet to find relevant and timely health information (eBizMBA – Rank, 2010), (See Table 1).

Table 1. Top six most popular health websites (2010) – Visitors / month

Website Name	URL	Visitors / Month
Yahoo!Health	http://health.yahoo.com	21 500 000
National Institute of Health	http://www.nih.gov/	20 000 000
WebMD	http://www.webmd.com/	19 500 000
Medicine Net	http://www.medicinenet.com/script/main/hp.asp	10 500 000
MayoClinic	http://www.mayoclinic.com/	7 000 000
Drugs	http://www.drugs.com/	6 000 000

Source: *eBizMBA Rank* – http://www.ebizmba.com/articles/health-websites.

Numbers vary and none are very accurate, but it is estimated that there are over 100,000 health-related websites on the Internet today (Risk & Dzenowagis, 2001), whilst health topics most often explored by young adults (17 – 25 years of age) include sexually transmitted diseases, diet, fitness and exercise and sexual behaviour (Borzekowski, 2001; Korp, 2006). From an American perspective, 80% of adults now have an 'always present' connection via wireless devices (Nielsen's Internet & Technology Report, 2010), with such increased Internet availability changing the behavior of health care consumers (Fox & Jones, 2009; Pew Internet & American Life Project, 2009).

The phenomena of modern communication technologies (i.e. the Internet) have been extensively researched throughout the world; especially undertaken in the United States and in European countries (Steptoe et al. 2002; American College Health Association, 2007; Laska et al. 2009), however, there is limited rigorous cross sectional research, investigating and comparing Australian university students' e-health knowledge management. From such an identified research gap, this study sought to determine the level of online health information usage trends by Australian university students.

METHOD

Data Collection

The survey was developed using the Lime Survey (www.limesurvey.org) on-line tool supported by the Griffith University Survey Research Centre. The survey was designed to collect both quantitative and qualitative empirical data and was hosted on the Griffith University website (Gold Coast campus, Australia). The survey was promoted via Facebook and 2 broadcast emails to students' email accounts who were attending Griffith University, Gold Coast, Australia (Arts, Education & Law). Questions were developed to achieve the stated research aim of the project. Ethics approval for the research was obtained through the Griffith University Office of Ethics (GU Ref No: EDN/18/11/HREC).

The main criterion to be included in the analysis was that participants needed to be currently living in Australia and they were a university student (either full or part time). A total of 365 responses was initially collected. Nevertheless, only 275 responses were included for analysis, with 90 responses being excluded due to either not meeting the selection criterion, limited detail associated with demographics or not a full survey completion.

Data Analysis

Data analysis was undertaken using Statistical Package for the Social Sciences (SPSS) (PASW18). Initial data preparation involved the development of 1 integrated SPSS file to incorporate all responses from the pilot and final survey undertaken. Initial data analysis used Frequencies to provide a profile of respondents by demographic characteristics (e.g. gender, age, course major, states where live) and questions relating to health / medical information used. Qualitative data were classified into groups and data analysis using Frequencies were performed. Chi-square tests were undertaken to assess factors that may differentiate females and males. Statistically significant differences were reported using $p < 0.05$.

RESULTS

Demographics of Participants

Two hundred and seventy-five (275) responses were received, with 82.5% of responses from female participants and 17.5% by male participants. The average of age of respondents was 24.45 (SD = 8.19). Participants were enrolled in a wide range of university programs, in which most of them majored in Education (41.1%), followed by Law / Criminology (13.5%) and Business (13.1%). Ninety-eight percent of participants lived in Queensland while 2.2% lived in New South Wales and 0.4% lived in Victoria. Table 2 summarizes the demographics of the participants, who are currently an Australian citizen and enrolled as a university student (either full time or part time).

Table 2. Demographic information of participants

		N	%
Gender	Female Male	227 48	82.5 17.5
Course Major	Education Law/Criminology Journalism Arts/Design Music Psychology Sociology Media/Communication Photography Environmental Science Languages/Linguistics Business	113 37 10 14 9 6 3 20 5 1 4 36 17	41.1 13.5 3.6 5.1 3.3 2.2 3.0 7.3 1.8 0.4 1.5 13.1 6.2
States Where Live	NSW QLD VIC	6 268 1	2.2 97.5 0.4
		M	**SD**
	Age	24.45	8.19

Trends of Online Health / Medical Information used Amongst Australian University Students

A question was proposed to participants in an attempt to ascertain whether they have ever used the Internet to access health / medical information. Among the 275 participants, 90.2% of them revealed that they have used the Internet for finding such information, while 9.8% indicated they had never done so. For the latter group of participants, 50.0% of them stated the reasons as to why they have never used the Internet to search for health / medical information. These included that they: 1) perceived the Internet as an unreliable source (50.0%), 2) did not see the need for it (37.5%), 3) had no interest or curiosity for the topic (8.3%) and 4) never thought of searching the Internet for such a topic (4.2%).

For participants (n = 248) who stated they have used the Internet as a means for sourcing health / medical information, they were then asked to rank the top 3 ways they used the Internet to find such information. The top 3 methods were:

1. A random search engine (Google, AltaVista, Yahoo) (83.3%),
2. A referral from media communications (television, magazine, radio, and social media) (27.0%), and
3. A referral from a friend (26.5%) (See Table 3).

Participants, who stated they have accessed online health / medical information (n = 248), were also asked to indicate how often they would search the Internet for health / medical information and how much time they spent reading it once they accessed the information. Interestingly, data from this study revealed that the majority of respondents searched for health information:

1. Every few months (44.6%),
2. At least once per month (15.7%) and
3. A few times per month (11.2%).

Table 3. Top 3 ways to search for health/medical information (Total response number for top 1 = 242, top 2 = 218, top 3 = 204)

	1st Method		2nd Method		3rd Method	
	N	%	N	%	N	%
A random search engine	**204**	**83.3**	12	5.2	13	5.8
A referral from family member	13	5.3	51	21.9	43	19.0
A referral from friend	1	0.4	31	13.3	**60**	**26.5**
A referral from lecturer	1	0.4	10	4.3	4	1.8
A referral from health professional	12	4.9	59	25.3	43	19.0
A referral from media	2	0.8	**63**	**27.0**	57	25.2
A referral from book	1	0.4	2	0.9	0	0
Other way	11	4.5	3	1.3	2	0.9
None	0	0	2	0.9	4	1.8

Further data also indicated that once they accessed the information, they would mostly spend:

1. More than 1-15 minutes (40.9%),
2. More than 15-30 minutes (33.1%) and
3. More than 30-60 minutes (19.4%) reading the information.

In addition, participants were asked to rank, from 6 core health categories (See Table 4), the top 3 types of health information they would mainly access and read from the Internet.

Among the 248 participants in the group (who had previously used online information), only 244 of them responded to this question. Table 4 identifies that the top 3 rankings were: 1) specific diseases (n = 97, 39.8%), 2) medical treatment (n = 62, 25.4%) and 3) health services (n = 52, 21.3%). Qualitative data identified those participants who indicated 'other information' revealed a curiosity about symptoms, diagnosis, nutrition / dietary, pregnancy and personal health issues.

Related to the 6 core health categories, participants were then asked to elaborate on each health category, providing further specific detail. On each of the 6 health categories, participants provided specific information which was then grouped into smaller categories, upon which the top 3 most often stated were chosen. The top 3 most often searched health topics, from each of the 6 core health categories, resulted in 18 sub-categories (See Table 5).

From these 18 sub-categories the top most often searched for information were issues pertaining to:

1. Mental health (depression and anxiety) (63.1%),
2. Medical services (56%),
3. Natural medicine / remedies (18.2%),
4. Sexually transmitted diseases (11.9%), and equally
5. Cancer (11.9%).

Participants were also asked about whether they had a favorite health website they used to obtain health / medical information (n = 226, 91.1%). Six percent (6.2%) of them said yes, while 93.8% said

Table 4. Top 3 types of health/medical information university students mainly access and read (total response number for top 1, top 2, top 3 each = 244)

	1st Type		2nd Type		3rd Type	
	N	%	N	%	N	%
1. Specific Diseases	**97**	**39.8**	36	14.8	32	13.1
2. Medical Treatment	49	20.1	**62**	**25.4**	43	17.6
3. Natural Therapy	34	13.9	42	17.2	18	7.4
4. Pharmaceutical Drugs	9	3.7	32	13.1	25	10.2
5. Health Services	18	7.4	42	17.2	**52**	**21.3**
6. Mental Health	23	9.4	18	7.4	31	12.7
Other	14	5.7	5	2.0	20	8.2
None	0	0	7	2.9	23	9.4

Table 5. Top 3 most frequent stated specific health information for the six groups

		N	%
1. Specific Diseases	**1.Sexual transmitted disease** **2.Cancer** 3.Mental illness	**17** **17** 10	**11.9** **11.9** 7.0
2. Medical Treatment	4.Treatment for skin problems 5.Treatment for flu/cold 6.Treatment for cancer	6 5 4	5.2 4.3 3.5
3. Natural Therapy	7.Natural medicine/remedies 8.Dietary tips 9.Herbal remedies	**14** 7 5	**18.2** 9.1 6.5
4. Pharmaceutical Drugs	10.Pain killers 11.Drugs for respiratory problems (e.g. asthma /anti-anxiety drugs) 12.Anti-depressants	5 4 (each) 3	9.8 7.8 (each) 5.9
5. Health Services	**13.Medical services** 14.Mental health services 15.Naturopath/ women health services	**47** 6 4 (each)	**56.0** 7.1 4.8 (each)
6. Mental Health	**16.Unipolar disorder (depression)** **17.Anxiety disorders** 18.Eating disorders	**28** **13** 4	**43.1** **20.0** 6.2

no to this question. For those who responded yes, they mostfrequently used such sites as 'Better Health' (a general health website -www.betterhealth.vic.gov.au), 'Beyond Blue' (a mental health website -www.beyondblue.org.au), and 'HealthInsite' (a general health website - www.healthinsite.gov.au).

Chi square analyses (with Yates continuity correction) were performed for gender and the question of whether they have ever searched for online health / medical issues. However, no significant difference was demonstrated between gender and history of health/medical information search (X^2 =.91, p =.34, phi =.07). Chi square analyses were also undertaken for gender across questions about the top 1 way of searching health / medical information, the top 1 information that most often being accessed, frequency of online health / medical information used and whether they have a favorite website for health / medical issues. Similarly, no significant results were found.

DISCUSSION OF RESULTS

This study opens a small window through which we can begin to study the opinions that Australian university students hold pertaining to the Internet and how they relate to it for health inquires. This Australian study mirrors similar earlier research by Kenneth (2005) and Fox & Raine (2006) upon which they conclude that the Internet is having a powerful influence on young adults, with 80% of those with Internet access, going online at least once a month for health information and that this information influenced their decisions about how to treat a specific disease (70%). Results from this study identify that every few months (44.6%), 90.2% of participants used the Internet for accessing health information and mostly spent more than 1-15 minutes reading (40.9%) about specific diseases (39.8%).

Interestingly, a majority of participants (n = 226, 91.1%) indicated that they *did not* have a favourite health website that they used to access health information and that a random Internet search (Google, AltaVista, Yahoo) (n = 204, 83.3%) was the main way that they obtained health information. Similarly, in a recent study, it was found that almost all of the respondents (n = 8,353) used search engines to find and access online health information (Head & Eisenberg, 2011). Boyer and Geissbuhler (2006) offer a possible explanation for such online information search behavior by stating that it seems that these mechanisms prevail mainly because they are easy, accessible, fast and contain a great deal of information. Hence, a recommendation from this study is to design avenues that will assist university students to develop critical appraisal skills associated with the retrieval, evaluation, and implementation of online health information. This is, perhaps, an initial step in improving the acceptance and adoption of e-health knowledge management by university students in a broader context (Mitra et al., 2005).

Furthermore, this study recommends that student health services should provide links that would direct university students to reliable health websites that address their identified health concerns. Issues related to the credibility of information on health websites are crucial considerations for students (Escoffery et al., 2005) and that the main problems reported in the search for e-health were the ignorance of good web pages (64.8%) and the lack of confidence or search skills (23.2%) (Head & Eisenberg, 2011). Similarly, Wood (2004) asserts that once university students have found information on the web, they lack the skills to critically analyse the information they have found, making the assumption that 'all information is equal, truthful, and has the same value'. He also found that students do not understand or appreciate the reasons for, and necessity of, accurately crediting the information source.

For those who had a favorite health website (6.2%), they most frequently used such sites as 'Better Health' (www.betterhealthvic.gov.au), 'Beyond Blue' (www.beyondblue.org.au) and 'HealthInsite' (www.healthinsite.gov.au). A closer inspection of these health websites revealed that they maintain and display many of the components that increase a health website's reliability levels (authority, accuracy, objectivity, currency, intended audience, coverage, confidentiality and justifiability) (Usher, 2009). Furthermore, these identified websites are Government designed, advertised and supported portals. These websites are becoming a more frequent and acceptable form of information exchange and health care delivery across all sectors of the health care landscape (Nielsen's Internet & Technology Report 2010). A further recommendation from this study would be to increase university students' knowledge pertaining to a health website's reliability components so as to encourage future access to reliable health websites. Increased levels of reliability are a major factor in, and motivation for, current and future Internet trends and patterns of online health information usage (Usher, 2009).

Another important consideration necessary for interpreting results from this study is the disproportional gender ratio of participants (female 227, 82.5% and male 48, 17.5%), whereby it could be assumed that the results obtained from this study is gender specific. Therefore, further research and cross-gender studies should be undertaken to determine e-health knowledge management trends by male university students, thus providing a heightened holistic approach to e-health care delivery (Horgan, et al., 2010; Head & Eisenberg, 2011; Jimenez-Pernett & de Labry-Lima, 2010). Current research supports such a recommendation stating that young men use the Internet more intensively for downloading news and entertainment, while young women use the Internet predominately for information about education and health-related information (ONS, 2009). Similarly, Escoffery et al. (2005) found differences in Internet use for health information by gender and by level of Internet experience.

Participants (n = 244) ranked 6 core health categories with further elaborations generating 18 subsequent sub-categories. Interestingly, these correspond with a number of Australia's identified National Health Priority Areas. Given these results, further research is warranted in an attempt to investigate the development and implementation of early preventative programs for Australian University students that address such issues as:

1. Mental health (depression and anxiety),
2. Medical services,
3. Natural medicine / remedies,
4. Sexually transmitted diseases, and
5. Cancer.

Justification for such a recommendation is supported by current research by Stallman (2011), who identifies that mental illness among Australian university students is five times higher than in the general population. Furthermore, it is understood that depression is commonly linked with a range of other health risk behaviours that Australian university students engage in, such as tobacco use, illicit drug use, alcohol misuse and dependence, eating disorders and obesity (MHS in Australia, 2010).

LIMITATIONS

The study had some limitations associated with the survey instrument, the major limitation being the initial online data collection method (LimeSurvey). There was an inability (due to an unbiased e-mail alert) to collect / identify equal sample sizes from male and female participants, resulting in a higher participation rate from Australian female University students. However, it was an expectation that given the nature of many of the University programs (i.e. Bachelor of Primary Education); a higher female participation rate was expected.

Secondly, the identified participation rates were only achieved via an email broadcast to Griffith University students (Arts, Education and Law). Due to regulations and privacy restrictions, only 2 e-mails were sent. This limited level of survey notification would have significantly affected participation rates. Future recommendations would include a need to establish a more concentrated avenue/s for the advertising of the survey, thus increasing participation rates. This could come in the form of further advertising the survey via Facebook (snowballing) and other Australian university health services. Future instrument designs may benefit from identifying and developing a data collection strategy that addresses the aforementioned limitations

FUTURE RESEARCH DIRECTIONS

Looking to the future, further research is needed around new initiatives that are underpinned by the Internet and provide opportunities for increased e-health knowledge management in the early 21st century. Findings from this study may help guide future research and policy and assist Australian university health services to develop the necessary e-health platforms for delivering effective health promotion. However, to date, there is little research indicating any substantial coordinated approach to addressing these recommendations (Australian Institute for Primary Care, 2008).

More importantly, the findings from this study indicate that future e-health initiatives (across all Australian universities) should include the development of e-health platforms that demonstrate practical e-healthcare delivery models for current and future Australian university students. The development and implementation of an e-health portal, designed to educate and reach Australian university students concerning the usage of reliable health websites for health care delivery and knowledge management would be one avenue. Given that young adults (primarily male) have been portrayed as reluctant to engage with traditional health services (Courtenay, 2000; White, 2006) this recommendation would seem plausible.

Comparable research, congruent with this study and its findings, has recognized that young people experience difficulties in accessing mainstream mental health services, particularly because of the stigma that remains associated with mental health problems (Horgan et al., 2010). One potential solution is to use the many interactive websites that are available and which offer information and support for mental health. Therefore, it seems conceivable that websites designed and managed by health services should have a predominant position among interventions which are specifically aimed at university students (Jimenez-Pernett and de Labry-Lima, 2010).

Furthermore, consideration should be directed towards newer forms of communication technology (i.e. SM – Web 2.0) which may present opportunities to engage with young adults pertaining to their health / medical issues. Social media (Web 2.0) technology allows its users to interact with other users or to change content, in contrast to non-interactive websites (i.e. the Internet - Web 1.0) where users are limited to the passive viewing of health information that is provided to them (Seeman, 2008). Young & Simon (2005) define social media technology as,

The literal fusion of multiple electronic, communications, computer, and media technologies. The art of listening, learning and sharing is being transformed through, for example, the development of social forums (Twitter, Facebook, Myspace), content sharing platforms (Wikis, Blogs, Diigo, Nigs, Google Docs) and high performance computing / advanced networking (Second Life, podcasts, instructional design, 3-D stereoscopic) (p. 14).

From such an identified research gap, further empirical data will be presented so as to highlight the shifting paradigms that have occurred over the past 5 years. This shift has been primarily caused by the increased technological advances when it comes to modern forms of communication technologies, namely wireless monitoring devices. Therefore, the forthcoming section will give specific reference to contemporary literature and research that goes to re-enforce and build on previous research in this field of investigation.

Web 2.0 or social media (SM) technology has become very popular among undergraduates, with usage rates upwards of 90% at most campuses (Lampe *et al.*, 2007; Stutzman, 2006). Specifically, there has been a great deal of recent research activity directed towards various aspects of Facebook use, such as the use of Facebook in academic settings (Hewitt & Forte, 2006). Steinfield *et al.*, (2008) suggest that more research on the role of social network sites among young adults is needed, since maintaining friendships through SNSs like Facebook may play an important role in psychological (emotional health) development. Social networking sites affordances help reduce barriers that lower self-esteem students might experience in forming the kinds of large, heterogeneous networks that are sources of bridging social capital (Steinfield *et al.*, 2008). Social capital is an elastic construct used to describe the benefits one receives from one's relationships with other people (Lin, 1999). Among young adults, relationships with peers are important both for generating offline benefits and for psychosocial development.

Moreover, Ellison et al., (2007) found evidence that self-esteem may operate as a moderator of the relationship between social network site use and social capital. That is, young people with lower self-esteem appeared to benefit more from their use of SNSs than those with higher self-esteem. As young adults are closely linked to social media as a way of communication (Seeman, 2008) and university students demonstrate higher mental health issues when compared to the general population (Stallman,

2011), further research that explores the use of Web 2.0 technologies for heightening e-health knowledge management and social capital would seem reasonable. Australian secondary schools have been seen more as a setting for promoting better mental health, but it hasn't occurred in the tertiary sector to the same degree (Higher Education, 2011).

Contemporary and future technologies (i.e. Web 2.0) which assist in generating, acquiring and disseminating health information will require new forms of literacy, to which this is another point of contention surrounding e-health knowledge management in the early 21st century (Usher, 2009). The concept of e-health literacy has been defined in terms of social action not just information processing as,

The ability to seek, find, understand and appraise health information from electronic sources and apply the knowledge gained to addressing or solving a health problem (Norman & Skinner, p., 57, 2006).

Social Media (Web 2.0) and University Students

O'Reilly (2007) identifies how the introduction of Web 2.0 technologies have created a new *'architecture of participation'*, emphasising that there is a growing nexus which has emerged between such communication platforms as the Internet (Web 1.0) and SM (Web 2.0) technologies. This relationship has co-operatively changed the way providers of 21st century healthcare and consumers alike, deliver, access and implement health services and access health information. Since their introduction, Web 2.0 technologies (Facebook, Twitter, Instagram, MySpace and Flickr have attracted millions of international users', with many integrating these platforms into their daily health and communication practices (Boyd & Ellison, 2007, p 9). Boyd and Ellison (2007) comment:

While their key technological features are fairly consistent, the cultures that emerge around SNSs (Web 2.0) are varied. Most sites support the maintenance of pre-existing social networks, but others help strangers connect based on shared interests, political views, or activities. Some sites cater to diverse audiences, while others attract people based on common language or shared racial, sexual, religious, or nationality-based identities. (p. 12).

What is more, Hackworth and Kunz (2011) identify that "Web 2.0 technologies provide the means for health care providers and marketers alike to provide actual content—not just marketing to the consumer, but providing the consumer with valuable information about health care topics, concerns, issues and controversies" (p. 3). Currently, Twitter, YouTube and Facebook are the most popular social media for hospitals, and the most effective in driving traffic to a web site (Cummins, 2010).

A framework, by Usher (2011), identifies four important health enabling qualities that Web 2.0 technologies collectively promote. These enabling aspects promote and allow for individuals to manage personal health conditions – by heightening the access and implementation of health information. The four (4) health enabling qualities are:

1. Multimodality;
2. Networkability;
3. Temporal flexibility; and
4. Message tailoring capabilities.

The 'overlapping' of these 4 qualities, brings about a number of *'Health Outcome Commonalities'*, being:

1. An increase in self-efficacy;
2. The ability to communicate and control information either synchronously or asynchronously;
3. The ability to manipulate text; and
4. The ability to narrow/segment information for a particular audience, target group or individual (Usher, 2011).

Simililarly, research by Ernst and Young (2012) reported that such enabling technologies, as above, potentially, offer and support for individuals to become increasingly more connected into any health-care ecosystem and can deliver actionable information, overcoming the barriers of multiple data silos across many platforms. Such attributes create unique opportunities to promote positive and sustainable behavioral changes amongst various populations.

Usher *et al.*, (2015) investigated how SM platforms create pathways for accessing widely available information; particularly those favored by the younger generations. The aim was to investigate the way university students use communication technologies in an attempt to access health information. The results ($n = 696$) indicated that communication technologies were used to extensively search for health information which ultimately resulted in positive health behavioural changes in participants' health patterns; however they perceived lack of reliability of the information as a pressing issue. The results suggested that appealing, persuasive and reliable SM can be used extensively to promote health amongst Australian youth.

Interestingly, Usher et al., (2015) further identified that the most preferred technology platforms were identified as being:

1. Smartphones, and
2. Facebook.

Similarly, Ernst and Young (2012) maintain that the transformation in health information access is being driven by modern technology's unique capacity for increased convenience, access to information, social connectedness and diversity. It is further understood that smartphones have become widespread and for most youth indispensable (World Economic Forum 2011). What is more, in this study, participants indicated that Instagram was used as the most likely technology for distributing and storing pictures on health information related to topics as: dietary intake, recipes and menu choices (Usher et al., 2015). Hochman *et al.* (2012: 6) explained such a trend:

Individuals are increasingly seeking ways to visualise, analyse and discover concealed socio-cultural characteristics and trends in an ever-growing flow of visual information.

Current and past research identifies the potential for utilising a variety of SM network for disseminating health information and for improving dietary habits, in a timely and accurate manner, and as such warrants further research regarding its effectiveness in achieving positive behaviour modification. Similar claims by Wong, Merchanta and Morenoc (2014), maintain that SM networks can provide prospects to heighten adolescents' and young adults' engagement in health care delivery. However, further study is required to outline a clear value proposition and develop evidence-based frameworks for measuring the impact of SM networks (such as Instagram) on young people's health. Of most significance, were results from this study (Usher *et al.*, 2015) which indicated that health related topics, such as exercise or diet, were the most frequently accessed types of health information. Ernst & Young (2012) also state that given the increasing trend of many CD are occurring at an older age, this information is important establishing preventive measures and delivering tailored and timely health related information. To minimise future CD epidemics, further research is necessary to explore how modern forms of communication technologies can be better harnessed to both equip and enable young adults as a means of preventing lifestyle diseases and that will sustain positive health behavioral changes.

Whilst positive behavioural changes were observed in this study, due to use of Web 1.0 (Internet) and Web 2.0 (social media), it is important to note that a small negative behaviour change, as a result of accessing mobile wireless devices (smartphones) and SM was also observed. It is possible that the inherent nature of modern technologies that exposes individuals to pervasive product marketing, powerful social norms and mass media, could account for the acquisition of various negative health behaviours evident in this research (Usher *et al.*, 2015).

SOLUTIONS AND RECOMMENDATIONS

Important to this chapter are specific recommendations for future practices and policies surrounding youth health (Cheung, Yip, Townsend and Scotch; 2008). Specifically, it is predicted that mental health issues among the student population are likely to escalate as Australian universities attract more young people from disadvantaged backgrounds (Higher Education, 2011). Similarly, Stallman (2011) further highlighted a need for Australian universities to take a broad and proactive approach to the mental health and wellbeing of students, in addition to targeting specific problems such as alcohol abuse.

Importantly, this study raises several questions that need to be addressed if e-health amongst Australian university students is to be successful. Firstly, what structural / environmental supports are needed to engage with university students from disadvantaged socio-economic groups? Secondly, what critical appraisal and e-literacy skills, do young adults attending universities, need to acquire to successfully access, comprehend and implement online health information? Lastly, what initiatives are required to ensure that gender resistance to e-health knowledge management is understood and subsequently minimized? However, firm conclusions, about the relationship between race, gender, and Internet use, are difficult to draw (Jones et al., 2009).

An initial start for Australian university health services could come in the form of adopting rigorous practices which maintain high ethical standards concerning e-health promotion and information dissemination. Discussions surrounding the importance of online practices and ethical guidelines are cause for further research (Risk & Dzenowagis, 2001). Notwithstanding, contemporary international literature and findings from this research, do provide guidelines that should be a consideration by current and future Australian University health services. In brief, these include the:

1. Establishment of third-party rating systems that enable students to filter harmful health information and to identify and select high-quality information ("downstream filtering") through health website content labels.
2. Creation of enforcement infrastructures.

3. Introduction educational modules which address reliability scales and seals associated with health websites.
4. The active encouragement of health information providers / services to conform to ethical codes of conduct.
5. Development of health information that is trustworthy and up-to-date.
6. Establishment of health information via providers who possess a high quality of service delivery through the application of meta tags and labeling technologies.
7. Implementation of a broad and proactive approach to the mental health and wellbeing of students – these to include e-health knowledge management initiatives.
8. Provision of on-line health services that follow Hi-Ethical principles.

As this is the first Australian study that has examined e-health knowledge management by Australian university students, further research should be undertaken to investigate possible avenues for the successful design and implementation of future university wide e-health initiatives. Therefore, again, it would be assumed that a larger cross-cultural study should be advocated for and undertaken. Primary prevention campaigns and strategies should be aimed to assist university students to reduce major risk factors associated with tobacco consumption, poor diet, insufficient physical activity, being overweight or obese, mental health, unsafe alcohol use, infectious diseases and exposure to ultraviolet radiation (AIHW, 2011). Moreover, results from this study, albeit drawn from a relatively small sample size, have been found to mirror many of the findings from similar international studies and literature. The results and recommendations presented throughout this paper are an opportunity for Australian university health services to develop and implement future effective health promoting strategies and campaigns.

CONCLUSION

This chapter has explored and presented how Web 1.0 (Internet), Web 2.0 (SM) and to a further extent mobile wireless devices (smartphones), are used by Australian university students for accessing personal health information, particularly for enhancing social connectedness, personal health care management, and the access and dissemination of health related information. It further presents, more contemporary and broader research and a theoretical basis of claim, which investigates the impact Web 2.0 and mobile wireless devices (smartphones) has had on youth and their health information access. The information and knowledge generated from this research has provided insights through which it could be determined how Australian university students use modern forms of communication technologies in an attempt to access and implement health information. What is clear, is that young Australians are turning to SM and similar devices / tools for accessing and implementing health related information. It is suggested that a possible way forward is to design effective electronic platforms that culminate the e-technologies so as to have the maximum health benefits for this generation. Future studies should be aimed at exploring how the health of young Australians could be enhanced by developing e-health platforms that mitigate a number of identified SM tools and devices that are frequently used by Australian youth (Usher *et al.*, 2015).

Lastly, futurists in the area of health care delivery, are looking to explore the possibilities of utilising, a third generation of Internet-based services – Web 3.0. It is envisaged that 'The Semantic Web' (Web 3.0) will simplify human–computer interfaces by enabling computers to 'understand' the actual/ intended meanings of the content as they process it. When combined with such technologies as health apps (applications), smartphones, wireless devices and mobile technologies, an ecosystem will be created that will be useful to the medical and health related professionals because they are agile, handheld, easy to use and can be used on the move. A recommendation from this chapter is for further research and cross-cultural studies to be undertaken to investigate possible collaborative avenues which will explore how such a health ecosystem could better deliver health information to Australian youth. Lastly, such recommendations and predictions, as proposed in this chapter, offer opportunities rather than barriers and needs to be embraced with a degree of optimism for creating better health for all Australians.

REFERENCES

American College Health Association. (2007). National College Health Assessment Spring 2006 Reference Group data report. *Journal of Health.*, *55*, 195–206. PMID:17319325

Anderson, K. J. (2001). Internet use among college students: An exploratory study. *Journal of American College Health*, *50*(1), 21–26. doi:10.1080/07448480109595707 PMID:11534747

Arnett, J. J. (2000). Emerging adulthood: A theory of development from the late teens through the twenties. *The American Psychologist*, *55*(5), 469–480. doi:10.1037/0003-066X.55.5.469 PMID:10842426

Australian Bureau of Statistics (ABS). (2011). *Households using the Internet*. Retrieved September 12, 2012, from: http://www.abs.gov.au/ausstats/abs@.nsf/mf/8146.0

Australian Institute for Primary Care. (2008). *System reform and development for chronic disease management*. Australian Institute for Primary Care. Retrieved October 21, 2009, from: http://www.health.gov.au/internet/nhhrc/publishing.nsf/Content/038-aipclatrobe/$FILE/038%20Australian%20Institute%20for%20Primary%20Care,%20La%20Trobe%20University%20Attachment%20B.pdf

Australian Institute of Health and Welfare. (2011). *Authoritative information and statistics to promote better health and wellbeing*. Retrieved September 12, 2012, from: http://www.aihw.gov.au/cancer-control-health-priority-area/

Avendaño, C., Mata, A., Villanueva, A. M., Martínez, V. S., & Sarmiento, C. A. (2010). Laptop expositions affect motility and induce DNA fragmentation in human spermatozoa in vitro by a non-thermal effect: A preliminary report. *Journal of Fertility and Sterility*, *94*(4), 73. doi:10.1016/j.fertnstert.2010.07.284

Barker, E. T., & Galambos, N. L. (2007). Body dissatisfaction, living away from parents, and poor social adjustment predict binge eating symptoms in young women making the transition to University. *Journal of Youth and Adolescence*, *36*(7), 904–911. doi:10.1007/s10964-006-9134-6

Bernhardt, J., & Hubley, J. (2001). Health education and the Internet: The beginning of a revolution. *Health Education Research*, *16*(5), 643–645. doi:10.1093/her/16.6.643

Binkowska-Bury, M., & Januszewicz, P. (2010). Sense of coherence and health-related behaviour among University students--a questionnaire survey. *Journal of Public Health*, *18*(3), 145–150. PMID:21033609

Borzekowski, D. (2001). Adolescent cyber-surfing for health information: A new resource that crosses barriers. *Archives of Pediatrics & Adolescent Medicine*, *155*(7), 813–817. doi:10.1001/archpedi.155.7.813 PMID:11434849

Boyd, D. M., & Ellison, N. B. (2007). Social network sites: Definition, history, and scholarship. *Journal of Computer-Mediated Communication, 13*(1), 210–230. doi:10.1111/j.1083-6101.2007.00393.x

Boyer, C., & Geissbuhler, A. (2006). Health and the Internet for all. *International Journal of Medical Informatics, 75*(1), 1–3. doi:10.1016/j.ijmedinf.2005.07.039 PMID:16325462

Brodie, M., Flournoy, E., Altman, D., Blendon, R. J., Benson, J. M., & Rosenbaum, M. D. (2000). Health information, the Internet, and the digital divide. *Health Affairs, 19*(6), 255–265. doi:10.1377/hlthaff.19.6.255 PMID:11192412

Cain, J., Brent, I., & Fox, P. (2009). Web 2.0 and pharmacy education. *American Journal of Pharmaceutical Education, 73*(7), 1–11. doi:10.5688/aj7307120 PMID:19960079

Charles, S., Nicole, E., & Cliff, L. (2008). Social capital, self-esteem, and use of online social network sites: A longitudinal analysis. *Journal of Applied Developmental Psychology, 29*(200), 434–445.

Cheung, K., Yip, K., Townsend, J., & Scotch, M. (2008). HCLS 2.0/3.0: Health care and life sciences data mashup using Web 2.0/3.0. *Journal of Biomedical Informatics, 41*(5), 694–705. doi:10.1016/j.jbi.2008.04.001 PMID:18487092

Cormode, G., & Krishnamurthy, B. (2008). Key differences between Web 1.0 and Web 2.0. *First Monday, 13*(6). doi:10.5210/fm.v13i6.2125

Courtenay, W. (2000). Construction of masculinity and their influence on men's well-being: A theory of gender and health. *Social Science & Medicine, 50*(10), 1385–1401. doi:10.1016/S0277-9536(99)00390-1 PMID:10741575

Cummins, J. (2010). *Few hospitals use social media effectively, says study*. Health Leaders Media. Retrieved from October 13, 2011, from http://www.healthleadersmedia.com/content/TEC-245418/Few-Hospitals-Use-Social-Media-Effectively-Says-Study.html

Department of Health and Ageing. (2008). *Towards a National Primary Health Care Strategy: a discussion paper from the Australian Government*. Retrieved Feburary 6, 2009, from http://www.health.gov.au/primaryhealthstrategy

eBizMBA Rank. (2010). Retrieved March 13, 2010, from http://www.ebizmba.com/articles/health-websites

Ellison, N., Steinfield, C., & Lampe, C. (2007). The benefits of Facebook "friends:" Social capital and college students' use of online social network sites. *Journal of Computer-Mediated Communication, 12*, 1143–1168.

Ernst & Young. (2012). Mobile technology poised to enable a new era in health care. *EYGM Limited.* Retrieved April 5, 2013, from http://www.ey.com/Publication/vwLUAssets/mHealth_Report_January_2013/$FILE/mHealth%20Report_Final.pdf

Escoffery, C., Miner, K., Adame, D., Butler, S., McCormick, L., & Mendell, E. (2005). Internet use for health information among college students. *Journal of American College Health, 53*(4), 183–188. doi:10.3200/JACH.53.4.183-188 PMID:15663067

Fox, S., & Jones, S. (2009). *The social life of health information*. Pew Internet and American Life Project. Retrieved March 13, 2010, from http://www.pewinternet.org/Reports/2009/8-The-Social-Life-of-Health-Information.aspx

Fox, S., & Rainie, L. (2006). The Online Health Care Revolution: How the Web Helps American Take better Care of Themselves. *ElectronicHealthcare*, *8*(5), 110–113.

Fox, S., Rainie, L., & Horrigan, J. (2000). The online health care revolution: How the web helps Americans take better care of themselves. *Pew Internet and American Life Project*, *91*, 235–245.

Gehl, R. W. (2011). The archive and the processor: The internal logic of Web 2.0. *New Media & Society*, *13*(8), 1228–1244. doi:10.1177/1461444811401735

Hackworth, B. A., & Kunz, M. B. (2011). Healthcare and social media: Building relationship via social networks. Morehead State University. *Academy of Health Care Management Journal*, *7*(2), 34–45.

Head, A., & Eisenberg, M. (2011). How college students use the Web to conduct everyday life research. *First Monday*, *16*(4), 2. doi:10.5210/fm.v16i4.3484

Hendricks, C., Murdaugh, C., & Pender, N. (2006). The Adolescent Lifestyle Profile: Development and psychometric characteristics. *Journal ofNational Black Nurses' Association*, *17*(2), 1–5. PMID:17410753

Hewitt, A., & Forte, A. (2006). *Crossing boundaries: Identity management and student/faculty relationships on the Facebook*. Poster presented at the ACM Special Interest Group on Computer-Supported Cooperative Work, Banff, Canada.

Higher Education. (2011). *Mental health issues among students to escalate*. Retrieved October 5, 2012, from http://www.theaustralian.com.au/higher-education/mental-health-issues-among-students-to-escalate/story-e6frgcjx-1226111953584

Hitlin, P., & Rainie, L. (2005). Teens, technology, and school. *Pew Internet & American Life Project*, *93*, 124–201.

Hochman, N., & Schwartz, S. (2012). *Visualizing Instagram: Tracing Cultural Visual Rhythms AAAI Technical Report WS-12-03. Social Media Visualization*. Association for the Advancement of Artificial Intelligence. Retrieved June 11, 2012, from http://www.aaai.org/ocs/index.php/ICWSM/ICWSM12/paper/viewFile/4782/5091

Horgan, A., & Sweeney, J. (2010). Young students' use of the Internet for mental health information and support. *ElectronicHealthcare*, *17*(2), 117–123. PMID:20465756

Huang, T. T., Harris, K. J., Lee, R. E., Nazir, N., Born, W., & Kaur, H. (2003). Assessing overweight, obesity, diet, and physical activity in college students. *Journal of American College Health*, *52*(2), 83–86. doi:10.1080/07448480309595728 PMID:14765762

Jimenez-Pernett, J., & Olry de Labry-Lima, A. (2010). Use of the internet as a source of health information by Spanish adolescents. *BMC Medical Informatics and Decision Making*, *10*(1), 6. doi:10.1186/1472-6947-10-6 PMID:20113486

Johnson-Yale, S., Millermaier, S., & Seoane Perez, F. (2009). Everyday life, online: U.S. college students' use of the Internet. *First Monday*, *14*(10), 1.

Jones, S., Johnson-Yale, C., Millermaier, S., & Seoane Perez, F. (2009). Everyday life, online: U.S. college students' use of the Internet. *First Monday*, *14*(10), 5. doi:10.5210/fm.v14i10.2649

Kamel Boulos, M. N., & Wheeler, S. (2007). The emerging Web 2.0 social software: An enabling suite of sociable technologies in health and health care education. *Health Information and Libraries Journal*, *24*(1), 2–23. doi:10.1111/j.1471-1842.2007.00701.x PMID:17331140

Kenneth, B. (2005). *Internet Enhances Patient Education*. U.S Publications. Retrieved from http:www.uspharmacist.com/oldformat.asp

Korp, P. (2006). Health on the Internet: Implications for health promotion. *Health Education Research*, *21*(1), 78–86. doi:10.1093/her/cyh043 PMID:15994845

Lampe, C., Ellison, N., & Steinfield, C. (2007). A familiar face(book): Profile elements as signals in an online social network. *Proceedings of the SIGCHI conference on human factors in computing systems* (pp. 435–444). New York: ACM. doi:10.1145/1240624.1240695

Landsberg, B., Plachta-Danielzik, S., Lange, D., Johannsen, M., Seiberl, J., & Müller, M. J. (2010). Clustering of lifestyle factors and association with overweight in adolescents of the Kiel Obesity Prevention Study. *Public Health Nutrition*, *13*(10A), 1708–1715. doi:10.1017/S1368980010002260 PMID:20883570

Laska, M. N., Pasch, K. E., Lust, K., Story, M., & Ehlinger, E. (2009). Latent Class Analysis of Lifestyle Characteristics and Health Risk Behaviors among College Youth. *Preventative Science*, *5*, 12. PMID:19499339

Lin, N. (1999). Building a network theory of social capital. *Connections*, *22*, 28–51.

Lowery, R., Galuska, D. A., Fulton, J. E., Wechsler, H., Kann, L., & Collins, J. L. (2000). Physical activity, food choice, and weight management goals and practices among U.S. college students. *American Journal of Preventive Medicine*, *18*, 8–27. PMID:10736536

Madden, M., & Zickuhr, K. (2011). *65% of online adults use social networking sites*. Washington, DC: Pew Internet and American Life Project, Pew Research Centre. Retrieved March 8, 2012, from http://www.pewinternet.org/~/media//Files/Reports/2011/PIP-SNS-Update-2011.pdf

Mitra, A., Willyard, J., Platt, C., & Parson, M. (2005). Exploring Web usage and selection criteria among male and female students. *Journal of Computer-Mediated Communication*, *10*(3), 10.

Nielsen's Internet & Technology Report. (2010). Retrieved March 13, 2011, from http://www.emerchant.com.au/blog/nielsen%E2%80%99s-2010-internet-technology-report/

Norman, C., & Skinner, H. (2006). Ehealth Literacy: Essential skills for consumer health in a networked world. *Journal of Medical Internet Research*, *8*(2), 9. doi:10.2196/jmir.8.2.e9 PMID:16867972

Nöthlings, U., Ford, E., Kröger, J., & Boeing, H. (2010). Lifestyle factors and mortality among adults with diabetes: Findings from the European Prospective Investigation into Cancer and Nutrition–Potsdam study. *Journal of Diabetes*, *2*(2), 112–117. doi:10.1111/j.1753-0407.2010.00069.x PMID:20923493

O'Reilly, T. (2007). What is Web 2.0: Design patterns and business models for the next generation of software. *Communications & Stratégies*, *65*(1), 17.

Office of National Statistics. (2009). *National Omnibus Survey*. Retrieved April 23, 2012, from http://www.statistics.gov.uk/default.asp

Pew Internet & American Life Project. (2009). *Usage over time*. Retrieved April 4, 2012, from http://pewInternet.org//trends/UsageOverTime_Jan_2009.xls

Pullman, A. W., Masters, R. C., Zalot, L. C., Carde, L. E., Saraiva, M. M., & Dam, Y. Y. et al. (2009). Effect of the transition from high school to University on anthropometric and lifestyle variables in males. *Applied Physiology, Nutrition, and Metabolism*, *34*(2), 162–171. doi:10.1139/H09-007 PMID:19370046

Reddy, P., Rankins, D., Timoshanko, A., & Dunbar, J. (2011). Life! in Australia: Translating prevention research into a large-scale intervention. *Br J Diabetes Vasc Dis*, *11*(4), 193–197. doi:10.1177/1474651411410724

Risk, A., & Dzenowagis, J. (2001). Review Of Internet Health Information Quality Initiatives. *Journal of Medical Internet Research*, *3*(4), 8. doi:10.2196/jmir.3.4.e28 PMID:11772543

Seeman, N. (2008). Web 2.0 and chronic illness: New horizons, new opportunities. *ElectronicHealthcare*, *6*(3), 104–110. PMID:18326388

Stallman, H. (2011). *Mental illness running high among uni students*. The World Today. Retrieved from http://www.abc.net.au/news/2010-11-23/mental-illness-running-high-among-uni-students/2348772

Steptoe, A., Wardle, J., Cui, W., Bellisle, F., Zotti, A. M., Baranyai, R., & Sanderman, R. (2002). Trends in smoking, diet, physical exercise and attitudes toward health in European University students from 13 countries. *Preventive Medicine*, *35*(2), 97–104. doi:10.1006/pmed.2002.1048 PMID:12200093

Stutzman, F. (2006). *An evaluation of identity-sharing behavior in social network communities. Paper presented at the International Digital Media Arts*. Association and the Miami University Center for Interactive Media Studies CODE Conference, Oxford, OH.

Towards a National Primary Health Care Strategy: A discussion paper from the Australian Government. (2008). Department of Health and Ageing, Commonwealth of Australia. Retrieved October 6, 2011, from http://www.health.gov.au/primaryhealthstrategy

Uden-Kraan, C. F. (2009). Health-related Internet use by patients with somatic diseases: Frequency of use and characteristics of users. *Informatics for Health & Social Care*, *34*(1), 18–29. doi:10.1080/17538150902773272 PMID:19306196

Usher, W. (2009). Gold Coast general practitioners' understanding pertaining to reliability, interactive and usability components associated with health websites. *International Journal of Behaviour and Information Technology*, *28*(1), 39–44. doi:10.1080/01449290802187736

Usher, W. (2011). Types of social media (Web 2.0) usage by Australian Allied Health professionals' for early 21st century practice promotion and e-health care delivery. *Social Work in Health Care*, *50*(4), 305–329. doi:10.1080/00981389.2010.534317 PMID:21512953

Usher, W., Gudes, O., & Parekh, S. (2015). Exploring the use of technology pathways to access health information by Australian university students: A multi - dimensional approach. *Health Information Management Journal*, *4*, 1–12. PMID:26113541

White, A. (2006). Men's Health in the 21st Century. *International Journal of Men's Health*, *5*(1), 1–17. doi:10.3149/jmh.0501.1

Wong, C., Merchanta, R., & Morenoc, M. (2014). Using social media to engage adolescents and young adults with their health. *Health Care*, *31*(3), 56–58. PMID:25984444

Wood, G. (2004). Academic Original Sin: Plagiarism, the Internet, and Librarians. *Journal of Academic Librarianship*, *30*(3), 237–242. doi:10.1016/j.acalib.2004.02.011

World Economic Forum. (2011). *Personal Data: The Emergence of a New Asset Class*. Geneva, Switzerland: World Economic Forum.

World Health Organisation (WHO). (2010). *The social determinants of health*. WHO. Retrieved November 2, 2012, from http://www.who.int/social_determinants/en/

Yee, K. C., Miils, E., & Airey, C. (2008). Perfect match? Generation Y as change agents for information communication technology implementation in healthcare. *Studies in Health Technology and Informatics*, *136*, 496–501. PMID:18487780

Young, J., & Simon, W. (2005). iCon: Steve Jobs, the greatest second act in the history of business. *Studies in Health Technology and Informatics*, *23*, 45–50.

KEY TERMS AND DEFINITIONS

Web 1.0: An early stage of the conceptual evolution of the World Wide Web, where users could only view websites but could not contribute to the content of the website. Technically, Web 1.0 webpage's information is closed to external editing. Web 1.0 concentrated on presenting, not creating so that user-generated content was not available (Cormode & Krishnamurthy, 2008).

Web 2.0: Social media (SM), has been characterised as 'representing various forms of consumer-generated content such as blogs, virtual communities, wikis, social networks, collaborative tagging, and media files shared on sites like Facebook, Instagram, YouTube and Flickr' (Young & Simon, 2005).

Web 3.0: Viewed as the first-generation (convergence of the virtual and physical world) of web development layers that include TV-quality open video, 3D simulations, augmented reality, human-constructed semantic standards, and pervasive broadband, wireless, and sensors (Gehl, 2011).

Wireless Monitoring Devices: Technologies that allow an electronic device to exchange data wirelessly (using radio waves) over a computer network, including high-speed Internet connections (Avendaño et al., 2010). Examples include, activity monitoring arm brace, foot sensors and GPS positioning supported by Android phones / e-platforms and smartphones.

This work was previously published in Design, Development, and Integration of Reliable Electronic Healthcare Platforms edited by Anastasius Moumtzoglou, pages 49-71, copyright year 2017 by Medical Information Science Reference (an imprint of IGI Global).

Chapter 4
Using Wikipedia to Teach Written Health Communication

Melissa Vosen Callens
North Dakota State University, USA

ABSTRACT

Unlike first-year writing courses, upper-division writing courses often require students to engage in discipline specific writing. In the author's upper-division course, Writing in the Health Professions, students examine health literacy as it pertains to both oral and written patient-provider communication. Students edit and expand a Wikipedia article for the final course assignment. The advantages of this assignment are threefold. First, students write for an authentic audience, decreasing student apathy. Second, students engage civically, improving health information accessed by millions of people across the world. Finally, students improve content of existing articles and broaden the scope of new articles written, leading to more diverse content and perspectives. In this chapter, the author discusses the above assignment, providing descriptions of scaffolding activities. Potential drawbacks of using Wikipedia to teach students how to write using plain language is discussed, in addition to strategies that might limit these difficulties.

INTRODUCTION

At North Dakota State University (NDSU), a land-grant research institution, I teach several upper-division writing courses: *Writing in the Health Professions*, *Business and Professional Writing*, and *Visual Culture and Language*. Unlike first-year composition courses, upper-division writing courses at NDSU require students to engage in discipline-specific research and writing. These 300-level courses are meant to prepare students for the workplace and / or graduate school. The primary focus of my *Writing in the Health Professions* course is health literacy as it pertains to both oral and written patient-provider communication. According to Osborne (2004), nurse and health literacy advocate, health literacy is "a shared responsibility in which patients and providers each must communicate in ways the other can understand" (p. 2). I believe health literacy is an important and appropriate focus for the course, as it best simulates the writing my students will engage in as healthcare professionals. While I could ask students to review

DOI: 10.4018/978-1-5225-1928-7.ch004

and / or write journal articles, both common upper-division writing assignments, realistically, most of these students will not formally review or write a journal article after graduation.

For the foreseeable future, most of my students will not be attending graduate school or working in a lab in academia. Upon graduation, a majority of the students will enter the workforce as pharmacists or registered nurses. Some students will get promotions from their current employers as they already work as pharmacy technicians, licensed practical nurses, or certified nursing assistants. When in the workplace, most will be asked to write to inform, to educate both colleagues and patients on a variety of work and health-related issues. With either of the above audiences, these students will be expected to write in a clear and concise manner. They will be expected to communicate using plain language. In my course, students quickly learn that plain language does not mean changing the meaning of their message; rather, plain language is using words and concepts people already know and understand. If that is not possible, words and concepts should be clearly defined in a manner that the reader can understand (Osborne, 2004, p. 157). Last summer, I asked students to expand a Wikipedia article of their choosing to hone their ability to communicate in a clear and concise manner. In addition to learning more about how to use plain language, students sharpened their research skills and understanding of how social media can facilitate collaboration. This chapter explores that endeavor, explaining both the benefits and pitfalls of using Wikipedia in a writing course.

THEORETICAL FRAMEWORK

Wikipedia: An Educational Social Media Platform

Some may argue that Wikipedia is not a social media site; rather, as its name suggests, it is an online reference book, an encyclopedia. While it is an online encyclopedia, Wikipedia is also a social media platform because anyone can contribute and exchange information on the site; Wikipedia is a collaborative endeavor. Wikipedia has a community of users that has a common goal: a desire to educate and make knowledge available to every single person on Earth—or at least every single person with access to a computer and the Internet. All Wikipedians (what contributors to Wikipedia are called) have their own user talk pages where they are encouraged to share information about themselves and their personal editing philosophy. They are also encouraged to share their reasoning behind each of their edits and contributions.

In addition to user talk pages, each article on Wikipedia has a talk page in which users can discuss the article's content as well as any edits prior to publishing those changes. Wikipedia encourages discussion on talk pages before changes are made. For talk pages that generate a large amount of conversation, Wikipedia archives these discussions to help keep the talk page easy-to-read and up-to-date (Help: Using talk pages, n.d.). Archiving these discussions documents the collaborative process of contributing users and is a great way to see how an article evolved. Talk areas provide Wikipedians, including student Wikipedians, a chance to communicate, socialize, and learn from one another. In addition to learning about Wikipedia and the collaborative writing process, students working on Wikipedia can improve their editing and grammar knowledge, hone their research skills, and learn how to communicate using plain language.

Collaborative Writing and ELL Learners

If an instructor wants students to learn more about collaborative writing and the Internet, he/she might require students to become active on several articles' talk pages and work with other Wikipedians to develop and tweak content. Developing a relationship with other editors is particularly fruitful for English language learners (ELL) as they learn more about the English language from native speakers across the world. Furthermore, if an instructor wants ELL students to practice their newly acquired skills, he / she might ask the students to translate an article in English to their native language, adding it to their native languages' Wikipedia site. This gives students much needed practice, but also expands Wikipedia, likely introducing more diverse content to different language versions of the site. Similarly, Wikipedia is also a great site to study if one wants to discuss differences between languages and dialects of languages, such as British English and American English. An introductory linguistics course may find this exercise useful.

Editing and Grammar

If an instructor wants students to learn more about grammar, he / she might ask students to edit articles and explain their choices and their editing philosophy to the class. In addition to engaging in a dialogue with their classmates, students may also have to explain their editing choices to other Wikipedians. While this may initially be overwhelming for some students, it is a great exercise in community and collaboration. If the dialogue goes in a negative direction, and it sometimes does, this is a teachable moment. Students can learn more about trolling and how to respond to people who engage in this type of activity on the Internet.

Research

If an instructor wants students to learn more about researching and presenting material from a neutral point-of-view, he / she might ask students to write a new article on a topic of their choosing or develop a "stub" article. A stub article on Wikipedia is an article that has been started, but has been flagged because it lacks content and needs to be developed. Any registered user can start a stub article. Expanding a stub article is a great alternative to traditional reports often assigned in writing courses. Students are still expected to find credible information and summarize and synthesize it. The primary difference between a Wikipedia entry and a traditional report is that students are writing for an audience beyond the four classroom walls. Since students often lack motivation in required general education courses, including first-year and upper-division composition courses, one way to avoid student apathy is to involve students in a writing activity that has an authentic audience (Graham & Harris, 2007, p.124). Writing for people other than their instructor and classmates can be highly motivating for some students, which is what can happen when students contribute to Wikipedia.

Plain Language in the Health Professions

Finally, when I was first assigned to teach *Writing in the Health Professions,* I found it difficult to teach pharmacy and nursing students, who have been immersed in medical jargon and academese for at least three years, to communicate using plain language. Studying Wikipedia, however, was a helpful way for these students to understand what type of information their patients do comprehend and *are* accessing and reading prior to their visits with healthcare providers. For example, Tunick and Brand (2015) note that "an August 2013 Google search yielded over 2 billion hits for 'health information,' 774 million hits for 'cancer information,' and 7.5 million hits for 'pediatric cancer information'" (p. 346). This translates to an incredible number of people seeking written healthcare information on the Internet. Is that information, however, easy to read and medically accurate? In my course, the students explored this question from a variety of angles.

In their study on Web 2.0 use by junior physicians, Hughes, Joshi, Lemonde, and Wareham (2009) noted that all 35 participants mentioned Internet use by patients, "such as receiving and discussing Wikipedia printouts during a patient consultation" (p. 651). This study was a perfect starting point for class discussion, as it helped explain why we were studying social media and plain language in an upper-division writing course. The students' patients and future patients already use Wikipedia. As medical providers, it is in my students' best interest to learn more about the site.

Because of its wide use, I believe it is important for my students to know what information is available on social media. It is also important that they understand how sites like Wikipedia work, as this knowledge will better prepare them for conversations with patients. In addition, because of the wide use of social media, it is important to encourage students to improve information on these sites, as they are near experts in their field.

METHODOLOGY AND PEDAGOGY

Participants

Students enrolled in my asynchronous online *Writing in the Health Professions* were juniors and seniors at NDSU; while most lived in the immediate area, some of the students were three hours away at a satellite campus. All of the students who completed the Wikipedia assignment (14) had been accepted into the nursing professional program, which means they had a minimum GPA of 2.75. For most of the students, they were introduced to genre theory in their first-year writing course(s). After being immersed in their nursing classes for three years, however, most of my students had forgotten about genre theory and how it relates to writing. In addition, there were a small number (three) of non-traditional students, who had returned to school after years in the workforce. These students took first-year English years ago, and some even took the course when it focused more on literature. Because of this, at the beginning of the course, we spent time reviewing genre theory. What are the genre conventions of lab reports? What are the conventions of patient charts? At the start of each unit, we reviewed genre theory and discussed what genre they would be exploring next, including, at the end of the semester, Wikipedia articles.

Purpose

The culminating project required students to improve, by editing and expanding, a Wikipedia article related to healthcare. This was an appropriate culminating project for a variety of reasons. First, by contributing to Wikipedia, students contributed to their field in a large and meaningful way—potentially educating hundreds of thousands of people—as many people use Wikipedia to obtain information. When writing for Wikipedia, students wrote for the general public, which helped them better understand audience and voice. Anyone with a computer and an Internet connection—family, friends, potential employers, and strangers—could see their work. Whether we, as instructors, like it or not, many people use Wikipedia as one of their primary go-to places for information on just about any topic. There were 8,524,715 views per hour during May 2015 on Wikipedia (Wikimedia, 2015). From a medical standpoint, these views were not simply from patients, but also providers. In their study on Web 2.0 use in the medical field, Hughes, Joshi, Lemonde, and Wareham (2009) found that tools like Google or Wikipedia are being "regularly employed in clinical practice by junior physicians" (p. 654). Not only would my students encounter patients using Wikipedia and other Web 2.0 technologies, but they also would likely end up using these resources as medical professionals.

Second, and most importantly for upper-division writing instructors, my students learned how to research a topic, find appropriate and credible sources, and present that information from a concise and neutral point-of-view. Third, students learned how to communicate using plain language. They were required to identify and consider the literacy levels of the general public. Finally, students learned (or relearned) how to properly cite sources and produce grammatically correct documents. As a secondary benefit, but one worth noting, this assignment also brought different and varied voices to the Wikipedia community. Student writers in a variety of disciplines can help make Wikipedia more diverse in regard to content *and* perspective. Based on a survey of 58,000 self-selected Wikipedians, "23% of contributors have completed degree-level education, 26% are undergraduates and 45% have secondary education or less. 87% are men and 13% women" (Wikipedia: Wikipedians, n.d.). In my course, 13 of the 14 students were female; by asking these students to complete this assignment, new female voices were introduced to the site.

Building up to Wikipedia

My students completed several scaffolding activities to ensure they not only understood the nuts-and-bolts of editing and contributing to Wikipedia, but also the community aspect of Wikipedia and how knowledge could be generated collaboratively. It was important to explain clearly why they were being asked to undertake this assignment, as many of my students had been told that Wikipedia is not a resource they should use in the classroom or otherwise. More of this will be discussed in a later section of this chapter, "Pitfalls."

Prior to the Wikipedia assignment, students completed several assignments that helped them think about how their patients find health-related information as well as if they comprehend it. For one of their first assignments, students identified a healthcare-related topic currently covered in the media and compared the popular media stories to peer-reviewed medical research on the same topic. The primary purpose of this assignment was so students learned how to evaluate health information from a variety of sources and see firsthand how accurate the media was at presenting health information. They also learned how to critical analyze a medical report, which is an important skill to have if they are going to take complex medical information and summarize it using plain language for their patients.

By understanding how to analyze medical research as well as how the media informs or misinforms the public, my students are better prepared to have conversations with their patients about evaluating medical information obtained on the Web. Health News Review (http://www.healthnewsreview.org/) provided my students with a set of ten criteria to use when analyzing popular media stories. The criterion helped students perform a systematic review and analysis of the media stories. Their review and analysis ultimately led to an evaluation, an evaluation similar to the ones they would likely have to provide in the workforce and an evaluation they would have to make before adding content to Wikipedia.

In addition, before moving to the Wikipedia assignment, students completed one other systematic review of health information. Students analyzed a healthcare document from a facility of their choosing using Helen Osborne's plain language checklist. These documents were typically patient-education brochures, handouts, or posters hung in pharmacies or clinics. Both of the above assignments helped students understand where patients currently get their information and how accessible and accurate that information might be. It helped them get a better understanding of plain language and how it is or is not used effectively in a healthcare setting. At this point the course, students evaluated Wikipedia articles on the same topic or related topics and chose an article to expand. Since they had already explored the topic in medical journals, popular media stories, and clinic literature, they had a good understanding of the information that was available to patients and what information was correct and what information was being misrepresented.

Resources

The WikiEd Foundation (https://wikiedu.org/) has great resources available to instructors, most of which I used. First, it offered an assignment generator that produced a course schedule for me to use, complete with scaffolding activities. It also offered several brochures related to planning a course, in addition to brochures that could be given to students. In an attempt to create an assignment that met my needs, when completing the assignment generator, I was asked to identify what type of project I was interested in assigning as well as how much time I wished to devote to the assignment. In addition to those questions, I also answered a series of questions that helped generate scaffolding activities that might be appropriate for the class. After I completed the generator, a schedule and rubric for the assignment was produced as well as a course page on Wikipedia. The WikiEd Foundation recommended a course page as it provided a space for my students to converse on Wikipedia, and it also made tracking student work much simpler. Without this function, it would have been difficult to determine what changes students made to articles, particularly if other Wikipedians removed those changes. In addition to the course page, the WikiEd Foundation also had a dashboard for me to use, which made tracking student activity and contributions even easier.

Scaffolding Activities

In my course, students completed several activities prior to editing and expanding an article. These scaffolding activities were required and graded on a complete / incomplete basis. After a brief introduction of the assignment, I led a discussion on Wikipedia use and asked how many students were familiar with it and use it. While most of the students used Wikipedia regularly in their personal lives, not one had edited or added to a Wikipedia entry. None of them had accounts, prior to the course. Because they were used to being consumers, I felt it was important to give them time to explore Wikipedia from the role of critical consumer and producer. Most of the students were surprised they were being asked to use Wikipedia in the classroom, as most had been told not to use it for course assignments. These comments prompted a discussion on our discussion board when is it okay to use Wikipedia as well as why I asked them to contribute to it for a class. First, students completed an online training offered by the WikiEd Foundation. I believe this is imperative step, as it introduced students to Wikipedia as a community, explained the editing process, and described the five pillars for contributing to Wikipedia. In addition to the online training, as mentioned, the WikiEd Foundation also provided handouts for students to use. I required students to read and discuss these handouts on the discussion board. Some of the handouts I used: Editing Wikipedia, Citing Sources on Wikipedia, Evaluating Wikipedia, and Illustrating Wikipedia. These handouts were of high quality and were great resources. It was one less document that I had to create. After completing the training, I asked my students to search for articles related to healthcare. They then evaluated those articles using criteria outlined in the Evaluating Wikipedia brochure provided by the WikiEd Foundation. Students posted their first evaluation to a safe space—on our course management site, Blackboard. This allowed them to obtain feedback from me as well as their peers in the class, honing their analysis skills. It also helped them hone their understanding of the five pillars of Wikipedia before engaging with other Wikipedians. This step was helpful because it also allowed me to answer any questions or concerns students had about the assignment *before* they moved to working on Wikipedia.

This particular activity was also useful because it helped students understand what makes a "good" article to edit. Some articles are already well-developed, particularly in the medical field. They do not need to be expanded. On the other hand, other articles, especially on obscure or relatively new topics, are difficult to edit and expand. I found that it takes a good amount of practice to find articles that need to be edited and can be edited without tremendous difficulty. Next, students were required to learn about the rules for editing medical content. Wikipedia has guidelines established to ensure that appropriate and accurate information is being published. One guideline, for example, reminds Wikipedians editing medical content to avoid medical jargon and to use plain language. This was particularly helpful for my students as they needed practice writing (and speaking) in a manner that all patients can understand. Not all guidelines, however, were as easy for my students to understand and follow. While the strict guidelines are there for good reason, they took some time for students to learn. For example, my students struggled to understand why they could not cite primary sources, likely because they were used to citing these sources in academic papers. They have been taught that peer-review journal articles, and rightfully so, are credible. Unfortunately, they are not appropriate for Wikipedia, an encyclopedia, and it took some time for my students to understand why that was. At this point, we again discussed genre, and students generated genre conventions of a Wikipedia entry.

After they practiced evaluating several different articles, students moved to working on Wikipedia. First, students communicated with one another on their personal user talk pages. This was also a safe space where they could converse with others and learn how to sign their comments, an important part of Wikipedia talk pages. Next, they worked in their own space, their sandbox, to draft article contributions before engaging others. Unlike Blackboard, both of those spaces gave them practice using the Wikipedia editor. Even the students who completed the online training several times (as an instructor, I could see who did) needed time to work in their sandbox to feel comfortable with the Wikipedia editor. After working in their sandbox, I asked students to suggest an edit for an article on the article's talk page. On the talk pages, some students received feedback from other Wikipedians; some did not. I wish I could have waited longer, to see if more students got feedback, but because this was a summer course, I had to keep the unit moving.

At this point, students were ready to make an actual edit. In my eight-week summer class, students only had time to add a few sentences to an article and suggest surface-level edits. In a longer 16-week course, I believe it would be possible for students to expand an article, two or three fold. Whatever the assignment objective, I also believe it is important to provide students with enough time to learn about the Wikipedia community and the guidelines for contributing. Because Wikipedia is a community of volunteers, volunteers who are proud of their work and proud of the value of Wikipedia, it is important—and respectful— for students to learn more about Wikipedia and the Wikipedia community before making any "live" changes to the site.

RESULTS AND DISCUSSION

By editing and expanding an article, my students were able to write for an authentic audience as well as participate actively in the larger community, to help create a better world.

Benefit: Authentic Writing

When writing for Wikipedia, my students wrote for an authentic audience, an audience beyond me, the classroom instructor. According to the Council of Writing Program Administrators (2011):

Effective instruction approaches writing as a whole and varied activity, by its nature including feedback from peers and experts that aims to create authentically communicative results. Most isolated drills and decontextualized instruction have shown no value in improving student writing in large part because authentic writing is always embedded in complex rhetorical situations. (Effective teaching practices in general studies writing classes section, para. 4)

In the assignment, students received feedback from other Wikipedians as well as their classmates and myself. I believe all these relationships were valuable to my students. The Wikipedians helped the students understand the importance of genre, purpose, voice, and audience.

For those unfamiliar with Wikipedia, it may seem as though they are no guidelines, no genre conventions, and no complex rhetorical situations. When I introduced this assignment to my students last summer, nearly all of them said just that. Most of them thought that anything goes on Wikipedia. In reality, all Wikipedia articles must adhere to a set of content guidelines, making a Wikipedia assignment a great way to teach or reinforce genre theory. All Wikipedia articles must be written from a neutral point-of-view, include only information that is verifiable, and contain no original research (Wikipedia: Policies and guidelines, n.d.). When discussing these guidelines with students, I reminded students of how each piece of writing can be categorized by genre. In addition, other Wikipedians also reminded students if they did not adhere to one of the guidelines.

Before the unit, all of my students were unaware of how Wikipedia worked and that professionals, in a variety of fields, were using Wikipedia and contributing to it. One student remarked about her contribution:

Seeing it on the Wikipedia page was really cool, and I felt like the information I contributed was useful. Before this course, I had no idea that anyone could edit Wikipedia articles let alone contribute to them. This is something that even if I had known I would not have done on my own.

In addition, many other students commented that they appreciated learning more about how the site worked, even if they were still unsure if they would use it or call it a credible source. One student commented:

Although it was a good experience to use Wikipedia and post on the site so I gained an understanding of how exactly the information is obtained by Wikipedia, I still will not count it as a reliable and will not be using it.

In addition to providing my students with an authentic audience and the opportunity to learn more about the site itself, one of the other benefits of incorporating the Wikipedia assignment was that my students were able to meaningfully contribute to their discipline.

Benefit: Civic Engagement

By assigning a Wikipedia project, my students had a chance to impact hundreds of thousands of lives. Civic engagement is when students participate actively in the community to "improve conditions for others or to help shape the community's future" (Adler & Goggin, 2005, p. 236). While editing and writing for Wikipedia may not be considered civic engagement in the traditional sense, when my students contributed to Wikipedia, they were improving content area knowledge for everyone in the world. According to Dr. Amin Azzam, a health sciences associate clinical professor at the U.C.S.F. School of Medicine, "If we want to get high-quality information to all the world's population, Wikipedia is not just a viable option, but the only viable option" (Cohen, 2013, para. 8). Dr. Azzam teaches a course for medical students on writing for Wikipedia at his institution.

In my course, one student reflected on contributing to Wikipedia as a form of civic engagement:

This assignment allowed me to write information that I felt was important on a topic and post it to a well-known and highly used website. Posting information for anyone in the world to read about a topic in my field that I wrote is pretty cool.

This is a sentiment I heard from a handful of students in my course evaluations.

Pitfalls

This assignment, however, was not without its challenges. When adopting a similar assignment, prepare for some resistance. My students had been told by previous instructors, and even their parents, that Wikipedia is not a legitimate source of information. Many students told me they were taught in middle school and high school that Wikipedia had no place in the classroom. It was clear that these students believed that writing for Wikipedia was not something they should learn how to do in an upper-division writing course. Some students also struggled to see how this particular assignment related to their chosen profession, immediately dismissing the assignment.

When I shared articles and statistics outlining how Wikipedia was currently being used in the medical profession, many remained skeptical. I remained positive and continued to share resources with them that showed how Wikipedia was being used in a variety of different settings. If assigning a similar assignment, I would encourage instructors to find articles to share with their class that show how Wikipedia is being used in their disciplines, using these articles as a starting point for discussion. These articles can be a great way to "sell" the assignment to students.

In addition to some resistance, some of my students were confused with the editing process and the Wikipedia editing interface. While the Wikipedia editor is much easier to use then it used to be, some of my students found the interface complicated, which is why I believe mandatory training is important. In addition to the mandatory online training, I found it helpful to complete the training myself, so I understood how the Wikipedia editing interface works. In addition to being a resource, I also provided my students with contact information for our university Technology Learning and Media Center.

Because my course was online, I found it extremely difficult to explain the project in general as well as the editing process. I ended up recording video lectures to explain the project and screencasts that walked students through the editing process. When creating screencasts, I would recommend free apps like Jing or Screen-cast-o-matic; both are easy to use. Adopting the scaffolding activities outlined above helped encourage my students to start the project early. Particularly with assignments that require an extensive contribution, I believe it is important that students are not only working on learning the Wikipedia editor, but also developing their content. As an instructor, it is important to provide time for drafting, peer review, and practice, like any other writing assignment. Small, but required, weekly contributions helped my students master the Wikipedia editor interface.

Finally, it is possible for a student's work to be taken down by Wikipedia editors. Sometimes, taking down the material is justified (the student failed to follow the content guidelines), and other times, the reason for taking the material down is not quite as clear. This can lead to difficult conversations with students. While having work taken down would undoubtedly be frustrating, it can also be a great learning moment. It is important to encourage students to engage in a dialogue with the editors that removed their contribution. Learning how the community works is a great secondary lesson of this assignment. Unfortunately, there are a few rogue, rude editors, but this, too, can be a learning experience. Even if work is taken down, it will appear on the edit page of the article the student was working on, so if an instructor was trying to grade a contribution, the instructor would be able to see the work and grade it accordingly. In my course, I did not experience this, but was warned about the possibility by the people at the WikiEd Foundation.

In addition, the people at the WikiEd Foundation told me they are more than willing to step in and indeterminate between students and other Wikipedians. They ensured me that problems do not happen regularly, but I found it reassuring, knowing they are a resource for instructors. The WikiEd Foundation was highly supportive of my students working on Wikipedia. They understood what a powerful learning experience this was for students and that these students can contribute greatly to Wikipedia.

IMPLICATIONS

Despite the difficulties in assigning a Wikipedia project, there are still many reasons to assign a Wikipedia project. More and more schools across the country are asking their students to edit Wikipedia to ensure that high-quality content in a variety of disciplines is available to the English-speaking population of the world. With the supervision of a professor, an expert in a given discipline, the impact one class can have is quite large. According to Heilman et al. (2011), those in the healthcare-related fields should contribute to Wikipedia for a variety of reasons:

- *It may be personally satisfying to provide an important educational service for individuals looking for health information, and to see articles grow that one created or improved.*
- *While not having a high scientific impact, Wikipedia's articles have a high social impact due to its broad readership. In the experience of the authors, a newly created article can often be found*

among the top Google results within a day, often outperforming review articles in highly regarded medical journals.

- *Editing or adding information helps contributing students or professionals master the subject matter and learn more about the evidence underpinning it.*
- *Translating complex ideas into accessible concepts and language is an interesting intellectual challenge, which can help in everyday nontechnical communication with patients.*
- *Writing for Wikipedia teaches modern online communication.*
- *WikiProject Medicine offers participation and recognition in a Web-based international community.*
- *Writing for Wikipedia teaches modern online communication (A call to action section, para. 2)*

If students learn how to contribute to Wikipedia in an educational setting, they may be more likely to continue to contribute after their class or schooling is over.

As mentioned earlier, Wikipedia noted that nearly 90% of Wikipedia editors are white males, which can lead to systematic bias in articles (File: Editor survey report, 2011). By requiring students to complete an assignment such as this one, more female voices will be introduced to Wikipedia and possibly other minority voices as well. This is tremendously important, as different voices improve the content of existing articles and broaden the scope of new articles written. A good experience in the classroom, may lead to students editing Wikipedia on their own time, providing more diverse perspectives and content on the site. At the end of my course, one student expressed her interest to continue editing. She wrote, "I have a new outlook on Wikipedia. I may even spend some time looking at ways of improving article information. I did not know this was an option prior to this class."

CONCLUSION

Wikipedia is a great way to provide students with an authentic writing opportunity as well as engage them civically. For my *Writing in the Health Professions* students, it gave them a chance to improve health information that is accessed by millions of English speaking people around the world. It also gave them practice writing using plain language, a skill they will need in their careers from both a written and oral communication perspective. This is a skill that is needed by not only healthcare professionals, but also professionals in a variety of fields, making Wikipedia an appropriate assignment for students across all majors. While the assignment is not without its problems, I believe the benefits outweigh them tremendously. My students were able to see how a community can work collaboratively to generate knowledge. They also better understood how important it is to making Wikipedia a place with accurate information from diverse perspectives.

REFERENCES

Cohen, N. (2013, September 29). Editing Wikipedia for med school credit. *The New York Times*. Retrieved from: http://www.nytimes.com

Council of Writing Program Administrators. (2011). WPA network for media action. *Effective teaching practices in general studies writing classes.* Retrieved from: http://wpacouncil.org/nma

File: Editor survey report. (2011). *Wikimedia foundation.* Retrieved from https://wikimediafoundation.org/

Graham, S., & Harris, K. R. (2007). Best practices in teaching planning. In S. Graham, C. A. McArthur, & J. Fitzgerald (Eds.), *Best practices in writing instruction* (pp. 119–140). New York: The Guilford Press.

Heilman, J. M., Kemmann, E., Bonert, M., Chatterjee, A., Ragar, B., Beards, G. M., & Laurent, M. R. et al. (2011). Wikipedia: A key tool for global public health promotion. *Journal of Medical Internet Research, 13*(1), e14. doi:10.2196/jmir.1589 PMID:21282098

Help: Using talk pages (n. d.). In *Wikipedia.* Retrieved from https://en.wikipedia.org/wiki/Help:Using_talk_pages

Hughes, B., Joshi, I., Lemonde, H., & Wareham, J. (2009). Junior physician's use of Web 2.0 for information seeking and medical education: A qualitative study. *International Journal of Medical Informatics, 78*(10), 645–655. doi:10.1016/j.ijmedinf.2009.04.008 PMID:19501017

Tunick, R. A., & Brand, S. R. (2015). Social media and health care. In L.S. Wiener, M. Pao, A.E. Kazak, M.J. Kupst, & A.F. Patenaude (Eds.), Pediatric psycho-oncology: A quick reference on the psychosocial dimensions of cancer symptom Management (pp. 345-357).

Wikimedia Foundation. (2015). *May 31, 2015 Wikipedia Statistics.* Available from the Wikimedia Foundation website: http://stats.wikimedia.org/EN/Sitemap.htm

Wikipedia. Policies and guidelines. (2015, July 18). *Wikipedia.* Retrieved from https://en.wikipedia.org/wiki/Wikipedia:Policies_and_guidelines

Wikipedia. Wikipedians. (2015, December 18). In *Wikipedia.* Retrieved from https://en.wikipedia.org/wiki/Wikipedia:Wikipedians

This work was previously published in Engaging 21st Century Writers with Social Media edited by Kendra N. Bryant, pages 247-258, copyright year 2017 by Information Science Reference (an imprint of IGI Global).

Chapter 5
Gamification to Improve Adherence to Clinical Treatment Advice:
Improving Adherence to Clinical Treatment

Deborah Richards
Macquarie University, Australia

Patrina H.Y. Caldwell
University of Sydney, Australia

ABSTRACT

This chapter looks at how gamification of existing technology can be used to incorporate the factors that have been found to improve patient adherence. Lack of adherence to medical advice is a major problem because it reduces the likelihood of improved health outcomes and is a waste of costly and scarce resources. To provide intrinsically motivating game mechanics we discuss the use of an embodied virtual character to build an ongoing therapeutic alliance with the patient. Extrinsically motivating game mechanics are added via a game based on the token economy. The intention is to empower, engage and encourage the patient to adhere with the medical advice. A case study is provided for the condition of paediatric incontinence.

INTRODUCTION

eHealth interventions have the potential to significantly improve the quality and safety of healthcare processes and outcomes. However, without adherence to the guidance provided by the health professional via the eHealth system, these benefits will not be realised. Fenerty, West, Davis, Kaplan, and Feldman (2012) report that "up to 30%-50% of patients are expected to demonstrate poor adherence to medication use" (2012 p.128). Similar figures are reported for eHealth systems (Donkin et al., 2011). Lack of adherence is a major problem because the intended outcomes of the advice, that is, improved health outcomes, are not likely to be achieved, and the costs associated with providing that advice are

DOI: 10.4018/978-1-5225-1928-7.ch005

wasted (Fenerty et al., 2012; Stinson, Wilson, Gill, Yamada, & Holt, 2009). The problem is exacerbated when long wait times in receiving the advice are involved because of the possible further deterioration of the situation for those waiting and the additional costs involved in managing the condition. While adherence is a multifaceted problem and the context will differ for each patient (Karoly, 1993), we will focus on eHealth solutions that provide a therapeutic alliance and help overcome health literacy barriers.

A therapeutic alliance encompasses the degree to which the helper and client agree on the goals of the therapy and tasks to be performed, and the extent to which a trusting and empathetic bond between the helper and client is established (Horvath & Luborsky, 1993). Limited literacy (health and other forms) has been found to negatively impact the efficacy and success of eHealth systems that provide information and interventions, and promote treatment adherence (T. W. Bickmore, Pfeifer, & Jack, 2009). Limited health literacy affects over one third of American adults (Paasche-Orlow, Parker, Gazmararian, Nielsen-Bohlman, & Rudd, 2005), nearly two-thirds of Australians (ABS, 2006) with worse figures for vulnerable populations such as children and the socially disadvantaged (Williams et al., 1995).

Games and virtual world technologies can help overcome health literacy barriers by improving medical knowledge and encouraging healthy behaviours. More importantly, gamification, "the process of game-thinking and game mechanics to engage users and solve problems" (Zichermann & Cunningham, 2011), can be used to provide therapy, treatment advice and support similar to that provided in clinical practice. We see that game elements such as goals, rules, challenges, interaction and rewards have a role to play in this context, but the relational nature of therapy requires the development of a working alliance in order to deliver lasting positive outcomes for the patient. We propose that "relational agents" are most suitable for this purpose. According to Bickmore, "relational agents are computational artifacts designed to build long-term socio-emotional relationships with users, including trust, rapport and therapeutic alliance, for the purpose of enhancing adherence to treatment" (T. W. Bickmore, Puskar, Schlenk, Pfeifer, & Sereika, 2010) p.7.

The conversational and social nature of the intelligent agent will seek to overcome barriers for patients, adults and children, who have low health literacy skills. For these cohorts, solutions involving online medical advice and treatment plans may be unattractive and do little to improve their situation. The familiar format of face-to-face conversation using a simplified and explicit method of interacting provides increased and tailored levels of engagement needed for repeated and ongoing adherence, and reduces confusion and misunderstandings (T. Bickmore, Gruber, & Picard, 2005).

The key goals of this chapter are to present the literature on relational agents for clinical practice and to present a relational agent for chronic paediatric conditions designed to improve treatment adherence and overcome health literacy barriers.

The background section covers: technology for empowerment and behaviour change; behaviour change and games; serious games and adherence; understanding adherence; increased patient agency to improve adherence and building a therapeutic alliance. We then look at the use of relational agents to build a working alliance and improve adherence specifically considering the limitations of technology, identify the right perspective and role of games, present the use of games to overcome social, health literacy and adherence barriers; present the use of agents to aid human agency and adherence, and discuss how agents can be designed to intrinsically motivate. We present a case study to explore how gamification can address the burden and health consequences of urinary incontinence in children. We explain how an existing treatment advice system was redesigned by integrating relational agents to improve intrinsic motivation and by adding gamification elements to provide extrinsic motivators. Finally we offer future directions and our conclusions for the use of gamification in clinical practice.

BACKGROUND

In this section, we review the history of technology that supports patient empowerment, illustrate how ongoing usage and adherence continue to be challenging in this domain, discuss how games may assist in overcoming these challenges. We then discuss adherence and explore the notion of a good therapist and working alliance.

Technology for Empowerment and Behaviour Change

The broad adoption of Web 2.0 technologies and approaches and the subsequent emergence of Personal Health Application (PHA) Platforms and Personally Controlled Health Records (PCHR) represent "tectonic shifts in the health information economy" (Mandl & Kohane, 2009) with far-reaching consequences for patient involvement, as the locus of control shifts away from health care providers as the sole custodian of medical data. With the emergence of Web 2.0 applications, the expectations of users have changed as well as the ways users interact with these applications. The changes in the architecture, appearance, usability, and spread of Web applications played their part in changing expectations. According to Eysenbach (2008), users expect the applications to be openly accessible, preferably free and interoperable. Open Web standards improve the collaboration and communication across applications. Collaboration between users is especially popular in social networking approaches. Users can communicate with each other, connect to other users in the network, and can find helpful information. Web 2.0 technologies like AJAX improve the Web interfaces and transform web applications into desktop like applications with real-time responsiveness (Eysenbach, 2008). The concept of Medicine 2.0 (Eysenbach, 2008) is a natural outgrowth of these developments.

Medicine 2.0 applications, services and tools are "Web-based services for health care consumers, caregivers, patients, health professionals, and biomedical researchers, that use Web 2.0 technologies and/or semantic web and virtual-reality tools, to enable and facilitate social networking, participation, apomediation, collaboration, and openness within and between these user groups" (Eysenbach, 2008). The three main user groups of Medicine 2.0 are consumers/patients, health professionals and biomedical researchers. While the "formal" training of these users differs, consumers and patients (i.e. end users) are recognized as experts as well, because according to the philosophy of Web 2.0, their collective wisdom can and should be harnessed (Eysenbach, 2008). Hughes, Joshi, and Wareham (2008), after conducting an extensive literature review of Medicine 2.0, concluded that healthcare systems need to move away from the traditional, hierarchical, closed structure within health care and hospital-based medicine, and should focus on promoting health, provide healthcare in people's own homes, and empower consumers to take responsibility for their own health instead.

The empowerment of users via Web 2.0, social media technology and Medicine 2.0 has influenced and encouraged the use and design of games for medical purposes. Games by nature are interactive and require participation. There are a number of reasons why games provide appropriate technology to support empowerment. In the context of education, games give players freedom to create their own learning pathway by providing cognitive flexibility (Spiro, Feltovich, & Jacobson). Game mechanics such as the progression dynamic (Priebatsch, 2010) and supportive feedback loop (Salen & Zimmerman, 2004) provide a form of educational scaffolding that can ensure learning outcomes are achieved while making the experience more coherent and provide a sense of game 'flow'.

Behaviour change is usually achieved via the use of an intervention. This notion revolves around bringing about change in inappropriate behaviours, beliefs or outcomes, such as disruptive classroom behaviour or holding misconceptions in the educational context. In the health context, an intervention may seek to break a habit such as smoking, drug or alcohol addiction or promote healthy behaviours such as exercise, eating right or taking prescribed medications or change health beliefs. Key theories that have influenced researchers and practitioners include self-determination theory (Ryan & Deci, 2000), social cognitive theory (particularly self-efficacy) (Bandura, 2001), and the transtheoretical model (Prochaska & Velicer, 1997).

Behaviour Change and Games

Game technology provides a suitable vehicle for the implementation of these theories, particularly as they relate to patient empowerment (C. Caldwell et al., 2013). For example, the transtheoretical model can be used for designing appropriate activities to perform in the game according to the state of the player (precontemplation, contemplation, preparation, action and maintenance). In line with self- determination theory, a game can trigger both intrinsic and extrinsic types of motivation by offering incentives, rewards and forms of recognition as the player increases in competence, autonomy and relatedness with others. The setting and attainment of goals in a game allows the player to achieve a sense of self-efficacy as they achieve performance outcomes and receive feedback on their successes and failures when faced with a challenge.

Games can be used not only to improve motivation, but also to measure motivation and understand cognitive processing as was done by Inchamnan and Wyeth (2013) using the Player Experience Needs Satisfaction (PENS) questionnaire (Ryan, Rigby, & Przybylski, 2006). PENS is able to measure in-game competency, autonomy, relatedness, presence, and intuitive controls and evaluates aspects of the game experience such as Goals, Challenges, Action and Interaction.

Despite the compelling argument for eHealth technology, including games, to empower, inform and help patients make good health decisions, users do not seem to persist in their use of eHealth intervention systems. Donkin et al. (2011) conducted a systematic review of 69 eHealth intervention studies across different disease states and found that intervention dropout, i.e. where the user stops using the intervention before the goal is met, is common for both physical and psychological health conditions, such as weight loss, smoking cessation or depression. In another systematic review of 83 web-based health interventions by Kelders, Kok, Ossebaard, and Van Gemert-Pijnen (2012) it was found that non-adherence was not predicted for a specific health area but rather by differences in technology and interaction.

Serious Games and Adherence

Games seek to be challenging and engaging. The experience can be further intensified when the game is part of an immersive virtual world. Serious games seek to leverage these benefits to increase the users' motivation and desire to participate in activities that are useful or necessary for their employment, education, health and well-being. The first serious games were training simulations for the military and first responders. Military examples include: Virtual Battlefield Simulator (VBS1) by Interactive Bohemia[1], and Joint Conflict and Tactical Simulation (JCATS) by the United States Joint Forces Command[2]. Simulations in the civilian sector covers all simulations working outside the law enforcement and military sphere but commonly involves emergency first responder training, e.g. the HazMat[3] training simulation for firemen, or the Weapons of Mass Destruction Decision Analysis Center (WMD-DAC) simulation by Sandia National Laboratories[4] which trains city administration officials to handle terrorist incidents or natural disasters.

Though a late starter, the recent sharp rise in interest in games for medical and health applications is apparent. For example, the proceedings of the 9th Australasian Interactive Entertainment Conference for 2012 contained one paper out of 22 on occupational health and safety (OH&S) in the construction industry. This single paper was written from the perspective of training and education, rather than a health application. In stark contrast, the 2013 proceedings contained 11 out of 33 papers on health-related games, categorised as follows: physical wellbeing (6), emotional or psychological health (5), cognitive health (1), specific medical condition (3); note that two papers covered two categories and one paper covered three categories.

Increasing awareness and interest in the use of games for the purpose of encouraging adherence is apparent, even if evidence of their efficacy is still scarce. For example, in Proceedings of the 3rd European conference on gaming and playful interaction in health care - Games for Health 2013 (Schouten, Fedtke, Bekker, Schijven, & Gekker) there was a track on Games For Care, Cure and Medicine Adherence. While this track included 3 papers, none of them used the word adherence or discussed it. The three papers concerned: a feasibility study on low back pain patients (Bonnechére et al., 2013), training motor skills (de Greef, van der Spek, & Bekker, 2013); and a game at the dentist to distract the user from their discomfort (Bidarra et al., 2013). Within the same proceedings, adherence was on the radar for games relating to therapy. Mert et al. (2013) suggest that "the problem with conventional therapy is that the therapy is intrusive, intense and in general experienced as boring. Hence therapy adherence is quite low. Virtual reality in combination with gaming principles might offer an engaging, compelling and challenging therapeutic environment that enhances therapy adherence and therefore also better therapeutic results."(p.248). Mert et al. (2013) are concerned with Posttraumatic Stress Disorder (PTSD) and following standard therapy have created a virtual reality game that combines cognitive behaviour theory and eye movement desensitisation and reprocessing (EMDR). Players reported a sense of control; attributed to the player's need to walk on a motion platform as part of the game. As a one off study, they were able to confirm that participants found the interactive "Achilles Initiative" game engaging, and participants expressed interest to play the game/perform the therapy again, but ongoing adherence could not be measured. In a different study, Khalil (2013) analysed the emotional aspects of the "Re-Mission" game that has been shown in randomized controlled trials to increase knowledge and medication adherence among young cancer patients. Of potential relevance to adherence, a number of authors considered empathy, and Guðmundsdóttir, Wille, and Savu (2013) specifically discussed how to design for empathy.

In a 2014 book on Future Trends of Virtual, Augmented Reality, and Games for Health the key future trends identified are Location-Based Excergaming, Mobile Apps, and Social Media Gaming for Public Health. Due to the influence of social and emotional factors, the latter trend is identified as playing a role in improving adherence. Two chapters explicitly discuss adherence, but one of those chapters is concerned with health managers adhering to changes in practice. Only one chapter looks at adherence in the context of game play to promote change to healthy behaviours (Durga et al., 2014) by including rewards and incentives in exergames. It is important to note that in all of the health and gaming books and proceedings abovementioned, we found no mention of agent technology.

At this point in time, games are an emerging technology with some promise that they may motivate adherence to a treatment plan or intervention. To better understand whether games are likely to face the same fate as many other eHealth intervention systems with respect to non-adherence to the treatment advice, let us seek to better understand adherence.

Understanding Adherence

Earlier research into adherence more commonly used the term compliance. Karoly (1993) defines compliance as the "goodness of fit between a program of health/illness management designed primarily by a health professional and the program-specific behaviours enacted by a patient (or patients) and/or those individuals in a caretaking role". p.12

In recent times, consistent with changes in medical practitioner thinking and consumer-driven technology such as Web 2.0 and specifically Medicine 2.0 as described earlier, the term "adherence" has become more acceptable as it is more focused on the patient's choices and decision-making than following the health professional's rules. The movement away from the concept of compliance towards adherence reflects the earlier mismatch between who designs the program (i.e. the health professional) and who must enact it (i.e. the patient). This mismatch is probably key to why compliance is such an issue. As the literature we present spans three decades and the terms have evolved over that time, we will use the terms adherence and compliance interchangeably. Note that persistence is another concept that is concerned with long term and ongoing adherence. While we do not use the term persistence, our discussions relating to adherence encompass persistence as we are interested in ongoing adherence in order to deliver improved patient health outcomes; ad-hoc or one-off adherence is not likely to achieve that goal. In support of our terminology usage, in a systematic review of the adherence literature, Barbosa, Balp, Kulich, Germain, and Rofail (2012) notes that the terms compliance and adherence were used interchangeably and they describe adherence as "intention to persist", thus closely linking the notions of adherence and persistence.

Firstly, we note that lack of adherence to medical advice is not a recent problem; it is a common phenomena that occurs in technology and non-technology-mediated interventions at similar rates (Donkin et al., 2011). Dunbar-Jacob, Dunning, and Dwyer (1993) conducted a review of the literature between 1970 and 1989 and found that the average adherence rate was around 50%. Their review included 91 intervention studies reporting compliance. Most studies focused on whether patients complied with taking prescribed medication, rather than other forms of adherence such as attending appointments or monitoring intake, outputs, insulin levels, etc. They noted over time a reduction in studies reporting compliance, making it even harder for knowledge to advance in this area. They also noted from the 80s a growing interest in correlational studies involving a single case. In the 70s, compliance studies concerned children of all ages, but the 80s saw a shift to a predominantly adolescent focus with less than 20% focused on pre-school aged children and infants. In line with that trend, in the 70s the parent was the target of intervention but this moved in the early 80s to the child or parent-child dyad and in the late 80s to the parent-child dyad. There has been growth in the number of educational and behavioural interventions, while behavioural interventions have been studied more.

Dunbar-Jacob et al. (1993) noted that in the studies analysed, none had considered adherence strategies and 79% of the adherence studies presented were atheoretical. Of those that drew on theory, the most commonly used theory was the Health Belief Model which is concerned with the mother's health beliefs. Less prominent was discussion of Social Learning Theory and Theory of Reasoned Action

(Fishbein, 1979). Dunbar-Jacob et al. (1993) also note that studies in the 70s focussed on acute diseases, but the 80s saw a shift to studies on chronic diseases such as diabetes and asthma. This trend continues.

A lack of focus on adherence and recognition of its importance is also evident in the 2009 Cochrane Review of Interactive Health Communication Applications (IHCAs) (Murray, Burns, See, Lai, & Nazareth, 2005) which sought to determine the effects of IHCAs on patients in terms of: knowledge; social support; self-efficacy; emotional outcomes; behavioural outcomes; clinical outcomes; and to determine the effects of IHCAs on economic outcomes, in terms of resource utilisation, but did not measure or even mention the term adherence or compliance.

More recently, Barbosa et al. (2012) conducted a search of articles assessing compliance, adherence or persistence and treatment satisfaction published between January 2005 and November 2010, resulting in a review of 20 studies. All studies found a positive association, sixteen were statistically significant, between treatment satisfaction and adherence, compliance, or persistence. Barbosa et al. state that "There are a number of elements that determine a patient's adherence to their treatment, including dosing complexity and frequency, convenience, and satisfaction" (Barbosa et al., 2012), p. 40). While the study did not investigate enjoyment, we conjecture that if a treatment were made fun through creating a game-like challenge this may increase the level of satisfaction with the treatment.

Krasnegor, Epstein, Johnson, Yaffe, and Epstein (2013) identify three models used to describe compliance: componential, contextual and experiential. The componential model is concerned with the mechanisms an individual uses to manage the illness. The contextual model is concerned with the patient's cognitive functions and their environment, which can be seen as enabling or disabling. The experiential model is concerned with motivation and evaluative feedback that drive the processes leading to compliance or non-compliance. We consider the usefulness and relevance of these models in the games and relational agent context later.

Of relevance when dealing with paediatric compliance and the influence of enabling or disabling situational factors in the contextual model, Anderson and Coyne (1993) have identified the "miscarried helping model" where a power struggle over autonomy between parent and child occurs concerning the child caring for his/herself with the result that the situation changes from an illness-related problem to a relationship problem (Iannotti & Bush, 1993). It is also interesting to consider that the nature of the illness itself may contribute to the problem (Iannotti & Bush, 1993). For example, the child may comply but if results are not delivered, the parent may accuse the child of noncompliance. This occurs if the parent has an incorrect view of the level of control the child has of the disease. This may lead to reduced interaction with the healthcare system and deterioration in communication about what is realistic.

Increased Patient Agency to Improve Adherence

Karoly (1993) notes that the mismatch between designer and enactor produces a fundamental struggle of determinism versus free will, comprising agency, self-determination and internal control, that would allow the patient to select, monitor and modulate their own goals. Elaborating further "the widespread tendency of patients (both young and old, informed and uninformed, with either serious or mild medical problems) to appear "non-compliant" results from the conceptual and technical failures of a *coercive (social power-based) model* – that is, a model built upon the necessity of nonagentic mechanism." Karoly (1993) p.12.

The alternative offered by Karoly is a control systems model involving internal and external sources of influence. While Karoly notes that children are "rule-oriented" he believes compliance must be more than just rule following. Compliance in the context of children may mean compliance by the child, the parent or a shared responsibility according to their ability to accept, preserve, recognise applicability and modify the medical regimen. Karoly warns that this could result in mental overload due to the need for measurement of performance in various primary and secondary tasks using a combination of self-report and physiological instruments. However, Karoly (1993) is not advocating reductionism where compliance is just a mental representation. Compliance includes behaviour around the dynamic between the clinician's prescription and patient's intention and requires a "flexibility-centered perspective based on inductive reasoning and dynamic problem solving." p. 16. He further argues that compliance "is a thing that happens" (p.18) where compliance is an emergent characteristic of a dynamic system. Karoly suggests the use of control systems theory to overcome or avoid the issues of reductionism. He defines a possible open system with dynamic equilibria (steady states), reference standards, feedforward and feedback. The actors in the system are in a reciprocal relationship with other significant persons where "no source is primary, even when the other is a powerful, authoritative physician and the actor is a 10-year-old diabetic child." p.21. He argues that in place of an outside-in model that states X increases compliance and Y decreases it, an inside-out model that is mediational, constructivist and time intensive lets us stand in the patient's shoes. The approach acknowledges that adherence includes motivation that is based on internal (self-generated), interpersonal (doctor-patient-parent) and social (normative) pressures. We suggest that agent-based modelling (Gilbert, 2008) could be used to reduce the complexity and simulate compliance by modelling expectancy, goal, need, value, preference, and the like leading to activation of action. Further exploration of this idea is outside the scope of this chapter.

Perhaps the first medical interactive agent-based virtual world or serious game was *Carmen's Bright IDEAS* (Marsella, Johnson, & LaBore, 2003) that sought to help the mothers of paediatric cancer patients to consider and deal with the social dilemmas they might face. The user plays the mother while a non-player or virtual character is a counsellor. The system is based on the simulation of agents who are able to dialog with each other via recorded sentences and who express emotions via facial expression and body gestures. The extent of agency on the part of the user is limited to a few choices in the story. As pioneer work in the field, the project was not focussed on addressing the issue of adherence.

More recently, researchers have used a number of techniques, with mixed outcomes, to reduce intervention dropout rates in eHealth systems. These techniques include: task support (e.g. self-monitoring, tailoring), dialogue support (e.g. reminders, suggestion), and social support (e.g. social comparison, social facilitation) (Kelders et al., 2012). In their study of internet based interventions, Kelders et al. (2012) found that "increased interaction with a counselor, more frequent intended usage, more frequent updates and more extensive employment of dialogue support significantly predicted better adherence" (p. 8). In particular, past studies have indicated the use of empathy and social dialogue in the computer program can lead to increased program usage (Watson, Bickmore, Cange, Kulshreshtha, & Kvedar, 2012), and that accountability to a coach who is seen as trustworthy, benevolent, and having expertise may increase one's adherence to the program (Mohr, Cuijpers, & Lehman, 2011).

Building a Therapeutic Alliance

The phenomena of a supporting, caring and trusting relationship between the patient and health provider has been referred to as a "therapeutic alliance" and has been shown to improve health outcomes and medication adherence (Chue, 2006). Other terms used include working alliance, therapeutic working alliance and helping alliance. The terms helping and working reflect that the therapist and client or patient are working together to help the client. In psychotherapy research, the quality of the therapeutic alliance has been shown to be the most robust predictor of treatment success (Safran & Muran, 2000). In a meta-analysis of the data from 79 studies (58 published, 21 unpublished), Martin, Garske, and Davis (2000) found that the overall relation of therapeutic alliance with outcome was "moderate, but consistent, regardless of many of the variables that have been posited to influence this relationship" (p. 438).

In a study of 79 alliance profiles, profiles that were characterized as V-shaped (i.e. relationships got off to a good start but were ruptured and then repaired) produced more satisfying patient outcomes (Stiles et al., 2004). From a study of the emergence of the concept of the therapeutic working alliance in psychotherapy to its current pantheoretical formulations, Horvath and Luborsky (1993) considered the relation between a positive alliance and success in therapy, what factors influence a positive alliance, how the alliance changed over time and what variables may predispose an individual to develop a strong alliance. To support measurement of the existence of a therapeutic alliance, Horvath and Greenberg (1989) developed the Working Alliance Inventory.

A good therapist is able to create and maintain a good therapeutic alliance, and to grasp the client's perspective and 'world view' (Ackerman & Hilsenroth, 2003). Achievement of this alliance will require the therapist to acknowledge the importance of achieving a good relationship and consensus over the goals of the therapy and the methods comprising the therapy. There are certain personal attributes which will affect the likelihood of forming a positive alliance (Ackerman & Hilsenroth, 2003). These include: flexibility and allowing the client to discuss the issues of importance to them; being respectful, being warm, friendly and affirming, being open, alert and active; being able to show honesty through self-reflection, being trustworthy. Factors that are likely to negatively impact the alliance include rigidity, criticism, inappropriate self-disclosure, being aloof or distracted and misuse of silence (Ackerman & Hilsenroth, 2001). The therapist will need to manage the conversation through active and empathic listening that aids the patient to express their concerns and fears about the treatment without judgement while gauging the degree of congruence in the aims of the client and therapist and dealing with any "alliance ruptures" (Safran & Muran, 2000) that threaten the progress of therapy.

The ground breaking work on human attitudes and behaviours towards computers by Reeves and Nass (1996) opened the way for research investigating how many human-human situations could be simulated by human-computer interactions. At around the same time computer-generated animations emerged as a new field and animation researchers observed that graphic realism was less important than believability (via simulation of emotion) in making viewers willing to suspend disbelief and fully engage with the characters (Bates, 1994).

Researchers have found that computer-mediated interactions can have advantages over face-to-face interactions. Lisetti (2012) outline the following 10 advantages of using avatars in patient-centered computer-based interventions for behaviour change: increases accessibility, increases confidentiality and divulgation, tailors information, diminishes variability, avoids righting reflex with infinite patience, addresses low literacy, lowers attrition rates, allows patient-physician concordance/matching, provides a working alliance and expresses empathy. Lisetti et al. (2012) seeks to gain these advantages by creating a personalized On-Demand VIrtual Counselor (ODVIC) to provide computer-delivery of Brief Motivational Interventions (BMIs) for behaviour change.

In early work on the use of computers for interviewing, Servan-Schreiber (1986) found that humans tended to report more to a computer than to a human interviewer. Studies dealing with individuals suffering from post-traumatic distress disorder found that there were population differences in distressed individuals for both non-verbal behaviour (Scherer et al., 2013) and verbal behaviour (DeVault et al., 2014). Based on anticipated benefits such as anonymity, increased disclosure and less fear of judgment,

Gratch, Lucas, King, and Morency (2014) developed models of these population differences and applied them in clinical interviews they conducted with 239 participants exposed to either a human or virtual interviewer. Gratch et al. (2014) found that the automated virtual humans (VHs) were able to reduce fear of self-disclosure and improved impression management. The VH was able to establish a relationship and build rapport through social dialog as in the human-human situation but gain the benefits of reduced fear of disclosure and sense of judgment associated with computer-administered assessments (Servan-Schreiber, 1986). Gratch et al. (2014) found that people were perceived as more judgmental. Thus, participants were more comfortable talking about personal matters with a VH. The SimSensei VH used by Gratch et al. (2014) was able to achieve increased disclosure due to a feeling of being unobserved and rapport.

RELATIONAL AGENTS TO BUILD A WORKING ALLIANCE AND IMPROVE ADHERENCE

We propose that gamification can be employed to improve all three adherence factors suggested by Barbosa et al. (2012) (i.e. complexity, convenience and satisfaction). The game mechanics we propose to achieve adherence, include but go beyond the more well-known awards, badges and points aimed at making the experience more engaging and fun. We believe, that merely making adherence/compliance more fun or at least less unpleasant does not quite achieve the definition of adherence as "the extent to which a patient participates in a treatment regimen after he or she agrees to that regimen" (Balkrishnan, 2005). Treatment adherence is related to the therapeutic alliance between the patient and the clinician. The use of a "relational agent" may be a viable alternative to provide an (semi-)automated supportive interpersonal relationship. We make a case below that agent technology can play an important role in creating the sense of a working alliance including achieving a mutually satisfactory treatment plan and providing an appropriate level of agency in the process. Before making our case, we first consider what technology in general and games in particular may or may not offer in the medical and particularly clinical context. The section concludes with consideration of a specific example for the condition of urinary incontinence in children.

Recognising the Limitations of Technology: Some Lessons from Education

Technology may offer solutions in many areas concerning health and wellbeing including: isolation and keeping physically active for aging populations; the increasing costs of providing healthcare; the shortage of specialists; growing waiting list; accessibility and availability issues for non-metropolitan dwellers; pandemic societal issues such as obesity, addictions and mental health illness; and the ongoing need to provide advice and support for chronic medical conditions. When the intervention or treatment involves motivational aspects, game technology seems particularly relevant. However, technology does not provide a silver bullet and will only be effective if designed and deployed appropriately.

Any technology aimed at dealing with adherence must be evaluated to ensure initial benefits are not due to the novelty of the technology. This phenomena is recognised as the 'novelty effect' associated with significant differences in outcomes when the technology is used for the first time, but these differences are less or non-observable on subsequent uses (Clark, 1983). In many cases the studies reported are one-off events and no data is reported on their subsequent use. We need to be careful to have appropriate expectations for game technology and the gamification of other technologies.

Based on compelling arguments for using games to improve motivation, enjoyment and engagement (Gee, 2005; Prensky, 2003), an interest in the use of games for education began over two decades ago with games like word rescue[5] and math rescue[6]. While these games have helped many children, including our own, learn their multiplication tables, spelling and math, the predicted digital education revolution (Buchanan, 2011) or transformed classroom of the 21st century (Lever-Duffy, McDonald, & Mizell, 2002) is still a long way from realisation. We believe there are parallel lessons that can be learned from the experience of games in education in terms of issues, barriers and appropriate expectation management for the use of games in clinical practice. Where the purpose of the medical game is for education, the parallel is obvious.

In a meta-analysis of 40 years of research in the use of technology in education, Tamim, Bernard, Borokhovski, Abrami, and Schmid (2011) stress that the nature of the technology intervention is less of a factor in achieving successful learning outcomes than the goals of instruction, pedagogy, teacher effectiveness, subject matter, age level and fidelity of technology implementation. Similarly, Ross, Morrison, and Lowther (2010) state that "educational technology is not a homogeneous 'intervention' but a broad variety of modalities, tools, and strategies for learning. Its effectiveness, therefore, depends on how well it helps teachers and students achieve the desired instructional goals" (p. 19). This also applies to game technology for health and wellbeing. We propose that technology in the medical domain will not deliver automatic benefits. Benefits derived, or not, will be due to multiple factors including the appropriateness of fit to the goal, patient and caregiver.

While the games industry might have billions of dollars, huge budgets to pay for graphic artists and games developer and many eager players willing to pay for upgrades to the next release, this is not the case in education or health. Games in education may seem to make perfect sense for the current generation of 'digital natives' (Prensky, 2003), however, many obstacles exist. These obstacles include lack of alignment of games with the curriculum to be delivered; inadequate technical skills and time for teachers to create their own game or even make use of existing games; resistance or reluctance from parents for their children to use games and virtual worlds in the classroom and/or at home; inadequate resources for education departments or bodies to develop appropriate content; and potential issues around cybersecurity and cyberbullying. The development of games in medicine have even greater safety concerns and requirements usually involving lengthy and costly clinical trials (C. Caldwell et al., 2013).

A key difference between games for pleasure or leisure and those for educational or health purposes is that the latter have specific, usually real world, outcomes and it can be difficult to measure whether they have been achieved. Educational games have learning outcomes; achievement of these needs to be monitored and often structured so that content is learnt in the right order. Even if learning outcomes are achieved in a specific context, there is often a lack of learning transfer that seeks to go beyond memorisation of facts to deeper learning of concepts and relationships between them so that they can be applied to new problem situations. As the literature has found, there are differences in cognitive and learning styles and personality that will affect the efficacy of the learning program (Honey & Mumford, 1986). Similarly, we read earlier that different characteristics of the therapist and/or the client will affect the quality of a therapeutic alliance (Ackerman & Hilsenroth, 2001, 2003; Horvath & Luborsky, 1993).

Identifying the Right Perspective and Role of Games

Following Salen and Zimmerman (2004) *Roles of Play* we can view a game and its purpose in different ways. Choosing which role of play is appropriate in a given context is one of the design decisions to be made. Games as *Social Play* is a common concept associated with games and commences early in childhood. There is no set goal to be achieved or challenges to be taken. Instead the focus is on learning how to interact in socially acceptable ways. Social play is not restricted to children. Simulations of fictitious and yet engaging and thought provoking experiences are particularly relevant for learning how to behave in social situations. This is fundamentally what Carmen's Bright Ideas (Marsella et al., 2003) was seeking to achieve, i.e. how do I respond to questions of others that relate to my terminally ill child?

When using a game or social simulation to make sense of what is happening, potentially understanding triggers and cause and effect, games provide *Play of Meaning*. Social simulations can do more than provide experience and transfer current best practice; they may be used to transform current social realities. Thorngate and Tavakoli (2009) note that simulations are conducted in order to form or change the beliefs and policies of policy makers. As a "rhetorical device" they become a "tool of social influence" (p. 513).

Game can be seen as a *Systems of Conflict*. The conflict can be seen as the disagreement between the current (unhealthy) situation and the desired healthy situation. The latter is the goal. The challenge is to achieve the goal. Levels with appropriate rewards can be set up to encourage the user to continue progressively towards the goal. Conflict often involves multiple players competing with one another to achieve a goal and is a key element of games (Vorderer, Hartmann, & Klimmt, 2003). It is not clear that competition in the health context is desirable, certainly not between the health care giver and receiver. More along the lines of achieving one's personal best, the competition could be with oneself. There are, however, potential pitfalls if framing the session as a conflict. There could be a sense of competition to achieve (perceived) societal norms (smoking or being overweight is not cool). But this means the system is making or supporting judgements on what is good or bad and this is contrary to studies that have shown that being non-judgemental is important for development of an open and satisfying relationship. While some individuals thrive on competition, for some, a sense of competition may overwhelm or demotivate.

Potentially one can weave the elements of each of these views together by viewing games as *narrative systems*. A scenario-based virtual world can provide an environment where the patient is the protagonist in an unfolding drama. Bruner (1991) considers stories as a unique way people structure their own knowledge. Laboratory experiments have shown that in a story, elements belonging to the main causal chain of events were better memorized than events not causally connected (Gerrig, 1993). Over a period of time, the pattern of interaction within the game records the patient's progress, even if small, and becomes the story of their successes and failures. This can be used to seek to encourage and motivate further improvement or maintenance of their success. The game could include a replay feature or a function to allow checking incidents at a given point in time. These incidents and the story flow can provide the basis of discussions between the patient and practitioner and allow a sense of sharing in the patient's life outside the clinic.

Drama and storytelling tend to be associated with fiction (Richards & Szilas, 2012). When using a game to gain or practice knowledge or skills, it may be useful to view games as the *Play of Experience*. As many educationalists, organizations and researchers are finding (e.g. (Davis, Murphy, Owens, Khazanchi, & Zigurs, 2009), there are many potential benefits of using a Virtual World for social simulations. Virtual Worlds (VWs) allow difficult situations to be safely explored. A virtual training simulation may allow the user to get involved in a believable environment to test out their knowledge and responses and to learn appropriate responses at more convenient times and/or locations. Furthermore, there can be less risk of embarrassment or social inhibition in a VW than in a live role play involving others with whom you work, study or live when VW participants are able to maintain anonymity while taking on a role, particularly an unfamiliar one.

Games to Overcome Barriers: Social, Health Literacy, Adherence

Learning social behaviours requires social interaction. In most current VWs for social simulation, a human selects an 'avatar', typically a humanlike graphical representation that they control, to play his/her role. However, requiring humans to play the roles in social role-playing games, places limits on when such training can occur and relies on adequate knowledge and role-playing skills of the humans involved. Also, for experimental or other purposes which require careful control of the environment and situational factors, humans may be less desirable than an environment in which the variables are managed by the computer/researcher. Thus, we are interested in VWs which support intelligent social interactions between humans and computer-based non-player characters (NPCs) known as intelligent virtual agents (IVAs), embodied conversational agents (ECAs), artificial intelligences (AIs), or simply *agents*. These agents behave autonomously, unlike an avatar that does not have its own intelligence but is controlled by a person or software script.

In the case of medical applications and websites, education of the user, however, is a secondary goal or means of achieving the primary goal: improved health or lifestyle. Education includes providing information concerning why certain questions are asked and why certain recommendations are made. Electronic games have been found to be effective for learning in complex or boring contexts (Prensky, 2003). Due to the increased level of engagement associated with games, they may motivate deeper learning (Gee, 2005). The value of using game technology for education is often associated with the learning theories of constructivism (Duffy & Jonassen, 1992) and constructionism (Kafai & Resnick, 1996) due to the active engagement of learners in constructing their own knowledge and the use of artifacts to achieve this, respectively. These theories are particularly relevant for the use of virtual worlds for learning due to their experiential and exploratory nature.

Games are typically associated with play and play is often associated with children as an important vehicle in their development to adulthood though we acknowledge that adults play games and there are different forms of games and play. In a similar developmental and educative capacity, we believe that games can play an important formative role in educating patients of any age by providing a more enjoyable and meaningful or memorable way of gaining learning building blocks such as the key health terms and concepts relevant to their medical condition and its treatment. Without this preparatory play (education), the patient may not be at the right stage of development to benefit from the advice delivered by a computer or a human. For example, eHealth systems that rely on good reading, numeracy, technology and health literacy skills are not likely to be useful for users without these skills. According to the Australian Bureau of Statistics (ABS, 2006), health literacy is defined as: "the knowledge and skills required to understand and use information relating to health issues such as drugs and alcohol, disease prevention and treatment, safety and accident prevention, first aid, emergencies, and staying healthy" (p. 5). The prevalence of poor health literacy is alarming. As part of an international study, the Adult Literacy and Life Skills Survey conducted in 2006 in Australia, found that only 43% of Australian participants aged 15 to 74 years achieved health literacy Level 3 or above (ABS, 2006). Skill Level 3 is regarded by the survey developers as the 'minimum required for individuals to meet the complex demands of everyday life and work in the emerging knowledge-based economy' (Desjardins, Murray, & Tuijnman, 2005). We propose that a game with levels, challenges, rewards that encourage recognising and remembering the meaning of a medical concept can act as an introduction or warm up before the actual intervention or advisory system is used. However, the design of a health literacy game is outside the focus of this chapter.

Games could be used to address the adherence factors of complexity, convenience and satisfaction identified by Barbosa et al. (2012). Dosing complexity and frequency relates to understanding of what needs to be done (eHealth) and can potentially be addressed by using reminders that have reduced the complexity. For example, some medication or procedure must be done at a certain time (e.g. before sleeping or 2 hours after food). This however requires a very rigid routine and for the patient to be aware of their circumstance. Devices and software that are able to monitor what is happening may be able to determine the best time and recommend when the medication should be taken or a treatment followed. Convenience includes the equipment, location, procedure length, possible collection and recording of data and timing (e.g. during a school day or every four hours). If a reminder system is being used, it will need to be convenient also and fit with the regimen. A small device (such as a smart phone or automatic and wearable insulin pumps) provides portability and is easy to carry. Satisfaction is more related with happiness or agreement with the treatment and is likely to be affected by complexity and convenience. The more complicated and inconvenient the treatment is, one could expect less satisfaction. However, if there is adequate understanding and agreement, then the patient may be satisfied with the treatment regardless of its complexity or (in)convenience.

The three adherence models suggested by Krasnegor et al. (2013), i.e. componential, contextual and experimental can be used to add game elements to a system designed to aid medical adherence. For example, reminders involving fun characters or graphics and dialogue, together with rewards for remembering and/or responding positively to the reminder can be useful mechanisms for managing one's condition. The contextual model reminds us of the importance of tailoring and personalisation of the program to the individual and their family. This means there should be age appropriate language and context and the requests should be appropriate for the developmental level in line with zone of proximal development (ZPD) theory (Vygotsky, 1987). Also, understanding, for example, in a split family that the child lives half of the time with their mother and the other half with their father and a certain medical device is only available or encouraged by one parent, will require the program to be able to identify the current context and adapt accordingly.

We suggest the experiential model aligns most closely to the inclusion of gamification elements due to the motivational and experiential nature of most games. We believe all three models are relevant and should be incorporated into the design of a game-like application to support adherence. Similarly, Leventhal (1993) takes a holistic approach to adherence, suggesting the need to take into account the individual's motivation and knowledge base. To this end, Leventhal offers a self-regulation framework involving the use of framing and combining elements of all three models of compliance.

While interest in games for healthcare has been growing over the past decade, their long term usefulness for clinical practice is still an emerging area. As found in the human-human context, we believe that technology-delivered therapy programs and medical advice will need to build and maintain a therapeutic alliance between the virtual clinician and the patient if it is to encourage adherence and deliver improved health outcomes. We highlight that the use of a relational agent has been found to effectively build and maintain a therapeutic alliance irrespective of the health literacy of the user (Bickmore et al., 2009).

Agents to Aid Human Agency and Adherence

Karoly (1993) suggested that adherence could be modelled as a control system that dynamically adapts to internal and external influences. We propose that agent-based modelling, where each actor and object are different types of agents defined by its properties and the rules of interaction and behaviour, can be used to create this control system. An agent is a software program that is capable of performing autonomous actions in response to the input it receives from the environment in which it is situated as it seeks to achieve its design objectives or goals (Jennings & Wooldridge, 1998). Agents are often characterised as being autonomous, reactive, proactive and having social ability. An autonomous characteristic means that agents can operate without the direct intervention of humans. Reactivity means that agents can perceive their environment and respond in a timely fashion to changes that occur in it. Pro-activeness enables agents to not simply act in response to their environment, but be able to exhibit goal-directed behaviour by taking the initiative. Social ability means that they can interact with other agents. Agents are currently being applied in domains as diverse as computer games and interactive cinema, information retrieval and filtering, user interface design, electronic commerce, autonomous vehicles and spacecraft, and industrial process control. Their use for medical applications, particularly clinical practice, is a recent but strong current focus. Most of this work is concerned with software agents and multi-agent systems that, among other purposes, may assist with decision making or monitor the patient's environment (e.g. (Corchado, Bajo, De Paz, & Tapia, 2008)) but they do not interact with the human in a humanlike way. We are interested in agents that not only plan, reason, make recommendations, perform tasks, etc., but which build a relationship with the human.

In contrast to a software agent that can be seen as something under the hood or behind the scenes that achieves the functionality of the system, a relational agent can be seen as additionally providing a human-like face and means of interaction that has been found important in building a "therapeutic alliance" between the patient and health provider, and is associated with improved adherence to treatment (Garrity, 1981). The use of animated characters further aids humanlike interaction through providing embodiment and congruent non-verbal communication, such as body gestures (e.g. pointing or nodding) and smiling or concerned facial expressions. We refer to these IVAs as relational agents to emphasis their main goal: relationship building. Relational agents are often developed using 3D modelling and game technology and deployed in virtual worlds (VWs) created using game engine technology, such as Active Worlds or Unity3D. These characters and the environments they inhabit seek to be immersive and engaging, often involving problem-solving and exploration of the virtual world, a scenario or even of the player herself.

In the context of a virtual world that allows patients to interact with a virtual health professional, technology known as agent-based virtual worlds (ABVWs) can be used. To support dynamism, an inherent part of the control system suggested by Karoly (1993), we propose that a society of agents could be employed to handle the complexity of interactions. An architecture for such a 3D virtual world using a multi-agent system or society of agents was proposed by Smith, Maher, and Gero (2003). Their solution offered a number of alternative implementations including the use of the game engines and virtual world platforms such as Active Worlds and provided an example of an agent that embodies the properties and behaviour of a wall, comprised of many other objects also modelled as agents that are aware of and able to respond to the environment as it changes (Maher & Gero, 2002). These triggers can encompass movements, conversations, thoughts, feelings, facial expressions or any of the changes in the properties or behaviours of the objects in the world including the avatars that represent the real and virtual humans involved in a session.

A relational agent seeks to change the power model and assist human agency by providing the patient with a greater sense of control and self-efficacy, in line with Bandura (2001). Using relational agents to communicate health information or interventions have been assessed as acceptable and easy to use by patients (Bickmore, Pfeifer, et al., 2010), even for users with inadequate reading, technology and/or health literacy skills (Bickmore et al., 2009).

Designing Agents to Intrinsically Motivate

Gamification elements such as competition, fast feedback/response, transparency, onboarding and orientation (involving introductions, bonding, customised individual and exciting group activities to get buy-in and commitment), goals, collaboration and community (Zichermann & Cunningham, 2011) can be found in most VWs and in many ABVWs. Interestingly, the features more commonly identified with gamification such as badges, levels and points (Zichermann & Cunningham, 2011) are less apparent in ABVWs; perhaps because these elements are primarily extrinsic motivators and the agent is seeking to intrinsically motivate the user. Based on the importance of patient agency in adherence, a focus on strategies that are intrinsically motiving seems more appropriate.

To address possible issues around agency and power-balance we will use a patient-centred communication style in which the physician shows concern for the patient and shares the conversation. In our design we use a female avatar to portray the therapist because, female physicians typically exhibit this style of communication as they tend to:

... have more positive talk (e.g., reassurance, encouragement), show more partnership building behaviors (e.g., eliciting rationale for visit and shared decision making), ask more psychosocial questions (e.g., how the disease affects the patient's daily activities), and focus more on emotions (e.g., empathy, eliciting patient concerns). (Schmid Mast, Hall, & Roter, 2007 p.17)

We will need to design both the verbal and nonverbal behaviours of our agent. Following Bickmore et al.'s (2005) verbal behaviours used to help create a working alliance (trust and belief) between the patient and agent, our dialogue will seek to demonstrate: empathy for the user; social dialogue; reciprocal self-disclosure; humor [sic]; meta-relational communication (talk about the relationship); expressing happiness to see the user; talking about the past and future together; continuity behaviors [sic] (appropriate greetings and farewells and talk about the time spent apart); reference to mutual knowledge; inclusive pronouns, politeness strategies and greeting and farewell rituals indicative of a close relationship. Nonverbal behaviours will include: close body distance, face and body directed towards the other party, facial expressions that are pleasant and congruent to the conversation content, gesturing such as nodding (Bickmore et al., 2005).

Finally, we will use the features of the alliance and of the healthcare provider as presented in the background section on the therapeutic working alliance (Ackerman & Hilsenroth, 2001, 2003) to design the verbal and non-verbal behaviours of our relational agent. The attributes can additionally be used as a checklist to validate the design and ensure the attributes have been included or avoided depending on whether their influence has been found to have a positive or negative influence.

A CASE STUDY/EXAMPLE

In 2012, researchers from Harvard Medical School demonstrated in a randomised controlled trial with 70 overweight or obese individuals that a virtual coach helped maintain their physical activity levels, calling for further additional applications of this technology (Watson et al., 2012). In answer to this call and to provide a concrete example of how a relational agent could intrinsically motivate a patient to be adherent, we present the design of an agent developed for the paediatric urinary incontinence context. While various projects are underway involving the use of buddies and coaches to encourage healthy behaviours, to our knowledge, no studies have attempted to use a relational agent to build a therapeutic alliance between the agent, paediatric patient and his/her family and guide parents and the family doctor on 'what-to-do' for their children with chronic conditions during the long waiting time for their specialist appointment.

We first introduce the condition, followed by brief description of an existing online system to assist with treatment of the condition while patients are awaiting a specialist appointment. We then suggest how the system can be modified to provide

1. Intrinsically motivating game elements via the use a relational agent, and
2. Extrinsically motivating game elements via the implementation of a currently paper-based reward system.

These additions are targeted at improving the adherence of both parents and children to the treatment advice.

The Burden and Health Consequences of Urinary Incontinence in Children

Urinary incontinence (daytime urinary incontinence (DUI) and nocturnal enuresis (NE)) is a common, stigmatizing condition that occurs in 20% of school-aged children which can progress to adulthood (Forsythe & Redmond, 1974), (Fitzgerald et al., 2006; Kuh, Cardozo, & Hardy, 1999), with up to 3% of adults remaining incontinent. Despite its apparent benign nature, urinary incontinence is associated with recurrent urinary tract infections (Hooton, 2001), depression (Macaulay, Stern, & Stanton, 1991), sexual dysfunction in adult life (Temml, Haidinger, Schmidbauer, Schatzl, & Madersbacher, 2000) and lower quality of life (Hägglöf, Andren, Bergström, Marklund, & Wendelius, 1998; Hunskaar & Vinsnes, 1991). Childhood sufferers are often socially isolated, avoiding school excursions and sleep overs, and live in fear of their "secret" being discovered.

Treatment is constrained by limited health care resources. Successful treatments for urinary incontinence in children are available from specialist services. After several months of treatment, there is usually improvement or alleviation of the incontinence and increased self-esteem and quality of life (Hägglöf et al., 1998). However, there are currently insufficient healthcare resources to address the needs of children with urinary incontinence, with many families desperate for help. Continence services are available in some tertiary centers, with no services in rural or remote areas of Australia. The Children's Hospital at Westmead (CHW) Continence Service provides a service for children from all over the Australian state New South Wales, with a waiting time of over 24 months. Urinary incontinence is ideal for testing new technology because the condition is common but relatively benign, face-to-face interactions are not essential, diagnosis is largely based on history and management involves a limited number of behavioural, psychological and pharmacological strategies.

The management of urinary incontinence at the CHW Continence Service follows an evidence-based algorithm, which incorporates the child's medical history and calculations using the child's data (P. Caldwell, Edgar, Hodson, & Craig, 2005; Chase, Austin, Hoebeke, & McKenna, 2010; Hoebeke, Bower, Combs, De Jong, & Yang, 2010) to determine the best treatment protocol. Algorithms have been developed and published for managing paediatric daytime urinary incontinence and nighttime enuresis (C. Caldwell et al., 2013; Deshpande, Craig, Smith, & Caldwell, 2012). Success depends on an accurate diagnosis (based on thorough history taking) (McGrath, Caldwell, & Jones, 2008; Sureshkumar, Caldwell, & Craig, 2010), education of the child and family, appropriate treatment advice and adherence to advice, frequent follow up and support and monitoring of progress (Chase et al., 2010; Neveus et al., 2010).

Funded by a Foundation for Children Grant and donations from individuals, CHW has built a prototype interactive eHealth program known as eADVICE (electronic Advice and Diagnosis Via the Internet following Computerised Evaluation), which can be accessed on a mobile device, which transfers the exchange of information between the parents and specialists following the algorithms for managing incontinence. Families are encouraged to seek support from their General Practitioner (GP) while using eADVICE. eADVICE follows the interaction pattern used in clinic-based consultations by first gathering the patient's history (e.g. "How often does your child wet themselves?") which the program uses to offer basic tailored specialist advice to the family and their primary care doctor while the child is awaiting their specialist appointment. The system is locked for two weeks to ensure that there is adequate time for the child to use the suggested treatment and for this to affect their incontinence. This is similar to waiting for your next face-to-face appointment. When parents and children revisit eADVICE the session commences with some follow-up questions to first determine the extent of adherence to the treatment plan, then gather up to date information about the patient's current condition and provide an updated treatment plan for the next two weeks. During the course of interaction the user may switch between the parent or child versions of the question, or ask for more information about why the question has been asked. The program liaises with the child's GP, and shares the data collected directly from the patient and parents, to aid decision-making and provide education. The program's feedback to the patients and doctor further strengthens the established doctor-patient relationship and communication channels.

However, in assessing the first 10 patients who piloted eADVICE, we found adherence to the treatment plan was quite low, with 50% of patients reporting poor adherence. Adherence was determined by self reported responses from families at follow up when our research team asked whether each component of the treatment advice was followed (yes/no). Parents reported being less likely to adhere to enuresis alarm training and medication use, due to their lack of trust of the computerised advice, and did not even seek clarification with their doctor despite being advised by eADVICE to do so. Consistent with the adherence literature, the specialist reported that in her experience face-to-face/personal contact (e.g. via weekly email chats) had higher adherence and better health outcomes compared to the reported adherence to the eADVICE program. We were thus encouraged to change the interface of eADVICE from a standard website to become a more conversational like interaction with a human face.

Giving eADVICE a Facelift: Intrinsically Motivating Patients

The current implementation of eADVICE is text based, using a traditional question- answer survey-style mode of interaction. To improve adherence, we want to add gamification elements into eADVICE that will intrinsically motivate patients and their families to follow the recommended treatment plan. As face-to-face communication has been found to offer the best support (Garrity, 1981), we are adding a new face to eADVICE in the form of an embodied relational agent with the intention that it provides a conversational mode of communication and potentially builds a therapeutic alliance with the patient, as other studies have found (e.g. (Bickmore et al., 2009) (Bickmore, Puskar, et al., 2010). The notion of a therapeutic alliance that underpins the design of our relational agent is consistent with self-determination theory and social cognitive theory by engaging the patient in setting their own goals and planning together with the healthcare provider. Our relational agent will incorporate the gamification elements of responsiveness, transparency, onboarding and orientation, goals, collaboration and community.

Gamification can be seen as putting a different (inter)face on a program. As Zichermann and Cunningham (2011) note when speaking about the DevHub website before and after it was gamified "make no mistake, the core work is unchanged and nothing has fundamentally shifted in the mechanics of designing a website. Only the perceptions of DevHub's users has been altered – for the better." P.xv" (Zichermann & Cunningham, 2011). Our agent is called Eadvice Virtual agent for Incontinence and Enuresis (EVIE). A screenshot of the current system and the agent version are shown in Figure 1.

As eADVICE's primary focus is on providing a treatment plan for the care seeker, we do not perceive a need for the experiential, exploratory or experimental elements often associated with games and virtual worlds (Kolb, 1984). eADVICE is not designed as a source of information and education that allows care seekers to come up with their own hypotheses or treatment plan or explore alternative scenarios before making a final choice, as other serious games typically allow (Davies & Dalgarno, 2009).

To manage the complexity of diagnosing the causes of a medical condition and suggesting a treatment plan, as with most electronic games (Gee, 2005) and in line with how the task is achieved in the actual clinical setting, eADVICE is interactive and highly structured commencing first with capture of the medical history where certain answers close off further inquiry or open up a new set of questions, drilling down from general to specific, avoiding unnecessary questions and providing a context in which the current question can be understood. Confirmation and, if requested, clarification and explanation are provided along the way. However, unlike many computer games (Gee, 2005) but again consistent with clinical practice, eADVICE does not provide immediate and ongoing feedback to the responses given by the care seeker but waits until the full patient history has been collected before offering a diagnosis. The way that the agent takes the history will be important because studies have shown that there are differences in the way that patient histories are taken and this will affect the diagnosis and treatment

Figure 1. a) eADVICE website screenshot. b) Agent version of the same screen.

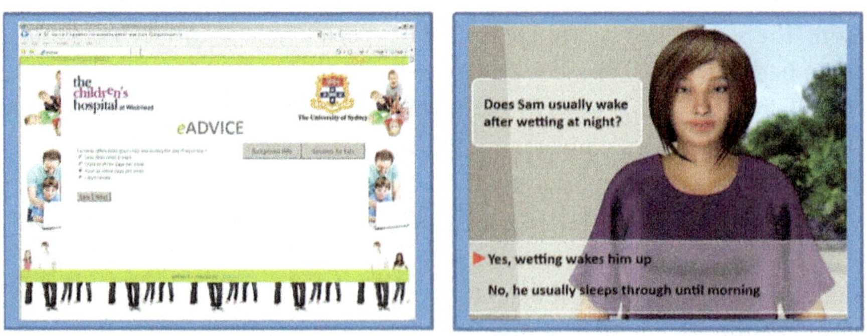

plan (McGrath et al., 2008; Sureshkumar et al., 2010). To improve the quality of the history taken we must ensure appropriate use of questions, feedback and backchannels (i.e. a supportive cues). Relational agents have been shown to aid the history taking process (Bickmore et al., 2009).

The development methodology and design for the agent follows a process similar to that established by other researchers (e.g. (Coyle & Doherty, 2009) (Bickmore, Puskar, et al., 2010)). Firstly, the design process involves an interdisciplinary team of Human-Computer Interaction (HCI) and medical specialists, comprising incontinence specialists, computer scientists and biostatistician. The conversations to be developed will be designed for engagement and will take into account any ethical and practical concerns relevant to our population. For example, dialogues for children will involve simple, familiar and concrete language.

The system is being developed using the UNITY3D[7] game engine. The unity 3D Player/Browser is free and can run as a standalone application or be accessed via the internet. A thin-client web-based architecture will allow users to access eADVICE using any machine that is connected to the Internet. A server to host the game engine and handle all processing will be maintained. Where a participant may not have access or sufficient bandwidth to handle the graphics, we will provide a downloadable installable application that can run on their computer. Data, which will require minimal bandwidth, can be stored on the local machine and uploaded automatically following the consultation, or other alternative arrangements could be made such as installation on a machine available at a community health clinic/library. The University of Southern California's Virtual Human Toolkit [8] is being used to create the relational agent and their dialogue.

As indicated in Figure 1(b), interaction with the agent involves responding to a question posed by the agent. The dialogues are provided as text within a speech bubble and also as audio. The user may ask the agent to repeat what has been said. The user is even able to choose not to interact with the agent and to be taken to the original website interface shown in Figure 1(a). The agent dialogue has been developed by the medical specialist team and designed to follow the structure and language used in the clinical setting. To date we have designed and recorded dialogue to collect the patient history and six dialogues concerning each type of treatment that a patient may be recommended to follow. The dialogues seek to be caring and empathic, while also being informative and allowing the patient or their caregiver to make the final decisions regarding their adherence to the treatment.

Adding Extrinsic Motivators to eADVICE: Building a Token Economy

In the process of gamifying eADVICE to improve adherence, we realised the potential of adding extrinsic motivators along the lines of badges, levels and points. On reflection of her current clinical practice, the incontinence specialist identified the similarity between these game elements and a paper-based activity she had been using with great success to improve adherence with recommended treatment behaviours such as going to the toilet, using a bedwetting alarm and changing fluid intake. The activity seeks to motivate children to perform the behaviours that are intended to help them achieve the goal of becoming dry. While it is this goal (i.e. dry child) that had motivated the parent to seek professional help, it is too abstract for the child. The activity involves creation of a shop that has three types of items: rewards (like lollies or toys); activities (usually outside the home) and privileges (like staying up late or screen time). Each identified item is worth a specified number of tokens. Each time the child does the desired behaviour they receive a token. Some behaviours are worth more tokens than others. For example, going to the toilet after repeated nagging is likely to earn only one token; after being reminded might earn two tokens and going without being asked might earn three tokens. Thus, the tokens themselves are small rewards that allow the child to build towards purchase of an item in the shop.

The behaviour modification strategy in the activity uses the notion of a token economy, first suggested by psychiatrists (Ayllon & Azrin, 1968). Since that time, the Skinnerism-based approach has been used by health professionals, teachers and parents as a means to bring about positive behaviour change. In many contexts this behaviour change concerns compliance with norms of acceptable classroom, institutional or societal behaviour. An assessment of the token economy by Liberman (2000) four decades after its inception acknowledged that while controlled research had provided an evidence-base for the success of the token economy in a wide variety of settings and for many patient populations, the past three decades of deinstitutionalization have seen an erosion in the efficacy of the token economy approach. Issues identified by Liberman (2000) include changes in mental health professional attitudes towards the causes of abnormal behaviour, lack of training and consistency by those needing to manage the reward system, resistance from managers to reduce the effort and associated cost of providing individualised treatment programs and finally the difficulty of designing programs for non-institutional settings due to lack of natural reinforcers in the wider community.

Similar issues relating to ideology, consistency, management, costs and persistence have been reported by parents in their use of the token economy as a discipline-related reward system[9] and also by the incontinence specialist in her clinical use of the approach. While the shop activity consistently delivers noteworthy improvements in adherence behaviours and was loved by children and adolescents, the two main challenges identified by the specialist were 1) ensuring that the child and parent worked together to agree upon what will earn a token (i.e. the expected behaviour) and what tokens can be redeemed for and 2) getting parents to be consistent and persistent (i.e. adherent) in managing the program. The first challenge relates to appropriately motivating and empowering each party. The parent wants the child to get dry but can't control the child's behaviour; the child wants to earn the reward. When the parent does not understand that the child must achieve his/her goals first before they can achieve theirs, they are unlikely to persevere and both parties become non-adherent.

An electronic game that implements the shop-based token economy and runs on a smart phone is likely to solve many of the parent's problems relating to management of the behaviours, tokens and rewards, potentially transferring much of the responsibility to the child. The App can do much more than the paper-based version or even an electronic document or spreadsheet. The App can remind, reward, monitor and motivate. The tokens themselves could have a favourite song or clip attached to them, perhaps ones that differentiate between rewards, activities and privileges, which play when one is earned.

At the start, when enthusiasm is high, the parent and child can enjoy together the activity of setting up their shop that will involve talking, selecting images, assigning values and sounds to the items the child wants to include in each section. This fun and positive activity will help to mitigate the risks of conflict and communication breakdown around the unavoidable discussion of the required behaviours. Once established, the child can take the leading role. Since the child is motivated to earn the reward, there will be little chance of them forgetting to hit a button on the App on their mobile phone to record the event. The App can be used to assist the child to remember the appropriate behaviour and adherence to this reminder would be scored as highly as a behaviour managed solely by the child without the parent.

The child-recorded event does not translate into a token until verified by the parent, probably involving the use of a parent-only password. This is not only to prevent the child from being tempted to enter false events, but also to ensure that both parent and child remain engaged in the goal to get the child dry. In the paper-based system, parents had increasing difficulty as time went on to remember to add a star to the paper-based chart/shop each time a behaviour was exhibited. In this electronic version, the child in wanting to obtain their token, can bring the phone to the parent, perhaps once a day. Unlike the paper-based version, the App will be able to store and display the successes of the child in a variety of different ways and allow the child to collect badges that provide recognition of total tokens awarded even if they have been redeemed for items in the shop. As a final benefit, due to the portability of a smart phone, the child can share their successes with the specialist when they visit, allowing further positive reinforcement to the child from the parent and the doctor.

FUTURE RESEARCH DIRECTIONS

Our next step is to evaluate our relational agent version of eADVICE. If successful in increasing adherence levels, it will not only reduce the burden of urinary incontinence but also contribute to reduced waiting times and medical costs associated with specialist visits. We anticipate that eADVICE could be adapted for adult incontinence, as adults with stigmatizing conditions are more likely seek treatment advice online (Berger, Wagner, & Baker, 2005). Furthermore, we anticipate that similar treatment systems could be developed for other common chronic paediatric conditions (such as wheezing in children, allergies and sleep disorders), where waiting times are long and early treatment advice can improve health outcomes.

The viability of using relational agents is closely tied to whether solutions are found to reduce the effort of authoring of these systems. Without such solutions, the paradigm is not likely to be scalable because of the need for costly and effort intensive collaboration between technical and domain experts to capture the knowledge around appropriate empathic behaviours and dialogues. Towards addressing these knowledge acquisition and authoring bottlenecks, we have offered two alternative approaches: one which enables the domain expert to create numerous alternative training scenarios by modifying a base scenario by changing selected characters, dialog, objects and actions (Richards and Taylor, 2011); the other allows knowledge to be captured as the expert experiences a scenario as a means to tap into their tacit knowledge as they exercise knowledge-in-action (Richards and Taylor, 2010). These approaches offer initial and simple solutions to this complex issue by reducing authoring and knowledge acquisition to modifying the story, dialogue or the domain knowledge in the context of the situation on hand. However, more sophisticated solutions are needed.

The widespread use of relational agents in healthcare is also dependent on advancements in human-computer interaction. The work on empathic agents (e.g. McQuiggan and Lester, 2006, Ochs, Pelachaud and Sadek, 2008, Niewiadomski, Ochs and Pelachaud, 2008, Paiva et al, 2004) is relevant and found to deliver improved interactions. Another emerging area is the notion of listening agents in recognition that virtual agents need to do more than passively sit or stand when a human user speaks since listener behaviour will impact the speaker. Maatman, Gratch and Marsella (2005) note that current speech understanding systems are limited because they are unable to process and respond to input until the utterance is complete. While we agree that listening behaviours are important for authentic human-agent interactions, the focus in this body of work is on simulating believable behaviour, rather than actual understanding of what the human is saying. Such approaches re-open the debate on whether AI technologies should/could replicate human behaviours or simply mimic them.

The use of a relational agent to take on the role of the therapist raises some issues around the desirability and consequences of substituting a person with a machine. In an article concerning the ethics of social robots – emotional agents, Becker (2006) warns that viewing social robots (such as humanoid robots and emotionally embodied agents) as independent actors is "highly questionable" and anthropomorphisation of such agents is "irrelevant". Instead, Becker suggests that instead of viewing:

... virtual agents, ECAs and robots as human-like interaction partners ... they could take on specific tasks with a relational behavioural concept, which would accord them an empowerment to act which is limited to this task. This would do justice to the potential of these supposedly "intelligent" artefacts while allowing their limitations." (Becker, 2006), p. 44.

In addition to addressing questions such as *what* should an agent be allowed to do and *why* (i.e. addressing the ethical concerns), *how* should the agent do it (i.e. addressing technical concerns), further research is needed to understand *when* an agent is appropriate and *who* would benefit. Some individuals are more likely than others to develop a strong alliance (Horvath & Luborsky, 1993). Understanding why and who these people are may help us to identify which patients can benefit most from a relational agent. For mental health conditions conversation with a relational agent can be less stressful and difficult than conversation with a human, however, agents used with psychotic patients will need to be designed to help patients maintain reality rather than believe the agent is in fact a person (Bickmore, Puskar, et al., 2010).

Growing interest in the effect of personality in intelligent virtual agent and human interaction will assist in answering related questions. In addition to understanding individual differences, due to observed differences in how girls and boys play and engage in computer-based games, further research into gender differences and age difference as they may relate to the efficacy or adaptation of relational agents should be explored. For example, (Schmid Mast et al., 2007) found that females have a more socio-emotional communication style compared to men who use a more directive communication style. Whether this also applies to children would be an important finding for relational agents in the paediatric context.

CONCLUSION

This chapter has specifically been concerned with gamification for the purposes of encouraging and supporting adherence to clinical treatments. The growing interest in gamification follows the trend of technology as a tool for empowerment. In our focus on adherence we reviewed the related literature and found that development of a therapeutic alliance was a key indicator in treatment success and factor in adherence. We proposed the use of a relational agent, which embodies a range of gamification elements that can be described as intrinsically motivating, to provide this therapeutic alliance and overcome health literacy barriers. We provided a brief case study in the incontinence domain that described how a relational agent could be used to provide a new way of interacting with a current web-based system. Further, we described the implementation of a token economy game that would add extrinsically motivating game elements.

As a final remark, we wish to emphasize that we do not see technology as a replacement for human expertise or caring. A computer-based counsellor can provide a more acceptable alternative in situations where there is fear of the consequences of disclosure, such as punishment or judgement, or the more likely situation that a human caregiver is not accessible. In both situations, solutions should be designed that keep the human clinician in the loop to ensure that the patient is receiving adequate care and support and risk situations are identified and handled appropriately.

REFERENCES

Ackerman, S. J., & Hilsenroth, M. J. (2001). A review of therapist characteristics and techniques negatively impacting the therapeutic alliance. *Psychotherapy (Chicago, Ill.)*, *38*(2), 171–185. doi:10.1037/0033-3204.38.2.171

Ackerman, S. J., & Hilsenroth, M. J. (2003). A review of therapist characteristics and techniques positively impacting the therapeutic alliance. *Clinical Psychology Review*, *23*(1), 1–33. doi:10.1016/S0272-7358(02)00146-0 PMID:12559992

Anderson, B. J., & Coyne, J. C. (1993). Family context and compliance behavior in chronically ill children.

Ayllon, T., & Azrin, N. (1968). The token economy: A motivational system for therapy and rehabilitation.

Balkrishnan, R. (2005). The importance of medication adherence in improving chronic-disease related outcomes: What we know and what we need to further know. *Medical Care*, *43*(6), 517–520. doi:10.1097/01.mlr.0000166617.68751.5f PMID:15908845

Bandura, A. (2001). Social cognitive theory: An agentic perspective. *Annual Review of Psychology*, *52*(1), 1–26. doi:10.1146/annurev.psych.52.1.1 PMID:11148297

Barbosa, C. D., Balp, M.-M., Kulich, K., Germain, N., & Rofail, D. (2012). A literature review to explore the link between treatment satisfaction and adherence, compliance, and persistence. *Patient Prefer Adherence*, *6*, 39–48. doi:10.2147/PPA.S24752 PMID:22272068

Bates, J. (1994). The role of emotion in believable agents. *Communications of the ACM*, *37*(7), 122–125. doi:10.1145/176789.176803

Becker, B. (2006). Social robots-emotional agents: Some remarks on naturalizing man-machine interaction. *International Review of Information Ethics*, *6*(12), 37–45.

Berger, M., Wagner, T. H., & Baker, L. C. (2005). Internet use and stigmatized illness. *Social Science & Medicine*, *61*(8), 1821–1827. doi:10.1016/j.socscimed.2005.03.025 PMID:16029778

Bickmore, T., Gruber, A., & Picard, R. (2005). Establishing the computer–patient working alliance in automated health behavior change interventions. *Patient Education and Counseling*, *59*(1), 21–30. doi:10.1016/j.pec.2004.09.008 PMID:16198215

Bickmore, T. W., Pfeifer, L. M., Byron, D., Forsythe, S., Henault, L. E., & Jack, B. W. et al. (2010). Usability of conversational agents by patients with inadequate health literacy: Evidence from two clinical trials. *Journal of Health Communication*, *15*(sup2S2), 197–210. doi:10.1080/10810730.2010.499991 PMID:20845204

Bickmore, T. W., Pfeifer, L. M., & Jack, B. W. (2009). *Taking the time to care: empowering low health literacy hospital patients with virtual nurse agents.* Paper presented at the proceedings of the SIGCHI Conference on Human Factors in Computing Systems. doi:10.1145/1518701.1518891

Bickmore, T. W., Puskar, K., Schlenk, E. A., Pfeifer, L. M., & Sereika, S. M. (2010). Maintaining reality: Relational agents for antipsychotic medication adherence. *Interacting with Computers*, *22*(4), 276–288. doi:10.1016/j.intcom.2010.02.001 PMID:20628581

Bidarra, R., Gambon, D., Kooij, R., Nagel, D., Schutjes, M., & Tziouvara, I. (2013). *Gaming at the dentist's–serious game design for pain and discomfort distraction Games for Health* (pp. 207–215). Springer.

Bonnechére, B., Jansen, B., Omelina, L., Da Silva, L., Mouraux, D., Rooze, M., & Van Sint, J. S. (2013). *Patient follow-up using Serious Games. A feasibility study on low back pain patients Games for Health* (pp. 185–195). Springer.

Bruner, J. (1991). The narrative construction of reality. *Critical Inquiry, 18*(1), 1–21. doi:10.1086/448619

Buchanan, R. (2011). Paradox, Promise and Public Pedagogy: Implications of the Federal Government's Digital Education Revolution. *Australian Journal of Teacher Education, 36*(2), 67–78. doi:10.14221/ajte.2011v36n2.6

Caldwell, C., Bruggers, C., Altizer, R., Bulaj, G., D'Ambrosio, T., Kessler, R., & Christiansen, B. (2013). *The intersection of video games and patient empowerment: case study of a real world application.* Paper presented at the Proceedings of The 9th Australasian Conference on Interactive Entertainment: Matters of Life and Death. doi:10.1145/2513002.2513018

Caldwell, P., Edgar, D., Hodson, E., & Craig, J. C. (2005). Bedwetting and toileting problems in children. *The Medical Journal of Australia, 182*(4), 190–195. PMID:15720177

Chase, J., Austin, P., Hoebeke, P., & McKenna, P. (2010). The management of dysfunctional voiding in children: A report from the Standardisation Committee of the International Children's Continence Society. *The Journal of Urology, 183*(4), 1296–1302. doi:10.1016/j.juro.2009.12.059 PMID:20171678

Chue, P. (2006). The relationship between patient satisfaction and treatment outcomes in schizophrenia. *Journal of Psychopharmacology (Oxford, England), 20*(6suppl), 38–56. doi:10.1177/1359786806071246 PMID:17046986

Clark, R. E. (1983). Reconsidering research on learning from media. *Review of Educational Research, 53*(4), 445–459. doi:10.3102/00346543053004445

Corchado, J. M., Bajo, J., De Paz, Y., & Tapia, D. I. (2008). Intelligent environment for monitoring Alzheimer patients, agent technology for health care. *Decision Support Systems, 44*(2), 382–396. doi:10.1016/j.dss.2007.04.008

Coyle, D., & Doherty, G. (2009). *Clinical evaluations and collaborative design: developing new technologies for mental healthcare interventions.* Paper presented at the proceedings of the SIGCHI Conference on Human Factors in Computing Systems. doi:10.1145/1518701.1519013

Davies, A., & Dalgarno, B. (2009). Learning fire investigation the clean way: The virtual experience. *Australasian Journal of Educational Technology, 25*(1), 1–13.

Davis, A., Murphy, J., Owens, D., Khazanchi, D., & Zigurs, I. (2009). Avatars, People, and Virtual Worlds: Foundations for Research in Metaverses. *Journal of the Association for Information Systems, 10*(2).

de Greef, K., van der Spek, E. D., & Bekker, T. (2013). *Designing Kinect games to train motor skills for mixed ability players Games for Health* (pp. 197–205). Springer.

Deshpande, A. V., Craig, J. C., Smith, G. H., & Caldwell, P. H. (2012). Management of daytime urinary incontinence and lower urinary tract symptoms in children. *Journal of Paediatrics and Child Health, 48*(2), E44–E52. doi:10.1111/j.1440-1754.2011.02216.x PMID:22050540

Desjardins, R., Murray, T., & Tuijnman, A. (2005). *Learning a living: First results of the Adult Literacy and Life Skills survey*. OECD.

DeVault, D., Artstein, R., Benn, G., Dey, T., Fast, E., Gainer, A., et al. (2014). *SimSensei kiosk: a virtual human interviewer for healthcare decision support*. Paper presented at the proceedings of the 2014 international conference on Autonomous agents and multi-agent systems, Paris, France.

Donkin, L., Christensen, H., Naismith, S. L., Neal, B., Hickie, I. B., & Glozier, N. (2011). A systematic review of the impact of adherence on the effectiveness of e-therapies. *Journal of Medical Internet Research, 13*(3), e52. doi:10.2196/jmir.1772 PMID:21821503

Duffy, T. M., & Jonassen, D. H. (1992). *Constructivism and the technology of instruction: A conversation*. Psychology Press.

Dunbar-Jacob, J., Dunning, E. J., & Dwyer, K. (1993). Compliance research in pediatric and adolescent populations: Two decades of research. *Developmental aspects of health compliance behavior*, 29-51.

Durga, S., El-Nasr, M. S., Shiyko, M., Sceppa, C., Naab, P., & Andres, L. (2014). Leveraging Play to Promote Health Behavior Change: A Player Acceptance Study of a Health Game *Virtual* [Springer.]. *Augmented Reality and Serious Games for Healthcare, 1*, 209–230. doi:10.1007/978-3-642-54816-1_12

Eysenbach, G. (2008). Medicine 2.0: Social networking, collaboration, participation, apomediation, and openness. *Journal of Medical Internet Research, 10*(3), e22. doi:10.2196/jmir.1030 PMID:18725354

Fenerty, S. D., West, C., Davis, S. A., Kaplan, S. G., & Feldman, S. R. (2012). The effect of reminder systems on patients' adherence to treatment. *Patient Prefer Adherence, 6*, 127–135. doi:10.2147/PPA.S26314 PMID:22379363

Fishbein, M. (1979). A theory of reasoned action: some applications and implications.

Fitzgerald, M. P., Thom, D. H., Wassel-Fyr, C., Subak, L., Brubaker, L., Van Den Eeden, S. K., & Brown, J. S. (2006). Childhood urinary symptoms predict adult overactive bladder symptoms. *The Journal of Urology, 175*(3), 989–993. doi:10.1016/S0022-5347(05)00416-7 PMID:16469599

Forsythe, W., & Redmond, A. (1974). Enuresis and spontaneous cure rate study of 1129 enuretics. *Archives of Disease in Childhood, 49*(4), 259–263. doi:10.1136/adc.49.4.259 PMID:4830115

Garrity, T. F. (1981). Medical compliance and the clinician-patient relationship: A review. *Social Science & Medicine. Part E, Medical Psychology, 15*(3), 215–222. doi:10.1016/0271-5384(81)90016-8 PMID:7323842

Gee, J. P. (2005). Learning by design: Good video games as learning machines. *E-learning, 2*(1), 5–16. doi:10.2304/elea.2005.2.1.5

Gerrig, R. J. (1993). *Experiencing narrative worlds: On the psychological activities of reading*. Yale University Press.

Gilbert, N. (2008). Agent-based models. *Sage (Atlanta, Ga.)*.

Gratch, J., Lucas, G. M., King, A. A., & Morency, L.-P. (2014). *It's only a computer: the impact of human-agent interaction in clinical interviews.* Paper presented at the Proceedings of the 2014 international conference on Autonomous agents and multi-agent systems.

Guðmundsdóttir, K., Wille, A. L., & Savu, A. (2013). *Designing games for children with cerebral palsy Games for Health* (pp. 99–116). Springer.

Hägglöf, B., Andren, O., Bergström, E., Marklund, L., & Wendelius, M. (1998). Self-esteem in children with nocturnal enuresis and urinary incontinence: Improvement of self-esteem after treatment. *European Urology*, *33*(Suppl. 3), 16–19. doi:10.1159/000052236 PMID:9599731

Health Literacy, Australia. (2006ABS. Canberra: Australian Government.

Hoebeke, P., Bower, W., Combs, A., De Jong, T., & Yang, S. (2010). Diagnostic evaluation of children with daytime incontinence. *The Journal of Urology*, *183*(2), 699–703. doi:10.1016/j.juro.2009.10.038 PMID:20022025

Honey, P., & Mumford, A. (1986). *Using your learning styles*. UK: Peter Honey Maidenhead.

Hooton, T. M. (2001). Recurrent urinary tract infection in women. *International Journal of Antimicrobial Agents*, *17*(4), 259–268. doi:10.1016/S0924-8579(00)00350-2 PMID:11295405

Horvath, A. O., & Greenberg, L. S. (1989). Development and validation of the Working Alliance Inventory. *Journal of Counseling Psychology*, *36*(2), 223–233. doi:10.1037/0022-0167.36.2.223

Horvath, A. O., & Luborsky, L. (1993). The role of the therapeutic alliance in psychotherapy. *Journal of Consulting and Clinical Psychology*, *61*(4), 561–573. doi:10.1037/0022-006X.61.4.561 PMID:8370852

Hughes, B., Joshi, I., & Wareham, J. (2008). Health 2.0 and Medicine 2.0: Tensions and controversies in the field. *Journal of Medical Internet Research*, *10*(3), e23. doi:10.2196/jmir.1056 PMID:18682374

Hunskaar, S., & Vinsnes, A. (1991). The quality of life in women with urinary incontinence as measured by the sickness impact profile. *Journal of the American Geriatrics Society*, *39*(4), 378–382. doi:10.1111/j.1532-5415.1991.tb02903.x PMID:2010587

Iannotti, R., & Bush, P. (1993). Toward a developmental theory of compliance. *Developmental aspects of health compliance behavior*, 59-76.

Inchamnan, W., & Wyeth, P. (2013). *Motivation during videogame play: analysing player experience in terms of cognitive action.* Paper presented at the proceedings of The 9th Australasian Conference on Interactive Entertainment: Matters of Life and Death. doi:10.1145/2513002.2513010

Jennings, N., & Wooldridge, M. J. (1998). *Agent technology: foundations, applications, and markets.* Springer. doi:10.1007/978-3-662-03678-5

Kafai, Y. B., & Resnick, M. (1996). *Constructionism in practice: Designing, thinking, and learning in a digital world.* Routledge.

Karoly, P. (1993). Enlarging the scope of the compliance construct: Toward developmental and motivational relevance. *Developmental aspects of health compliance behavior*, 11-27.

Kelders, S. M., Kok, R. N., Ossebaard, H. C., & Van Gemert-Pijnen, J. E. (2012). Persuasive system design does matter: A systematic review of adherence to web-based interventions. *Journal of Medical Internet Research, 14*(6), e152. doi:10.2196/jmir.2104 PMID:23151820

Khalil, G. E. (2013). *Fear and Happiness in" Re-Mission": Teasing Out Emotional Gaming Events Responsible for Cancer Risk Perception Games for Health* (pp. 27–44). Springer.

Kolb, D. A. (1984). *Experiential learning: Experience as the source of learning and development* (Vol. 1). NJ: Prentice-Hall Englewood Cliffs.

Krasnegor, N. A., Epstein, L., Johnson, S. B., Yaffe, S. J., & Epstein, L. H. (2013). *Developmental aspects of health compliance behavior*. Psychology Press.

Kuh, D., Cardozo, L., & Hardy, R. (1999). Urinary incontinence in middle aged women: Childhood enuresis and other lifetime risk factors in a British prospective cohort. *Journal of Epidemiology and Community Health, 53*(8), 453–458. doi:10.1136/jech.53.8.453 PMID:10562862

Leventhal, H. (1993). Theories of compliance, and turning necessities into preferences: Application to adolescent health action. *Developmental aspects of health compliance behavior*, 91-124.

Lever-Duffy, J., McDonald, J., & Mizell, A. (2002). *The 21st-Century Classroom: Teaching and Learning with Technology*. Addison-Wesley Longman Publishing Co., Inc.

Liberman, R. P. (2000). The token economy. *The American Journal of Psychiatry, 157*(9), 1398–1398. doi:10.1176/appi.ajp.157.9.1398 PMID:10964853

Lisetti, C. L. (2012). 10 advantages of using avatars in patient-centered computer-based interventions for behavior change. *SIGHIT Record, 2*(1), 28. doi:10.1145/2180796.2180820

Lisetti, C. L., Yasavur, U., de Leon, C., Amini, R., Visser, U., & Rishe, N. (2012). *Building an On-Demand Avatar-Based Health Intervention for Behavior Change.* Paper presented at the FLAIRS Conference.

Macaulay, A. J., Stern, R., & Stanton, S. (1991). Psychological aspects of 211 female patients attending a urodynamic unit. *Journal of Psychosomatic Research, 35*(1), 1–10. doi:10.1016/0022-3999(91)90002-6 PMID:2023138

Maher, M. L., & Gero, J. S. (2002). Agent Models of 3D Virtual Worlds1.

Mandl, K. D., & Kohane, I. S. (2009). No small change for the health information economy. *The New England Journal of Medicine, 360*(13), 1278–1281. doi:10.1056/NEJMp0900411 PMID:19321867

Marsella, S., Johnson, W. L., & LaBore, C. (2003). *Interactive pedagogical drama for health interventions.* Paper presented at the 11th International Conference on Artificial Intelligence in Education, Sydney, Australia.

Martin, D. J., Garske, J. P., & Davis, M. K. (2000). Relation of the therapeutic alliance with outcome and other variables: A meta-analytic review. *Journal of Consulting and Clinical Psychology, 68*(3), 438–450. doi:10.1037/0022-006X.68.3.438 PMID:10883561

McGrath, K. H., Caldwell, P. H., & Jones, M. P. (2008). The frequency of constipation in children with nocturnal enuresis: A comparison with parental reporting. *Journal of Paediatrics and Child Health*, *44*(1-2), 19–27. PMID:17854414

Mert, A., Buirma, R., van Luijk, J., Melkonian, G., Pels, J., & Vermetten, E. (2013). *Development of a theory-based applied game for the treatment of Post-Traumatic Stress Disorder: proof of feasibility Games for Health* (pp. 247–253). Springer. doi:10.1007/978-3-658-02897-8_19

Mohr, D. C., Cuijpers, P., & Lehman, K. (2011). Supportive accountability: A model for providing human support to enhance adherence to eHealth interventions. *Journal of Medical Internet Research*, *13*(1), e30. doi:10.2196/jmir.1602 PMID:21393123

Murray, E., Burns, J., See, T. S., Lai, R., & Nazareth, I. (2005). Interactive Health Communication Applications for people with chronic disease. *Cochrane Database of Systematic Reviews*, 4. PMID:16235356

Neveus, T., Eggert, P., Evans, J., Macedo, A., Rittig, S., & Tekgül, S. et al. (2010). Evaluation of and treatment for monosymptomatic enuresis: A standardization document from the International Children's Continence Society. *The Journal of Urology*, *183*(2), 441–447. doi:10.1016/j.juro.2009.10.043 PMID:20006865

Paasche-Orlow, M. K., Parker, R. M., Gazmararian, J. A., Nielsen-Bohlman, L. T., & Rudd, R. R. (2005). The prevalence of limited health literacy. *Journal of General Internal Medicine*, *20*(2), 175–184. doi:10.1111/j.1525-1497.2005.40245.x PMID:15836552

Prensky, M. (2003). Digital game-based learning. [CIE]. *Computers in Entertainment*, *1*(1), 21–21. doi:10.1145/950566.950596

Priebatsch, S. (2010). The game layer on top of the world. *TEDx Talks*.

Prochaska, J. O., & Velicer, W. F. (1997). The transtheoretical model of health behavior change. *American Journal of Health Promotion*, *12*(1), 38–48. doi:10.4278/0890-1171-12.1.38 PMID:10170434

Reeves, B., & Nass, C. (1996). *How people treat computers, television, and new media like real people and places*: CSLI Publications and Cambridge university press.

Richards, D., & Szilas, N. (2012). *Challenging reality using techniques from interactive drama to support social simulations in virtual worlds.* Paper presented at the Proceedings of The 8th Australasian Conference on Interactive Entertainment: Playing the System. doi:10.1145/2336727.2336739

Ross, S. M., Morrison, G. R., & Lowther, D. L. (2010). Educational Technology Research Past and Present: Balancing: Rigor and Relevance to Impact School Learning. *Contemporary Educational Technology*, *1*(1).

Ryan, R. M., & Deci, E. L. (2000). Self-determination theory and the facilitation of intrinsic motivation, social development, and well-being. *The American Psychologist*, *55*(1), 68–78. doi:10.1037/0003-066X.55.1.68 PMID:11392867

Ryan, R. M., Rigby, C. S., & Przybylski, A. (2006). The motivational pull of video games: A self-determination theory approach. *Motivation and Emotion*, *30*(4), 344–360. doi:10.1007/s11031-006-9051-8

Safran, J. D., & Muran, J. C. (2000). *Negotiating the therapeutic alliance: A relational treatment guide*. Guilford Press.

Salen, K., & Zimmerman, E. (2004). *Rules of play: Game design fundamentals*. MIT press.

Scherer, S., Stratou, G., Mahmoud, M., Boberg, J., Gratch, J., Rizzo, A., & Morency, L.-P. (2013). *Automatic behavior descriptors for psychological disorder analysis*. Paper presented at the Automatic Face and Gesture Recognition (FG), 2013 10th IEEE International Conference and Workshops on. doi:10.1109/FG.2013.6553789

Schmid Mast, M., Hall, J. A., & Roter, D. L. (2007). Disentangling physician sex and physician communication style: Their effects on patient satisfaction in a virtual medical visit. *Patient Education and Counseling*, *68*(1), 16–22. doi:10.1016/j.pec.2007.03.020 PMID:17482418

Schouten, B., Fedtke, S., Bekker, T., Schijven, M., & Gekker, A. Games for Health.

Servan-Schreiber, D. (1986). Artificial intelligence and psychiatry. *The Journal of Nervous and Mental Disease*, *174*(4), 191–202. doi:10.1097/00005053-198604000-00001 PMID:3514790

Smith, G. J., Maher, M. L., & Gero, J. S. (2003). *Designing 3D virtual worlds as a society of agents*. Paper presented at the Proceedings of CAADFutures.

Spiro, R., Feltovich, P., & Jacobson, M. & Coulson, RL (1992). Cognitive flexibility, constructivism, and hypertext: Random access instruction for advanced knowledge acquisition in ill-structured domains. In T.M Duffy, & D.H. Jonassen (Eds.), *Constructivism and the technology of instruction: A conversation*, 57-76.

Stiles, W. B., Glick, M. J., Osatuke, K., Hardy, G. E., Shapiro, D. A., & Agnew-Davies, R. et al. (2004). Patterns of alliance development and the rupture-repair hypothesis: Are productive relationships U-shaped or V-shaped? *Journal of Counseling Psychology*, *51*(1), 81–92. doi:10.1037/0022-0167.51.1.81

Stinson, J., Wilson, R., Gill, N., Yamada, J., & Holt, J. (2009). A systematic review of internet-based self-management interventions for youth with health conditions. *Journal of Pediatric Psychology*, *34*(5), 495–510. doi:10.1093/jpepsy/jsn115 PMID:19029142

Sureshkumar, P., Caldwell, P. H., & Craig, J. C. (2010). Diagnosing daytime bladder symptoms in children with nocturnal enuresis: A comparison of brief parental questionnaire with in-depth, physician-elicited, assessment. *Journal of Paediatrics and Child Health*, *46*(11), 636–641. doi:10.1111/j.1440-1754.2010.01821.x PMID:20796179

Tamim, R. M., Bernard, R. M., Borokhovski, E., Abrami, P. C., & Schmid, R. F. (2011). What forty years of research says about the impact of technology on learning a second-order meta-analysis and validation study. *Review of Educational Research*, *81*(1), 4–28. doi:10.3102/0034654310393361

Temml, C., Haidinger, G., Schmidbauer, J., Schatzl, G., & Madersbacher, S. (2000). Urinary incontinence in both sexes: Prevalence rates and impact on quality of life and sexual life. *Neurourology and Urodynamics*, *19*(3), 259–271. doi:10.1002/(SICI)1520-6777(2000)19:3<259::AID-NAU7>3.0.CO;2-U PMID:10797583

Thorngate, W., & Tavakoli, M. (2009). Simulation, rhetoric, and policy making. *Simulation & Gaming, 40*(4), 513–527. doi:10.1177/1046878108330539

Vorderer, P., Hartmann, T., & Klimmt, C. (2003). *Explaining the enjoyment of playing video games: the role of competition.* Paper presented at the Proceedings of the second international conference on Entertainment computing.

Vygotsky, L. (1987). Zone of proximal development. *Mind in society: The development of higher psychological processes*, 52-91.

Watson, A., Bickmore, T., Cange, A., Kulshreshtha, A., & Kvedar, J. (2012). An internet-based virtual coach to promote physical activity adherence in overweight adults: Randomized controlled trial. *Journal of Medical Internet Research, 14*(1), e1. doi:10.2196/jmir.1629 PMID:22281837

Williams, M. V., Parker, R. M., Baker, D. W., Parikh, N. S., Pitkin, K., Coates, W. C., & Nurss, J. R. (1995). Inadequate functional health literacy among patients at two public hospitals. *Journal of the American Medical Association, 274*(21), 1677–1682. doi:10.1001/jama.1995.03530210031026 PMID:7474271

Zichermann, G., & Cunningham, C. (2011). *Gamification by design: Implementing game mechanics in web and mobile apps.* O'Reilly Media, Inc.

KEY TERMS AND DEFINITIONS

Adherence: Performing a task or behaviour in accordance with a rule, recommendation, directive or norm based on the wilful agreement of the performer.

Agent: An agent is a software program that is not only autonomously reacts to its environment, it is proactive and socially capable.

Compliance: Following a rule, standard, guideline, recommendation, directive or norm.

Gamification: The use of game-thinking and game mechanics to enhance user motivation, enjoyment and engagement with the software.

Health Literacy: The knowledge and skills needed to be able to access, understand and apply health-related information in order to manage one's health and wellbeing.

Medicine 2.0: The application of Web 2.0, semantic web and/or virtual-reality technologies for health care consumers, caregivers, patients, health professionals, and biomedical researchers.

Relational Agents: Relational agents are virtual characters that seek to develop trust, rapport and an emotional relationship with the human user through believable and empathic behaviours.

Therapeutic Working Alliance: A therapeutic alliance encompasses the degree to which the helper and client agree on the goals of the therapy and tasks to be performed, and the extent to which a bond between the helper and client is trusting and empathetic.

Working Alliance Inventory (WAI): WAI is a self-reported 12-item Likert scale questionnaire produces a composite score based on three measures: WAI goal, WAI task, WAI Bond to measure the extent of a Therapeutic Working Alliance.

ENDNOTES

1. http://www.bistudio.com/
2. http://www.jfcom.mil/about/fact_jcats.htm
3. www.hazmat.com
4. http://www.sandia.gov/mission/homeland/wmd.html
5. http://www.classicdosgames.com/game/Word_Rescue.html
6. http://www.classicdosgames.com/game/Math_Rescue.html
7. http://unity3D.com
8. https://vhtoolkit.ict.usc.edu/
9. http://discipline.about.com/od/decreasenegativebehaviors/tp/5-Common-Problems-With-Token-Economy-Reward-Systems-For-Kids.htm.

This work was previously published in the Handbook of Research on Holistic Perspectives in Gamification for Clinical Practice edited by Daniel Novák, Bengisu Tulu, and Håvar Brendryen, pages 47-77, copyright year 2016 by Medical Information Science Reference (an imprint of IGI Global).

Chapter 6
Content Elements for Web-Based Health Promotion

Marwan Noman
Multimedia University, Malaysia

Ah Choo Koo
Multimedia University, Malaysia

Sim Hui Tee
Multimedia University, Malaysia

ABSTRACT

This paper provides an analysis of the basic elements required for health promotion based on digital content. It covers the feedback from the respondents involved in a pilot study type; content interventions were examined among the respondents to analyze the most required content elements for health promotion programs for workplace community. These elements should be focused on to highlight the importance of content quality and interactivity features for health promoters using technology solutions to provide digital content. The findings of this research has attracted the interest of policy makers associates in Malaysia to engage with the research team to enhance the quality of content provided to the Malaysian society.

INTRODUCTION

Information Communication and Technology tools have been accessible nowadays almost by everyone, the content creation and dissemination have been rapidly changing from the traditional methods to better modern methods such as using interactive multimedia and media based content. In correlation with health communication; the ICT tools have been used widely between healthcare professionals and health communication societies to ensure better info transmitting, which will lead to knowledge sharing atmosphere. "The concept of eHealth has gained momentum within health care in recent years, but surprisingly little has addressed the issue of health promotion within eHealth" (Evers, 2006), the ICT tools have been used a lot among health care industries to ensure better health care delivery services but it hasn't been used utilized with sufficient strategy into health promotion approach. Evers (2006) has also mentioned

DOI: 10.4018/978-1-5225-1928-7.ch006

how the Internet should serve as an information hub in America. However, it was mentioned that the Americans who are looking for health information online increased from 46 million to 73 million in December 2002. World Health Organization has determined the role of IT tools into health promotion and healthcare delivery quality. "The internet has become a powerful global communication method for health interventions, providing public access to a wide range of health promotion programs" (Levac, and O'Sullivan, 2010). Eventually, Media tools are still the fastest in terms of becoming the future tools for health promotion "A recent study by the Centre for Health Promotion found that social media was fast becoming a powerful tool in delivering health promotion" (HNC, 2013).

Background Study

WHO (2010) states the health problems in Malaysia reside in NCDs (Non-Communicable Diseases). The World Health Organization and the Malaysian Ministry of Health have collaborated into developing a strategy to address the opportunities and challenges of Malaysia's Public health. "This includes, adding lifelong wellness to disease prevention and control, by emphasizing health promotion and consumer empowerment" (WHO-Malaysia, 2009). Health promotion strategies need a lot of planning due to community changes and human behaviors as well, therefore the content is really important since it is the core object that will draw an effect on the behaviors.

Ragunath (2013) has stated that the Ministry of Health in Malaysia has prioritized the focus on promoting health at the workplace environment as a partial contribution of the overall health promotion initiative. This step is implemented in collaboration with Mysihat (Malaysia Health Promotion Board) in order work on the strategies and plans, *"Continuous effort with intersectoral collaboration e.g. Malaysian Health Promotion Board"* (Ragunath, 2013). The role of multimedia content is also missing in the Malaysian society due to the loads of informative content, which only focuses on documentation rather than content quality and methods. Myhealth (2011) is a portal application powered by the Ministry of

Table 1. Malaysian country cooperation strategy

First Arm: WHO support for Malaysian priority areas	**Second Arm:** Malaysia's participation in-and contribution to- regional and international collaboration with WHO support towards mutual learning
Development and strengthening of the health system and health policy related to: • Health reform and health care financing • Inter-sectoral action in addressing health inequities • Strategic planning and coordination for human resources • Capacity building for evidence based policy and practice • Health information and knowledge management	• Health system governance • Improved quality of care • Integrated Primary Health Care (PHC) • Maternal, newborn, child, adolescent and reproduction health • Nutrition • Food safety and Quality • Pharmaceuticals • Environmental health • Harm Reduction Programmes for Injecting Drugs Users
Prevention and control of NCD, their risk factors and promotion of healthy lifestyles	
Communicable disease control focusing on: • HIV/AIDS and STIs • Surveillance and response to outbreaks, IHR including APSED and 'Beyond' • Prevention and Control of Dengue, Malaria Elimination and Lymphatic Filariasis Elimination	

WHO-Malaysia (2009)

Health in Malaysia, the portal is very good in terms of information bowls and categories, but unfortunately the portal does not have any sort of interactive/creative content even though they provide media elements such as videos, illustration, animation and audio; but the content of all these elements are not presented in a method that will ensure community participation or awareness.

For instance, when creating content to a specific niche of the community, the content has to be developed based on this niche preference and what can impact them mostly. When thinking to implement e-health promotion, there are some interventions to be considered as mentioned by Barretto et al (2010). The interventions can be inherited for theory-based phases such as: Best Practices, Design, Content, Construct, and Finalize. It is vital that the best practices are done in the first phase since they will help determine the health issues/problems to be covered, and the most appropriate programs to be deployed. Based on that, it will assist to set a change for a specific target behavior; which will be the metric factor during the evaluation. Next, is to analyze the best practices and conduct data collection among the target audience and examine their results. Once the practices are defined, the next phase will be to design the material. "Evidence suggests that health promotion programs are more effective if they are theory-based" (Barretto et al, 2010). Therefore, the initial phase in outlining any health promotion intercession is to build up the framework, which will structure the concepts, definition and related behavior change as stated by Barretto et al (2010). When it comes to Design, it is recommended to state the expected objectives of the health promotion tool, such as increase awareness, positive change in behavior, and better dietary programs and so on. Based on these objectives, the design will set its conceptual framework. The figure below demonstrates how Barretto et al (2010) defined the domain of the objectives for the health promotion; it helped the research to have a conceptual framework that the ehealth application will be built based upon.

Building the eContent items rely on the delivery mode as stated by Barretto et al (2010), whether it is audiovisual materials (audiotapes, instructional television, video), computerized instruction (World Wide Web, CD-ROM, Web-based tools), or written materials. It was suggested to follow three general steps to construct ehealth application regardless the mode of delivery: (1) Mockups to be designed by creative people, which is done using CSS, HTML, XML and other development/design tools; to be shared with the project team and to be interfaced with the participants. (2) The functionality of the mockups are to be analyzed by audience members as an iterative process, (3) The materials are re-written by the project team, and mockups are revised by creative people based on the feedbacks. At the last stage of Barritto et al (2010), is the pretesting and finalizing stage. A minor experiment is done through inviting college students to have a review web-based application; after that there is survey given to gather their feedback. Based on the results, the development team could figure out whether the content was related, whether the website is useful in general, and whether the website is interactive enough with the members. As a conclusion, it was a summary evaluation phase to determine what the interventions covered well, and what was missing on the other hand.

Problem Statement

Health promotion strategies are available in different methods, but content design and presentation is becoming the hot topic since it relies on behavioral change. The study will focus mainly on Content Interventions that can be useful in health promotion through investigation of the content analysis and how it affects the human behavior intention as well.

Health issues have become one of the important and critical topics in Malaysia; the public is not really educated enough of the major health facts and issues, which has grabbed the attention of Malaysian Governmental entities and bodies towards strategically plans solutions; the issue is the lack of health awareness and knowledge; "Malaysians suffer of lack of awareness of importance of proper diet" (Rasol & Yusof, 2011). Shocking news was announced from Health Minister Datuk Seri Liow Tiong Lai, who mentioned that Malaysia currently is the fattest country in ASEAN. In addition, Petch (2004) identified four elements to be considered when developing health information website despite the medium of delivery; Focus, Audience, Accessibility and Quality. "The lack of research applying content analysis to web sites is partially a results of the complexity of web-based information" (Petch, 2004). Kanina has also mentioned the importance of good content. Overall, Most of the health promotion websites are neither ground based on content interventions, nor human behavior theory.

However, it was indicated that the researchers who have not shown the right combination across these models have been the most successful. The research gap contains in the lack of promoting health awareness using ICT tools and applications for better commitment, however there is also a gap into designing these applications and websites because it should be relying on grounded theories and content intervention theories that shall drive the intention level.

Study Objectives

This study has two objectives: The ability of health promotion based on website Content; to lead to positive health behavior intention. In addition, the study aims to discover most appropriate content elements for web-based health promotion for Workplace community in Malaysia

The study will investigate the criteria of content elements of multimedia and ICT into health promotion, as an output; the research will result into evaluating the Content Elements and analyzing how content is the most critical when influencing behavioral change. The study will help organizations establish a health promotion framework that is based on health digital content in order to affect the knowledge workers in the organization environment. The research aims to highlight the importance of content elements analysis into presenting health information using multimedia elements; which will play an important role into how people react and respond to health resources based on the produced web content; since it relates to behavioral change even though it is more to do with individualism issues.

LITERATURE REVIEW

It is important to have a review of content interventions and analysis methods for health promotion in general, and specifically into web-based resources. The study will explore case studies and samples of multimedia-content health promotion websites. In the meantime, it will keep looking to distinguish the relationship between content creation and human behavioural changes, with the consideration of Mysihat (2013) model. The combination of these literature will contribute into a major understanding of the role of web-based content and multimedia content for health promotion and workplaces.

Content Strategies

Many studies prove that content writing and design of any material relies on several factors, these factors can differ from user perspectives, behavioral approaches, and objectives of the item. When it comes to health promotion plan, content theories should be studied at first in order to determine the most suitable content for the targeted audience. "Theories range from behavior theory through change theory (at individual, organizational and community levels), to community development and policy theory" (Green, 2000).

e-Health promotion is becoming one of the largest spots nowadays due to the large number of users accessing the internet. "According to a 2006 survey, 80 percent of Internet users have looked for health information on the Web. As a result, both public and private institutions are using the Internet to streamline the delivery of health information and connect people and services in exciting new ways" (Department of Health and Human Services, 2010). DHHS (2010) has provided guidance on how to design web-based health information based on several researches done. These guidelines will help the web developers, as they are acting as the designers; and content producers, as their role is to create the content and produce it in interactive methods.

Moreover, the literacy issue will remain the biggest challenge whilst developing web-based health promotion since there are many people who do not have medical backgrounds, although they have a basic knowledge in health issues. "The aim of creating easy-to-use health Web sites is to reach as many Web users as possible, especially those adults who are overwhelmed by everyday literacy tasks" (DHHS, 2010). It was also highlighted that most people when accessing the website to view the health topics, face difficulties when trying to read/understand the content due the fact that the content was created in an informative method rather than interactive and audience-focused method. "They struggle not only with reading the content on the page, but also with retaining and managing new information as they move through a Web site" (DHHS, 2010).

Case Studies for Web-Based Health Promotion

This section will cover variety of health promotion websites, and will explore the features provided by each.

Figure 1. Common behaviors of using web health information (DHHS, 2010)

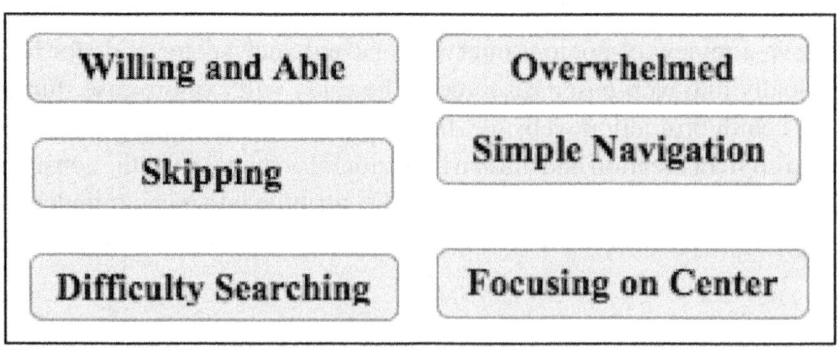

Mayo Clinic

Mayo Clinic (2013) has implemented a smart idea, which is a blog for patients, doctors and staff; the portal enables the users to post text supported with image/video upload. The portal is very powerful method to support storytelling activities, and they also created experts blog for medical and diet experts to post regarding various topics. It is a good example of health communication that is blog based, but is still in need of a stronger presentation of multimedia objects to add more value.

National Health Services (NHS-UK)

NHS (2014) is a website for health information supported from UK government. The website works as a health knowledge hub focusing on improving health awareness and lifestyle of individuals based on national level. The website is considered very rich and vast due to the tons of information, services and news available, it covers all health issues among different genders, and it also interacts with audience through health tools such as fitness assessment, healthy dietary assessments and many more.

Having surverys will always encourage people to suggest new features and content in order to improve the quality of the content. Moreover, NHS (2014) published the concept of "Online Clinics", with their health providers and partners for short periods. This process will enhance the communication between people and health professionals. The website is enriched with thousands of videos that cover several health problems. These videos also are supported by comments section for members to post.

Healthier Scotland

Healthier Scotland – Scottish Goverment: Healthier Scotland (2014) promotes healthy lifestyles through activities and clean eating. It provides several types of healthy meals and it offers easy recipes for those who would like to cook themselves. Moreover, it provides real stories and testimonials from real people who shared their ideas through the website. Healthier Scotland (2014) is offering simple games to motivate people to join these activates on a weekly basis through family trips. These offers are available online through the website and all they have to do is print the vouchers to enjoy their liberties.

Talk to Frank (TTF)

It is a website that is used to spread awareness about all kinds of drugs, and it demonstrates the promotion by using animated videos to show how these drugs affect the mind. The good thing is that TTF (2014) is offering facts about almost all the drugs indexed from A-Z. In addition, it lets users share their stories. People share their stories and any user can just simply share their story while supported by comments from others.

Moreover, TTF (2014) offers several choices to contact them; it can be via phone, live chat, email and even hotline for emergency texting. Another positive feature, is the advices provided if you are under the influence of drugs, or you want to help a member of your family, all the tips and advice, and even the drug treatment method was provided as part of the guidelines.

Figure 2. Activities list (Healthier Scotland, 2014)

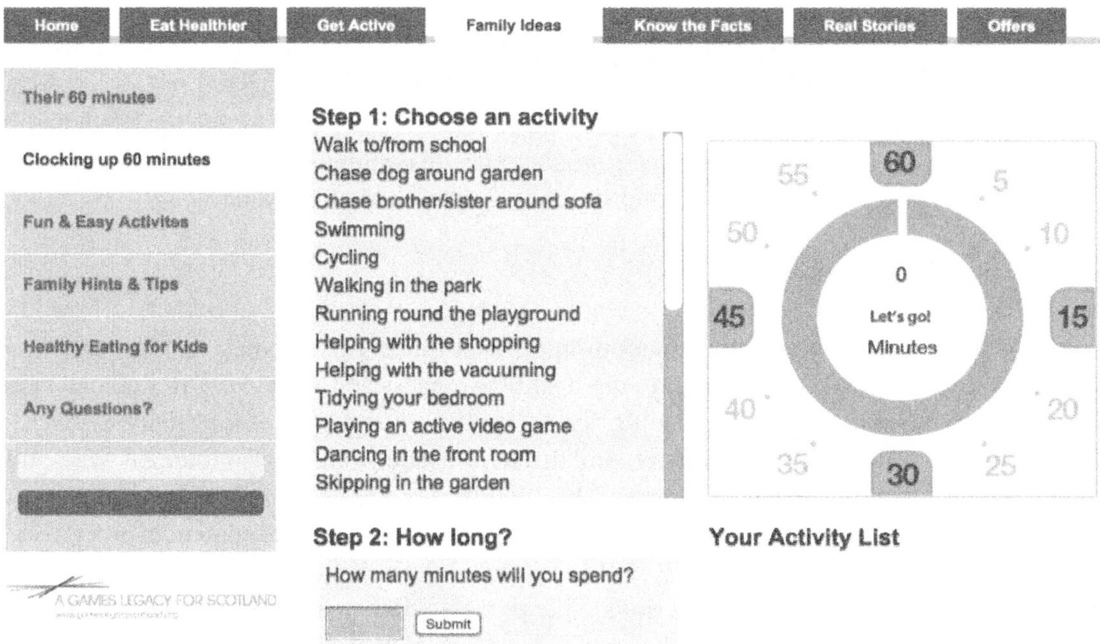

Health Promotion Board – Singapore (HPB)

HPB (2014) is a website implemented by the Singaporean government for health promotion purposes. The website offers a range of health promotion programs and users will need to register for these programs accordingly.

One good feature is the mutiple resources, which means the website doesn't depend on one single resource. The reseources differ from Media, Tools and Gaming, Published Articles and Educational Materials. In addition, HPB (2014) has categorized the information to be provided based on the role, if you are a workplace health faciliator you can just select the category under "I am A.." as a workplace health faciliator. Next, all related information regarding Workplace health promotion will be listed on the page. Events related to workplace health awareness will be also presentable, and tools that are related to work environment as well.

Health Promotion Board – Malaysia (Mysihat)

Mysihat has developed a portal (MyHealth), which is rich of information but unfortunately has a lack of interactive elements or media elements such as videos, infogrpahics, and pictures. Moreover, the portal suffers of unknown structure of the info or main sections of the portal; which led the users to be confused while browsing the portal. Another issue is the lack of interactive tools or apps which should have encouraged the intention level of the users.

The Role of Digital Technologies

Kalnina (2010) did a study about web based interventions and the role of digital technologies into tempting the level of changes in the health behavior. "Web based interventions can support self-directed behavior change" (Kalnina, 2010). It highlighted the important relationship between Internet intervention and health behavioral change; since it stated there is a necessity to tie the web-based health promotion tools with at least one single theory, "Behavior change is surrounded by theories and models. Web based interventions are shown to have often applied an individual model to programme designs, however researchers have not shown which combination across these models have been the most successful" (DHHS, 2010). It was stated that several researches suggest using IIM (Internet Interventions Model); because this model combines different content disciplines together within various human behavior theories. It was also mentioned that the most important factor of web-based application; is user engagement.

DHHS (2010) concluded based on the previous studies that general informative health websites are not sufficient enough to promote change of behavior even if these websites are information rich. "Early studies have discovered that people who received behaviorally based self-help materials did better than those who received only general advice" (Kalnina, 2010). As mentioned earlier, interactivity tools or features will lead to better engagement, these interactivity features might be able to monitor, assess, manage the users' progress since it involves routine feedback from the users. Kalnina (2010) has clarified that there are two basic aspects of Internet interventions; credibility and content. Internet content should be based on trusted resources with accurate data so believability factors will be increased. "Therefore, when interactive applications are developed it is strongly recommended that all aspects are evaluated to ensure credibility (accurate data, credible message sources, 'believability' factors, attractiveness, etc)" (Kalnina, 2010). On the other hand, Content is considered the most important component among the Internet interventions, "Content is one of the factors securing credible perception and in various cases content would serve as the most important component" (Kalnina, 2010).

Health Promotion Theories and Models

It is important to highlight the health promotion theories and models, and how these theories can be integrated with content creation and presentation.

MySihat – Malaysian Health Promotion Board

Mysihat (2013), Malaysian health promotion board has identified four main keys for its missions: Community Empowerment, healthy lifestyles promotion, operational governance, and healthy public policy. Each of these areas has specific strategies. The common factor of these areas will lead to one unique objective, which is quality of life. "Enhancement of health literacy through educating individuals and communities with adequate knowledge and skills for self care" (Mysihat, 2013). Back to the health behavior, Mysihat always takes this topic into consideration when it comes to organizing some programs or campaigns "Mysihat will focus on the specific behaviors and their long term effects on lifestyles, this approach will provide knowledge and facilitate the enhancement of skills for community to adopt the healthy behavior" (Mysihat, 2013).

Health Belief Model

It is based on many elements such as barriers, actions, seriousness, susceptibility and self-efficacy. Seriousness is about how individuals take the health issue seriously in order to reduce the risk level, while susceptibility is about how individuals take a commitment to take care of their health status. Barriers are the difficulties faced by individuals to maintain their health issues, while benefits contribute to how individuals make a judgement of the potential impacts of their positive health status.

Each of these concepts have been applied to the Ecological framework in order to understand the factors that play a role into changing human behavior towards health issues. Redding et al (2000) have mentioned that Health Belief Model has the longest history among the other theories and models, "The model's our key components are conceptualized as perceived: (1) susceptibility, 2) severity, 3) effectiveness, and 4) cost" (Redding et al, 2000).

Social Cognitive Theory (SCT)

For interpersonal factors, Parker et al (2004) has used two theories: Social Cognitive Theory and Social Supports. The Social Cognitive Theory (SCT) was developed by Bandura (Redding et al, 2000) to be divided into four areas: self-observation, self-evaluation, self-reaction and self-efficacy.

"The key concepts within SCT are categorized into major determinants of behavior, including environment, outcome expectations, self-efficacy, behavioral capability, and methods for behavior change, including observational learning and reinforcement" (Parker et al, 2004). The environmental determinants can be social such as friends and family members, or even physical such as place to exercise, neighbourhood and workplace.

Health Promotion Model (HPM)

Pender (2011) has developed a health promotion model (HPM) specifically for nurses to understand the major determinants of health behavior in order to motivate people into healthy lifestyles. The study was based on previous proposed theories/models since the last twenty-seven years, "The model identifies background factors that influence health behavior" (Pender, 2011).

Internet Intervention Model (IIM)

It has been recommended to be applied as a theoretical framework for health promotion based on Internet features. Internet interventions are the factors that can play roles into drawing an impact on behaviors, or leading to the intention to change the behavior, "These Internet interventions are usually behavioral treatments that have been operationalized and transformed for delivery over the Internet" (Ritterband et al, 2010). Even though there is a clear evidence of the benefits of using internet as a health promotion channel, yet not a single model was published to highlight these programs based on any theory, this indicates a need for further research in this area of internet interventions to explain how health behaviors can be improved through the use of internet for health promotion purposes (Ritterband et al, 2010).

A model of internet elements has to be applied in health promotion based on internet in combination with foundations and theories of human behavior. In addition, there are many benefits of using the internet as a health promotion tool such as: "Online treatments can reduce traditional face-to-face treatment barriers, increase adherence, and reduce treatment time and costs" (Ritterband et al, 2010). As a result, (IIM) was formed based on multiple theories and clinical researches, Ritterband et al (2010) have indicated that no single theory is believed to fit the purpose, "In designing this Internet intervention model, multiple theories from numerous disciplines were integrated to help conceptualize behavior change, measure the change, and identify the factors that might contribute to symptom improvement" (Ritterband et al, 2010). Internet Interventions Model (IIM) is considered the most suitable theory to be applied for internet-based health promotion since it combines theories from various perspectives such as: theories of motivation, other psychological models, social marketing/advertising strategies, Web-based design/development techniques, information architecture and design, models of knowledge transfer and behavior change, and general research and clinical experience. The main objective of this model is provide a framework to help in improving behavior change and symptom development.

RESEARCH METHODOLOGY

The research is based on Evaluation research. The research is through qualitative methods mostly since data collection is applied to knowledge workers for content elements analysis and the use of interactive features; therefore interview when possible, and survey questionnaire is applied to gather the inputs from users and applied into Web-based health promotion prototype trial.

Figure 3. Internet Intervention Model (Ritterband et al, 2010)

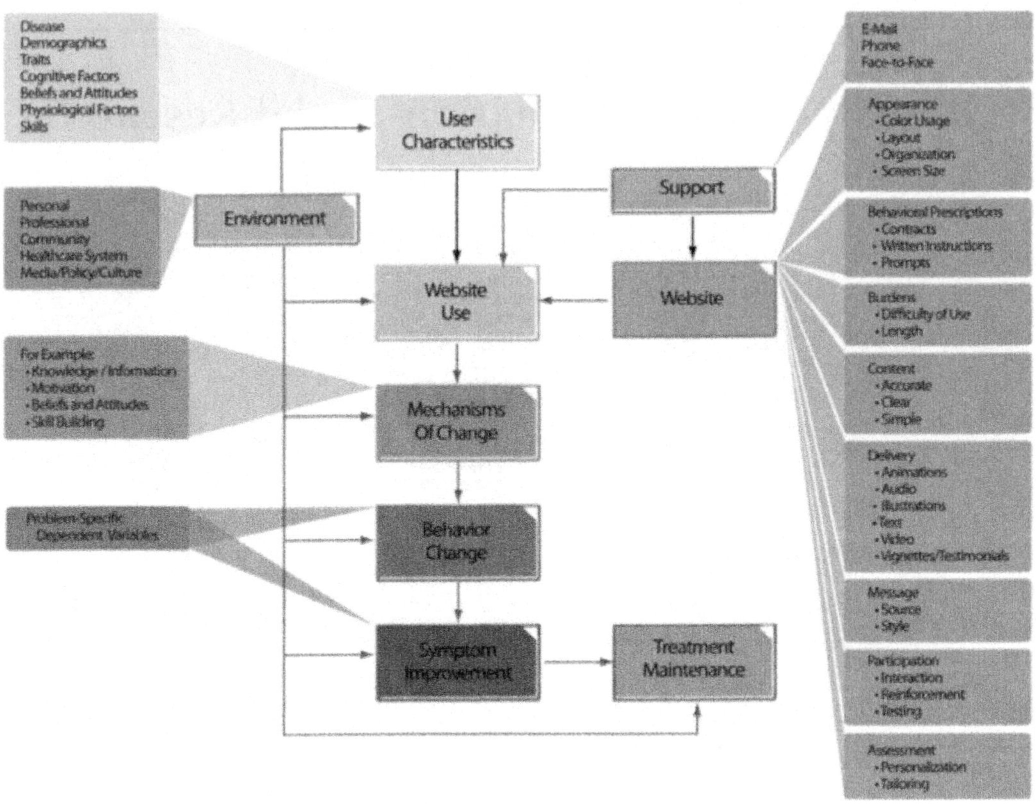

Based on the study, the users' interactions with the prototype, change behavior intention levels are measured. Basically, the study follows evaluation research approach; the approach is generally relies on two main phases: Survey and Evaluation. The study will use purposive samples with systematic selection of the samples. The research approach goes through five steps; Figure 5 shows the overall research cycle. The first stage is to identify key issues and problems, and this step is aimed to set the survey questionnaire: health literacy and Barriers & Attitudes. This is to understand how much knowledge the selected samples have, and their barriers and attitudes towards health promotion. The second stage is action planning, which is planning and developing the web-based health promotion prototype; the research uses the existing content discovered through the review of existing websites, and apply them in the prototype in different forms and methods of delivery. In addition, the design of the content, the delivery, and overall implementation is based on the IIM (Internet Intervention Model) as proposed by Ritterband et al (2010). The third stage is taking action, which means the prototype has to be examined through the selected samples participated in Stage 1. The website prototype is be produced in different content delivery formats, and to be rich of interactive features to encourage participants' engagement rate. After this stage; the researcher conducted the fourth stage, studying and evaluating the intention level rate changes, and feedback given from the audience regarding the content from all interventions' aspects. In this last stage, which is considered the analysis stage of Evaluation Questionnaire; the researcher will need to validate the data, and ensure the prototype was reliable to enhance the intention level of behavior change of the audience.

Figure 4. Evaluation Research Cycle (Parker et al, 2004)

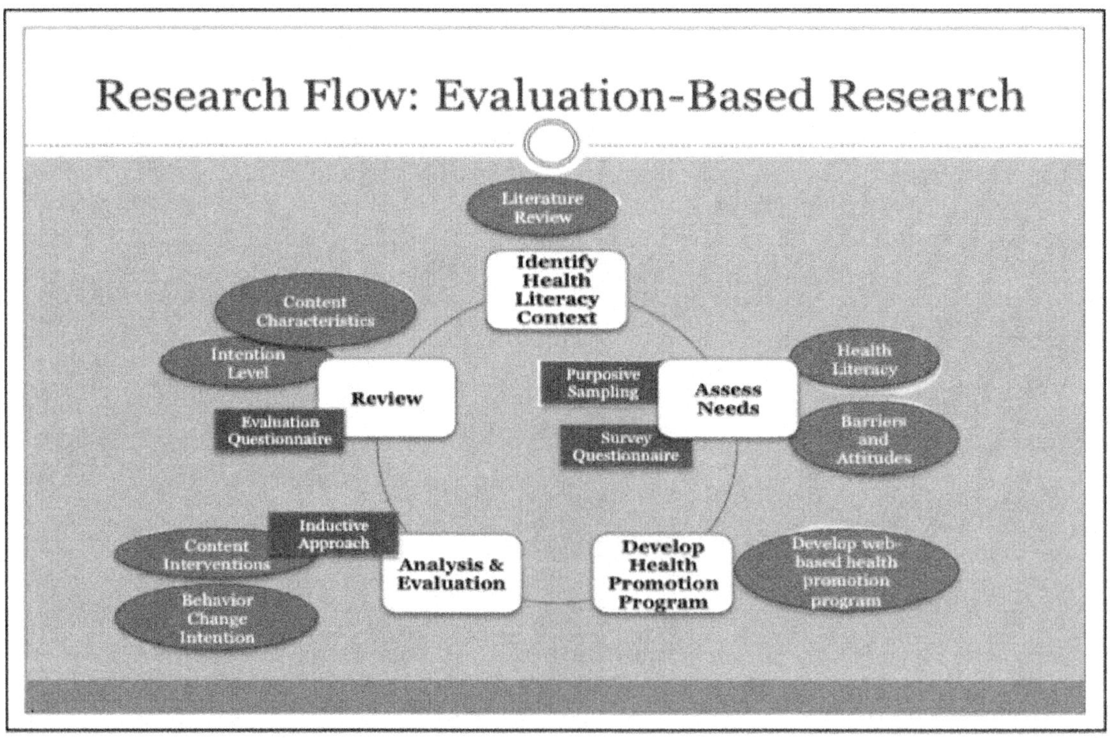

Research Framework

The study aims to evaluate the content elements as described by Ritterband et al (2010). Interactivity elements are analyzed based on how the users can interact with the web-based portal and in which perspectives and events, it also highlights how the user would prefer to have an interaction and how the user would prefer to have an interaction with the web-based health promotion references.

Interactivity can be established through routine tests, progress monitoring, updated information and advice from the website. Multimedia elements will include images, videos, and audio affects and any sort of multimedia objects that will be participated during the web-based portal development. Multimedia objects are considered very important for the research analysis since they will help the researcher to understand what type of content should be involved in the health promotion. Content presentation will be another important area; which investigates how data, information, news, advices, and guidance should be presented and delivered through the website.

Data Collection

The study is based on qualitative and quantitative data; therefore, the involved data collection methods will be questionnaires based on quantitative and qualitative approaches (Survey & Evaluation) and face-to-face interviews for the participants who agree to do so. Data collection will be done twice; the first time will be applied upon engaging with selected samples during the Survey Questionnaire. Moreover, the questionnaire will be distributed using systematic selection to ensure the validity of data collected and to represent the views from intended group of users.

Survey questionnaire will be completely quantitative based; it includes adapted quantitative questions from Pender (2011) regarding (A) Demographics, (B) Beliefs/Attitude and (C) Barriers. The additional section is the (D) intention level; will adapt some quantitative questions from Ritterband (2010). Demographics include questions about gender, age, status, academic qualification, status, and race. For section (B) Beliefs/Attitude, there are 10 questions, and for section (C) Barriers, there are 6 question, and section (D) Intention level, there are 8 questions about physical activity and healthy lifestyle. However, the scale used for sections (B) and (C) is arranging from 1-4 (strongly disagree-strongly agree), but section (D) is ranging from 1-5 (definitely No- definitely Yes).

After the Survey Questionnaire, the research will move into the action planning stage based on the Survey Questionnaire results that will guide the study to determine the basic fundamentals of the samples' health literacy and required content to be considered in the prototype. As an outcome, the prototype will be initially developed and provided to the samples so the users can interact with the prototype and give their feedbacks. The prototype trial period will be for a month, then the second data collection round will take place; the researcher will distribute the Evaluation Questionnaire to the same participants who were involved in the Survey Questionnaire, and they will be expected to have used the website. The evaluation questionnaire will have mixed types of questions, one section is the intention level in quantitative based, it works as a comparison of the intention level results between Survey Questionnaire and Evaluation Questionnaire (Before Vs After) of the samples. For the second section is qualitative based, where open-ended questions will be provided in order to have the ability to evaluate the impact of content used through the prototype.

Sampling

Local samples were selected among ICT companies in Malaysia, where a lot of IT and multinational companies are based. However, the samples should have different factors such as age, gender, culture and interpersonal skills to ensure research reliability. The research team managed to get twenty samples to accept joining the study. The twenty users were introduced to the study objectives and the reasons of this study, and they started with answering the survey questionnaire.

Data Analysis

For the quantitative data, there were two main tests to be applied to the data. Descriptive analysis will be used to analyze the demographic data, and also the other sections of the first questionnaire (Survey Questionnaire). The second test is

Mean difference, which will be used to compare the intention level results during the first and second questionnaires.

For the qualitative data, the four qualitative questions in the second data collection round (Evalution Questionnaire) focus on several areas of content as follows: (1) Design & Appearance, (2) Content Quality, (3) Delivery & Interactivity and (4) Motivation Factors. The questions were structured in a way to capture the content interventions model developed by Ritterband et al (2010). The questions would help the research to distinguish the most important elements for web-based health promotion for knowledge workers in Malaysia, as a response to the second research question

Verification Process

The verification process to ensure validity of the research will be measured and monitored through advices and consultations from SME (Subject Matter experts), who have the knowledge and experience in the field of health promotion and content experts too, based on their outputs the prototype shall be adjusted as well. This was done through engaging with Msyihat team (Malaysian Health Promotion Board), the research team had several sessions to evaluate the content.

Reliability

It is important to examine the questions reliability, therefore the research team have done a reliability test for the Survey Questionnaire. Intention level questions that concern physical activity results' was.831 (The alpha coefficient for the four items is.831), suggesting that the items have relatively high internal consistency. The same test was applied to the intention level questions that concern healthy lifestyle, beliefs and attitudes, and the results were was.847 and.800 respectively. While the barrier questions were weakly reliable with a.593 rate.

Study Material

The website prototype was influenced by Internet Interventions model proposed by (Ritterband et al, 2010). Moreover, it was guided through the guidelines published by US Department of Health and Human Services, DHHS (2010). The below description will demonstrate the relationship between "Be

Figure 5. Research framework

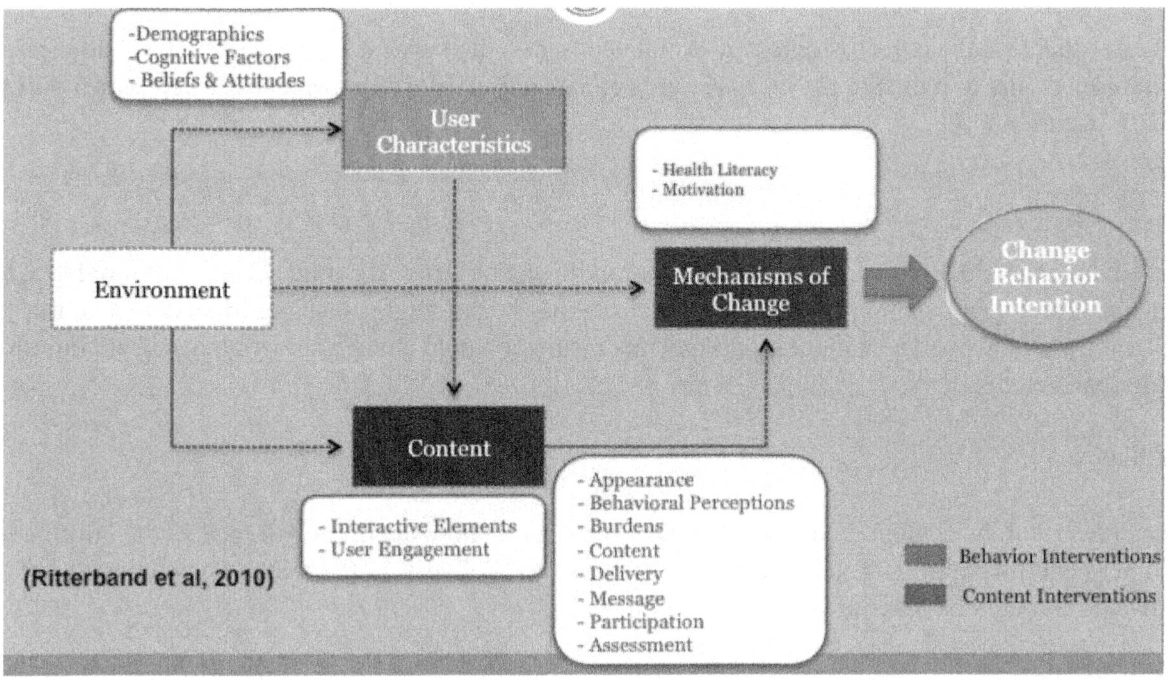

Healthy - Malaysia" website and how it was influenced by Internet Intervention model proposed by Ritterband et al (2010). The website (BeHealthyMalaysia) was developed after the research team have analyzed the websites that was studied in the literature review, and the most important components to be included in the website were analyzed based on grounded theory given by the model developed by Ritterband et al (2010).

Appearance

The appearance should cover four elements as suggested by (Ritterband et al, 2010), Color, theme, size and organization. In addition, the design of the theme/template was following the guidelines provided by DHHS (2010), to have white spaces and crispy web page. "Clean, crisp Web pages are easier to read".

Burden

Ritterband et al (2010) have also highlighted that length of the content might lead to low rate in impact behavior change since users might lose interaction with the website if the content is lengthy and it doesn't provide what they want.

Message

It is also advised to provide content that contain information about the targeted audience to reflect the content on their daily routine and lifestyle

Behavior Perceptions

Features that lead the users to address some related issues, the purpose of these features are to increase commitment and to motivate the users towards enhancing their health awareness level, which will increase intention level.

Content

Ritterband et al (2010) have covered the content in three elements: Accurate, Clear, and Simple. "Content, the actual treatment information, of the website may be the single most important component of the program. Without good content, it is unlikely that behavior would change or symptoms would improve" (Ritterband et al, 2010).

Delivery

The delivery of the content is important since it plays a role how the users will receive the information and get benefits out of it. Ritterband et al (2010) defined delivery as the method how content will be delivered through the website features.

Participation

Participation is meant to engage the users through the website interactive features such as sharing stories or assessing themselves. DHHS (2010) has mentioned that including interactive content such as online tools or surveys can increase the engagement level.

Analyzing Stage

The twenty samples were ten Males and ten Females. Therefore, the survey questionnaire was distributed equally. Moreover, the majority of samples were falling in the category 31-40 Years (nine samples), while the lowest was for 41-50 Years (three samples). In addition, the majority of samples were Single (ten samples), while there were only two samples who are Divorced, and the other 8 are were married. For the academic qualification, there are 10 samples that have Undergraduate qualification, while there were six samples with Postgraduate qualification. However, eleven samples were from Malay race, and there are four samples with Chinese race, and three samples from Indian race.

In addition, Mean different was conducted in the intention questions for both sections, physical activity and healthy eating; to compare the means for the period before the samples use the website (BeHealthyMalaysia) and after they use it. For physical activity questions, the intention level mean before was 3.66 with standard deviation of 0. 97, while the physical activity intention level mean after using the website was 3.95, with standard deviation of.64, these results conclude a difference in the mean of.28 which represents the increment of the intention level regarding the physical activity. Moreover, for healthy eating questions, the intention level mean before was 3.45 with standard deviation of.96, while the healthy eating intention level mean after using the website was 4.26, with standard deviation of.52, these results conclude a difference in the mean of.81250 which represents the increment of the intention level regarding the healthy eating as well. Since the second questionnaire (Evaluation Questionnaire) has open-ended questions for the content interventions analysis, therefore the research team has used ATLAS.ti software.

The document represents the data to be analyzed such as image, video, audio, text, article, survey and other types. While quotation, mostly represents the responses, and it can be segments of document as well. Code, is the most important thing, which is how the researcher wants to code each segment, and at the end the researcher can construct theoretical assumptions by connecting these codes and determine the linkage between them.

Basically, the findings will be presented based on two aspects: the first aspect is to represent the most important elements of content required for web based health promotion for knowledge workers; and that was done by analyzing the responses and discover the most highlighted elements as per the participants. The second aspect will be analyzing and explaining how web-based health promotion can affect the intention and commitment in the health behavior, and what are the factors that should be considered.

Design and Appearance

According to Participant 1" Overall, it's nice and the color is calm to look at", while Participant 2 has answered "I find the site is not a professional site, or appears to be health related site. The navigation is simple very direct, and not nested, so users may have to go to the specific page to have access to the related links, for example user won't know that there's a "Start Now" link in "Healthy Eating" page, which I feel like it should've been highlighted on the landing page". However, it seems Participant 4 also agreed by stating "The color combination makes the site seems comforting". In addition according to Participant 6, "The visual aspect of the website is appealing and it is most importantly user-friendly". While Participant 8 expresses his opinion saying, "It's simple and very direct. Easy reading for the viewers to go through it at it has a clear explanation on what being healthy is all about". Participant 9 explains how the website was attractive, "I really liked the appearance such as the color of the page and it was user-friendly. Good design too with nice pictures on each segment. Overall a nice website that keep you interested to continue scrolling". On the other hand, Participant 10, Participant 11 and Participant 13 have responded respectively with minor words "It is Okay, nothing much to say", "Excellent design and appearance" and "Nice and simple". Participant 14 has suggested some enhancements "The website has a nice choice of color scheme and site navigation is good since it is not complex. However, the information is often repeated and can be found through multiple menus". However, Participant 17 and Participant 18 have answered respectively, "The design in neat and nice to see" and "I find it very interesting and user-friendly".

The content elements in terms of Design and Appearance. Based on the responses given from the participants, these are the most highlighted elements in terms of design and appearance of "BeHealthy-Malaysia" (Figure 7). However, these are all the elements mentioned by all the participants, but some of them were highlighted so often, which gives an impression about which elements are the most needed for design. The elements are: interesting design, user friendly, navigation, multimedia objects, responsive design, simple design, attractive website, easy to use website, and the color of the website. In addition, ATLAS ti can generate a report for the codes count compared to each participant. It is shown that "easy to use" feature has been mentioned the most with 10 times, next is the "simple" feature. These two elements are almost similar since "easy to use" is considered in terms of the website is easy for sections accessibility, and the feature "simple" represents how the design was simple for users and it doesn't cause any burden to the users during browsing the website. As mentioned before by DHHS (2010), it was mentioned that there are common behaviors of using web-based health information, overwhelming and simple navigations are from these elements. Moreover, DHHS (2010) mentioned that simplified content is one of the Six Strategies for Writing and Designing Health Websites. However, there is the "multimedia" feature, which got 8 times mentioned in the quotations among the participants, and it covers the user of videos, images and other multimedia objects. According to some researchers, "Interactivity can be achieved by using various technology applications and multimedia experiences" (Kalnina, 2010).

Content Quality

According to Participant 1 and Participant 2, they have not agreed on the website clearness, they have commented respectively, "Not very clear as there is no clear instruction what to do after you click the get started button" and "The site is not that clear as it doesn't highlight what the site is about, and user has to go through the site to know what's in store for them. But on the other hand, Participant 3, Participant 8 and Participant 9 have disagreed with that and they highlighted respectively, "Very clear contents beside its logical and it leads to good health" and "It's clear understanding as it elaborates the things that we needed to know" and "It was very clear to me because like I said the website is user-friendly, the content relevant and simple to use". According to Participant 4, "The content are relevant and informative however perhaps there should be an a bit of an explanation who these resources are and what are their main purpose". Participant 6 and Participant 7 have commented respectively, "It is rather interactive and insightful. Find the health assessments and quizzes really a good reminder in practicing healthy lifestyle and habits" and "The contents should be systematically arranged, bold, concise, and clearer. What I see, it's unstructured". But Participant 14 said, "The contents of the website are clear and reliable, since they are mostly common sense". However, Participant 12 and Participant 13 have agreed on the clearness and knowledge value of the content. Participant 15 and Participant 16, they have responded respectively, "It was clear contents. Would be more nice if the language could be more simple and easy understanding, less jargons and terms." and "Useful".

Participant 17 has responded, "Its pretty clear after taking the assessments cause I know what is wrong and what is needed to be improved". Participant 19 highlighted his answer by saying, "The contents were very clear and yes I find them reliable as the references were from the UK NHS and other official guidelines". At the end, Participant 20 has commented with some suggestions, "The contents were clear, but however it will be better to have more customized content that touch the Malaysian society ".

For Content Quality, The elements are: clearness, interesting content, knowledge, relevancy, reliability and the provided trusted resources in the website. But the top elements that were highlighted in terms of content Quality is clearness of the content, most of the participants have indicated that the clearness of the content was there. The participants mentioned the "clearness" feature 14 times. While the second feature is "knowledge", it was mentioned 11 times. However, some participants have also highlighted how the "simple" element was helpful for them since the content provided was simple and easy to be understood since it covers the basic information. Omar (2013) has mentioned earlier the important role of health promotion to strengthen the knowledge value among the population, and to open their eyes for basic information that can help prevention from early stages. Petch (2004) identified four elements to be considered when developing health information website despite the medium of delivery; Focus, Audience, Accessibility and Quality. Therefore, the content was focused to deliver quality-based information to enhance the basic knowledge of the participants, and with easy accessibility and clear structure. In addition, Kalnina (2010) has clarified that there are two basic aspects of the Internet interventions; credibility and content.

Delivery and Interactivity

According to Participant 1, "Quite interactive. I have gained new knowledge about healthy lifestyle". While Participant 2 responded "The delivery methods are highly rely on tools, then the text which is not sufficient to deliver the information needed for user to use the site. As for the "Personalized Profile", the tools are great, but user has no guidance on how to start or what to do when they're on this page. Maybe Facebook experience can be applied on this page". However, Participant 3 has highlighted the idea of the customized profile, "I like the interactive contents and it deliver the information easier and faster". While Participant 5 expressed his opinion regarding the tools provided, "The tools of the website page is more interesting to me since it shows me the way of taking care of my health with only few clicks there are many links that direct me to many tools". Participant 6 and Participant 7 have responded respectively, "It is engaging in a not judgmental fashion. It is especially more encouraging with some of the healthy lifestyle recommendations included in the interactive media" and "It was nice. Add on a little bit flavor of simpleness, it will be great". On the other hand, Participant 9 has given comments the cover all the website aspect, "I liked that the text given to you in the website were short but very informative. The links provided were also easy to use and not too long". According to Participant 10, Participant 11 and Participant 13, they have commented respectively, "It was very good", "Excellent delivery methods and very interactive" and "Good and Interesting". While Participant 12 described how the website is helpful, "All very helpful, even though it's still beta, I guess it's very helpful for others who want to start a healthy way, or that already start their diet or programs". Participant 15, Participant 16 and Participant 17 have commented with minor words respectively, "Useful, compact. Information needed are there", "Attractive and fascinating. Not too crowded" and "OK". Meantime, Participant 18 explained the content preference, "When I inquire about subjects on the web, I would go with the text based content rather than content with a lot of multimedia as it's simpler to read for me. Participant 19 responded, "The personalized profile was use friendly and easy for me to monitor". However, Participant 20 mentioned the importance of having content of videos "More videos will be better since videos and images deliver the message faster than text".

Based on the responses given from the participants, these are the most highlighted elements in terms of Delivery and Interactivity of "BeHealthyMalaysia". Delivery and Interactivity elements cover the aspects of interaction with users, attraction, engagement, personalized content. The elements are: tools, videos, interactive features, customized content, personalized content, ordinal content, instructional delivery, knowledge value and the attraction points of the website. But the top element that was highlighted in terms of interactivity is the tools. Most of the participants have expressed their likeness and preferences to have more tools and interactive applications such as the self-assessments through questionnaires. The second feature was the personalization method used as a part of the tools. DHHS (2010) has highlighted the role of interactive applications or tools within the health information websites; this will avoid the burden of reading only, and avoid leading to boredom. "They struggle not only with reading the content on the page, but also with retaining and managing new information as they move" (DHHS, 2010). In addition, Muray (2012) has identified the three main areas that are targeted by web-based interventions, which are: self-management, health promotion, and mental health. For Self-Management, ehealth tools are being used to empower the users with self-efficacy.

Motivation Factors

According to Participant 1, "Now I'm more aware about my health and will be more conscious when eating food etc. I will try to exercise more in the future". But Participant 2 has suggested some tips, "The site provides a lot of tools for user to use, and the result/information the user get are very reliable as most of the tools came from NHS". Moreover, Participant 4 mentioned some enhancement for the website, "The website provides all kinds of tests that would allow me to measure my current health conditions. However, the website goes to the affiliated sites (the resources relevant to the website) from the same page, it would be better if these links are opened on a different tab browser". Meantime, Participant 5 responded, "The website help me maintain my physical activities in order to what I need to be healthy since my requirement is to be healthy not to build up hence".

Participant 6 and Participant 7 have mentioned how the website encouraged them, they commented respectively, "It provides encouragement as well as some of the ways to kick-start someone to a healthy lifestyle" and "It provides encouragement as well as some of the ways to kick-start someone to a healthy lifestyle". However, Participant 10 and Participant 11 have suggested respectively, "Yeah, but website needs to be more informative, having like rss feed" and "More practical interactions or live sessions". In addition, Participant 13 responded, "Check what I'm eating and exercise regularly". According to Participant 12, "Many trusted source that been provide by the website, I guess they can improve it by really making it a real live world wide website, at least in Malaysia globally first. Interactive chat with the health professional would be a great addition for the website, and less cost for the visitor for consultation". But Participant 14 has mentioned some suggestions for the website to increase motivation factors, "The website did not quite motivate me enough. The actual intention of the website is rather indistinguishable".

Participant 15, Participant 16 and Participant 17 have responded respectively, "Personally, I love the website to be more fancy. Full of colorful notes and interesting charts, pictures and also interesting interface", "To suggest menu of food for breakfast, lunch and dinner, to include healthy meal recipes. To add on food calories guide" and "maybe can improve the site by providing the information without having to go through the assessment first". In addition, Participant 19 explained how the assessment tools are motivating, "After checking my BMI it especially motivated me to do some exercise and eat more healthily. It gave me motivation to keep checking my BMI to see when I am in the normal range".

Based on the responses given from the participants, these are the most highlighted elements in terms of Motivation of "BeHealthyMalaysia". Motivation elements cover the areas that will motivate the users towards engaging in physical activity or organizing their daily routine towards healthy lifestyles. However, looking through the responses and analyzing the motivation reasons, there were several factors for motivation to enhance the intention level. That is because the world is full of people with different behaviors; which accordingly will require different strategies. "Different behaviors will require different strategies, different methods of intervening" (SHPC, 2010).

However, these are all the motivation elements mentioned by all the participants: intention level, encouragement, engagement, website guidance, and "avoid burden" elements of the website. But the two top elements that were highlighted in terms of motivation are: "avoid burden" and "intention". Moreover, that has increased their intention level, especially with the tools, which provided self-assessment features. It shows the motivation themes attached to each participant based on the segments of data analyzed. However, some participants have also highlighted how the website was helpful enough for them, but they would like to have more and more engagement features similar to the tools or live sessions. "The

Figure 6. Content elements

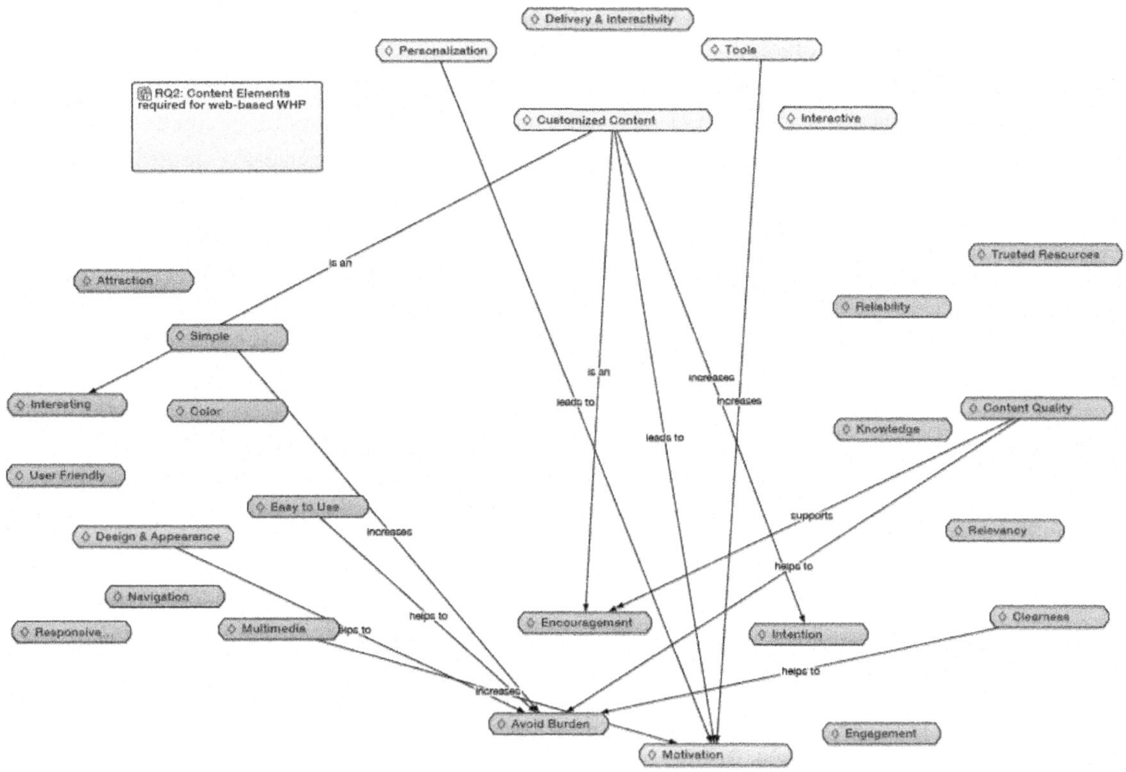

eHealth researcher's responsibility is not limited to developing and evaluating effective Web-based interventions, the main cost-benefits of such interventions tend to be achieved with large numbers of users" (Muray, 2012)

RESULTS AND RECOMMENDATION

Based on findings of this study, the research could dSetermine some recommendations based on the findings' analysis. These findings have answered the second aspect of the study, which is enabling web-based helth promotion to have better intention and commitment in the health. Moreover, the results have indicated the factors that should be considered during developing web-based health promotion reference:

- "BeHealthyMalaysia" should be accommodated with localized content that touches the local context
- "BeHealthyMalaysia" needs more tools and interactive applications to attract the users
- "BeHealthyMalaysia" should present more in depth content to deliver wider content

In terms of Multimedia, "BeHealthyMalaysia" website should have more videos and infographic elements to increase the motivation among the users. Many users have mentioned that videos and graphics deliver the message faster. However, the resources used in "BeHealthyMalaysia" website needs to highlight the resources used, and their main contribution. The users have indicated that it will be important and positive to have an introduction about these resources or at least highlight their main roles. While many have suggested that "BeHealthyMalaysia" should be accommodated with localized content that provide local context of the Malaysian society such as providing health meals based on local ingredients.

In addition, for the interactivity level of "BeHealthyMalaysia" website; it needs more tools and interactive applications to attract the users. Tools grabbed most of the users' attentions, and they all highlighted that these tools were quite useful with regards to self-assessments agendas. Lastly, many users have mentioned the content created for the website were too simple, therefore it should present more in depth content to deliver wider content in terms of knowledge and value. Most of the participants mentioned that there should be some knowledge out of the basic information box, so they can get more knowledge about ideas or things they don't recognize.

REFERENCES

Barretto, A., Bingham, C., Goh, K., & Shope, J. (2010) Developing a Web-Based Health Promotion Intervention: A Case Study From a Brief Motivational Alcohol. *Department of Health and Human Services US (DHHS), Office of Disease Prevention and Health Promotion*. Retrieved from http://www.health.gov/healthliteracyonline/

Evers, K. (2006). eHealth Promotion: The Use of the Internet for Health Promotion, The Art of Health Promotion. *American Journal of Health Promotion*, 2006, 1–7. PMID:16555803

Green, J. (2000). The Role of Theory in Evidence-based Health Promotion Practice. *Oxford Journals.*, *15*(2), 125–129. PMID:10751371

Health Promotion Board (HPB). (2014). Health Promotion Board Singapore. Retrieved from http://www.hpb.gov.sg/HOPPortal

Healthier Scotland. (2014). Take Life On. Retrieved from http://www.takelifeon.co.uk/

Healthy North Coast (HNC). (2013). Social Media and Health Promotion. Retrieved from http://healthynorthcoast.org.au/social-media-and-health-promotion/

Iacquire. (2014). Quantitative Data Analysis Techniques for Data-Driven Marketing. Retrieved from www.iacquire.com/blog/quantitative-data-analysis-techniques-for-data-driven-marketing-2

Kalnina, R. (2010). The role of digital technologies when designing web-based interventions as effective self-help platforms for people who drink at increasing and high-risk levels. Retrieved from http://www.d2digital.co.uk/publications/Web-based-interventions-and-Technology-Use-in-Public-Health-UK.pdf

Levac, J., & O'Sullivan, T. (2010). Social Media and its Use in Health Promotion, Interdisciplinary. *Journal of Health Science*, *1*(1), 49–57.

Malaysian Health Promotion Board (Mysihat). (2013). Strategic Plan 2013-2017.

Mayo Clinic. (2013). Patient Stories. Retrieved from http://www.mayoclinic.org/patientstories/

Muray, E. (2012). Web-Based Interventions for Behavior Change and Self-Management: Potential, Pitfalls, and Progress. *Medicine*, 1(2), 1-6.

MyHealth-Ministry of Health Malaysia (MyHealth). (2011). Background. Retrieved from http://www.myhealth.gov.my/v2/index.php/en/about-us

National Health Service (NHS). (2014). NHS Choices. Retrieved from http://www.nhs.uk

Nottingham Trent University (NTU). (2011). Assessing The Impact of Social Media in Delivering Health Promotion campaigns. Retrieved from http://www.ntu.ac.uk/apps/news/11101015/Assessing_the_impact_of_social_media_in_delivering_health_promotion_campaig.aspx/

Omar, Z. (2013). *Healthy Lifestyle Programmes and other Government Efforts in Combating NCDs in Malaysia, National Strategic Plan for Non-Communicable Disease*. Malaysia: Ministry of Health.

Parker, E., Baldwin, G., Israel, B., & Salinas, M. (2004). Application of Health Promotion Theories and Models for Environmental Health Education and Behavior. *Health Promotion Practice*, *31*(4), 491–509.

Pender, N. (2011). *The Health Promotion Model*. University of Michigan.

Petch, T. (2004). *Content Analysis of Selected Health Information Websites – Final Report*. Simon Fraser University.

Ragunath, P. (2013). *Workplace Health Promotion: Evidence and Practice in Malaysia*. Malaysia, Ministry of Health. Retrieved from http://sehat.perkeso.gov.my/panelclinichtml/APS2013/10_DR%20PRIYA.pdf

Redding, C., Rossi, J., Rossi, S., Velicer, W., & Prochaska, J. (2000). Human Behavior Models. *International Electronic Journal of Health Education*, *3*, 180–193.

Ritterband, L., Thorndike, F., Cox, D., Kovatchev, B., and Gonder-Frederick, L. (2010). A Behavior Change Model for Internet Interventions. *National Institute of Health (NIH)*, 38(1), 18–27.

Steno Health Promotion Center (SHPC). (2010). Workplace Health Promotion: Bridging Towards Version 2.0.

Talk To Frank (TTF). (2014). Friendly, Confidential Drugs Advice. Retrieved from http://www.talktofrank.com/

World Health Organization – Malaysia (WHO-Malaysia). (2009). Country Cooperation Strategy 2009-2013.

World Health Organization (WHO). (2009). Milestones in Health Promotion: Statements from Global Conferences.

This work was previously published in the International Journal of E-Health and Medical Communications (IJEHMC), 7(2); edited by Joel J.P.C. Rodrigues, pages 50-69, copyright year 2016 by IGI Publishing (an imprint of IGI Global).

Chapter 7
A Computational Perspective of Knowledge Empowerment for Healthcare Decision Making:
Computational Perspective of Knowledge Empowerment

Timothy Jay Carney
University of North Carolina, USA

ABSTRACT

People in a variety of settings can be heard uttering the phrase that "knowledge is power" or the relatively equivalent concept that "information is power." However, the research literature in particular lacks a simple and standardized way to examine the relationship between knowledge and power. There is a lack operational quantitative definitions of this relationship to adequately support the building of complex computational models used in addressing some longstanding public health and healthcare delivery issues like differential access to care, inequitable care and treatment, institutional bias, disparities in health outcomes, and eliminating barriers to patient-centered care. The objective of this discussion is to present a relational algorithm that can be used in both conceptual discussions on knowledge empowerment modeling, as well as in the building of computational models that want to explore the variable of knowledge empowerment within computer simulation experiments.

INTRODUCTION

To begin we start by asking a series of simple questions: How does knowledge lead to empowerment? How and under what conditions does empowerment reduce health disparities and promote health equity? The common expression "knowledge is power" and the less common equivalent "information is power" express the value of knowledge as key resource in social and organizational arrangements. Knowledge dependent social and organizational arrangements—as seen from the perspective of the primary of user

DOI: 10.4018/978-1-5225-1928-7.ch007

of knowledge—focuses largely on knowledge as a key driver of decisions/choices and tasks/actions in the pursuit of some set of personal or collective goals. We will assume in this discussion that knowledge is also used to foster learning that is typically leveraged to maximize gain and minimize harm in meeting public health and healthcare delivery objectives.

The overarching research goal that generated this targeted discussion focuses on the role of knowledge in helping public health and healthcare delivery system stakeholders at all levels support informed choices and actions, manage uncertainty, and engage in meaningful communication and knowledge exchange. We want to view this topic through the lens of a complex multilevel health system facing the challenging issue of health disparities—where the users of knowledge such as health consumers, patients and caregivers; providers; healthcare organizational representatives; community leaders; policy makers; and researchers—must operate with adequate knowledge to facilitate delivery of guideline concordant care. We want to explore the extent to which knowledge, in the form of both individual-tacit (that which is typically housed in the mind of individual—what I know) and collective-explicit (that which is typically displayed in an array of knowledge products and artifacts used by others—what we produce and share), can be leveraged as a tangible asset resulting in quantifiable empowered versus disempowered states (Nonaka, 1994). We want to support the building of computational models that can more closely examine the ability of stakeholders to make informed choices, take informed actions, operate under uncertain and risky conditions, and communicate among and between stakeholder groups. The goal of this discussion is to move a step closer in actually quantifying this dynamic in computational terms to support complex multilevel modeling and complex mathematical algorithm design of multilevel stakeholder social and organizational knowledge use to address issues like health disparities.

The underlying concept of this approach is based on the following statement:

Knowledge is a neglected commodity in [urban] regeneration. It can be seen as the 'new currency'—the element in modern society which very largely distinguishes the empowered from the disempowered. But while much attention is paid to developing sustainable communities in contemporary settings, very little is paid to the flow and accumulation or acquisition of knowledge or knowledges which might inform and empower them. (Burrage, 2009)

We argue here that while knowledge can be viewed as a precursor to some more desirable expression of power, research typically fails to place a concrete, generalizable, and standardized measurement of what a state of empoweredness might mean throughout all levels of our healthcare system in simplistic binary terms.

Additionally, the Burrage statement suggests that the factors that shape the evolution of empowerment as a by-product of the knowledge life cycle—which ranges from the generation of knowledge to knowledge use and dissemination there of— have been relatively understudied. Despite the wide usage and agreement on the value of knowledge and its corresponding impact on self-reported states of health empowerment in healthcare delivery, there are few, if any, models to express the empowerment value of knowledge for health system stakeholders in quantifiable terms. Existing studies of empowerment are typically linear in nature and defined in terms highly specific to localized interventions. Typical intervention strategies might focus on: patient engagement and/or confidence in decision making to support patient behavior change; provider decision support to effectively manage changing conditions within their patients' course of care; community-level awareness campaigns to foster screening; healthcare organization care management programs to manage cost, safety, and quality; and policy maker management of population burden of disease in a given geopolitical boundary. However, the design of models that accurately reflect the social and organizational dynamics of complex health objectives, like eliminating health disparities and achieving equity in care delivery, as well as articulating the corresponding impact knowledge may have in addressing them requires a more fundamental view of knowledge and empowerment as core variables within a complex adaptive and at times chaotic healthcare system (Roosaar, Johansson, Sandborgh-Englund, Axéll, & Nyrén, 2008). Currently no standardized assessment instrument exists in the realm of health disparities that effectively measures knowledge as a resource and its corresponding role in shaping multilevel stakeholder networks arrangements to support high-level complex multilevel computational modeling exercises. Such exercises are critical in shaping our understanding and generating hypotheses on the:

- Root causes of health disparities;
- Most effective intervention strategies;
- Monitoring and evaluation of healthcare system knowledge-dependent choices and actions that are critical to maintaining guideline concordant care;
- Mitigating health disparities trigger events in a timely manner (Resnicow & Vaughan, 2006).

This discussion provides a basic relational algorithm for knowledge empowerment that can be used in as a precursor to the modeling of any healthcare setting or stakeholder perspective in clear and easy to understand layman's terminology and also support the design of higher order mathematical modeling algorithms.

The existing disease prevention and health promotion literature is highly reliant on subjective qualitative measures of empowerment, rarely presenting concrete objective and quantifiable measures of empowerment through knowledge (Uphoff, 2005). According to Uphoff and colleagues:

Empowerment is commonly understood as the condition of having power and of being able to exercise it and obtain the benefits thereof. This means that empowerment cannot be properly measured or achieved without a valid and practical understanding of what constitutes power. The term power, however, has long been one of the most perplexing and contested concepts in the social sciences, even though the word gets used continuously in academic discourse and even more often in everyday discussions. (Uphoff, 2005)

This research seeks to fill this gap in the literature through the computational modeling of knowledge empowerment for health disparities stakeholders centered on our presentation of knowledge understood as a function of power. These goals align with those articulated within the National Institutes of Health (NIH) Health Disparities Strategic Plan and Budget Fiscal Years 2009-2013, which calls for a greater and enhanced "health disparities informatics capacity" and demands that we evolve health disparities research from qualitative to quantitative approaches through the develop and use of new computational tools, increased interconnectedness, and design of a knowledge environment that maximizes collaboration both within and across institutional boundaries (National Institutes of Health & Health, 2012).

The more analytically objective, quantitative, and computational conceptualization of knowledge provided within this paper offers additional parameters for the modeling of multilevel stakeholders' empowered states. These states of empowerment can be examined within the complex multilevel networks of individuals and organizations engaged in health disparities reduction and elimination healthcare strategies and interventions and improve health outcomes. We first present the background literature on chronic disease (here we choose to focus on colorectal cancer as illustrated case example) and health disparities, health disparities and knowledge, and knowledge and empowerment. Next, we introduce the application on the computational modeling of the nature of health knowledge and empowerment. Finally, we discuss the value of the research through the lens of the knowledge gap hypothesis and health empowerment theory, its application in health disparities research, and the next steps of the research.

LITERATURE REVIEW

Health disparities, such as those found in cancer screening, incidence, treatment, and mortality, are commonly related to the knowledge and empowerment of vulnerable populations (Finney Rutten, Nelson, & Meissner, 2004; Lisovicz, Wynn, Fouad, & Partridge, 2008).

Cancer health disparities among preventable cancers are primarily attributed to low cancer-screening rates, which increases cancer incidence and mortality, as well as decreases the five-year survival rates (Haggstrom, Taplin, Monahan, & Clauser, 2012; Taplin et al., 2008; U.S. National Institutes of Health, 2009). Cancer health disparities patterns emerge within race/ethnicity, gender, and socioeconomic status (SES).

The intersectionality framework provides that these identities cannot be viewed as independent of each other as they are often combined to facilitate or restrict healthcare access and usage (Williams et al., 2012). There are complex and confounding associations between cancer rates and race/ethnicity, gender, and SES. Although cancer health disparities have been extensively studied in terms race/ethnicity, gender, research is lacking on the interdependent and reinforcing knowledge gap between these predictors as variations in health (Hesse, 2012; Viswanath et al., 2006).

Vulnerable populations show variation in health and health services utilization, as well as health knowledge. Healthcare marginalization is often the result of knowledge gaps, including language, communication, and more general cultural barriers (Viswanath et al., 2006; Williams et al., 2012). Health disparities may result from the marginalization of stakeholders engaging in various scenarios throughout the course of care. Common health topics of health disparities include sexual health, cancer, cardiovascular disease, and preventative health (Heiman, Haynes, & McKee, 2015). The knowledge gap hypothesis is commonly used to postulate that knowledge is a form of wealth and that it (knowledge) is differentially distributed throughout society (Tichenor, Donohue, & Olien, 1970). Specially, the hypothesis provides that groups of higher socioeconomic status acquire more information and they acquire new information faster (Tichenor et al., 1970). These widening disparities in knowledge may serve as major contributing factors toward widening disparities in health (Viswanath et al., 2006). This in our estimation provides that differential knowledge (access, use, dissemination, etc.) translates into differential states of empowerment. Where empowered is conceptually understood to represent the ability to leverage knowledge to mitigate the undesirable elements that disproportionately harm populations of a certain race/ethnicity, gender, and socioeconomic status (SES).

Health empowerment theory provides that health empowerment arises from personal and social-contextual resources, such as knowledge (Shearer, 2009). The resources result in empowerment related patterns of well-being. Knowledge is derived from both self-capacity and through the support of social networks and social support systems. This knowledge results in health empowerment when it is used to facilitate "one's awareness of the ability to participate knowingly in health and health care decisions. Health empowerment theory is expressive of a human health pattern of well-being and is viewed as a relational process that emerges from the recognition of personal resources and social contextual resources (Shearer, 2009). This process facilitates purposeful participation in the attainment of health goals and the promotion of individual well-being" (Shearer, 2009). Therefore, building capacity—facilitating empowerment—entails cultivating transferable health knowledge, skills, and resources both at the individual [tacit] and community [explicit] level (Griffith et al., 2010).

APPLICATION

Computational models are commonly used to provide information on scenarios in which traditional methods of data collection are not possible, suitable, or ethical (Carley, 1999; Carney et al., 2015). Computational models can be used to conceptualize the core components that directly and indirectly impact on complex healthcare issues like cancer health disparities in a variety of organizational and social settings (Burton & Obel, 2004; Kling, 1993). Computational models enable the virtual design and computerized simulation of a system, which can be used to study outcomes under various conditions. This goal of this research is to develop a hypothesis generating and predictive computational model of knowledge and its varying relationship factors. Traditional statistical applications are not fully equipped to study the conceptualization of knowledge in complex adaptive environments, but computational models are able to fill the gap and generate more robust hypotheses on the relationship between knowledge and empowerment. Many but not all computational models are tools for explanation, as opposed to prediction (Harold & Ken, 2012). Computational models provide a framework on decision behavior and learning in dynamic and evolving networked environments (Ilgen & Hulin, 2000).

The widely accepted adage, "knowledge is power," is axiomatic to health empowerment theory. The computational modeling of knowledge empowerment in this presentation begins with the acceptance of this premise as true. This research does not seek to prove or disprove the premise. Rather, the purpose of the discussion is to express knowledge as a function of power in quantitative relational terms as a necessary first step in higher order mathematical algorithm development. First, we present the complete argument (indicating the separation of statements by S1-S8) and then we present it through eight computational statements.

CONCEPTUALIZATION OF ARGUMENT

We start with the understanding that knowledge is power or more precisely that power (in the sense of empowerment) is a function of knowledge (S1). Power, however, can be redefined in terms of its component parts to expand our understanding of knowledge with respect to power. Knowledge is expressed in terms of power in hopes of yielding a more precise definition (Uphoff, 2005). Borrowing from the realm of physics and mathematics, power can be defined as a function of work over time. By transitive property of equality, this also provides that knowledge can be defined as a function of work done over time (S2).

Operationally, for multilevel cancer and other disease-specific health disparities (e.g. cardiovascular, diabetes, HIV, etc.) stakeholders' knowledge empowerment—expressed as a function of this equivocation of knowledge and power—serves as a necessary first step in our efforts to be make the construct concrete and quantifiable. For our purposes, we might want to examine the level of work over the course of time that is expended on the knowledge management (production) side that involves the generation, storage, refinement, display/staging, and dissemination of knowledge. We might also want to examine the work expended over time on the user side with respect to knowledge acquisition, curation, absorption and understanding, as well as in the sharing of knowledge with others within ones' social network. These all become measurable rates of work over time with respect to knowledge and may serve as proxy measures of power in the context of (S2).

If we consider knowledge empowerment to be measured in terms functional capabilities for leveraging the "knowledge currency" (Burrage, 2009) for informed decision making, managing uncertainty and risk, and participating in high quality communication and knowledge exchange—which we will later refer to as health-specific knowledge commerce—then these three empowerment criteria essentially become de facto measures of a high-performance knowledge environment. We hypothesize that the relative rates of our proxy measures of power—as expressed above in terms of production-side and user-side knowledge measures of work over time—will display correlations to knowledge environment quantified levels of informed decision making, uncertainty/risk, and communication quality. This algorithm can assist in the design and evaluation of such studies. Such a representation of a knowledge environment would represent a practical implementation, in accordance with the enhanced health disparities informatics capacity, called for by the NIH strategic plan to eliminate health disparities. These knowledge environment performance measures of power (or work over time) are also hypothesized as being strong influencing agents on the decisions made and the actions performed by multilevel stakeholders in the course of their social and organizational interactions and engagements. Herein, we will use the term "actionable intelligence" to refer to these knowledge-driven decisions and actions. Furthermore, "knowledge performance" measures of health disparities are herein categorized into two main categories for stakeholders:

1. Performance (represents knowledge applied to action/task);
2. Judgment or discernment (represented knowledge applied to choice/decision) (S3).

Knowledge performance is more commonly understood in the context of intelligence and wisdom. Here, we attempt to contextualize knowledge in terms of its use within some setting (e.g., healthcare organization, home, clinical encounter, work environment, etc.) as a tool to generate actionable intelligence. Knowledge, knowledge users, and the overall knowledge environment are not only measured in terms of the sum of all knowledge within a given knowledge-base, but also in how well said knowledge is applied to inform decisions and actions. The act of applying knowledge to decisions and actions is operationally defined as *intelligence* and the act of displaying increasing levels of intelligence over time in the face of multilevel healthcare system challenges is called *wisdom* (S4).

For our purposes intelligence is not a concrete measure of the sum total of what is known but by how well what is known is used and applied in problem solving and can be thought of as a collective, organizational, or social I.Q. of sorts, understood in to the context of shared values, goals, and objectives. While wisdom is much more abstract and harder to define we simply assume it to be a measure of intelligence over time. Knowledge empowerment is, therefore, conceptualized in terms of knowledge performance and/or actionable intelligence and wisdom. This is then applied to conceptualize the typical knowledge of stakeholders in disease management strategies such as to cancer care delivery. Here we highlight an example of the typical multilevel knowledge cancer care delivery stakeholders and their respective decisional or actionable challenges where knowledge can be applied. These stakeholders and their informational needs are provided in Table 1.

Table 1. Cancer care delivery knowledge needs by stakeholder category

Stakeholder	Knowledge Need
Cancer Health Consumers	To know about individual or community level cancer risk and risk prevention strategies
Cancer Patients	To know about treatment options, clinical trials, support resources, and navigating the health system
Cancer Care Givers	To find the cancer resources for care and treatment of family, friends, or loved ones
Providers	To know best evidence-based care and treatment available to patients, monitor and track patient health status, and of the implementation and dissemination of innovations in cancer care
Health Care Organizations	To provide the best cancer care services at the highest quality, safety, and cost-effective levels of delivery to patient population served
Community Groups	To protect and empower community members through continued awareness, advocacy, and engagement
Researchers and Policy	To mine the evidence to determine the best possible intervention and programmatic strategy to improve outcomes; to monitor and track population burden of disease in the general population

From the perspective of cancer health disparities, the computational modeling challenge would be to identify the factors that account for multilevel stakeholder knowledge needs being met or unmet in a timely manner using such measures as the:

1. Rate of knowledge generation;
2. Rate of knowledge transfer;
3. Rate of knowledge absorption within any knowledge environment.

Additionally, how individual- and/or institutional-level bias, discrimination (racial, ethnic, sexual, etc.), differentials in SES, variations in geography, and lowered health literacy in cancer care might serve as degrading factors that artificially increase workload in the knowledge flow (e.g., generation, access, use, and dissemination and sharing of knowledge) in cancer care delivery. We hypothesize that the more prevalent the degrading factors are in any given social and organizational setting, the more difficult it will be in meeting multilevel stakeholder knowledge needs. Additionally, the greater the prevalence of these degrading factors, the greater the adverse impact they will have on multilevel stakeholder use of actionable intelligence to inform choice and actions. The presence of degrading factors may contribute to the environment conditions that foster cancer health disparities related to unmet knowledge needs and inadequate levels of actionable intelligence (Kreps & Sivaram, 2008).

Cancer health disparities stakeholders often make decisions and take actions in cancer care under uncertain conditions that include, but are not limited to the following:

1. Patients' uncertainty regarding medications;
2. Patient care givers' uncertainty regarding medication dosage, side effects, and affordability;
3. Providers' uncertainty on how to incrementally improve minority enrollment in cancer clinical trials, identifying eligible patients for screening, and the effectiveness of treatment protocols;
4. Healthcare organizations' uncertainty regarding meeting accreditation standards for navigating patients through gaps and barriers to quality of care and eliminating disparities;

5. Community groups' uncertainty regarding how to engage healthcare systems as an advocate for empowerment and equitable care and treatment of their community members (Epstein & Street, 2007).

Despite operational constructs for knowledge, power, intelligence, and wisdom, the construct of "empowerment" specifically through knowledge remains to be precisely defined. Thus, the next step is to propose a clear, operational definition for knowledge empowerment to assist health professionals and researchers (e.g., informaticians, computational engineers, researchers, etc.) in modeling transitions of multilevel stakeholders in modeling complex knowledge environments from disempowered to empowered states or vice versa.

Two concepts of significant importance to the direction of this argument are that:

1. There is a subtle but distinct difference in our modeling between power and empowerment;
2. Power is described in the realm of physics as a force and with any force there comes the potential for counter force.

Regarding the first concept, power can be viewed as a binary state of existence or a condition that represents two mutually exclusive possibilities of either having something or not having something. One can compare this to the idea of light switch or automobile being turned on or off. While empowerment provides us with a transitional state where there may be a range of possibilities between being fully empowered or fully disempowered. Thus, in our model power is considered binary and empowerment occurs on a continuum. These two distinctions in the model allow us to design a matrix of potential stakeholder conditions where an individual-, group-, organizational-, or system-level entity may have access to a vast supply of knowledge (recall that knowledge is power and the two terms are used interchangeably) and be utterly disempowered (displaying low levels of intelligence and wisdom in the application of knowledge to their choices and actions). Such can be the result of low literacy, poorly designed or constructed knowledge resources (e.g., displays, texts, colors, language or cultural barriers, etc), low levels of knowledge absorption due to pace and style of content curation, learning or communication styles, and poorly designed workflows, etc. Conversely, a person can have limited access to knowledge resources, yet display exceptional ability to process and convert raw knowledge resources into usable applications of intelligence and wisdom. This type of knowledge empowerment is displayed in environments where the translation of available knowledge and its corresponding rates of absorption and use occur at highly efficient rates.

Thus, in our models we assume that having access to knowledge does not automatically equate into empowerment, any more than tuning on a light switch makes one enlightened. Knowledge "wealth" as described by Burrage implies in our model that one has the capacity to convert knowledge into usable assets—that can overcome degrading factors and exercise necessary levels of knowledge performance and discernment—to maximize health and wellness and minimize harm, uncertainty, and risk. Our model assumes that populations typically faced by disproportionately higher levels of conditions commonly associated with health disparities are ill equipped to fully engage in equitable and empowering knowledge-commerce and operate under we term we introduce as knowledge-poverty. We further assert the traditional interventions that focus largely on bombarding health consumers, patients, and communities with social-messaging, informational campaigns, and knowledge resource portals without addressing the corresponding factors of knowledge degradation, knowledge performance, and knowledge judgment/

discernment are likely to have either no impact, a limited impact, or positive impact that is unsustainable and/or not generalizable to other communities. We believe this is one of the major reasons why disparities persist despite massive amounts of resources dedicated toward their elimination. However, the testing of this assertion is beyond the scope of this discussion and is intended to be explored in a future study. Our model seeks to design a more precise way of quantifying conditions of knowledge-poverty, expressed as poor management of uncertainty and risk among all stakeholder levels.

Regarding the second concept, we recognize that power is described in the realm of physics as a force and with any force there comes the potential for counter force and it is here where we'll discuss the counter force, "friction," and its impact on knowledge empowerment. As stated above, if power is viewed as a function of knowledge and power is work over time, then knowledge can be understood as a function of work over time. Work itself can then be restated to refer to force over distance, which is treated in our model as "effort" (S5). In the context of force and counter force, knowledge can be understood as degrees of effort over time in the presence or absence of some counter force. We express the counter force of friction in our computational models as knowledge degradation. We discussed above how for example factors such as individual- and/or institutional-level bias in cancer care can serve as sources of degradation (friction) with any social and organizational setting. We can now express any given knowledge environment and its corresponding measures of efficiency in knowledge-production side and/or knowledge-use side as a function of effort over time in the presence or absence of knowledge degradation (S6).

Here, knowledge-efficient environments are those where knowledge degradation within the knowledge environment from beginning (knowledge generation) to end (knowledge dissemination and use) and all points throughout the knowledge life cycle have levels of knowledge degradation at or approaching zero. Thus, knowledge degradation can serve as an indirect measure of knowledge efficiency in any given knowledge environment. However, efficiency requires additional elements for true evaluation, including:

1. Measures of utility or value attached to the knowledge applied to tasks and decisions;
2. Contextual factors that can serve to provide boundaries on the unlimited array of possibilities.

Both utility and context now makes the evaluation of knowledge empowerment or knowledge efficiency squarely as understood from the perspective of the knowledge stakeholder him- or herself, the environmental conditions, and the factors that determine the boundaries of possibility and measures of success. In the absence of these factors of utility, knowledge empowerment and efficiency can only be measured in abstract and subjective terms.

In other words, in order to answer how effective stakeholders are in demonstrating knowledge discernment (or knowledge applied and decisions/choices) and knowledge performance (knowledge applied to actions/tasks) in the management of uncertainty for instance, we would need to understand the relative value of the knowledge elements, based on the relative complexity and level of importance (criticality) placed upon the decision and actions. For example, the knowledge required to support an array of decisions and actions to cooking one's breakfast is valued much less than the knowledge required to support the array of choices and actions related to landing a space probe on Mars. Factors, such as acceptable margins of error, the rate of supply and demand of knowledge (i.e., elasticity), and the factors shaping cognitive processing (typically in real-time) all play a part in helping us to assign value to any knowledge-commerce activities.

Correspondingly, knowledge context forces us to also limit the possibilities from the infinite to come to some concrete set of boundaries or conditions. Here, the forces and counterforce of knowledge generation and degradation retrospectively can be defined with respect to some pre-defined system boundaries, some set of system stakeholders and organizations, and how they change over time within a network of social or organizational interactions. In this context, uncertainty and knowledge degradation serve as constant protagonists that compromise the idealized state of perfect knowledge, which we assume in our modeling is unobtainable in absolute terms. As such, we define boundaries and limits to allow us to conceptualize perfect or idealized knowledge states in relative terms in the presence of varying degrees of uncertainty and knowledge degradation (S7, S8).

It should be noted that determination of both the relative utility/value and contextual factors that shape how critical a body of knowledge is or is not is typically performed by a review of literature or a panel of subject matter experts. The literature on cancer health disparities related knowledge is still maturing in this space and the development of such an array of experts to inform our assumptions is ongoing and out of scope for this discussion and our mock scenario example below will assume this has been completed. As such, (S7 and S8) represent our best approximation of these relationships with respect to our modeling of (S1-S6).

COMPUTATIONAL STATEMENTS

We first re-state the notion that knowledge (K) is power (P) in by saying that power (in the sense of empowerment) is a function of knowledge and present statement one as follows:

S1: $P_e = f_1(K)$

Power is then defined as work (W) over time (t), which also provides the expanded expression of knowledge in terms of power. If power is a function of knowledge and $(P) = \left(\frac{W}{t}\right)$, then we can say that:

S2: $K \infty \frac{W}{t} = f_2\left(\frac{1}{t}\right)$

Knowledge defined in actionable terms leads to concept of knowledge performance (K_{perf}), which consists of a measure of performance (or knowledge applied to tasks) (K_T) and that of discernment (knowledge applied to decisions) (K_D). Furthermore, the sum total of individual and/or collective environmental uncertainty among multilevel stakeholders is represented as (U). Acceptable levels of knowledge performance, therefore, represents states where the sum of performance and discernment is greater than the stakeholders' environmental uncertainty. That is knowledge (K) can be parameterized in terms of work (W) and the inverse of time (t). Furthermore, we can introduce intelligence (I) as the following:

S3: $I = K_{perf} = K_T + K_D$ subject to $I > U$

We bring in the concept of wisdom Ω and how it relates to a rate of intelligence (I):

$$\textbf{S4: } \Omega = \frac{I}{t} = \frac{K_D + K_T}{t}$$

subject to: $\Omega > \frac{U}{t}$

Finally, the following series of statements relies on the concepts that knowledge (K) is power (P) (or more precisely that K is a function of P), and knowledge over time (t) is work (W). Work is commonly defined as force (F) over distance (D) or what we more commonly refer to as Effort. Therefore, the following statements are provided: Now, we introduce the concept of effort:

$$\textbf{S5: } K \propto \frac{F \times D}{t} \text{ or } \frac{Effort}{t}$$

Thus, knowledge can now be presented as degrees of effort over time. Knowledge efficiency (K_{EF}) is considered to be a function of effort over time in the presence or absence of K_{DEG}:

$$\textbf{S6: } K_{EF} \propto f_3\left(Effort, \frac{1}{t}, -K_{DEG} \right)$$

This concept can be expanded in terms of knowledge and efficiency to account for actionable intelligence (I). Statement seven's (S7) computational modeling of intelligence is joined with the additional elements of utility (U_T) and contextual (C) factors and accounts for knowledge degradation (K_{DEG}). Furthermore, statement eight's (S8) computational modeling of wisdom (Ω) is joined with these same additional elements:

$$\textbf{S7: } I = f_4 (K_T + K_{D,} U_T + C, - K_{DEG}) \text{ subject to } K_T + K_D > U$$

$$\textbf{S8: } \Omega = f_5 (K_T + K_{D,} U_T + C, \frac{1}{t}, -K_{DEG}) \text{ subject to } K_T + K_D > U$$

Thus, actionable intelligence or simply intelligence is now being defined as the degree to which adequate task-specific and decision-specific knowledge is available to offset the level of inherent uncertainty within any social or organizational environment making up a system boundary. The level of complexity of the task and associated level of importance (typically derived from external subject matter expert panels regarding the phenomena in question), determines the relative number of discrete knowledge elements (bits or chucks) of the knowledge content that will be required to perform. For example, in our scenarios above of landing a space craft on Mars versus cooking breakfast one can imagine that the years of didactic training and relative bits of information contained in instruction manuals for those two events to be drastically different in size, detail, scope, and complexity. A recipe for breakfast may contain 50 discrete bits of instructional knowledge and the landing of a space craft may contain 50,000 discrete instructional bits of knowledge. This, concept of utility and context are further shaped by the stakeholders' own level of aptitude and ability to absorb said instructional bits of knowledge.

As such, we are asserting that intelligence (I) can be expressed in terms of the ability to leverage available task-specific knowledge bits (K_T) and decision-specific knowledge bits (K_D) required to:

- Overcome environmental uncertainty;
- Meet the cognitive demands (need-to-know)—of expertly-defined measures—associated with stakeholder-specific value and complexity, to mitigate or eliminate individual or collective forms of knowledge degradation (K_{DEG}).

Intelligence (I) is the measure of this in absolute terms and wisdom (Ω) is this same capability with the added dimension of time (t).

CASELET: THE COLORECTAL CANCER (CRC) HEALTH DISPARITIES MOCK SCENARIO

A Patient Perspective: Calculating Knowledge Baselines for (P) Power, (KD) Knowledge Discernment, and (KT) Knowledge Performance

A community-based organization within tri-city is holding a community health fair relying on the local professional football team to help market the event throughout the region. The event will be held at the stadium and is expected to draw people from each of the three partnering cities that make up the coalition. The intent of the health fair is to raise awareness of risk, educate and inform on measures of prevention, healthy lifestyle choices, and encourage patients to get screened for diseases where early detection has proven effective. Colorectal Cancer (CRC) is listed as the top priority for this coalition and efforts were made to ensure that this well represented at the fair. At the start and end of the event participants were given CRC awareness level tests that measured their self-perceived and actual level of knowledge on CRC related topics as seen in Table 2.

Here in this caselet we are able to explore two dimensions of our knowledge empowerment algorithm with respect to uncertainty and friction. We will explore scenarios for effort, intelligence, wisdom, and learning in subsequent manuscripts. Here were are interested in seeing the extent to which available knowledge is properly accessed by both patients and providers, and the factors that help to degrade the use of that knowledge in decision making and task performance. The event CRC testing of CRC awareness campaign participants revealed the scoring results (all scores reports in terms of knowledge bits) in Table 3.

In very simply terms we were able to show that of the 35 discrete bits of knowledge for patients and general health consumers—based on some predefined inventory of what should be knowledge-task and knowledge-decision about CRC according to our hypothetical expert guidelines—that our audience all assumes they knew more than they actually did about CRC and that both males and females were operating at a CRC-specific knowledge deficit and as a result bound to make decisions about CRC screening, level of person risk, and places to get tested under uncertain conditions. Males exhibited an uncertainty score of 24 versus 15 for female participants. This implies that women were making CRC-related decisions and actions with a little more than half of the knowledge they are expected to have to inform them, while men were doing the same with less than one third of the knowledge they should have available. In this case, we can create a proxy measure of patient-level CRC Uncertainty as a function of the total available minus the actual number of knowledge bits on average. For men, this would be 35-11 or 24 Uncertainty Units and for women 35-20 or 15 Uncertainty Units.

Table 2. Patient-level assumptions, tasks, and key artifacts

Key Assumptions	Key Tasks	Provides
Assume a knowledge, task, and decision inventory has been conducted and verified by existing literature or panel of subject matter experts. In this mock scenario assume: • 100 total CRC knowledge bits o 65 providers (30 task bits and 35 decision bits) o 35 patients (20 task bits and 15 decision bits)	Model the clinical pathways for screening, treatment, and survivorship. • Task bits can be related to screening tests, scheduling, interviewing to determine eligibility for screening, review lab results, referrals, patient tracking, treatment plans, etc. • Decision bits can be related to decision to get screened, interpretation of lab results, communication strategy, treatment options, to adhere to medication regimen, to complete referrals, to enroll in clinical trials, to keep scheduled appointments, etc.	Library of key tasks, decisions, and knowledge resources used at each step of any clinical pathway
Patients - Assume total number of bits is 35 and assumes 15 bits related to key decisions and 20 bits related to key tasks	Assess Self-Perceived (SP) CRC Knowledge Empowerment at start	Baseline K (self-perceived) expressed as # of bits
Assume expert panel has defined the core knowledge elements in required in CRC clinical pathway (e.g., screening, treatment, and survivorship) and their relative importance in *task performance* and *decision making*	Assess Self-Perceived Knowledge Empowerment at end	Comparative K (self-perceived) expressed as # of bits
All numbers are hypothetical	Assess Actual (ACT) CRC Knowledge Empowerment at start	Baseline K (actual) expressed as # of bits
Assumes barriers to care – identified as friction factors have been listed and weighted by an expert panel	Assess Actual Knowledge Empowerment at end	Comparative K (self-perceived) expressed as # of bits

Table 3. Scoring results in terms of knowledge bits of CRC awareness campaign participants

	Average Male Participant	Average Female Participant
Initial $K_{(Self\text{-}Perceived)}$	22 bits	30 bits
Initial $K_{(Actual)}$	11 bits	20 bits
$K_{D\,(Actual)}$	6 of 15 KD bits	9 of 15 KD bits
$K_{T\,(Actual)}$	5 of 20 KT bits	11 of 20 KT bits
Uncertainty	35 – 11 = 24 bits	35 – 20 = 15 bits

A Provider's Perspective: Calculating Knowledge Baselines for (P) Power, (KD) Knowledge Discernment, and (KT) Knowledge Performance

One information session and panel discussion featuring providers, health plans, and community groups took on an unexpected tone of seriousness when someone named Patricia from the audience recounted her father's experience with the health care system. Patricia went on to say that her father was a relatively healthy African-American man but suddenly became ill at the age of 53. He had severe abdominal pain and was presenting with related gastrointestinal system distress. He did not have a primary care physician, no health insurance, and decided to go the emergency department. He was treated for a severe stomach infection and given antibiotics, evaluated for ulcers, and given over-the-counter medications to assist with persistent indigestion. No further tests were determined to be needed. She explained how her father never seemed to get any better and over the course of a few months became increasingly worse. Her father eventually collapsed and was taken back the emergency and admitted to the hospital. Her father was later diagnosed with late stage colorectal cancer following a full battery of tests and the prognosis was not encouraging. Despite aggressive forms of treatment for the cancer her father eventually passed away within 8 months of initial diagnosis.

While the audience sat in silence one of panelists, a Caucasian-American internal medical physician referred to as Dr. Carol, offered words of comfort and provided a testimony of her own. Dr. Carol expressed how hard it must have been for Patricia but suggested that there is probably a lot we can learn from her own father's experience. She explained that her father was much the same in that he too was fairly healthy for most of his life. And, following some news that her father was also feeling some sharp pains in both in his abdominal and rectal area she proceeded to make an appointment for him to see a primary care provider the very next day. Her father was interviewed extensively on his family history and it was determined that her dad might have been at an increased risk for CRC. The doctor referred him for an immediate CRC screening and decided to wait in treating the abdominal and rectal pain until after the tests were completed. The CRC screening test results revealed a cluster of adenomas (or polyps) in his colon, which were removed during the screening procedure. Because her father had more than 10 adenomas during his exam the gastroenterologist recommended that her father be screened again in three years instead of the typical 5 or 10 year time periods for others that present with 1 to 2 or no adenomas respectively. Dr. Carol went on the report that her father was doing well and was really lucky.

She went on to contrast the two situations and said outlines factors made a difference in the decisions about care and treatment:

1. **Access to Health Insurance:** Allowed her father to be more selective in identifying his provider whereas those without are typically limited to resources of their local emergency department once symptoms reach acute or severe stages;
2. **Interview on Family History:** Versus her counterpart's father which was probably evaluated only for acute care and treatment. Dr. Carol stated that this more extensive evaluation probably resulted in her father's long-term risk for chronic conditions to be assessed while Patricia's father only got treatment for the acute symptoms in an attempt to eliminate immediate pain and discomfort;
3. **Access to Specialty Care:** For additional evaluation versus Patricia's father who was sent home to treat the immediate symptoms and wait and see if more care was warranted;
4. **Services of a Curator or Advocate:** Who understood medical terminology as well as the culture of health care and assisted him in the decision making process about screening and treatment options. While Patricia was not well versed on these same health system concepts and merely trusted that her father was getting adequate care.

Table 4 lists the full set of provider-level assumptions informing this portion of our case discussion.

Let's also assume that both providers of Patricia's and Dr. Carol's fathers were given the CRC knowledge provider-level awareness test as a CRC quality improvement effort at their hospitals and clinics. Each provider's scores were captured in a database and a hospital administrator present at the event was able to search on these results following the Tri-City. They were tested on recognizing the signs and symptoms of CRC, determining eligible population for screening, testing options, managing patient anxiety of about testing, treatment options, testing, sites, the cost of testing, types of insurance coverage

Table 4. Provider-level assumptions, tasks, and key artifacts

Key Assumptions	Key Tasks	Provides
Assume Patricia's father is being treated by Provider A and Dr. Carol's father by Provider B and that this experience represents the realm of possibility for this tri-city event audience	Model provider-specific community and action pathways same as above	Provide overview of provider-based decisions and tasks informed by specific knowledge resources
Assume total number of CRC knowledge bits is 65 and assumes 30 bits related to key tasks and 35 bits related to key decisions	Examine opportunities how providers perform relative to establish guidelines for CRC screening, treatment, and survivorship	Provide basis for studies that evaluate the correlation between knowledge-task and knowledge-decision couplings with that of performance and outcomes
Assumes that the literature or an expert panel has identified friction points or "things that can go wrong" represented as deviations from guideline concordant care and provide numerical weights for their level of negative impact on outcomes.	Identify a list of issues or friction points and use assigned numerical weights in calculating degradation in CRC knowledge	Friction elements here are measured in terms of the percentage of degradation from 100% perfect transmission or use of knowledge. For example, a score of 75 means that 75% of potential knowledge was lost or went unused.

associated with CRC testing and treatment, prognosis and stages of CRC. Someone also did a follow-up interview of each provider to examine and compare conditions under which CRC related decisions were made to determine how efficiently knowledge was used throughout the process (here labeled as Friction Elements). Their respective scores are reported in Table 5 and Table 6.

This assessment of provider uncertainty and system-wide friction elements reveals that both Provider A and Provider B were well versed on CRC screening procedures, protocols, and guidelines. However, as an emergency room physician priority is given to assessing and remediating acute conditions and

Table 5. Scores reported for Patricia's father and Dr. Carol's father

	Provider A (Patricia's Father)	Provider B (Dr. Carol's Father)
Initial $K_{(Actual)}$	50	62
$K_{D\,(Actual)}$	25 of 35 KD bits	32 of 35 KD bits
$K_{T\,(Actual)}$	25 of 30 KT bits	30 of 30 KT bits
Uncertainty	65 – 50 = 15	65 – 62 = 3

Table 6. Friction elements

CRC Risk Assessment	10	90
Family History Evaluation	15	100
Patient Literacy	30	30
Differential Diagnosis (treating lesser conditions first)	35	70
Time Restraints	15	95
Knowledge Curator/Advocate	0	100
Level of Insurance	0	100
Sub-Total Friction	105	585
Total Friction	700 -105 = 595	700 – 585 = 115

preventive evaluation skills may have eroded somewhat over time revealing that Provider A had an uncertainty score of 15 as compared to only 3 for Provider B.

We were also able to observe the relative degree of friction during the patient-provider encounters and the initial stage of diagnosis upon presenting with symptoms. Here the fundamental question is what if any factors might prohibit the full expression of guideline concordant screening, early-detection, risk assessment, and transference into treatment upon a positive testing. As stated in Table 2 an expert panel has assigned weights to a full list of potential friction points within the CRC clinical pathway and we have scored this scenario accordingly. Our hypothetical assessment reveals that conditions in an emergency room settings (typically chaotic) for what are traditionally low literacy, low income, and uninsured patients revealed that a frication factor of 595 represents that up to 85% (or 595/700 =.85) of available knowledge was compromised to inform CRC-related guideline concordant care for Patricia's father. In the case of Dr. Carol's father only 16% (or 115/700 =.16) of available knowledge was compromised to inform CRC-related guideline concordant care. Factors that greatly advanced CRC care for Dr. Carol's father were a thorough review of family history to assess CRC risk level, having adequate insurance and access to primary care, and having a knowledge curator/advocate that helped to broker the best care and a more thorough diagnosis that included immediate referral for testing.

We are therefor able to apply our knowledge empowerment algorithm and summarize the relative experiences in more quantitative terms. Let's assume that patient-level K_D and K_T for both Patricia's and Dr. Carol's fathers are relatively the same (as taken from our male patients above). We arrive at the following.

We are representing CRC knowledge performance or K_{Perf} as a function of used knowledge ($K_D + K_T$) minus unused knowledge (Uncertainty) to gauge a measure of effectiveness in the use of knowledge. In other words, how much is used relative to how much is available to satisfy individual cognitive demand (or the need to know), within the context of friction events (F) during a clinical encounter (space and time).

Patricia: $(K_D + K_T) - U = (6 + 5) - 24 = (-13)$; Prov A $(25 + 25) - 15 = 35$
Overall $(K_D + K_T) - U = (-13) + 35 = 22$
Dr. Carol: $(K_D + K_T) - U = (6 + 5) - 24 = (-13)$; Prov B $(30 + 32) - 3 = 59$;
Overall $(K_D + K_T) - U = (-13) + 59 = 46$

We can thus say that the clinical encounter for Dr. Carol's father leveraged twice as much of the total knowledge available to support decisions and task than did the clinical encounter for Patricia's father. Additionally, of those knowledge bits accessed and used there were a series of contextual factors that shaped the access, use, and absorption levels as reflected in the following statement on friction below.

We are representing CRC knowledge performance or K_{Perf} as a function of used knowledge ($K_D + K_T$) within the context of friction events (F) during a clinical encounter (space and time) to gauge a measure of efficiency in the use of knowledge. This assessment recognizes that there are 100 CRC related knowledge bits available in total and that the Friction for clinical encounter between Patricia's father and Provider A yielded a frication factor of 85% or that the use of up to 85 knowledge bits were compromised due to contextual factors within the clinical encounter. Comparatively speaking the clinical encounter for Dr. Carol's father and Provider B experienced a friction factor of only 16% or 16 knowledge bits potential use being comprised.

Patricia: Overall ($K_D + K_T$) – (F) = 22 – 85 = (-63)
Dr. Carol: Overall ($K_D + K_T$) – (F) = 46 – 16 = 30

This suggests that even in the presence of frictional factors within the environment the cumulative knowledge in the second case of Dr. Carol acting as knowledge curator/advocate, her father's limited knowledge of CRC-related materials, and her primary care doctor (Provider B) was sufficient to guide him to a favorable outcome. In the first case Patricia's father's limited knowledge, lack of advocacy and knowledge curation to question the provider, and Provider A's orientation toward acute disorders and less so on preventive care were not enough to account for the knowledge deficit. This situation would have either called for the infusion of new knowledge from a second opinion, a curator, advocate, or family member, or called for an immediate follow-up visit to a primary care provider in a community health center setting that typically serves patients like Patricia's father having no insurance, low income, and low health literacy.

With the help of measures like Actual Knowledge (K_{ACTUAL}), Perceived Knowledge ($K_{Self\text{-}Perceived}$), Task-Specific Knowledge (K_T), Decision-Specific Knowledge (K_D), Uncertainty (U), and Friction (F) we are able to calculate baseline measures and statistics that can be used to inform more complex statistical and computational experiments (e.g., network analysis, computer simulation, and predictive modeling) that examine knowledge as an agent of change in health outcomes. Topics related to wisdom, intelligence, learning, effort over time require additional modeling and assumption building that go beyond the scope of this manuscript. We are designing real world and hypothetical scenarios to examine them in more detail. The intent of this manuscript was to present the entire algorithm and offer a simple case example using one scenario highlighting the application of a few statements.

DISCUSSION AND PRACTICAL APPLICATIONS

One may ask why is it necessary to create a relational algorithm expression for knowledge and/or empowerment when the former is rather tangible in nature as something one either has or does not have, while the latter is a condition that either one feels or does not feel. As such, why go through the added effort to design something to express it in formulaic terms. Our response is predicated on the notion that there are really no universal standardized definitions for knowledge-driven smart, intelligent, and learning health systems. There are also no consistent definitions for it means to function as stakeholders in such systems engaging in what we call health-related knowledge commerce. Health-related knowledge-commerce refers to something we reiterate from above as the pursuit of knowledge to inform decision/choice and action/tasks carried out to maximize gain/benefit and minimize harm/risk. This pursuit is valid from each level of the socio-ecological framework from patient- to policy-level. Our model draws from theory from a variety of fields that include communication theory ((ORISE), 2012), network theory (Borgatti & Foster, 2003; Carley, 1999), social learning theory (Bandura, 1977), and organizational information-processing-entity theory (Burton & Obel, 2004). These theories help us to construct computational models that examine dynamic interactions of multi-level health system stakeholders, in complex social and organizational network arrangements, engaging in knowledge-commerce to carry out a series of health-related objectives and solve complex health-related problems. Within this network the knowledge life-cycle operates as an intentional or unintentional construct where knowledge is generated, processed, stored, accessed/used, managed, analyzed, distributed, and converted into actionable intelligence. Out relational algorithm assumes the following:

1. That degradation can occur at any stage of the knowledge life cycle;
2. That not all knowledge is the same in form/structure/type, level of importance, and degree of complexity;
3. That external factors such as culture impact patterns of knowledge sharing and learning;
4. That the rate of knowledge absorption differs among intra- and inter-stakeholder levels;
5. That knowledge synthesis is in part largely dependent upon the rate of conversation of knowledge from individual-tacit forms of knowledge (what is in one's mind, individual mental models) to collective-explicit forms of knowledge (what is produced, shared, and available for group problem solving, collective cultural models in codified into tangible knowledge products) (Nonaka, 1994);
6. That the access to knowledge as a commodity is not equal among all stakeholder classifications, as such the social and economic cost of knowledge results in tiers that range from highly informed (knowledge-wealthy) to uninformed (knowledge-impoverished) consumers; and
7. That the primary driver of all knowledge pursuits is the resolution of multilevel health-stakeholder cognitive demand (need-to-know) expressed as a direct function of uncertainty and risk, thus the higher the levels of uncertainty and risk the higher the levels of cognitive demand.

We believe the once knowledge is understood computationally we can better apply theory such as the knowledge gap hypothesis and the health empowerment theory in association with our series of assumptions. We can also construct conceptual models that can examine a series of complex health scenarios.

Our relational algorithm represents a necessary first step in designing complex computational experiments that examines the environmental contextual factors which shape cognitive demand and stakeholder engagement in health-related knowledge-commerce to address varying levels of stakeholder uncertainty and manage risk. We seek to build models that will allow us to better understand discrete changes of the knowledge life cycle within a defined health-system over the course of time (e.g., 1, 3, 5, 10, 25 years) (Carney et al., 2014, 2015). This is not unlike our previous research where we examined the rate of knowledge in a network of community health centers over a ten-year simulated period to compare high and low performance in breast, cervical, and colorectal cancer screening among vulnerable populations. We were able to use dynamic network analysis to reveal that health environment (e.g., patient characteristics, provider beliefs, and organizational factors) contributed to the ability of community health centers to leverage a knowledge dissemination tool such as clinical decision support (e.g. provider prompts at point-of-care, computerized reminders, electronic patient results, and information reporting to patients) to improve cancer screening performance. Our networks models revealed that knowledge absorption rates—expressed as the ability of community health centers to leverage clinical decision support to process and apply cancer screening practice guidelines and best practices—more efficient within higher performers than low performing health centers (Carney et al., 2014). Additionally, we found that network structural characteristics such as network symmetry, network clusters and cliques, and network connectivity were all positively correlated to performance level as well (Carney et al., 2015). Only network density proved difficult for our model to explain as a function of community health center performance. As a result, we felt the need to design relational algorithms of knowledge environments that more discretely measured degradation, knowledge application/use, uncertainty, and even the more abstract concepts like intelligence and wisdom over time. We intend to address learning in a subsequent manuscript.

We believe this relational algorithm for knowledge and empowerment can assist us in better exploring a variety of conditions that result in knowledge degradation such as treatment bias, provider processing and applying of a volume of clinical guidelines, policy changes, organizational practice procedure changes at the point-of-care, patients retention of medical-specific details and complex treatment plans, processing of community health status reports, national surveillance timeliness gaps, patients lost to referral and follow-up, shifting population dynamics, responsiveness to the emergence of new diseases, integrating new evidence into practice, and many more scenarios. We argue that the lack of a standardized way of measuring knowledge and the subsequent rates of degradation and empowerment can make modeling and managing complex knowledge environments extremely difficult. Our relational algorithm attempts to quantitatively represent a commonly used expression in both social and research settings and to later convert it into a mathematical expression to inform complex computational modeling.

CONCLUSION

New methods and techniques are needed to more fully examine the dynamics leveraging knowledge as an agent of changed in addressing complex health issues like health disparities research. We envision that our treatment of knowledge, power, empowerment, uncertainty, frication, as well as the more abstract concepts of intelligence and wisdom, as a proposed new approach in modeling, measuring, and managing any knowledge environment. We view this relational algorithm as a preliminary exercise in building complex computational models, network diagramming of knowledge, and even contributing to higher order mathematical algorithms needed to properly represent the social and organizational networks arranges that impact on the knowledge life cycle and subsequent levels of multilevel stakeholder empowerment. The chief aspect of this modeling approach that our algorithm exploits is in treating knowledge on the discrete elemental level. This also requires a comprehensive understanding of the total knowledge complement, decisions, and tasks as a part of any systems analysis which we called knowledge-task and knowledge-decision inventories. We also recognize that this modeling effort is co-dependent on either a sound subject specific literature or panel of subject matter experts to assist in the contextualizing of the relative value (utility and criticality) of said knowledge and the circumstances that help to shape is degree of complexity. Here we demonstrated how this modeling would be applied to a case example dedicated to colorectal cancer. We might also use these measures to compare populations on the basis of race/ethnicity, SES, and health literacy levels to understand the relationship between knowledge dynamics and health disparities. We can also leverage this to measure the overall application of clinical guidelines by comparing one provider to another to measure the ability to process this knowledge at the point-of-care. We view the building of inventories and contextualizing of knowledge, with respect to some set of system goals and objectives, is all part of a dynamic and adaptive knowledge culture and knowledge environment. Our goal was to take a necessary first step in moving from the more abstract construct that *knowledge is power* to something more concrete, measurable, and easy to model in computational terms. This computational argument achieves that goal.

REFERENCES

Bandura, A. (1977). *Social learning theory*. Englewood Cliffs, N.J.: Prentice Hall.

Borgatti, S. P., & Foster, P. C. (2003). The Network Paradigm in Organizational Research: A Review and Typology. *Journal of Management*, *29*(6), 991–1013. doi:10.1016/S0149-2063(03)00087-4

Burrage, H. (2009). From Regeneration to Sustainability: A northern take on knowledge. *Journal of Urban Regeneration and Renewal*.

Burton, R.M., & Obel, B. (2004). *Strategic organizational diagnosis and design: the dynamics of fit*. Boston: Kluwer. doi:10.1007/978-1-4419-9114-0

Carley, K.M. (1999). On Generating Hypotheses Using Computer Simulations. *Systems Engineering*, *2*, 69-77.

Carney, T. J., Morgan, G. P., Jones, J., McDaniel, A. M., Weaver, M., Weiner, B., & Haggstrom, D. A. (2014). Using computational modeling to assess the impact of clinical decision support on cancer screening improvement strategies within the community health centers. *YJBIN Journal of Biomedical Informatics*, *51*, 200–209. doi:10.1016/j.jbi.2014.05.012 PMID:24953241

Carney, T. J., Morgan, G. P., Jones, J., McDaniel, A. M., Weaver, M., Weiner, B., & Haggstrom, D. A. (2015). *Hypothesis Generation Using Network Structures on Community Health Center Cancer-Screening Performance*. YJBIN Journal of Biomedical Informatics.

Epstein, R., & Street, R. L. (2007). *Patient-centered communication in cancer care: promoting healing and reducing suffering*. U.S. Dept. of Health and Human Services, National Institutes of Health, National Cancer Institute.

Finney Rutten, L. J., Nelson, D. E., & Meissner, H. I. (2004). Examination of population-wide trends in barriers to cancer screening from a diffusion of innovation perspective (19872000). *Preventive Medicine*, *38*(3), 258–268. doi:10.1016/j.ypmed.2003.10.011 PMID:14766107

Griffith, D. M., Allen, J. O., DeLoney, E. H., Robinson, K., Lewis, E. Y., Campbell, B., & Reischl, T. et al. (2010). Community-Based Organizational Capacity Building as a Strategy to Reduce Racial Health Disparities. *J. Primary Prevent The Journal of Primary Prevention*, *31*(1-2), 31–39. doi:10.1007/s10935-010-0202-z PMID:20127281

Haggstrom, D. A., Taplin, S. H., Monahan, P., & Clauser, S. (2012). Chronic Care Model implementation for cancer screening and follow-up in community health centers. *Journal of Health Care for the Poor and Underserved*, *23*(3), 49–66. doi:10.1353/hpu.2012.0131 PMID:22864487

Harold, K., & Ken, K. (2012). The Potential Value of Computational Models in Social Science Research.

Heiman, E., Haynes, S., & McKee, M. (2015). Sexual health behaviors of Deaf American Sign Language (ASL) users. *Disability and Health Journal Disability and Health Journal*, 12.

Hesse, B., Galen, C. E., & Powe, B. D. (2012). *Partnering Against Cancer Today (PACT): A Blueprint for Uniting Action through Communication Science. National Cancer Institute (NCI), Centers for Disease Control and Prevention (CDC), American Cancer Society.*

Ilgen, D. R., & Hulin, C. L. (2000). *Computational modeling of behavior in organizations: the third scientific discipline*. Washington, D.C.: American Psychological Association. doi:10.1037/10375-000

Kling, R. (1993). Organizational Analysis in Computer Science. *The Information Society*, *9*(2), 71–87. doi:10.1080/01972243.1993.9960134

Kreps, G. L., & Sivaram, R. (2008). Strategic health communication across the continuum of breast cancer care in limited-resource countries. *Cancer*, *113*(8 Suppl.), 2331–2337. doi:10.1002/cncr.23832 PMID:18837025

Lisovicz, N., Wynn, T., Fouad, M., & Partridge, E. E. (2008). Cancer Health Disparities: What We Have Done. *The American Journal of the Medical Sciences*, *335*(4), 254–259. doi:10.1097/MAJ.0b013e31816a43ad PMID:18461726

National Institutes of Health. (2012). NIH Health Disparities Strategic Plan and Budget Fiscal Years 2009-2013. Rockville, Md.: National Institute on Minority Health and Health Disparities.

Nonaka, I. (1994). A Dynamic Theory of Organizational Knowledge Creation. *Organization Science*, *5*(1), 14–37. doi:10.1287/orsc.5.1.14

ORISE. (2012). The Role of Communication Across the Cancer Continuum: a Systematic Review of the Literature. American Cancer Society (ACS), Centers for Disease Control (CDC), National Cancer Institute (NCI).

Resnicow, K., & Vaughan, R. (2006). A chaotic view of behavior change: A quantum leap for health promotion. *The International Journal of Behavioral Nutrition and Physical Activity*, 3. PMID:16968551

Roosaar, A., Johansson, A. L. V., Sandborgh-Englund, G., Axéll, T., & Nyrén, O. (2008). Cancer and mortality among users and nonusers of snus. *International Journal of Cancer*, *123*(1), 168–173. doi:10.1002/ijc.23469 PMID:18412245

Shearer, N. B. (2009). Health empowerment theory as a guide for practice. *Geriatric Nursing (New York, N.Y.)*, *30*(2). PMID:19345857

Taplin, S. H., Haggstrom, D., Jacobs, T., Determan, A., Granger, J., Montalvo, W., & Calvo, A. et al. (2008). Implementing colorectal cancer screening in community health centers: Addressing cancer health disparities through a regional cancer collaborative. *Medical Care*, *46*(Suppl. 1), S74–S83. doi:10.1097/MLR.0b013e31817fdf68 PMID:18725837

Tichenor, P. J., Donohue, G. A., & Olien, C. N. (1970). Mass Media Flow and Differential Growth in Knowledge. *Public Opinion Quarterly*, *34*(2), 159–170. doi:10.1086/267786

Uphoff, N. (2005). Analytical Issues in Measuring Empowerment at the Community and Local Levels. In D. Narayan-Parker (Ed.), *Measuring Empowerment Cross-Disciplinary Perspectives*. Washington, DC: World Bank.

U.S. National Institutes of Health. (2009). Cancer Screening Overview Retrieved from http://www.cancer.gov/cancertopics/pdq/screening/overview/HealthProfessional

Viswanath, K., Breen, N., Meissner, H., Moser, R. P., Hesse, B., Steele, W. R., & Rakowski, W. (2006). Cancer knowledge and disparities in the information age. *Journal of Health Communication*, *11*(sup001), 1–17. doi:10.1080/10810730600637426 PMID:16641071

Williams, D. R., Kontos, E. Z., Viswanath, K., Haas, J. S., Lathan, C. S., MacConaill, L. E., & Ayanian, J. Z. et al. (2012). Integrating Multiple Social Statuses in health disparities research: The case of lung cancer. *Health Services Research*, *47*(3 Pt. 2), 1255–1277. doi:10.1111/j.1475-6773.2012.01404.x PMID:22568674

This work was previously published in the International Journal of Civic Engagement and Social Change (IJCESC), 3(3); edited by Susheel Chhabra, pages 16-35, copyright year 2016 by IGI Publishing (an imprint of IGI Global).

Chapter 8
Personal Health in My Pocket:
Challenges, Opportunities, and Future Research Directions in Mobile Personal Health Records

Helen Monkman
University of Victoria, Canada

Andre Kushniruk
University of Victoria, Canada

Elizabeth Borycki
University of Victoria, Canada

ABSTRACT

Consumers' access to their health records is increasing, and one of the ways they can gain access and potentially contribute to their records is by using a mobile Personal Health Record (mPHR). mPHRs emerged as a combination of mHealth and Personal Health Records (PHRs). Despite the current shortage of evidence supporting mPHR use, these systems are already being deployed, and examples of currently available mPHRs are provided. mPHRs have an array of potential uses and different target user groups, but there are also several challenges impeding their success. The physical constraints of mobile devices, health literacy, and usability all create obstacles for mPHRs. However, mPHRs create opportunities due to the affordances of mobile devices and the potential to integrate consumer mHealth applications. The challenges and opportunities of these nascent systems are outlined in this chapter, as they inform research topics with respect to mPHRs.

INTRODUCTION

There are a number of important changes occurring in healthcare today. Perhaps foremost among these is a greater move towards involvement and empowerment of consumers (i.e., citizens and patients) in the self-management of their health. Indeed, over the past decade the concept of consumer access to their

DOI: 10.4018/978-1-5225-1928-7.ch008

records has moved from a pilot in the late 1990's (Cimino, Patel, & Kushniruk, 2002), when electronic access by consumers to their health data via the worldwide web (WWW) was being explored, to the current access by millions of patients and citizens to their own institutional health data today over the Internet (Halamka, Mandl & Tang, 2007; Protti, 2008). This movement has stemmed from a desire of consumers to have access to their own data, with the first manifestation of this appearing as the "stand-alone Personal Health Record (PHR)" (Tang, Ash, Bates, Overhage & Sage, 2006). This movement has included access by patients to health data contained in their own PHRs and it has also included a move towards increased access to their own data stored in hospital and even national databases. The objective of this chapter is to introduce the reader to the concept of mPHRs, provide examples of these systems, outline potential users and use environments, and discuss the challenges, opportunities and directions for future research.

What is a PHR?

According to the Medical Library Association (MLA) / National Library of Medicine (NLM) Joint Electronic Personal Health Record Task Force, a PHR is

a private, secure application through which an individual may access, manage, and share his or her health information. The PHR can include information that is entered by the consumer and/or data from other sources such as pharmacies, labs, and health care providers. The PHR may or may not include information from the electronic health record (EHR) that is maintained by the health care provider and is not synonymous with the EHR (Jones, Shipman, Plaut & Selden, 2010, p. 244).

In the past decade, several models for providing consumers with personal health have emerged. PHRs are available in three basic types based on their connectivity or integration with other health information systems. PHRs under the sole control of the consumer and which do not connect with any other health information systems are called stand-alone PHRs (Tang et al., 2006). In contrast, tethered PHRs allow patients to access their own personal information contained in their health provider's health information system (Tang et al., 2006). For example, the Epic health information system (used by many hospitals in the United States) has included in many implementations a component called MyChart that allows patients to access parts of their electronic record remotely. Interoperable PHRs are ideal, because they allow a variety of different health information systems to exchange data and thus, offer the most financial benefits (Kaelber & Pan, 2008) and utility (Tang et al., 2006). Yet another model for consideration are national portals, which allow citizens read-only access to their health data that is interconnected across regions and even nationally. This approach has emerged over the past ten years and examples include the Sundhed.dk patient portal in Denmark, which allows all Danish citizens to access their own health data over the Internet (Protti, 2008).

What is mHealth?

Concurrent with the trend towards PHRs has been a staggering increase in the use of mHealth applications (i.e., health applications running on mobile devices). mHealth is the use of mobile devices for healthcare, or "mobile computing, medical sensor, and communications technologies for health care" (Istepanian, Jovanov, & Zhang, 2004, p. 405). mHealth is revolutionizing the way health data is collected and how healthcare is delivered. A multitude of mHealth applications are available to clinicians and consumers. Consumer mHealth applications are a distinct subset of mHealth applications designed for use by health consumers, or laypeople, rather than healthcare professionals. Consumer mHealth applications have been developed for health promotion (e.g., exercise applications) and monitoring physical activities (e.g., pedometers), as well as more advanced applications used in conjunction with healthcare providers to monitor vital signs, such as heart rate and sleeping patterns (Househ, Borycki, Kushniruk, & Alofaysan, 2012). The devices used for such applications have varied, but cell phones, smartphones, and tablets are currently the most prevalent. Moreover, because mobile devices are becoming increasingly affordable, consumer mHealth applications are becoming viable options for facilitating healthcare in traditionally underserved populations.

What is an mPHR?

A mobile Personal Health Record (mPHR) is a Personal Health Record (PHR) integrated with a consumer mHealth application or mobile platform (See Figure 1). An mPHR is distinct from other consumer mHealth applications because it is integrated with the user's health records. Further, an mPHR can serve multiple purposes whereas a consumer mHealth application typically only serves a single purpose. Thus, an mPHR can be considered to be multiple integrated consumer mHealth applications, as well as a consumer mHealth application in and of itself. mPHRs are a potential forum for amalgamating various types of health information (e.g., allergies, family history, advanced directives, laboratory reports). The information in an mPHR therefore can be generated both by healthcare providers and consumers, within healthcare settings (e.g., hospital, clinic, laboratory) and also in naturalistic environments (e.g., consumer's home, workplace). Ideally, mPHRs are gateways to health information entered by healthcare providers, as well as repositories of complementary health information added by consumers. As is true for PHRs, mPHRs are often comprised of tools to facilitate self-management by helping consumers adhere to individualized care plans, graph their symptoms, collect physiological data, receive tailored instructions or motivational feedback, use decision aids, and receive reminders (Pagliari, Detmer & Singleton, 2007). Ideally, every mPHR should be customized to the user's specific needs, in order to streamline the user's experience and increase efficiency. Thus, an mPHR can be envisioned as a collection of independent consumer mHealth applications as component modules, or as a single application that amalgamates disparate applications with health information. Given that they have only been deployed recently, there is a dearth of research on mPHRs. However, consumer mHealth applications have been more extensively studied. If mPHRs are viewed as compositions of consumer mHealth applications integrated with electronic patient record information, evidence from these domains can be leveraged to inform the design and development of mPHRs.

Examples of mPHRs

A number of experiments have allowed healthcare providers to access to health data using mobile devices since 2000. For example at Columbia University the PalmCIS application was created that allowed healthcare providers to access patient records using smartphones (Chen, Medonca, McKnight, Stetson, Lei, & Cimino, 2003). Since then, this approach has taken off and mobile interfaces have been developed not only for healthcare providers, but also for consumers to access their health records (i.e., mPHRs) (see Table 1 for examples).

Figure 1. The mPHR

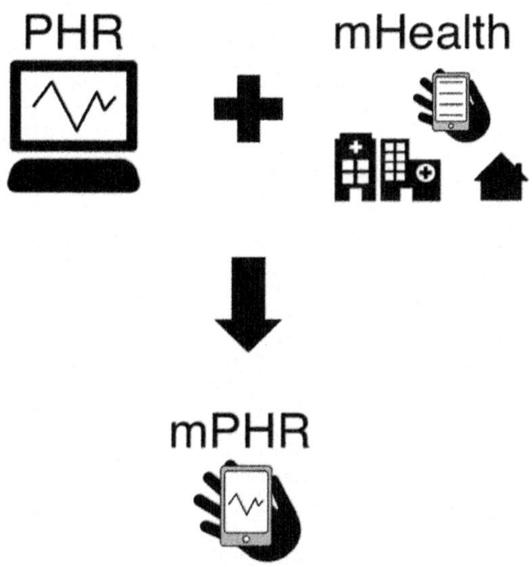

To date, the primary functions of mPHRs are oriented around accessing ones personal health information. In a comparison of 19 stand-alone mPHR applications, Kharrazi, Chisholm, VanNasdale, and Thompson (2012) found that the functionality available in mPHRs was highly variable. These authors evaluated mPHRs from three platforms (iOS™, BlackBerry®, and Android™) and they ranged in price from no cost to $9.99. Kharrazi and colleagues evaluated PHRs' functionality by using 10 data elements (problems/conditions, procedures, medications, providers, allergies, labs, immunizations, family history, emergency contact, and insurance) and four features (import/export, images, in case of emergency feature, and password) as indices.

Kharrazi and colleagues' comparison may be valid for the current landscape of mPHRs, which are in their infancy and primarily stand-alone systems; howevever, as with PHRs, the value of mPHRs is affected by the extent of their integration with other health information systems, or mPHR interoperability. That is, the usefulness of mPHRs increases with the number of health information systems it can exchange information with, from stand-alone, to tethered, and finally to interoperable. As described, mPHRs may be used to store, maintain and manage a variety of different personal health information as well as offer other features (see Figure 2a). In addition to containing information entered by healthcare professionals, in many circumstances it may be valuable to have consumers enter monitoring data into their mPHRs (see Figure 2b and c).

Depiction of possible mPHR information and features (a), potential mPHR data collected by consumers (b), mPHR blood pressure graph example (c).

WHO ARE mPHR USERS?

Identifying the needs and preferences of the users is an imperative process for any system that is designed, developed and deployed and mPHRs are no exception. It is estimated that approximately one in every seven people are currently using smartphones (Nmawston, 2012) and users may want to have

Figure 2. Example of an mPHR

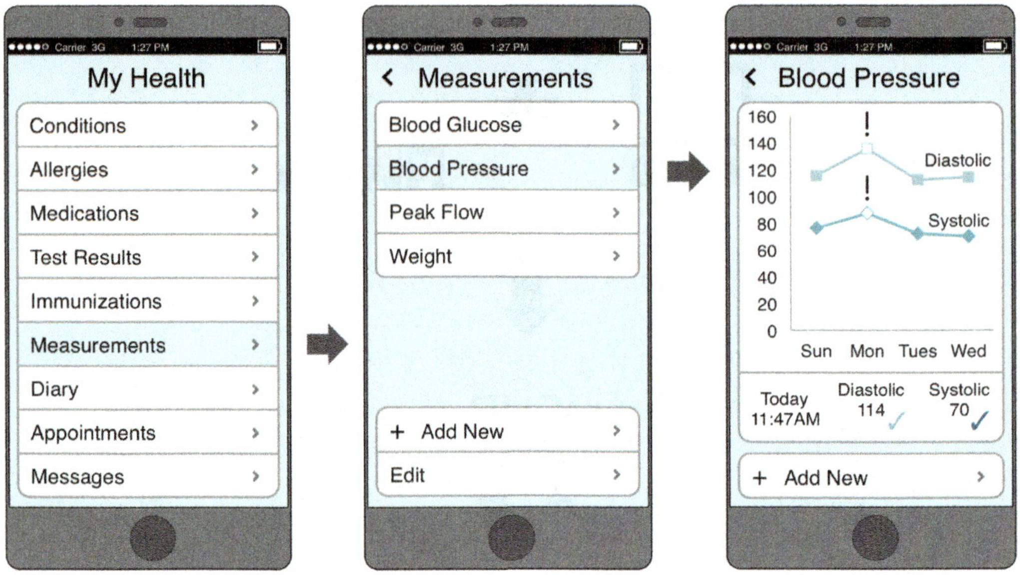

(a) (b) (c)

Table 1. Three Examples of Currently Available mPHRs

mPHR Name	Vendor Name	URL	Interoperability	Features
MyChart	Epic Systems Corporation (EPIC, 2013)	http://www.epic.com/software-phr.php	Tethered	• Viewing test results. • Viewing and scheduling appointments. • Uploading photos. • Updating medications and allergies. • Refilling prescriptions. • Filling out questionnaires. • Accessing chronic disease summaries. • Securely messaging providers.
motionPHR	Communication Software Inc. (CSI, 2013)	http://motionphr.com	Stand-alone or Interoperable	• Entering and storing information on medications, allergies, conditions, procedures, test results, advance directives & organ donation, emergency contact, and immunizations. • Medication and prescription refill reminders. • Managing information for multiple consumers (e.g., a family).
HealthTrak	University of Pittsburgh Medical Center (UPMC, 2013)	https://myupmc.upmc.com	Tethered	• Requesting appointments. • Tracking current health issues. • Renewing prescriptions. • eVisit digital house calls. • Viewing medical records. • Tracking medications. • Messaging providers.

access to their records via their smartphones. Although consumers are the primary users of mPHRs healthcare providers and caregivers may also access consumers' mPHRs. Providers have a distinct set of user and information needs with respect to mPHRs. Thus, the provider-facing component of mobile personal health applications should be designed differently to accommodate these users. For example, providers may need automatic notifications when consumers have hit critical thresholds of specific values consumers are monitoring. These notifications will help providers gauge whether consumers need more support or changes to their medication and management plans. However, it is important that mPHRs avoid inundating providers with daily information that is not indicative of a problem; providers will likely find more value in reviewing the general trends and being notified of episodes that require their attention. Alternatively, caregivers may only need access to certain types of information (e.g., appointments, medication allergies). Health consumers and caregivers often have limited, or no, clinical understanding, it is imperative that mPHRs are designed such that users with limited health literacy can evaluate, understand and apply the information contained in mPHRs. Thus, mPHRs may need changes in design to accommodate two or more different user groups.

Given that mobile devices are becoming increasingly affordable, mPHRs are becoming a viable medium for reaching traditionally underserved populations. Simon and Sneldon (2012) posited the feasibility of mPHRs use for people in developing countries. Evidence suggests that PHRs are beneficial in helping underserved populations self-manage their illnesses (Botts, Horan & Thoms, 2011), and it is reasonable to assume that mPHRs will have similar benefits. Consumer mHealth applications have been explored for homeless people with mental illnesses (Depp et al., 2010), low-income pregnant women (Evans, Wallace, & Snider, 2012), people who live in remote areas (Proudfoot et al., 2010), and indigenous people (Bramley et al., 2005). However, providing underserved populations with mPHRs could introduce the risk of theft of the mobile device, especially for consumers living in shelters (Depp et al., 2010). Mobile devices are gradually becoming less alluring to thieves, as they become more common and stolen devices can be deactivated and rendered unusable by anyone other than the owner. However, users might sell their devices, if they are in stressful financial situations. As mobile devices continue to become pervasive and affordable, loss of devices due to theft or sale will likely diminish. Thus, it is plausible that mPHRs will enable a broad range of previously underserved health consumers to access and share their health records.

Although there is vast potential reach for mPHRs, the unique needs of the different users groups must also be considered. For example, users with severe mental illness may feel that mPHRs with the capability of delivering interventions increase the physical and emotional distance between them and their providers (Depp et al., 2010). However, mPHRs designed for users with severe mental illness could also increase the continuity of care and expedite care provision during critical mental illness episodes (Depp et al., 2010). Thus, there are costs (e.g., creating distance in the patient-provider relationship) and benefits (e.g., opportunity to increase patient safety and quality of care) that need to be considered regarding mPHR deployment to people with severe mental illness.

Similarly, older adults may also reap the benefits of mPHRs, but these systems must adapt to their needs, capabilities, and preferences. Given that the prevalence of multiple chronic illnesses, or multimorbidities, increases with age (Health Council of Canada, 2010), it becomes increasingly important for personal health information to be kept current and comprehensive. Additionally, mPHRs may incorporate functions of consumer mHealth applications to allow older adults to live autonomously for longer by facilitating engagement in physical activity (Sunwoo et al., 2010), detecting and conveying information about falls (Lee & Carlisle, 2011), contacting emergency assistance, as well as tracking dementia patients when they wander (e.g., Miskelly, 2005). However, older adults appear to have more challenges learning how to successfully use mobile devices (Kurniawan, Mahmud, & Nugroho, 2006). Further, given generational differences (Leung, McGrenere, & Graf, 2011) as well as perceptual, cognitive and motor changes associated with aging, special design considerations (e.g., Leung et al., 2012) are imperative for mPHRs to accommodate elderly peoples' needs and capabilities.

In addition to the aforementioned groups of users, consumers may have specific reasons for needing mPHRs. For example, people who travel often may benefit from having mPHRs. Also, consumers with specific illnesses or conditions may also find having mPHRs worthwhile. Studies have found that consumers are receptive to using consumer mHealth applications for mental health (Depp et al., 2010; Proudfoot et al., 2010), recovery after kidney transplantation (McGillicuddy et al., 2013), and managing asthma (Cleland, Caldow, & Ryan, 2007). Further, mPHRs with these functions could facilitate early identification of problems and improve continuity of care (e.g., Cleland et al., 2007). As mPHRs integrate functions such as those previously mentioned, it is reasonable to assume there will be a demand for mPHRs from frequent travellers and users with specific health conditions.

Although mPHRs may be valuable for a variety of different user groups, each of these groups has unique needs that need to be identified and addressed in the respective mPHR designs. It is not prudent to assume that a single mPHR solution will be suitable for all different types of users. To identify their specific needs, preferences and usability challenges, target consumers should be included in the design process. Further, these investigations can also be used to reveal what functionality is most important to specific types of users and what contexts they are likely to use mPHRs in.

WHERE AND WHERE ARE mPHRs USED?

One of the main advantages of mPHRs is that they can be used almost anytime, anywhere. For example, users who travel or move frequently may find mPHRs particularly valuable. However, this ubiquity also presents novel design challenges. For example, privacy may present as an issue in certain circumstances. Historically, to enter personal health information, users logged-in from the privacy of their own homes, but mPHRs may send messages and reminders to users without any sensitivity or regard to the particular context the user is in. As such, if messages were sent to the consumer at an inopportune time (e.g., in a meeting, on a busy commuter bus) bystanders could potentially read sensitive information.

Although their constant availability is appealing, there will inevitably be fluctuations in mPHR use, as a reflection of a user's health status at a given time. Depp and colleagues (2010) argued that is unreasonable to expect participants to partake in mobile interventions for an infinite duration. Users' participation may decrease over time and/or become more sporadic, which is referred to as "fatigue effects" (Shiffman, Stone, & Hufford, 2008). Thus, instead of continuous intervention delivery, a more flexible approach that identifies critical periods and increases the frequency of intervention events during windows of opportunity should be developed (Depp et al., 2010). Similarly, mPHRs should identify critical time points for intervention delivery. For example, if a user is not ready to quit smoking currently, but indicates that she might be ready to consider it in a few months, the mPHR could store this response and query the consumer again after the indicated time has elapsed. Further, mPHRs should also give users the opportunity to participate in or withdraw from interventions as they see fit.

mPHRs have inherent possibilities for delivering tailored health information when users and providers need it most. That is, the delivery of information that is suited to the users' levels of health literacy can be triggered by specific events (e.g., disease diagnosis, pregnancy) to educate consumers when they are facing new health challenges or experiences and perhaps when they are most in need of credible, personalized, health information. For example, if an mPHR is populated with a positive pregnancy test, it could prompt the user to ask if she would like to receive information related to prenatal care and could activate a pregnancy module. Furthermore, in emergency situations, context-aware mPHRs could also make important health information (e.g., allergies, medications, pre-existing conditions) available to providers upon user arrival at the hospital and automatically notify to the user's emergency contact or caregiver. Thus, mPHRs have the potential to effectively deliver information to consumers and providers in such a way that will foster patient safety.

CHALLENGES FOR mPHRs

In addition to some of the advantages and disadvantages of mPHRs due to their nearly limitless use cases, there are a variety of other challenges that deploying these new systems to consumers present.

Constraints of Mobile Devices

Mobile devices have unique affordances and constraints that differ from computers. In order to optimize the human-mobile device system, designers must capitalize on the affordances and minimize the limitations by using human factors methods to evaluate design solutions. Understandably, the screen size of mobile devices plays a critical factor in mPHR design whereby the conciseness of content on smaller screens is imperative. Given that users understood significantly less content read on a phone-sized screen than on a desktop computer (Singh, Sumeeth, & Miller, 2011), limited display size increases the demand for succinct, actionable information in mPHRs. Additionally, text data may be more difficult to input due smaller keyboards and interacting with graphic user interface elements (e.g., menus, buttons) may be more challenging and error prone as a result of the limited screen size of mobile devices. Thus, the physical constraints of mobile devices generate a unique set of problems for mPHRs.

Health Literacy

Another challenge relevant to all consumer health information systems is making information appropriate for people with limited health literacy. The World Health Organization (WHO) endorses Nutbeam's (1998) definition of health literacy, which states that health literacy "represents the cognitive and social skills which determine the motivation and ability of individuals to gain access to, understand and use information in ways which promote and maintain good health" (p. 357). Consumers with limited health literacy present a challenge for healthcare. The Canadian Council on Learning (2008) argued that "without adequate health-literacy skills, ill-informed decisions may be taken, health conditions may go unchecked or worsen, questions may go unasked or remain unanswered, accidents may happen and people may get lost in the health-care system" (p. 5). Thus, it is not surprising that people with limited health literacy are more likely to report low health statuses (Canadian Council on Learning, 2008) and are prone to worse health outcomes (DeWalt, Berkman, Sheridan, Lohr, & Pignone, 2004).

The health literacy challenge cannot merely be reduced into increasing consumers' health literacy levels, as lowering the demands on health literacy is an equally important goal. Baker (2006) argued that health literacy is a combination of both the consumers' capabilities and the health literacy related demands of the healthcare system. Unlike the majority of health information systems, those designed for consumers are unusual because consumers often have limited or no health care experience (Segall et al., 2011). Thus, to optimize the value mPHRs, it is imperative that the demands mPHRs impose on consumers are aligned with the users' levels of health literacy.

Usability

Although mPHRs are being deployed rapidly and they have the potential to exceed the value of PHRs, mPHRs are inherently unique from their PHR counterparts due the medium they are delivered on (i.e., mobile devices). However, all of the possible opportunities associated with mPHRs, require research from a human factors perspective to confirm that consumers consider them useful and usable.

One of the most difficult problems facing mPHRs designers is creating an efficient user experience. First, the more seamlessly added functionality can be built directly into mobile devices and alleviate the need for additional external medical devices, the more likely these devices will be available (not forgotten or misplaced) when users need them. Second, as mPHRs develop and provide more diverse functions and inevitably become more complex, a simple, efficient means of using these systems must be preserved. Thus, a balance between complexity and ease of use must be achieved. Although mPHRs have considerable potential, consumers' adoption of mPHRs relies on their usability.

Several evaluation methods are available to identify usability issues and thus generate design solutions to make systems easier to use (Jaspers, 2009). Many of these methods are relevant for evaluating mPHRs, yet they remain to be applied. Resources that could inform usability focused user-centred design include Kushniruk (2002) and Årsand and Demiris (2008). Årsand and Demiris' (2008) provided advice for using these methods and when specific methods are most useful. Further, a resource focused on designing for users with limited health literacy is *Health Literacy Online* (U.S. Department of Health and Human Services, 2010). Årsand and colleagues' (2012) provided the following suggestions based on their research of consumer mHealth applications that could inform the design of mPHRs: whenever possible, data should be transferred automatically; user interfaces should be visual and motivational; effort exerted to use the system should be minimized and benefits from use should be maximized; and systems should be dynamic and adaptable.

Usability testing is considered the gold standard of usability evaluation methods because it identifies problems that typical users encounter and it is a promising method for evaluating mPHRs. Usability testing has been recognized as a valuable method for investigating usability problems in health information systems for well over a decade (Kushniruk, Patel, & Cimino, 1997). Despite that these methods have been used to investigate PHRs (e.g., Haggstrom et al., 2011; Segall et al., 2011) and mobile Web sites and applications (e.g., Nielsen & Budiu, 2013), to date, no usability testing of mPHRs was found.

An important research consideration for mPHRs are the physical settings for usability testing. mPHRs should be subjected to usability testing with different levels of naturalism, in order to reveal all of the potential usability problems. That is, mPHR usability testing may begin in a laboratory setting to identify obvious problems with the system, but additional testing should be conducted with mPHRs "in-situ" or in naturalistic environments. Due to the complexity of healthcare environments, this "in-situ" evaluation approach for health information systems is being promoted for identifying problems that may not be revealed due to the over simplified context of laboratory settings (Kushniruk, Borycki, Kuwata, & Kannry, 2011). Similarly, many issues that users encounter in specific contexts may go undetected if mPHR evaluation is limited to the confines of the laboratory. Thus, mPHRs could benefit from "in-situ" usability testing to identify problems that only occur in particular contexts, in users' day-to-day lives and activities; however, given the nearly limitless contexts in which mPHRs could be used, new data collection methods (e.g., the snippit technique developed by Brandt, Weiss, and Klemmer, 2007) may warrant exploration.

Challenges associated with usability testing of mPHRs also include mobile screen recording and inferring users' attention. Currently, mobile screen recording is less than robust, but the software is continuously improving. Inexpensive mobile screen recording applications exist, but they have limitations (e.g., brief maximum recording length, beta versions). Fortunately, there are alternative methods to collect data of users interacting with mobile devices. Presently, the most vigorous and reliable methods available for mobile screen recording are tethering or mirroring the mobile device under investigation to a computer and recording the computer screen. This can be accomplished with software such as Ashot (Sourceforge, 2013) for Android™, and Reflector (Squirrels, 2013) for iOS™ devices. Unlike screen recordings of computers, where users' attention may be inferred from the location of the cursor, there is no cursor on mobile devices so it is more important to have both screen recordings and scene camera recordings for mobile usability testing. One potential method for supplementing traditional usability test data for mPHR evaluations is collecting eye-tracking data. This technique has demonstrated utility in detecting usability problems in eBook readers (Siegenthaler, Wurtz, & Groner, 2010). Cheng (2011) argued for using both head-mounted (i.e., portable) and stationary (i.e., remote) eye-trackers to collect data for mobile device usability evaluations. It is expected that screen recording will become increasingly reliable and eye-tracking data may become increasingly viable for mobile usability tests such as those conducted on mPHRs.

In addition to usability testing, usability inspection methods (e.g., heuristic evaluation, cognitive walkthrough) may improve mPHR design through usability expert analyses. Heuristic evaluation is a popular usability inspection method because it is informal, rapid, inexpensive, and relatively easy to perform and it may be useful for investigating mPHRs. Given its advantages, it is not surprising that heuristic evaluation has been used to investigate PHRs (e.g., Monkman & Kushniruk, 2013b) and consumer mHealth applications (Monkman & Kushniruk, 2013a). Further, Monkman and Kushniruk's (2013a) method may be a viable option for identifying both usability and health literacy issues in mPHRs, given that their heuristics originate from evidence synthesized by the U.S. Department of Health and Human Services (2010).

There are undoubtedly challenges associated with mPHRs and usability evaluation of mPHRs; however, there are a variety of potential benefits to mPHRs over PHRs accessed traditionally on full sized computers. Some of the opportunities that mPHRs have yet to capitalize on will be outlined.

OPPORTUNITIES OF mPHRs

Despite the challenges associated with mPHRs, these systems introduce a wide range of new opportunities. Combining the advantages of PHR technology with mobile devices is beginning to be explored and promises even greater patient and citizen (i.e., consumer) access to their health data than was previously possible, through access to PHRs via smartphones, tablets, cell phones and other emerging pervasive computing devices that are wearable and portable (Bardram, Mihailidis, & Wan, 2007). Further, mobile device users, especially generations X and Y (i.e., born after 1965), are very receptive to the idea of accessing their health information using their mobile devices (Keckley, & Hoffman, 2010). Thus, the move towards mPHRs is an exciting trend that is likely to help promote health and ultimately empower healthcare consumers.

Leveraging the Affordances of Mobile Devices

mPHRs create unique opportunities for information to be delivered to consumers, as well as for consumers to enter data into their records. People have changed the method and frequency of their communication and information sharing as a result of the advent and proliferation of mobile devices. Short message service (SMS or text messages) for synchronous or asynchronous communication between individuals has rapidly increased in use, and many people prefer receiving text messages to phone calls (Smith, 2011). In addition to the propensity of users to text, text messaging is an appealing form of health communication for several other reasons. First, text messages can be asynchronous, the user decides whether or not, and when she will respond to a text message. Second, health topics are often sensitive in nature and texting provides a discreet way of health information exchange. Third, texting is often a relatively inexpensive way of communicating and likely entails minimal adaptation from existing paper-based materials. Given these potential advantages, it may be useful to explore text messaging as a method of information delivery and data entry into mPHRs.

With respect to information delivery, many mobile devices have Text-To-Speech (TTS), a development that could enhance the output of mPHRs. TTS generators convert written text into spoken language. Many mobile devices come equipped with TTS generators, which merely have to be activated. TTS generators have become increasingly more natural sounding and thus, are an appealing complementary method of delivering health information to people who may have challenges reading it (e.g., if the information is not in the user's native tongue, users with limited health literacy). Similarly, multimedia messaging system (MMS) (i.e., photograph and movie messages) and video clips also provide opportunities to increase understanding and enhance data entry accuracy. For example, Vargas, Robles, Harris and Radford (2010) found that reducing the amount of reading (i.e., by showing native language video clips) and writing (i.e., by providing questions with multiple choice answers) required by users with limited health literacy facilitated accurate reporting (Vargas et al., 2010). Thus, audio and audiovisual materials are viable complementary modes of delivering information through mPHRs to improve user comprehension and data entry accuracy.

Mobile devices are equipped with microphones, which create opportunities for both interacting and perhaps eventually entering data into mPHRs. Currently, touch (i.e., finger or stylus contact with the screen) is the predominant method for user interaction with smartphones and tablets. However, multi-touch gestures (e.g., pinch-to-zoom) broaden the number of commands available. Nielsen and Budiu (2012) provided an insightful comparison between mouse and fingers as inputs devices. Due to the limited size of keyboards on mobile devices, it important to limit the extent of typing required for all types of interaction (e.g., searching terms, booking appointments) with mPHRs. Typing can be reduced through strategies such as auto-complete, selection wheels, and more recently voice commands. Given the recent influx in the use of natural language user interaction (e.g., Siri for iOS™), and the increasing robustness of these systems, in the near future, users may simply speak into the microphone of their mobile devices perform mPHR tasks (e.g., find lab results, schedule appointments). Voice commands are a promising mode of interaction for users who can talk but have limited dexterity. Thus, natural language interaction should be explored with respect to how it can benefit mPHRs (e.g., data entry) and mPHR users.

Other recent advances in mobile device interaction may also benefit mPHRs. Specifically, the use of front facing cameras which track the eyes allow users to interact with onscreen information using their focal attention. For example, the Samsung GALAXY S4® enables users to scroll up or down by focusing their gaze on upper or lower portions of the screen. Similar techniques are also in early development for iOS™ devices (Pino & Kavasidis, 2012). The feasibility of blinking gestures to serve as button-clicks has also been explored (Miluzzo, Wang, & Campbell, 2010). Additionally, simply by swiping a hand in the air above the sensor, the Samsung GALAXY S4® allows users to check the display status, scroll through pages, browse forward and backward, and answer calls (Samsung, 2013). Eye movements and hand gestures for interacting with mPHRs is promising for users who have physical impairments, or limited fine motor skills, but whose gross motor and/or eye control is preserved.

Mobile devices are typically equipped with accelerometers and gyroscopes, which users' physical movements of a device (e.g., tilt, twist, rotate) to be translated into inputs. Initial exploration of this method of interaction has yielded evidence that gesture based mobile games have potential for engaging older adults in range of motion exercises (Sunwoo et al., 2010). Thus, it is reasonable to assume that accelerometers and gyroscopes could be valuable for such purposes as they are relevant to mPHRs.

A variety of possibilities are created because mPHRs are accessed through mobile devices. Some of these opportunities include delivering information to consumers through SMS, MMS, and TTS, as well as allowing consumers to enter information and interact with mPHRs through voice commands, gestures, eye movements and physically manipulating the mobile device.

Integrating Functionality from Consumer mHealth Applications

There is currently sparse evidence linking mPHR use to improved patient outcomes; however, the evidence is mounting in support using consumer mHealth applications for an array of purposes. Multiple independent consumer mHealth applications could demonstrate value if effectively incorporated into mPHRs. Further, given the commonalities between consumer mHealth applications and mPHRs, insight from research in the previous domain can be used to inform the latter.

Perhaps one of the most promising purposes for PHRs and mPHRs alike, as well as one of the most popular research topics for consumer mHealth applications, is the potential utility of scaffolding self-management and monitoring in people with chronic illnesses. Chronic illnesses (e.g., arthritis, cancer, chronic obstructive pulmonary disease, diabetes, heart disease, high blood pressure) cannot be cured and often occur in conjunction with other chronic illnesses. Management of chronic illnesses may benefit from frequent (i.e., several times a day) consumer reports of health and wellbeing (e.g., peak flow measurements, sleep quality). As consumers who have mobile devices are rarely without them, they are ideal for the collection of real-time personal health data and the delivery of information to facilitate self-management. In a review by Holtz and Lauckner (2012), trends of improved self-efficacy, hemoglobin A1c, and self-management behaviors were found in the studies of consumer mHealth applications for supporting diabetics. Given their demonstrated effectiveness, it is likely that mPHRs will adopt functionality to facilitate self-management of diabetes and other chronic illnesses.

If incorporated into mPHRs, other potential functionality that may benefit users include offering preliminary screening tools, providing educational resources, and facilitating access to healthcare services. These features have been already developed as independent consumer mHealth applications. For example, preliminary screening tools for hearing, vision, and sleep apnea are available (see Pope, Silva, & Almeyda, 2010). Preliminary screenings may be a rapid, cost-effective way to determine whether more robust, traditional screening methods are necessary. Additionally, the Detroit Medical Center (DMC) currently offers two consumer mHealth application educational resources aimed to educate parents and pregnant women (DMC, 2013). Both the DMC ER Wait Times application (DMC, 2013) and the Alberta Health Services (AHS, 2013) smartphone applications were launched to expedite access to emergency services by providing users with local hospital wait times, phone numbers, and directions. The AHS application also offers information about other nearby healthcare facilities, programs, services, and immunization clinics. By offering consumers different types of consumer mHealth applications, the DMC and AHS seek to engage and educate consumers, as well as help their users make better use of emergency services in critical situations. iTriage is a consumer mHealth application that has recently been integrated with Microsoft's HealthVault PHR (Microsoft, 2013). Several million patients previously used iTriage to view information on symptoms, procedures, medications, diseases, facilities, and healthcare providers. By integrating this application with Microsoft HealthVault, users of iTriage can also now view their records (stored on HealthVault) when using the iPhone application (Microsoft, 2013). It is expected that this trend for integrating consumer health applications with PHRs will continue and lead to greater usage of mPHRs by the general population.

mPHRs may a help extend the length of time older adults can live independently, by increasing physical activity, and providing alerts and information in case of emergency. Consumer mHealth applications have shown limited success for tracking dementia patients (Miskelly, 2005). However, using mobile devices to detect falls (e.g., Lee & Carlisle, 2011; Zhang, Wang, Liu, & Hou, 2006) and automatically contact emergency services (Sposaro, & Tyson, 2009) have shown promise and could be beneficial if incorporated into mPHRs. Consumer mHealth applications for fall detection and tracking are both ineffective, if the consumer is not wearing the mobile device at the time of the event (i.e., fall, or wandering). This may be exacerbated by some consumers' reluctance against carrying the mobile device continuously due to its size and weight (e.g., Miskelly, 2005) or simply forgetting to carry the device. Thus, it may be prudent to explore compact wearable devices that are more comfortable and less likely to be forgotten. Despite these potential limitations, developing mPHRs that can detect falls, contact the user's emergency contact and/or emergency services, as well as provide crucial health information upon arrival at the hospital have potential value.

From a telehealth perspective, mPHRs are very encouraging (Simon & Seldon, 2012). Telehealth aims to "maintain or improve the health of people outside the normal healthcare infrastructure" (Simon & Sneldon, 2012, p. 125). The University of Pittsburgh Medical Center offers an eVisit service that enables consumers to interact with their healthcare providers remotely, in real-time, which may be very valuable for users who have difficulty commuting to healthcare facilities due to the distance or mobility challenges (UPMC, 2013). Additionally, mPHRs may overcome data collection limitations. Specifically, Simon and Sneldon (2012) identified three key limitations of collecting biosensor information restricted to traditional healthcare facilities (e.g., clinics, hospitals) that could be overcome by mPHR monitoring in naturalistic, daily environments. Specifically, the limitations to monitoring solely within healthcare facilities are:

1. Failure to sample rare events.
2. Failure to measure physiological responses during normal periods of activity, rest, and sleep.
3. Brief periods of monitoring cannot capture rhythmic variations in physiological signals (Simon & Sneldon, 2012, p. 126).

Home telemonitoring, or collecting a consumer's physiological and/or biological data while at home and transferring the data to remotely located providers, overcomes some of these limitations, but mobile monitoring offers consumers even more flexibility and freedom. Evidence has shown that home telemonitoring improved clinical outcomes for diabetes, asthma, and hypertension (Paré, Moqadem, Pineau, & St-Hilaire, 2010). As biosensors (i.e., devices that collect physiological and/or biological data) become increasingly compact and portable, it is increasingly possible to monitor consumers beyond the confines of the home, in any location through mPHRs. Although mPHRs exhibit potential for monitoring, few available mPHRs are currently equipped with monitoring capabilities, and furthermore, no research was found identifying the benefits and challenges of mPHR monitoring.

A variety of biosensors are available that work in conjunction with mobile devices and the data they collect include: heart rate, pulse, blood oxygen saturation, blood glucose, temperature, and weight. Another recently developed biosensor is a phone case embedded with electrodes that works as a single lead electrocardiogram (ECG) (Lau et al., 2013). The developers of this mobile ECG suggest that it will facilitate large-scale community screenings to detect atrial fibrillation (Lau et al., 2013). Using mobile devices to collect continuous physiological information, which can be stored in an mPHR, is a valuable approach to providing baseline or prototypical consumer data that can used for comparison during healthcare events (e.g., diagnosis of chronic illness, acute injury). In addition to monitoring physiological data, it may be beneficial to use mPHRs to deliver questionnaires and monitor consumers' self-reported health status. Bielle and colleagues (2004) found some success administering quality-of-life questionnaires remotely to cancer inpatients, which led them to posit that this method could result in earlier detection of suffering and improved intervention timing. Thus, mPHRs may soon enable the collection and storage of physiological, biological, and self-reported health statuses, to facilitate care provision.

mPHRs may soon follow the lead of consumer mHealth applications as meands of delivering interventions. Mobile interventions have the potential to mitigate obstacles associated with "accessing, sustaining and benefiting from clinic-based services" (Depp et al., 2010, p. 2). Evidence suggests that mobile interventions may be viable options for health promotion to help users adopt healthy behaviours. Specifically, several studies supported using consumer mHealth applications to help consumers lose weight (Kubota, Fujita, & Hatano, 2004; Patrick et al., 2009; Wang, Kogashiwa, Ohta, & Kira, 2002), increase physical activity (Consolvo, Everitt, Smith, & Landay, 2006; Hurling et al., 2007), quit smoking (Bramley et al., 2005; Free et al., 2009; Free et al., 2011; Lazev, Vidrine, Arduino, & Gritz, 2004; Obermayer, Riley, Asif, & Jean-Mary, 2004; Rodgers et al., 2005; Vidrine, Arduino, & Gritz, 2006a; Vidrine, Arduino, Lazev, & Gritz, 2006b), as well as reduce drug use (Freedman, Lester, McNamara, Milby, & Schumacher, 2006) and alcohol consumption (Collins, Kashdan, & Gollnisch, 2003; Wilkins, Casswell, Barnes, & Pledger, 2003). In addition to health promotion, mobile interventions have been investigated for medication adherence (Brath et al., 2013), mental illness (Depp et al., 2010), and prenatal beliefs and behaviour (Evans et al., 2012). mPHRs could benefit from offering interventions such as these to consumers and allowing them to opt in (and out) of these programs at their discretion.

Perhaps unsurprisingly, most consumer mHealth applications have been developed to serve a single, isolated purpose (e.g., monitoring blood glucose). However, many individuals have an array of different conditions or needs that mPHRs have the potential to meet and further, these needs may vary over time. Depending on their unique condition(s), consumers may require a variety of specialized mobile applications to serve their individual health needs. Indeed, an mPHR has the potential to satiate user needs by providing a selection of tools that can be tailored to the individual and adapt to their changing needs over time. Furthermore, this type of mPHR is destined to provide a more comprehensive perspective of the user's health. However, added functionality is typically associated with added complexity making them more difficult to use; this obstacle must be overcome in order for mPHRs to reach their potential.

FUTURE RESEARCH DIRECTIONS FOR mPHRs

This next generation of PHRs delivered through mobile devices, or mPHRs, is expected to enable a new set of complementary capabilities for consumers to participate in their health and carry their health information wherever they go. Despite the vast potential of mPHRs, and their availability, there is currently very limited evidence to support their use. Throughout this chapter, different potential users, use contexts, and various opportunities and challenges associated with mPHRs were presented. All of the topics identified here require investigation.

Investigations should be devoted to identifying different types of target users' and their distinct characteristics and needs. It is encouraged that new studies aim to explore the needs of different potential mPHR user groups, what functions they want and will use, as well as where and when mPHRs will be used. Some conjunctures were made about how mPHRs could be valuable for different types of users; however, the needs of these groups may differ and should be investigated before and during development (i.e., adopt a user-centred, iterative, design process). It is unlikely that a single mPHR solution will meet the distinct needs and preferences of different user groups, or even the same user over time. Therefore, it is important to explore the different characteristics (e.g., age, illnesses) of mPHRs users and how their needs vary. Additionally, communicating with users who have different levels of health literacy should also be considered to ensure the information is understandable and to increase the accuracy of the data in the mPHR. Thus, flexible mPHRs, that can accommodate different user needs initially, as well as their evolving knowledge and skills over time, should be explored.

The advantages and disadvantages of having ubiquitous personal health records (i.e., mPHRs) should also be explored. That is, where and when mPHRs can demonstrate the most utility, and in what situations are they less useful or potentially problematic (e.g., compromising privacy) should be examined.

Several challenges associated with mPHR use require further attention. Not only are there the physical constraints associated with mobile devices, but consumers' levels of health literacy, and usability evaluation are issues that require investigation to reveal effective strategies to ameliorate these potential obstacles. Although the tools for collecting usability test data are becoming increasingly robust, there are still challenges associated with testing mPHRs "in situ". However, given their nearly limitless use environments, it is imperative to test these systems beyond the confines of the laboratory, to reveal usability problems that only arise in real world situations. A wide range of scenarios where users access their health records using mPHRs are possible and new usability challenges are likely to arise given this unprecedented accessibility. Further, users are not static and their needs may change over time; therefore, mPHRs should be designed to adapt to users' evolving needs.

Despite the challenges associated with mPHRs, there are many inherent opportunities created through these systems. New ways of delivering (e.g., TTS, MMS), entering (e.g., SMS, speech recognition), health information, as well as new methods of interacting (e.g., eye tracking) with mPHRs warrant exploration. These new methods may contribute to overcoming health literacy challenges, as well as difficulty entering data into an mPHR.

Although the features and functionality of mPHRs is generally limited at the moment, it is reasonable to expect the number of mPHR functions available will increase. Given the current expansion and success of consumer mHealth applications that could complement the information in mPHRs, it is anticipated that many of these functions will soon become integrated and offered through mPHRs. Some of the anticipated benefits of incorporating consumer mHealth applications into mPHRs include facilitating self-management of chronic illnesses, providing educational resources, pre-screening for health problems, expediting service delivery, monitoring conditions, complementing care for older adults, and delivering interventions. Further, the timing of information and how interventions are delivered are also important considerations for mPHRs, in order to maximize their opportunity for success. Moreover, whether mPHR use is actually related to user empowerment, enhanced understanding and participation, as well as improved self-management has yet to be empirically supported.

CONCLUSION

In this chapter, examples of currently available mPHRs were described and speculations were made regarding the potential users and use contexts of mPHRs. mPHRs are emergent consumer health information systems and there are a variety of different directions mPHRs may take in the future. Additionally, some of the challenges and opportunities regarding mPHR development, which constitute some of the future research directions, were discussed. Although PHRs are rapidly expanding into the mHealth environment, there is a dearth of research evidence supporting their use. Furthermore, most mPHRs currently available have limited value, because they are stand-alone systems (i.e., not integrated with a consumer's electronic health record) and/or do not offer tools that can be tailored to each user to foster health promotion and facilitate illness management. Thus, we anticipate that as mPHRs mature, more research will be focused on their efficacy, as well as how to integrate them with other health information systems and consumer mHealth applications to maximize their utility.

Given that mPHRs have recently been developed, it is not surprising that there is an array of topics requiring research. Future studies should aim to reveal how to optimize mPHRs by overcoming the obstacles and capitalizing on the opportunities inherent to mPHRs. Usability evaluation for mPHRs is critical to increase the likelihood of their adoption. That is, a successful mPHR will leverage the benefits of mPHRs and ensure that it can be used quickly and easily. mPHRs are bound to include more functionality to better serve their users and hopefully exchange information with other information systems. As these systems evolve, one of the biggest challenges facing mPHR designers is to conceal their complexity and provide a streamlined user experience.

REFERENCES

AHS. (2013). *Alberta Health Services*. Retrieved October 17, 2013 from www.albertahealthservices.ca/mobile.asp

Årsand, E., & Demiris, G. (2008). User-centered methods for designing patient-centric self-help tools. *Informatics for Health & Social Care*, *33*(3), 158–169. doi:10.1080/17538150802457562 PMID:18850399

Årsand, E., Frøisland, D. H., Skrøvseth, S. O., Chomutare, T., Tatara, N., Hartvigsen, G., & Tufano, J. T. (2012). Mobile health applications to assist patients with diabetes: Lessons learned and design implications. *Journal of Diabetes Science and Technology*, *6*(5), 1197–1206. doi:10.1177/193229681200600525 PMID:23063047

Baker, D. W. (2006). The meaning and the measure of health literacy. *Journal of General Internal Medicine*, *21*(8), 878–883. doi:10.1111/j.1525-1497.2006.00540.x PMID:16881951

Bardram, J., Mihailidis, A., & Wan, D. (Eds.), *Pervasive Computing in Healthcare*. New York: CRC Press.

Bielli, E., Carminati, F., La Capra, S., Lina, M., Brunelli, C., & Tamburini, M. (2004). A wireless health outcomes monitoring system (WHOMS), Development and field testing with cancer patients using mobile phones. *BMC Medical Informatics and Decision Making*, *4*(1), 7–7. doi:10.1186/1472-6947-4-7 PMID:15196308

Botts, N. E., Horan, T. A., & Thoms, B. P. (2011). HealthATM: Personal health cyberinfrastructure for underserved populations. *American Journal of Preventive Medicine*, *40*(5), S115–S122. doi:10.1016/j.amepre.2011.01.016 PMID:21521584

Bramley, D., Riddell, T., Whittaker, R., Corbett, T., Lin, R., Wills, M., & Rodgers, A. (2005). Smoking cessation using mobile phone text messaging is as effective in Maori as non-Maori. *The New Zealand Medical Journal*, *118*(1216), U1494. PMID:15937529

Brandt, J., Weiss, N., & Klemmer, S. R. (2007). txt 4 l8r: Lowering the burden for diary studies under mobile conditions. In *Proceedings of CHI'07 Extended Abstracts on Human Factors in Computing Systems* (pp. 2303-2308). ACM. doi:10.1145/1240866.1240998

Brath, H., Morak, J., Kästenbauer, T., Modre-Osprian, R., Strohner-Kästenbauer, H., Schwarz, M., & Schreier, G. (2013). Mobile health (mHealth) based medication adherence measurement – A pilot trial using electronic blisters in diabetes patients. *British Journal of Clinical Pharmacology*, *76*, 47–55. doi:10.1111/bcp.12184 PMID:24007452

Canadian Council on Learning. (2008). *Health Literacy in Canada: A Healthy Understanding*. Retrieved March 17, 2013, from http://www.ccl-cca.ca/pdfs/HealthLiteracy/HealthLiteracyReportFeb2008E.pdf

Chen, E., Medonca, E., McKnight, L., Stetson, P., Lei, J., & Cimino, J. (2003). PalmCIS: A wireless handheld application for satisfying clinician information needs. *Journal of the American Medical Informatics Association*, *11*(1), 19–28. doi:10.1197/jamia.M1387 PMID:14527976

Cheng, S. (2011). The research framework of eye-tracking based mobile device usability evaluation. In *Proceedings of the 1st International Workshop on Pervasive Eye Tracking & Mobile Eye-Based Interaction* (pp. 21-26). ACM. doi:10.1145/2029956.2029964

Cimino, J. J., Patel, V. L., & Kushniruk, A. W. (2002). The patient clinical information system (PatCIS), Technical solutions for and experiences with giving patients access to their electronic medical records. *International Journal of Medical Informatics*, *68*(1-3), 113–127. doi:10.1016/S1386-5056(02)00070-9 PMID:12467796

Cleland, J., Caldow, J., & Ryan, D. (2007). A qualitative study of the attitudes of patients and staff to the use of mobile phone technology for recording and gathering asthma data. *Journal of Telemedicine and Telecare*, *13*(2), 85–89. doi:10.1258/135763307780096230 PMID:17359572

Collins, R. L., Kashdan, T. B., & Gollnisch, G. (2003). The feasibility of using cellular phones to collect ecological momentary assessment data: Application to alcohol consumption. *Experimental and Clinical Psychopharmacology*, *11*(1), 73–78. doi:10.1037/1064-1297.11.1.73 PMID:12622345

Consolvo, S., Everitt, K., Smith, I., & Landay, J. (2006). *Design requirements for technologies that encourage physical activity*. doi:10.1145/1124772.1124840

CSI. (2013). *motionPHR*. Retrieved October 8, 2013, from http://motionphr.com/

Depp, C. A., Mausbach, B., Granholm, E., Cardenas, V., Ben-Zeev, D., Patterson, T. L., & Jeste, D. V. (2010). Mobile interventions for severe mental illness: Design and preliminary data from three approaches. *The Journal of Nervous and Mental Disease*, *198*(10), 715–721. doi:10.1097/NMD.0b013e3181f49ea3 PMID:20921861

DeWalt, D. A., Berkman, N. D., Sheridan, S., Lohr, K. N., & Pignone, M. P. (2004). Literacy and health outcomes: A systematic review of the literature. *Journal of General Internal Medicine*, *19*(12), 1228–1239. doi:10.1111/j.1525-1497.2004.40153.x PMID:15610334

DMC. (2013). *Detroit Medical Center*. Retrieved October 17, 2013, from www.dmc.org/apps

Epic. (2013). *Epic Systems Corporation: Mobile Applications and Portals*. Retrieved October 8, 2013, from http://www.epic.com/software-phr.php

Evans, W. D., Wallace, J. L., & Snider, J. (2012). Pilot evaluation of the text4baby mobile health program. *BMC Public Health*, *12*(1), 1031. doi:10.1186/1471-2458-12-1031 PMID:23181985

Free, C., Roberts, I., Knight, R., Robertson, S., Whittaker, R., Edwards, P., & Kenward, M. G. (2011). Smoking cessation support delivered via mobile phone text messaging (txt2stop), A single-blind, randomised trial. *Lancet*, *378*(9785), 49–55. doi:10.1016/S0140-6736(11)60701-0 PMID:21722952

Free, C., Whittaker, R., Knight, R., Abramsky, T., Rodgers, A., & Roberts, I. G. (2009). Txt2stop: A pilot randomised controlled trial of mobile phone-based smoking cessation support. *Tobacco Control*, *18*(2), 88–91. doi:10.1136/tc.2008.026146 PMID:19318534

Freedman, M. J., Lester, K. M., McNamara, C., Milby, J. B., & Schumacher, J. E. (2006). Cell phones for ecological momentary assessment with cocaine-addicted homeless patients in treatment. *Journal of Substance Abuse Treatment*, *30*(2), 105–111. doi:10.1016/j.jsat.2005.10.005 PMID:16490673

Haggstrom, D. A., Saleem, J. J., Russ, A. L., Jones, J., Russell, S. A., & Chumbler, N. R. (2011). Lessons learned from usability testing of the VA's personal health record. *Journal of the American Medical Informatics Association*, *18*(Suppl 1), i13–i17. doi:10.1136/amiajnl-2010-000082 PMID:21984604

Halamka, J., Mandl, K., & Tang, P. (2007). Early experiences with personal health records. *Journal of the American Medical Informatics Association*, *15*(1), 1–7. doi:10.1197/jamia.M2562 PMID:17947615

Health Council of Canada. (2010). *Helping patients help themselves: Are Canadians with chronic conditions getting the support they need to manage their health?* Toronto, Canada: Health Council of Canada.

Holtz, B., & Lauckner, C. (2012). Diabetes management via mobile phones: A systematic review. *Telemedicine Journal and e-Health*, *18*(3), 175–184. doi:10.1089/tmj.2011.0119 PMID:22356525

Househ, M., Borycki, E., Kushniruk, A., & Alofaysan, S. (2012). mHealth: A passing fad or here to stay? In Telemedicine and E-health Services, Policies, and Applications: Advancements and Developments. Hershey, PA: IGI Global.

Hurling, R., Catt, M., Boni, M. D., Fairley, B. W., Hurst, T., Murray, P., & Sodhi, J. S. (2007). Using internet and mobile phone technology to deliver an automated physical activity program: Randomized controlled trial. *Journal of Medical Internet Research*, *9*(2), e7. doi:10.2196/jmir.9.2.e7 PMID:17478409

Istepanian, R. S. H., Jovanov, E., & Zhang, Y. T. (2004). Guest editorial introduction to the special section on M-health: Beyond seamless mobility and global wireless health-care connectivity. *IEEE Transactions on Information Technology in Biomedicine*, *8*(4), 405–414. doi:10.1109/TITB.2004.840019 PMID:15615031

Jaspers, M. W. M. (2009). A comparison of usability methods for testing interactive health technologies: Methodological aspects and empirical evidence. *International Journal of Medical Informatics*, *78*(5), 340–353. doi:10.1016/j.ijmedinf.2008.10.002 PMID:19046928

Jones, D. A., Shipman, J. P., Plaut, D. A., & Selden, C. R. (2010). Characteristics of personal health records: Findings of the medical library association/national library of medicine joint electronic personal health record task force. *Journal of the Medical Library Association: JMLA*, *98*(3), 243–249. doi:10.3163/1536-5050.98.3.013 PMID:20648259

Kaelber, D., & Pan, E. C. (2008). The value of personal health record (PHR) systems. In *Proceedings of AMIA Annual Symposium*. American Medical Informatics Association.

Keckley, P. H., & Hoffman, M. (2010). *2010 Survey of Health Care Consumers: Key Findings, Strategic Implications*. Deloitte Center for Health Solutions. Retrieved October 10, 2013, from http://www.deloitte.com/assets/Dcom-UnitedStates/Local%20Assets/Documents/US_CHS_2010SurveyofHealthCareConsumers_050310.pdf

Kharrazi, H., Chisholm, R., VanNasdale, D., & Thompson, B. (2012). Mobile personal health records: An evaluation of features and functionality. *International Journal of Medical Informatics*, *81*(9), 579–593. doi:10.1016/j.ijmedinf.2012.04.007 PMID:22809779

Kubota, A., Fujita, M., & Hatano, Y. (2004). Development and effects of a health promotion program utilizing the mail function of mobile phones. *Japanese Journal of Public Health*, *51*(10), 862. PMID:15565995

Kurniawan, S., Mahmud, M., & Nugroho, Y. (2006). *A study of the use of mobile phones by older persons*. doi:10.1145/1125451.1125641

Kushniruk, A. (2002). Evaluation in the design of health information systems: Application of approaches emerging from usability engineering. *Computers in Biology and Medicine*, *32*(3), 141–149. doi:10.1016/S0010-4825(02)00011-2 PMID:11922931

Kushniruk, A. W., Borycki, E. M., Kuwata, S., & Kannry, J. (2011). Emerging approaches to usability evaluation of health information systems: Towards in-situ analysis of complex healthcare systems and environments. *Studies in Health Technology and Informatics*, *169*, 915. PMID:21893879

Kushniruk, A. W., Patel, V. L., & Cimino, J. J. (1997). Usability testing in medical informatics: Cognitive approaches to evaluation of information systems and user interfaces. In *Proceedings of the AMIA Annual Fall Symposium* (pp. 218). American Medical Informatics Association.

Lau, J. K., Lowres, N., Neubeck, L., Brieger, D. B., Sy, R. W., Galloway, C. D., & Freedman, S. B. (2013). iPhone ECG application for community screening to detect silent atrial fibrillation: A novel technology to prevent stroke. *International Journal of Cardiology*, *165*(1), 193–194. doi:10.1016/j.ijcard.2013.01.220 PMID:23465249

Lazev, A., Vidrine, D., Arduino, R., & Gritz, E. (2004). Increasing access to smoking cessation treatment in a low-income, HIV-positive population: The feasibility of using cellular telephones. *Nicotine & Tobacco Research: Official Journal of the Society for Research on Nicotine and Tobacco*, *6*(2), 281–286. doi:10.1080/14622200410001676314 PMID:15203801

Lee, R. Y. W., & Carlisle, A. J. (2011). Detection of falls using accelerometers and mobile phone technology. *Age and Ageing*, *40*(6), 690–696. doi:10.1093/ageing/afr050 PMID:21596711

Leung, R., McGrenere, J., & Graf, P. (2011). Age-related differences in the initial usability of mobile device icons. *Behaviour & Information Technology*, *30*(5), 629–642. doi:10.1080/01449290903171308

Leung, R., Tang, C., Haddad, S., Mcgrenere, J., Graf, P., & Ingriany, V. (2012). How older adults learn to use mobile devices: Survey and field investigations. *ACM Transactions on Accessible Computing*, *4*(3), 1–33. doi:10.1145/2399193.2399195

McGillicuddy, J. W., Weiland, A. K., Frenzel, R. M., Mueller, M., Brunner-Jackson, B. M., Taber, D. J., & Treiber, F. A. (2013). Patient attitudes toward mobile phone-based health monitoring: Questionnaire study among kidney transplant recipients. *Journal of Medical Internet Research*, *15*(1), e6. doi:10.2196/jmir.2284 PMID:23305649

Microsoft. (2013). *Microsoft HealthVault Personal Health Record Goes Mobile in 2012 with iTriage*. Retrieved October 8, 2013, from http://www.prweb.com/releases/2011/12/prweb9064141.htm

Miluzzo, E., Wang, T., & Campbell, A. (2010). *EyePhone: Activating mobile phones with your eyes*. doi:10.1145/1851322.1851328

Miskelly, F. (2005). Electronic tracking of patients with dementia and wandering using mobile phone technology. *Age and Ageing*, *34*(5), 497–499. doi:10.1093/ageing/afi145 PMID:16107453

Monkman, H., & Kushniruk, A. W. (2013a). A Health Literacy and Usability Heuristic Evaluation of a Mobile Consumer Health Application. *Studies in Health Technology and Informatics*, *192*, 724. PMID:23920652

Monkman, H., & Kushniruk, A. W. (2013b). Applying Usability Methods to Identify Health Literacy Issues: An Example Using a Personal Health Record. *Studies in Health Technology and Informatics*, *183*, 179–185. PMID:23388278

Nielsen, J., & Budiu, R. (2012). *Mobile usability*. Pearson Education.

Nmawston. (2012, October 17). Worldwide smartphone population tops 1 billion in Q3 2012. *Strategy Analytics*.

Nutbeam, D. (1998). Health promotion glossary. *Health Promotion International*, *13*(4), 349–364. doi:10.1093/heapro/13.4.349

Obermayer, J. L., Riley, W. T., Asif, O., & Jean-Mary, J. (2004). College smoking-cessation using cell phone text messaging. *Journal of American College Health*, *53*(2), 71–78. doi:10.3200/JACH.53.2.71-78 PMID:15495883

Pagliari, C., Detmer, D., & Singleton, P. (2007). Potential of electronic personal health records. *BMJ (Clinical Research Ed.)*, *335*(7615), 330–333. doi:10.1136/bmj.39279.482963.AD PMID:17703042

Paré, G., Moqadem, K., Pineau, G., & St-Hilaire, C. (2010). Clinical effects of home telemonitoring in the context of diabetes, asthma, heart failure and hypertension: A systematic review. *Journal of Medical Internet Research*, *12*(2), e21. doi:10.2196/jmir.1357 PMID:20554500

Patrick, K., Raab, F., Adams, M. A., Dillon, L., Zabinski, M., Rock, C. L., & Norman, G. J. (2009). A text message-based intervention for weight loss: Randomized controlled trial. *Journal of Medical Internet Research*, *11*(1), e1. doi:10.2196/jmir.1100 PMID:19141433

Pino, C., & Kavasidis, I. (2012). Improving mobile device interaction by eye tracking analysis. In *Proceedings of Computer Science and Information Systems (FedCSIS), 2012 Federated Conference on* (pp. 1199-1202). IEEE.

Pope, L., Silva, P., & Almeyda, R. (2010). i-Phone applications for the modern day otolaryngologist. *Clinical Otolaryngology: Official Journal of ENT-UK. Official Journal of Netherlands Society for Oto-Rhino-Laryngology & Cervico-Facial Surgery*, *35*(4), 350. doi:10.1111/j.1749-4486.2010.02170.x

Protti, D. (2008). A comparison of how Canada, England and Demark are managing their electronic health record journeys. In *Human, Social and Organizational Aspects of Healthcare Information Systems*. Hershey, PA: IGI Global. doi:10.4018/978-1-59904-792-8.ch012

Proudfoot, J., Parker, G., Hadzi Pavlovic, D., Manicavasagar, V., Adler, E., & Whitton, A. (2010). Community attitudes to the appropriation of mobile phones for monitoring and managing depression, anxiety, and stress. *Journal of Medical Internet Research*, *12*(5), e64. doi:10.2196/jmir.1475 PMID:21169174

Rodgers, A., Corbett, T., Bramley, D., Riddell, T., Wills, M., Lin, R., & Jones, M. (2005). Do u smoke after txt? Results of a randomised trial of smoking cessation using mobile phone text messaging. *Tobacco Control*, *14*(4), 255–261. doi:10.1136/tc.2005.011577 PMID:16046689

Samsung. (2013). How do I use Air Gestures to control my Samsung Galaxy S® 4? In *How to Guides*. Retrieved, November 1, 2013, from http://www.samsung.com/us/support/howtoguide/N0000003/10141/120552

Segall, N., Saville, J. G., L'Engle, P., Carlson, B., Wright, M. C., Schulman, K., & Tcheng, J. E. (2011). Usability evaluation of a personal health record. In *Proceedings of AMIA Annual Symposium*. American Medical Informatics Association.

Shiffman, S., Stone, A. A., & Hufford, M. R. (2008). Ecological momentary assessment. *Annual Review of Clinical Psychology*, *4*(1), 1–32. doi:10.1146/annurev.clinpsy.3.022806.091415 PMID:18509902

Siegenthaler, E., Wurtz, P., & Groner, R. (2010). Improving the usability of e-book readers. *Journal of Usability Studies*, *6*(1), 25–38.

Simon, S. K., & Seldon, H. L. (2012). Personal health records: Mobile biosensors and smartphones for developing countries. *Studies in Health Technology and Informatics*, *182*, 125. PMID:23138087

Singh, R. I., Sumeeth, M., & Miller, J. (2011). Evaluating the Readability of Privacy Policies in Mobile Environments. *International Journal of Mobile Human Computer Interaction*, *3*(1), 55–78. doi:10.4018/jmhci.2011010104

Smith, A. (2011, September 19). *Americans and text messaging*. Pew Internet & American Life Project: A Project of the Pew Research Center. Retrieved from http://www.pewinternet.org/~/media//Files/Reports/2011/Americans%20and%20Text%20Messaging.pdf

Sourceforge. (2013). *Android Screenshots and Screen Capture*. Retrieved November 8, 2013, from http://sourceforge.net/projects/ashot/

Sposaro, F., & Tyson, G. (2009). iFall: An Android application for fall monitoring and response. In Proceedings of Engineering in Medicine and Biology Society, (pp. 6119-6122). IEEE.

Squirrels. (2013). Reflector. In *Products*. Retrieved November 8, 2013, from http://www.airsquirrels.com/reflector/

Sunwoo, J., Yuen, W., Lutteroth, C., & Wünsche, B. (2010). Mobile games for elderly healthcare. In *Proceedings of the 11th International Conference of the NZ Chapter of the ACM Special Interest Group on Human-Computer Interaction* (pp. 73-76). ACM.

Tang, P. C., Ash, J. S., Bates, D. W., Overhage, J. M., & Sands, D. Z. (2006). Personal health records: Definitions, benefits, and strategies for overcoming barriers to adoption. *Journal of the American Medical Informatics Association*, *13*(2), 121–126. doi:10.1197/jamia.M2025 PMID:16357345

UPMC. (2013). *HealthTrak: Your health online – and on your schedule*. Retrieved November 2, 2013, from https://myupmc.upmc.com/

U.S. Department of Health and Human Services. (2010). *Health literacy online: A guide to writing and designing easy-to-use health Web sites.* Retrieved July 4, 2013, from http://www.health.gov/healthliteracyonline/

Vargas, P. A., Robles, E., Harris, J., & Radford, P. (2010). Using information technology to reduce asthma disparities in underserved populations: A pilot study. *The Journal of Asthma: Official Journal of the Association for the Care of Asthma*, *47*(8), 889–894. doi:10.3109/02770903.2010.497887 PMID:20846082

Vidrine, D. J., Arduino, R. C., & Gritz, E. R. (2006a). Impact of a cell phone intervention on mediating mechanisms of smoking cessation in individuals living with HIV/AIDS. *Nicotine & Tobacco Research: Official Journal of the Society for Research on Nicotine and Tobacco*, *8*(1), S103–S108. doi:10.1080/14622200601039451 PMID:17491177

Vidrine, D. J., Arduino, R. C., Lazev, A. B., & Gritz, E. R. (2006b). A randomized trial of a proactive cellular telephone intervention for smokers living with HIV/AIDS. *AIDS (London, England)*, *20*(2), 253–260. doi:10.1097/01.aids.0000198094.23691.58 PMID:16511419

Wang, D., Kogashiwa, M., Ohta, S., & Kira, S. (2002). Validity and reliability of a dietary assessment method: The application of a digital camera with a mobile phone card attachment. *Journal of Nutritional Science and Vitaminology*, *48*(6), 498–504. doi:10.3177/jnsv.48.498 PMID:12775117

Wilkins, C., Casswell, S., Barnes, H. M., & Pledger, M. (2003). A pilot study of a computer assisted cell phone interview (CACI) methodology to survey respondents in households without telephones about alcohol use. *Drug and Alcohol Review*, *22*(2), 221–225. doi:10.1080/09595230100100651 PMID:12850908

Zhang, T., Wang, J., Liu, P., & Hou, J. (2006). Fall detection by embedding an accelerometer in cellphone and using KFD algorithm. *International Journal of Computer Science and Network Security*, *6*(10), 277–284.

KEY TERMS AND DEFINITIONS

Consumer mHealth Application: A program for use by laypeople to educate and/or monitor and/or manage health information delivered on mobile platforms (e.g., smartphones, tablets).

Electronic Health Record (EHR): An integrated, longitudinal patient record curated by healthcare providers that is electronically stored and accessed.

Health Information System (HIS): An electronic system that enables the acquisition, storage, management and sharing of health information (e.g., laboratory reports, prescriptions, immunizations) for different health-related purposes (e.g., disease surveillance, clinical decision-making, development of management plans).

Health Literacy: The ability for consumers to find, acquire, and understand health information and use this information to guide health-related decisions.

Mobile Health (mHealth): The use of mobile platforms (e.g., smartphones, tablets) to deliver health information systems.

Mobile Personal Health Record (mPHR): A Personal Health Record (PHR) integrated with a consumer mHealth application or mobile platform.

Personal Health Record (PHR): A record accessed and/or curated by consumers' containing their own clinical health information.

Telehealth: Healthcare delivery or data collection conducted remotely, beyond the confines of traditional clinical environments (e.g., hospitals, primary care facilities).

Usability: The ease and efficiency with which a tool can be used to accomplish a given task.

This work was previously published in Social Media and Mobile Technologies for Healthcare edited by Mowafa Househ, Elizabeth Borycki, and Andre Kushniruk, pages 281-303, copyright year 2014 by Medical Information Science Reference (an imprint of IGI Global).

Chapter 9
Electronic Patient Records (EPR), Library Services (LS) and Multidisciplinary Team (MDT) Meetings:
Is It Not Time to Integrate Primary Care for the Better?

Shahid Muhammad
The Renal Patient Support Group (RPSG), UK

Malcolm Rigler
NHS North Somerset Clinical Commissioning Group (CCG), UK

Meshia Adams
Meshia's Hope, USA

ABSTRACT

Patients with Long-Term Conditions (LTCs) account for around 50% of General Practitioner (GP) appointments, 64% of outpatient appointments and 70% of hospital bed days. There needs to be a wider access to knowledge and understanding such as directories with information leaflets, documents, books on lifestyle, helpful contacts and sources to information that can support patients and the general public on the most important elements their health. This cannot be achieved just through patients accessing their health records in sole. The objective of this paper is to 1) highlight the importance of integrating General Practice (GP), Electronic Patient Records (EPR) with Library Services (LS) and 2) also explore why it would be advantageous to implement patient-centred Multidisciplinary Team (MDT) meetings in primary care for patients with Long-Term Conditions (LTCs). This article provides a UK glance and how primary care services can be improved, integrating for the better. Having access to Electronic Patient Records (EPR) alone will not help or encourage a patient to gain confidence and/ or understanding especially if patients are overwhelmed by their healthcare choices and Health Literacy (HL) complexi-

DOI: 10.4018/978-1-5225-1928-7.ch009

ties. Patients' whose first language is not English for example, approaching more methods to support HL is/ will be challenging. Library and Health Services partnerships should be initiated to allowing access to wider resources. In addition, patient-centred Multidisciplinary Team (MDT) meetings should be arranged at dedicated time points between a doctor and patient/ carer and these can take place in a private section within library setting involving wider participation in care plans. Given that more patients and the public will have opportunity to access their health records, a "Libraries and Health" partnership can help integrate primary healthcare better thus allowing all to access health-related literature, using books, leaflets and digital media in a comfortable environment in a setting that also has staff that can support with HL and technology. An EPR and MDT initiative should be supported with library and health partnerships; this needs to be encouraged.

KEY POINTS: WHAT THIS WORK ADDS

1. There is now a need for GPs to enter dialogue with and social services, to prompt tighter integrated services in primary care.
2. Electronic Patient Records (EPR) need to be supplemented by decision support, personalised care planning and self-management education from trained health professionals, as well as social support from family, friends and peers.
3. There needs to be a neutral environment where patients and health professionals can come together to provide more awareness of EPR in addition a neutral environment where patients and the public can source additional literature and context.
4. Patient-Centred Multi-Disciplinary Team (MDT) meetings will allow patient and carers to gain more EPR awareness and a tighter understanding of what their results actually mean.
5. GPs should look to pilot and implement rotation-based patient-centred MDT meetings in library environment, where one GP from a practice can rotate and call upon colleagues from primary and secondary care sectors to meet at library location where a patient is also called in for review. This should be at least piloted for patients with an LTC since they might have a number of co-morbidities and who might require further support with respect to EPR, HL and online support who would otherwise not know how to use facilities. A rotation system would allow more time for GPs to spend with patients in primary care.
6. Health Literacy (HL) is predominantly a skills-based construct that does not include motivational elements. Using modes to improve HL alone to determine the needs of patients and simplifying instructions for them as a result may be a barrier to that person, thus affecting patient and professional relationship.
7. There is an on-going need to support and work in partnership to increase awareness of local services in health and social care.

INTRODUCTION

Patients with Long-Term Conditions (LTCs) account for around 50% of General Practitioner (GP) appointments, 64% of outpatient appointments and 70% of hospital bed days (Department of Health 2012). Around 70% of total health and care expenditure in England is attributed to people with Long-Term

Conditions (LTCs) (Department of Health 2012). People diagnosed with an LTC are perhaps the most rigorous consumers of health and social care (Barnett et al. 2012).

Between 2010 and 2030, it is postulated that the number of younger adults with disabilities (aged 18–64) will increase by 32.2% from around 220,000 to around 290,000, and the number of younger adults with physical or sensory impairment by 7.5% from almost 2,900,000 to 3,100,000 (Snell et al. 2011).

In relating, coping too has an impact on how patients approach healthcare; responses used in challenge are referred to as problem-focused coping strategies. It appears palpable that what happens in one challenge that causes a person to exploit one coping approach may not automatically be the same specified for another hazard. It is evident that coping has to be observed from various implications since there are various archetypes to an individual within and outwardly, (Muhammad et al. 2012). Some coping strategies are associated with increases in positive actions and others increasing negative ones (Folkman & Lazarus 1988). Not being able to cope can make people feel excluded; have perceptions of vulnerability and outlooks of hopelessness against a backdrop of weakened health (Jones and Dutton, 2014; Luxford and Sutton, 2014; Wolf et al. 2014). Depending on how patients approach services, problem-focused coping may be one approach. This includes problem solving, information gathering, goal-setting and problem-orientation (for example, sourcing healthcare information and discussing with a professional) (O'Leary 1990).

An estimated 15 million people in England have at least one LTC with the prevalence of cancers, chronic kidney disease (CKD) and diabetes rising most quickly (Department of Health 2012). This consequently has an impact on access to lives, wider services and healthcare impact more generally (Barnett et al 2012). Already the 30% of the population with LTCs account for 70% of NHS spending (De Silva, 2011). Reducing the public's dependence on health professionals and increasing their sense of control and wellbeing is perhaps a more academic and efficient way of progressing (De Silva, 2011). Despite overwhelming evidence, patients face a number of challenges.

OBJECTIVE

The objective of this paper is to 1) highlight the importance of integrating General Practice (GP), Electronic Patient Records (EPR) with Library Services (LS) and 2) also explore why it would be advantageous to implement patient-centred Multidisciplinary Team (MDT) meetings in primary care for patients with Long-Term Conditions (LTCs). This article provides a UK glance and how primary care services can be improved, integrating for the better.

THE ISSUE WITH CURRENT PRACTICE

Living with a LTC can be viewed as a major stressful life event, characterized by a number of recurrent stressful situations that pose serious challenges to adaptation (Ridder et al. 1998; Moos and Schaeffer, 1984; Zautra, 1996). Patients have to cope with challenging situations and, depending on the results of their coping efforts; they may be able to maintain adequate levels of physical, social, and emotional functioning. Inspired by the stress-coping model of Lazarus (Lazarus 1974; Lazarus 1985; Lazarus, 1992; Lazarus, 1993a; Lazarus, 1993b), research has explored coping and adjustment of patients with illnesses (for a review see also Ridder and Schreurs, 1996; Maes et al. 1996).

Although research has provided valuable insights into the ways patients use healthcare services, it is difficult to determine the precise understanding of such a wealth of information across different illnesses. It is important to gain better insight into the type of stressors experienced by patients suffering from different diseases as information on the nature of disease-related stressors may contribute to a better understanding of patients and the general public. By implementing tighter integrated services in primary care and improving healthcare experiences, this can improve wellbeing and progress general healthcare, generally (Folkman et al. 1986; Folkman and Lazarus 1988; Folkman and Moskowitz 2000; Folkman and Moskowitz 2004;Harden et al. 2012). Understanding how patients and the public access information is thus important considering many may feel less positive about their own competencies, with some who may feel inadequately prepared about their healthcare; this places them at higher risk of poor healthcare when compared to their peers, (Ilic et al. 2005; GMC 2012; Giles 2012; Jones et al. 2014).

There needs to be a wider access to knowledge and understanding such as directories with information leaflets, documents, books on lifestyle, helpful contacts and sources to information that can support patients and the general public on the most important elements their health. This cannot be achieved through just patients accessing their medical records and general practice in sole. The issue with current practices is that there is a lack of integration not only between sectors of healthcare but also between sectors between primary care and integration in the community.

STATE OF HEALTHCARE SERVICES 'TODAY'

In the UK, the NHS and most modern health services know nothing about this way of offering "Health Services" but have been led astray by "big-pharma" and "the dominance of the medical model" into believing that it is perfectly fine for the GP to sit and wait in the consulting room for patients to come to see them when they are ill (often when the horse has bolted) or quite often these days when they have joined the ranks of "the worried well". As a profession Medicine has forgotten that the title "doctor" is derived from "docere – to teach".

GPs within the NHS and across the developed world where patients and carers have access to the internet, are increasingly finding that "internet searches" are being brought to the consultation to help patients explain their conditions to their GP to question and challenge their GPs and to seek the opinion of their GP about the information they have discovered. For many GPs this is the *"straw that breaks the camels back"* but for others this additional presence in the consultation is a great opportunity to develop the "Library and Health Partnership". Instead of trying to curb the patients' desire to study and learn about their conditions, their drugs and treatments and the ways in which they can avoid further problems it seems to some GPs to be better by far to encourage patients' and carers to become fully involved in decision making with the GP concerning matters such as diagnosis, treatment options, unwanted effects of drugs medicines and procedures, informed consent and options for self-care, self-help and home care.

LITERATURE REVIEW - HEALTH AND EDUCATION OFFER IN THE HIGH STREET

What patients and the public do in their everyday lives – what they eat, how much they exercise and how far they follow medical advice largely determines their health and their need for health care (WHO,

2005). The influence of patient behaviour on health outcomes can be seen in everything from preventing illness in the first place through to the management of LTCs. As 60 - 70% of premature deaths are caused by behaviours that could be changed (Schroeder 2007), it is essential that patients and the general public become more engaged with adopting positive health behaviours. *How can this be explored further?*

Town centres have become too reliant upon retailing. This 'function' needs to be rebalanced to provide a broader range of alternative purposes, including employment, commercial, leisure, community, residential, healthcare and education. Local authorities and public sector agencies have a key role to play in ensuring towns and cities do not lose public and private sector jobs to out-of-town locations, leaving a rotten and decaying core. Independent research organisation Centre for Cities *Beyond the High Street: Why our city centres really matter* report clearly demonstrates that where jobs are located can affect how well a city's economy performs. For example, for retail if a city has more jobs in out-of-town locations, it reduces the number of people who have to come to the city centre, (Beyond Retail, 2013).

The Longevity War Game programme on BBC Radio 4 demonstrated how Newcastle University war game was put together to identify ways to bridge the Longevity gap by 50% in ten years with no extra money. The programme highlighted that the UK faces various concerns in health services as the population ages and this is because there is a lack of healthcare integration, which should start from community and bottom-up; it is communities that need to be at the top of decision-making – not policy-makers (BBC, 2014).

Public libraries are a key social institution in many communities. They provide access to and assistance with diverse informational and recreational resources. Today especially, libraries play and will continue to play a vital role as community access points for computers, the Internet, and Internet-enabled services Bertot et al. 2012). These publicly accessible services are especially critical in an environment where a significant percentage of Internet users do not have access to the Internet at home, school, or work (Becker et al. 2010). The (2011-2012) Public Library Funding and Technology Access Study found that Bertot et al. 2010)

- 100% of public libraries offer free public Internet access
- 64.5% of public libraries report they are the only free provider of Internet access in their community
- 90.5% of public libraries offer Wi-Fi
- 60.2% of libraries reported increased usage of desktops over the previous year

HEALTHCARE INTEGRATION IN THE COMMUNITY

Almost all public libraries (99.3%) offer some form of free public Internet access. More significantly, public libraries are perhaps reported as being the only provider of free public access to computers and the Internet in 64.5% of communities. Some 90.5% of public libraries offer free wireless (Wi-Fi) access for users (Gibson et al. 2009). In addition to desktop and Internet connection, two-thirds of library computer users receive assistance in using the computer or Internet (Shuler, 1996).

Libraries provide access to and training for a range of technologies and online resources. These community access services include, but are by no means limited to, databases, homework resources, audio-visual content and e-books, and digital reference services. 99.1% of public libraries provide access to databases, and 81.9% provide access to homework resources.

To facilitate access to online resources, public libraries average 16.4 public desktop, a 2.5% increase over the past year. Almost half (45%) of all visitors to public libraries use the library's Internet access, making it one of the most-used public library services. (Jaeger et al. 2007). Opportunities for content generation are another area wherein public libraries play an important role. Almost all (93.2%) of public libraries allow the use of portable drives or other storage devices, and two-thirds (64.4%) support the use of digital cameras and other content manipulation options (Shuler, 1996).

A UK PERSPECTIVE

Although for most in the UK, the National Health Service (NHS) has been the only "Health Service" that is known and for a few people *The Peckham Experiment* in the District of Peckham in London is still within "living memory" (Pioneer Health Foundation, 2014). *The Peckham Experiment* was also known as a "Health Centre" but it offered health services vastly different from the NHS as it is today. The Health Centre was a place where near neighbours could meet each other on neutral ground, share a cup of tea or a meal together and watch their children and folk of all age groups learn to walk, to talk, to swim, to dance and play (Pioneer Health Foundation, 2014).

The key insight of *The Peckham Experiment* was that the guiding principle in the minds of the founders was that *"the environment is key to good health"*. By this the founders meant what we now call the *"psychosocial environment"*. Being able to sit around a table to share ideas and stories with other people who were from other families living in the terraced houses in the streets of Peckham surrounding the Health Centre was considered to be "vital for health and well-being". As people shared their stories of pregnancy and birth, child care and work, farm outings and seasonal events such as Christmas and seaside holidays friendships were formed, support networks were created and through the exchange of stories a great deal of shared learning took place. The "Health Professionals" at the Health Centre would join in the conversations when invited to help individuals, families and community groups to learn things that were not yet known to them such as how to access general and specialist medical services, how to pay the professional fees involved, how to encourage young people to be confident and to enjoy sport and exercise much more (Pioneer Health Foundation, 2014).

The Peckham Experiment continues to feature in BBC Radio programmes these days as an historical footnote. The building that was used is now a "listed building" in London and the 16 or more boxes of documents and research material sits waiting to be discovered in the archives of the Wellcome Foundation. The idea that the *psychosocial environment* needs attention and is important for health and well-being is now the subject of debate daily via various media streams and where people meet (Pioneer Health Foundation, 2014). There is now an increased understanding of how Information Communication and Technology (ICT) in addition to using SM can support the acquisition of knowledge and understanding for patients from varying conditions (Andersson and Lyttkens 1999; Iezzoni et al. 2000; Coughlin et al. 2002; Beatty et al. 2003). This has been demonstrated through a number of studies (Drainoni et al. 2006; Armstrong and Powell 2009; Barnett et al 2012). User-friendly ICT and SM platforms can be important for knowledge and resource acquisition integrating care. Contrast, it is important to appreciate that using ICT/ the internet for knowledge acquisition does not apply to all owing to complications of Health Literacy (HL).

THE IMPORTANCE OF HEALTH LITERACY (HL)

Whilst the Internet and Social Media (SM) usage has grown exponentially (Nielsenwire 2013), not surprisingly people are identifying new modes of sourcing information; for the technological savvy patient, the internet and SM offers advantages over standard forms of engagement/ education with wide accessibility (Xie B 2009), (Timimi 2012). The overwhelming penetration of SM into lives necessitates a renewed commitment to changing the way society addresses the use of accessing context relating to advice, awareness and knowledge on disease subject areas (Mendelsohn et al. 2008; Edyburn, 2000; Edyburn, 2004; Edyburn, 2005).

The use of the internet and SM use does not suit everyone, however. In contrast to the above, patients' whose first language is not English for example, approaching more methods to support Health Literacy (HL) is/ will be challenging. HL is predominantly a skills-based construct that does not include motivational elements. Using modes to improve HL alone to determine the needs of patients and simplifying instructions for them as a result may be a barrier to that person, thus affecting patient and professional relationship. As such, the patient may gain some of the understanding, however does not have the mind-set to take action (Smith et al. 2013). Work by (Salter et al. 2014) highlight what can be learned from patients living with chronic musculoskeletal conditions, health professionals and carers about the concept of HL using qualitative methods of inquiry. This team inform patients' desire predictable interactions and search for more than knowledge, empowerment and responsibility from their engagement with healthcare (Salter et al. 2014).

Several studies have shown that concerns that shared decision-making is only of interest to well-educated middle class people are unjustified (Nutbeam 2000; Lindquist et al. 2012; Protheroe et al. 2013; Salter et al. 2014). It is possible to inform and engage patients from all walks of life and educational backgrounds, if they are provided with well-designed information materials and given appropriate decision support by well-trained staff (King et al. 2011; O'Connor et al 2009). Importantly, more evidence has shed light that people with low HL tend to defer to health professionals to make decisions for them and also tend to have less good health outcomes than people who are more actively involved in their health. The temptation for health professionals faced with someone who has little knowledge of health matters and is not confident about asserting their views is to make the decision for them, thus further reinforcing their passive role and the tendency towards poorer health in the long term. All should be encouraged and supported to become active partners in care (Hibbard et al. 2009; Volandes et al. 2011). Library and Health Services partnerships should actively collaborate to ensure that there is a wider HL available for those who whose first language is not English and in addition information needs to be accessible for those with disabilities (Andersson and Lyttkens 1999; Iezzoni et al. 2000; Coughlin et al. 2002; Beatty et al. 2003; Drainoni et al. 2006; Armstrong and Powell 2009; Barnett et al 2012).

ELECTRONIC PATIENT RECORDS (EPR) – PATIENTS ACCESSING RECORDS

There is compelling evidence that patients who are active in managing their lives, accessing their health records have better outcomes than those who are passive service recipients (Stoves et al. 2010; Stoves et al. 2014). An NHS Future Forum was set up by the Government in 2011 to consult broadly on the future of the NHS. As part of their review, the NHS Future Forum examined the Government's information strategy and made several key recommendations which have been accepted in the Department of Health information strategy report. The commitment made by the Department of Health in General Practice is that by 2015:

- All NHS patients will have secure EPR
- All practices will be expected to make available EPR and cancelling of appointments, ordering of repeat prescriptions, and communication with the practice
- The Royal College of General Practitioners (RCGP) agreed to take forward this work, and the Patient Online Road Map highlighted some important principles.
  (The Patient Online, Road Map, 2011)

The Patient Online Information strategy report informs:

Practices that can already provide their patients with online access to their records are encouraged to do so as soon as possible. Practices are encouraged to extend the range of transactions that people can deal with online, for example: electronic booking and cancellation of GP/nurse consultations, repeat prescriptions, access to test results and online secure communication between GPs and patients.

(The Patient Online, Road Map, 2011)

Consistent with above context, research by Bertot et al. 2010; Bertot et al. 2012) inform:

- 86.5% of public libraries report offering classes on general Internet use
- 87.0% of public libraries report offering classes in general computer skills
- 82.7% of public libraries report offering point-of-use technology training
- 66.1% of public libraries report that technology training is important in their communities

One good example of joined up EPR between primary and secondary care environs is work by (Stoves et al. 2014) who look at EPR sharing between primary and secondary care to support renal pathways, however studies have also investigated doctors' attitudes towards EPR and shared-decision making with patients in an attempt to comprehend why it is not yet practised universally (Legare et al. 2008). Some commonly voiced objections include: *1) 'We already do it', 2) 'Patients don't want it', 3) 'Not appropriate for those with low health literacy', 4) 'Patients will want inappropriate/expensive treatments', 5) 'No time to do it', 6) 'It's irrelevant and ineffective' and 7) 'There's no incentive to do it'.*

The NHS Constitution (2010) and the NHS Care Record Guarantee (2011) enhance the guide of access to records by patients. These are highlighted in the RCGP guidance on EPR access. Service user-friendly Electronic Patient Record (EPR) technology should allow the delivery of understandable result interpretation, enhancing care quality across primary care, thus enabling better patient outcomes (Giles, 2012). It is also important to recognize that even if majority of patients and the public have EPR access; a bulk will require further awareness and support in the interpretation of test results etc. (Coulter and Collins 2011). This is presently not offered in the GP environment because of time constraints. This also means EPR alone is unlikely to be sufficient to motivate change (De Silva, 2011) and will not increase autonomy in the general population.

The chronic illness model is underpinned by a body of evidence highlighting that EPR and self-management support can make a real difference to health outcomes (Bodenheimer et al. 2002; Stoves et al. 2010; Stoves et al. 2014). Information is helpful, particularly if it is personalised. EPR needs to be supplemented by decision support, personalised care planning and self-management education from trained health professionals, as well as social support from family, friends and peers. There is evidence that this can improve patient and carers understanding and level of participation, as well as their coping skills and confidence to self-manage, leading to better health outcomes (Coulter and Ellins 2007; Loveman *et al* 2008). There thus needs to be a neutral environment where patients and health professionals can come together to provide more awareness of EPR in addition a neutral environment where patients and the public can source additional literature and context. EPR learning and development can be taught and achieved through a library partnership.

WHAT ADDITIONAL RESOURCES ARE REQUIRED IN DEVELOPING A LIBRARIES AND HEALTH PARTNERSHIP?

The need for the General Medical Practitioner to work in close partnership with education professionals was highlighted some years ago by John Macdonald in 'Occasional paper No 64 from the Royal College of General Practitioners' (Macdonald 1994) who says:

For patients to become fully engaged with their treatment and care there needs to be a huge and sustained educational programme .... developed within Primary Health Care.

The need for patients to be fully "engaged with their treatment and care" has more recently been highlighted in 'The Wanless Report' (Wanless 2004) which estimated that fully engaged patients and carers were likely to save the NHS millions of pounds of unnecessary spending. Similarly, the importance of supporting patient education and patient and carer learning was also emphasised in the report 'From the Rockies to the Rhondda' (The Welsh NHS Confederation nd, 2014).

The General Medical Council (GMC) in its updated document 'Good Medical Practice' (GMC 2013) insists that doctors MUST give information to patients in language and terms that they can understand. This information should relate to their conditions and treatments available, together with possible adverse effects of medicines and procedures, so that patients, following GP or Consultant consultations, can truly give "informed consent" to their treatments, procedures and operations. This is clearly quite impossible in the time available during the average GP consultation of between 7 and 11 minutes; even more impossible when the language and culture of the patient is not shared by the doctor.

Just as community access has become an important component of public library services, so too has patron technology training. Although public libraries face many challenges in their efforts to provide access and instruction services, they are embracing their role bridging the digital divide, and they continue to expand their services and innovate in their practices (Becker et al. 2010).

In spite of the importance of these services, public libraries face a number of challenges in their efforts to provide access to and instruction in digital resources. Increased use of technology training classes coincides with increased use of library resources internationally, representing an increase in demand on library resources and staff (Chicago: American Library Association, 1989). Over half (65.4%) of libraries report they have insufficient public access to meet patients' needs during at least some part of a typical day. Most libraries (60.2%) report an increase in the usage of public access Internet in the last fiscal year. Increasing demand means many libraries have established time limits for patrons using public access desktops, which has a significant impact on people who lack other means of access this information. Technology training competes with other library services in its importance to the community. Job seeking services and E-government services are consistently ranked amongst the most important services to the community provided by libraries. That the public library is the only or one of few, community resources addressing these issues means librarians often must combine Health Literacy (HL) instruction with health care services.

WHAT ABOUT LIBRARY HEALTH PARTNERSHIPS WITH PATIENT-CENTRED MULTIDISCIPLINARY TEAM (MDT) MEETINGS?

For a long time, Multidisciplinary Team (MDT) meetings have traditionally taken place in secondary care with health professionals in a particular specialty coming together to discuss a proposed care plan for a particular patient. These meetings have always taken place in the background. Whilst it would still be a challenge to perhaps have patient-centred MDT meetings in secondary care, this should be explored at the primary care level to increase health care integration and further EPR awareness. The notion of patient-centred MDT meetings would increase knowledge and understanding of health at various stages of care and where health professionals within a practice can/ should physically involve a patient they would like to discuss care further.

One example is a programme aimed at increasing the activation of patients attending a clinic for people on a low income in USA. The programme focused on teaching patients how to draw up and prioritise questions regarding their health care concerns and treatments before their meetings with health care professionals. The programme was evaluated as part of a randomised controlled trial, and found that the patients who were placed in the intervention group had significantly increased patient activation scores. In addition, they asked more questions during their meetings with doctors and were more likely to use decision aids (specially designed information resources) than those who did not receive the intervention (Deen et al. 2011).

Many patients with LTCs do not see a role for themselves in managing their health, or are ineffective at doing so because they lack the skills (e.g. health literacy) or confidence. As patients' confidence levels increase, they gain a greater sense of control over their health and feel empowered to take action. Another important factor in the proposal of patient-centred MDT meetings at primary care level is the use of strategies that stimulate autonomous motivation. There should be a call for proposals to physically involve patient perspectives and encourage shared-decision making. Having access to EPR alone will not help or encourage a patient to gain confidence and/ or understanding (Ryan and Deci 2000), especially if they are overwhelmed by their healthcare choices and HL complexities. Patient-Centred MDT meetings will allow patient and carers to gain more EPR awareness and a tighter understanding of what their results actually mean.

MDT meetings can be arranged at dedicated time points between a doctor and patient/ carer and these can take place in a library setting, which would be a inviting environment. A patient/ carer will also be able to access additional sources of information to support their decision-making. Individual consultations may indeed take a little longer, but time spent engaging/ involving the patient in the decision may reduce the overall time spent dealing with patients who are unsure or unhappy about a decision in which they were not involved (Bekker et al. 2004). Shared decision-making may involve re-thinking clinical pathway design to incorporate time for information provision and care.

Almost all (93.2%) of public libraries allow the use of portable drives or other storage devices, and two-thirds (64.4%) support the use of digital cameras and other content options. Overall, IT technologies (the Internet, smart devices) today allow accessing online library resources at any convenient location. GP surgery partnerships should contemplate on implementing 'rotation-based' patient-centred MDT meetings in libraries, where one GP from a practice can rotate and call upon colleagues from primary and secondary care sectors to meet at library location where a patient is also called in for review. This should be at least piloted for patients with an LTC since they might have a number of co-morbidities and who might require further support with respect to EPR, HL and online support who would otherwise not know how to use facilities. A library-centred service would also allow access to wider resources and information post MDT meetings in a public environment.

PATIENT-CENTRED MDT MEETINGS AND THE MID-ATLANTIC RENAL COALITION (MARC) EXAMPLE

The Mid-Atlantic Renal Coalition (MARC) is one of 18 Medicare-funded organizations in the USA responsible for improving the quality of care delivered to patients with CKD. MARC is a non-funded organization specifically supporting the District of Columbia, Maryland, Virginia, and West Virginia. MARC recognizes that the success of efforts to empower patients, their families, and/ or caregivers, is dependent on collaborations between these patients and health professionals. The driving force of this collaboration is at the facility level; family and caregiver engagement is patient-centred, and not a 'tick-box exercise'.

Patient-centred care is not characterized by a particular programme or practice, but rather by the core values and attitudes that drive changes to improve practices. Involving patients, families, and caregivers in the care of a patient means engaging the hearts and minds of the people with whom MARC work and the patients for whom are cared for. MARC introduced MDT meetings and implemented an ENGAGE programme as a means for health professionals and patients engaging to share knowledge and as a means of support in clinical decision-making. When CKD management involves the patient experience through MDT meetings and considers their perspective, patients become more active in their management and health outcomes improve. MARC MDT meetings thus allow a great opportunity for shared-decision making. The Centres for Medicare and Medicaid Services (CMS) has tasked the District of Columbia, Maryland, Virginia, and West Virginia renal community to engage patients, families, and caregivers in a more MDT model of care involving patients. MARC works at community level and is another good example opening its doors to implementing a MDT methodology (The Mid-Atlantic Renal Coalition - MARC, 2014).

DISCUSSION

Against a background of impossible demands being placed on the GP and the hospital consultant within the NHS, a high profile national charity 'The Patients' Association (PA)' has now adopted the strap line "no decision about me, without me" in light of the influential paper by (Coulter and Collins 2011) concerning "shared decision making in medical practice". Similarly, the British Medical Journal has begun a campaign to encourage doctors to form "partnerships" with their patients.

Doctors recognize both the moral importance and desirability of the idea of an expert patient. However, in terms of compliance with treatment regimens and awareness of health conditions, professionals suggest that due to the practical pressures of time and resourcing placed on the GP, the cultural barriers potentially created by differences in language use and background knowledge between the GP and the patient, it is unreasonable to expect the GP to make available time and to acquire further complex communication skills in order to enable a patient to enter into dialogue and acquire expertise of the condition and treatment possibilities.

Among the plans set out in the strategy document published by the National Information Board, (which brings together all bodies in England with responsibility for health), is a move to digitize the *"red book"* given to all new mothers in which to record their baby's information. After a successful scheme in London, terminally ill patients will have digital records detailing how they wish to die, which will be accessible to ambulance services, A&E departments and the NHS 111 helpline. Tim Kelsey, NHS England's director for patients and information, says:

These are a series of quite radical steps to modernize healthcare by making it much more digitally supported.

Tim Kelsey adds:

We must embrace modern technology to help us lead healthier lives, and if we want, to take more control when we are ill. Our ambition is to make the NHS a digital pioneer for our patients and citizens.

CONCLUSION

Within the existing financial limits of the NHS in the UK - and no doubt in other "developed" countries - resources for this kind of activity are not available but within the context of a "Libraries and Health Partnership Development *"much might be achieved for the benefit of patients, carers, families and communities including the whole professional community of GPs and Practice Nurses"*.

By encouraging partnerships and inviting patient and public involvement with "expertise", who can effectively and efficiently add to this important discussion, there is now a need for GPs to enter dialogue with and social services, to prompt tighter integrated services in primary care. Such partnerships would not merely enable an individual patient to better understand their health and treatment, thus realising the model of the 'Expert Patient', but would also bring about a deeper public understanding of, and engagement in primary care. INVOLVE have set out a document highlighting strategies for diversity and inclusion in public involvement (INVOLVE, 2012). A shared decision-making partnership should be PPI-driven to ensure policy is all inclusive. There is an ongoing need to support and work in partnership to increase awareness of local services in health and social care.

Given that more patients and the public will have opportunity to access their health records, a "Libraries and Health" partnership can be an enhanced methodology that integrates primary healthcare better thus allowing all to access health-related literature, using books, leaflets and digital media in a comfortable environment in a setting that also has staff that can support with HL and technology.

There must be more unilateral thinking to ensure diversity and inclusion of different populations when developing/ improving healthcare services. Partnership working can also allow reliable professional help and advice that patients and the public need at a time that suits them and in a language or format that they can understand and from which they can learn. An EPR and MDT initiative should be supported with library and health partnerships; this needs to be encouraged and to happen now.

REFERENCES

American Library Association. (1989). *Presidential Committee on Information Literacy. Final Report.* Chicago: American Library Association.

Andersson, F., & Lyttkens, C. H. (1999). Preferences for equity in health behind a veil of ignorance. *Health Economics*, *8*(5), 369–378. doi:10.1002/(SICI)1099-1050(199908)8:5<369::AID-HEC456>3.0.CO;2-Q PMID:10470544

Armstrong, N., & Powell, J. (2009). Patient perspectives on health advice posted on Internet discussion boards: A qualitative study. *Health Expectations*, *12*(3), 313–320. doi:10.1111/j.1369-7625.2009.00543.x PMID:19555377

Barnett, K., Mercer, S., Norbury, M., Watt, G., Wyke, S., & Guthrie, B. (2012). 'Epidemiology of multimorbidity and implications for health care, research, and medical education: A cross-sectional study'. *Lancet*, *380*(9836), 37–43. doi:10.1016/S0140-6736(12)60240-2 PMID:22579043

Radio, B. B. C. 4 The Longevity War Game (http://www.bbc.co.uk/programmes/b03k2k7y) (accessed November 2014)

Beatty, P. W., Hagglund, K. J., Neri, M. T., Dhont, K. R., Clark, M. J., & Hilton, S. A. (2003). Access to health care services among people with chronic or disabling conditions: Patterns and predictors. *Archives of Physical Medicine and Rehabilitation*, *84*(10), 1417–1425. doi:10.1016/S0003-9993(03)00268-5 PMID:14586907

Becker, S., Crandall, M. D., Fisher, K. E., Kinney, B., Landry, C., & Rocha, A. (2010). Opportunity for all: How the American public benefits from Internet access at U.S. libraries. (IMLS-2010-RES-01). Washington, D.C: Institute of Museum and Library Services; Available http://cis.washington.edu/usimpact/

Bekker, H. L., Hewison, J., & Thornton, J. G. (2004). 'Applying decision analysis to facilitate informed decision making about prenatal diagnosis for Down syndrome: A randomised controlled trial'. *Prenatal Diagnosis*, *24*(4), 265–275. doi:10.1002/pd.851 PMID:15065100

Bertot, J. C., McDermott, A., Lincoln, R., Real, B., & Peterson, K. (2012). 2011-2012 Public Library Funding & Technology Access Survey: Survey Findings & Report. College Park, MD: Information Policy & Access Center, University of Maryland College Park; Available at http://www.plinternetsurvey.org, accessed May 2015.

Bertot, J. C. (2010). Community-based E-government: Libraries as E-government partners and providers. *Electronic government: 9th IFIP WG 8.5 International Conference, EGOV 2010 Lausanne, Switzerland, August/September 2010 Proceedings.* Maria A. Wimmer, et al. (Eds.) Germany: IFIP International Federation for Information Processing 2010.

Retail, B. (2013). Redefining the shape and purpose of town centres is the final report from the Distressed Town Centre Property Taskforce (www.bcsc.org.uk) (accessed November 2013)

Bodenheimer, T., Wagner, E. H., & Grumbach, K. (2002). 'Improving primary care for patients with chronic illness: The chronic care model, Part 2'. *Journal of the American Medical Association*, *288*(15), 1909–1914. doi:10.1001/jama.288.15.1909 PMID:12377092

Coulter, A., & Ellins, J. (2007). 'Effectiveness of strategies for informing, educating, and involving patients'. *British Medical Journal*, *335*(7609), 24–27. doi:10.1136/bmj.39246.581169.80 PMID:17615222

Coughlin, T. A., Long, S. K., & Kendall, S. (2002). Health care access, use, and satisfaction among disabled Medicaid beneficiaries. *Health Care Financing Review*, *24*(2), 115–136. PMID:12690698

Department of Health. (2012), Long Term Conditions Compendium of Information, 3rd ed. London: Department of Health. (www.dh.gov.uk/prod_consum_dh/groups/dh_digitalassets/@dh/@en/documents/digitalasset/dh_134486.pdf)

Department of Health. Public Health England, Healthcare UK, (www.dh.gov.uk/health/category/policy-areas/nhs/constitution/) (Accessed November 2014)

De Silva, D. (2011). The Health Foundation - Helping People help Themselves, The Health Foundation - Helping People help Themselves (http://www.health.org.uk/media_manager/public/75/publications_pdfs/Helping%20people%20help%20themselves.pdf)

Drainoni, M. L., Lee-Hood, E., Tobias, C., Bachman, S. S., Andrew, J., & Maisels, L. (2006). Cross-disability experiences of barriers to health-care access. *Journal of Disability Policy Studies*, *17*(2), 101–115. doi:10.1177/10442073060170020101

Coulter A and Collins (2011). Shared Decision Making A Reality, No Decision about me Without Me

http://www.kingsfund.org.uk/sites/files/kf/Making-shared-decision-making-a-reality-paper-Angela-Coulter-Alf-Collins-July-2011_0.pdf

Deen, D., Lu, W.-H., Rothstein, D., Santana, L., & Gold, M. R. (2011). 'Asking questions: The effect of a brief intervention in community health centers on patient activation'. *Patient Education and Counseling*, *84*(2), 257–260. doi:10.1016/j.pec.2010.07.026 PMID:20800414

Edyburn, D. L. (2000). Assistive technology and students with mild disabilities. *Focus on Exceptional Children*, *32*(9), 1–24.

Edyburn, D. L. (2004). Measuring assistive technology outcomes in reading. *Journal of Special Education Technology*, *19*(1), 60–64.

Edyburn, D. L. (2005). Assistive technology and students with mild disabilities: From consideration to outcome measurement. In D. Edyburn, K. Higgins, & R. Boone (Eds.), *Handbook of special education technology research and practice* (pp. 239–269). Whitefish Bay, WI: Knowledge by Design, Inc.

Folkman, S., Lazarus, R. S., Gruen, R. J., & DeLongis, A. (1986). Appraisal, coping, health status, and psychological symptoms. *Journal of Personality and Social Psychology*, *50*(3), 571–579. doi:10.1037/0022-3514.50.3.571 PMID:3701593

Folkman, S., & Lazarus, R. S. (1988). Coping as a mediator of emotion. *Journal of Personality and Social Psychology*, *54*(3), 466–475. doi:10.1037/0022-3514.54.3.466 PMID:3361419

Folkman, S., & Moskowitz, J. T. (2000). Positive affect and the other side of coping. *The American Psychologist*, *55*(6), 647–654. doi:10.1037/0003-066X.55.6.647 PMID:10892207

Folkman, S., & Moskowitz, J. T. (2004). Coping: Pitfalls and promise. *Annual Review of Psychology*, *55*(1), 745–774. doi:10.1146/annurev.psych.55.090902.141456 PMID:14744233

General Medical Council. (2012). (http://www.gmc-uk.org) (accessed November 2014)

General Medical Council. (2013). Good Medical Practice. London: GMC (www.gmc-uk.org/guidance/good_medical_practice.asp. (Accessed July 2013)

Gibson, A. N., Bertot, J. C., & McClure, C. R. (2009). Emerging role of public librarians as E-government providers. *Proceedings of the 42nd Hawaii International Conference on System Science*. R. H. Sprague, Jr. (Ed.), 1-10. (Available: http://mcclure.ii.fsu.edu/publications/2009/; Beker et al. (2010)

Giles, R (2012). Viewpoint paper, Envisioning the digital hospital – The Future of Healthcare

Guidance for health professionals. London: RCGP; (2010) (www.rcgp.org.uk/clinical-and-research/practice-management-resources/health-informaticsgroup/~/ media/Files/CIRC/Health%20Informatics%20Report.ashx) (Accessed November 2014)

Harden, P. N., Walsh, G., Bandler, N., Bradley, S., Lonsdale, D., Taylor, J., & Marks, S. D. (2012). Bridging the gap: An integrated paediatric to adult clinical service for young adults with kidney failure. *BMJ (Clinical Research Ed.)*, *344*, e3718. PMID:22661725

Hibbard, J., Greene, J., & Tusler, M. (2009). 'Improving the outcomes of disease management by tailoring care to the patient's level of activation'. *The American Journal of Managed Care*, *15*(6), 353–360. http://healthforum.brandeis.edu/about/grant-pages/univ-oregon-grant.html accessed March 2014 PMID:19514801

Jones, A., & Dutton, K. (2014). "Patients and families as partners in safety, quality, and experiences of care," Patient Experience, Journal: Vol. 1: Iss. 1, Article 8

Iezzoni, L. I., Davis, R. B., Soukup, J., & O'Day, B. (2000). Satisfaction with quality and access to health care among people with disabling conditions. *International Journal for Quality in Health Care*, *14*(5), 369–381. doi:10.1093/intqhc/14.5.369 PMID:12389803

Ilic, D., Maloney, S., & Green, S. (2005). Guiding users to quality information about osteoarthritis on the Internet: A pilot study. *Telemedicine Journal and e-Health*, *11*(6), 703–706. doi:10.1089/tmj.2005.11.703 PMID:16430390

Institute for Healthcare Improvement. (www.IHI.org) (accessed November, 2014).

Involve (2012). Strategies for Diversity and Inclusion in Public Involvement: Supplement to the briefing notes for researchers (http://www.invo.org.uk/wp-content/uploads/2014/10/INVOLVE_Inclusion_Supplement_links-updated-July-2014-WEB.pdf) (accessed November 2014)

Jaeger, P. T., Langa, L. A., McClure, C. R., & Bertot, J. C. (2007). The 2004 and 2005 Gulf Coast hurricanes: Evolving roles and lessons learned for public libraries in disaster preparedness and community services. *Public Library Quarterly*, *25*(3/4), 199–214.

King, J. S., Eckman, M. H., & Moulton, B. W. (2011). 'The potential of shared decision making to reduce health disparities'. *The Journal of Law, Medicine & Ethics*, *39*, s30–s33. doi:10.1111/j.1748-720X.2011.00561.x PMID:21309892

Legare, F., Ratte, S., Gravel, K., & Graham, I. D. (2008). 'Barriers and facilitators to implementing shared decision-making in clinical practice: Update of a systematic review of health professionals' perceptions'. *Patient Education and Counseling*, *73*(3), 526–535. doi:10.1016/j.pec.2008.07.018 PMID:18752915

Loveman, E., Frampton, G. K., & Clegg, A. J. (2008). 'The clinical effectiveness of diabetes education models for type 2 diabetes: A systematic review'. [iii.]. *Health Technology Assessment*, *12*(9), 1–116. doi:10.3310/hta12090 PMID:18405469

Luxford, K., & Sutton, S. (2014). "How does patient experience fit into the overall healthcare picture?" Patient Experience Journal: Vol. 1: Iss. 1, Article 4

Lazarus, R. S. (1974). Psychological stress and coping in adaptation and illness. *International Journal of Psychiatry in Medicine*, *5*(4), 321–333. doi:10.2190/T43T-84P3-QDUR-7RTP PMID:4618837

Lazarus, R. S. (1992). Coping with the stress of illness. *WHO Regional Publications. European Series*, *44*, 11–31. PMID:1514969

Lazarus, R. S. (1993a). Coping theory and research: Past, present, and future. *Psychosomatic Medicine*, *55*(3), 234–247. doi:10.1097/00006842-199305000-00002 PMID:8346332

Lazarus, R. S. (1993b). From psychological stress to the emotions: A history of changing outlooks. *Annual Review of Psychology*, *44*(1), 1–21. doi:10.1146/annurev.ps.44.020193.000245 PMID:8434890

Lazarus, R. S. (1985). The psychology of stress and coping. *Issues in Mental Health Nursing*, *7*(1-4), 399–418. doi:10.3109/01612848509009463 PMID:3854019

Lindquist, L. A., Go, L., Fleisher, J., Jain, N., & Elisha Friesema, B. A. C. (2012). Relationship of health literacy to intentional and unintentional non-adherence of hospital discharge medications. *Journal of General Internal Medicine*, *27*(2), 173–178. doi:10.1007/s11606-011-1886-3 PMID:21971600

Macdonald, J. (1994). *Community Participation in Primary Health Care, RCGP Occasional paper no. 64*. London: Royal College of General Practitioners.

Maes, S., Leventhal, H., & de Ridder, D. T. D. (1996). Coping with chronic diseases. In M. Zeidner & N. Endler (Eds.), *Handbook of Coping: Theory, Research and Applications* (pp. 221–251). New York: Wiley.

Mendelsohn, S., Edyburn, D. L., Rust, K. L., Schwanke, T. D., & Smith, R. O. (2008). Using assistive technology outcomes research to inform policy related to the employment of individuals with disabilities. *Assistive Technology*, *20*(3), 139–148. doi:10.1080/10400435.2008.10131941 PMID:18939654

Moos, R. H., & Schaeffer, J. A. (1984). The crisis of physical illness. An overview and conceptual approach. In Moss, R.M. (Ed.), Coping With Physical Illness, Vol. 2, New Perspectives, Plenum Press, New York, pp. 3–39 doi:10.1007/978-1-4684-4772-9_1

Muhammad S, Banks P, Martin C, (2012) Coping: is this the foundation of wellbeing? A narrative review. British Journal of Mental Health Nursing Winter 2012 Vol 1 No 4

Nutbeam, D. (2000). Health literacy as a public health goal: A challenge for contemporary health education and communication strategies into the 21st century. *Health Promotion International*, *15*(3), 259–267. doi:10.1093/heapro/15.3.259

O'Connor, A. M., Bennett, C. L., Stacey, D., Barry, M., Col, N. F., Eden, K. B., & Rovner, D. et al. (2009). 'Decision aids for people facing health treatment or screening decisions'. *Cochrane Database of Systematic Reviews*, (3): CD001431. PMID:19588325

O'Leary, A. (1990). Stress, emotion, and human immune function. *Psychological Bulletin*, *108*(3), 363–382. doi:10.1037/0033-2909.108.3.363 PMID:2270233

Patients told to go online in radical NHS reform, Health News, The Times, (http://www.thetimes.co.uk/tto/health/news/article4266243.ece) (accessed November 2014)

Pioneer Health Foundation. (www.thephf.org, 2014) (accessed November 2014)

Protheroe, J., Brooks, H., Chew-Graham, C., Gardner, C., & Rogers, A. (2013). 'Permission to participate?'A qualitative study of participation in patients from differing socio-economic backgrounds. *Journal of Health Psychology*, *18*(8), 1046–1055. doi:10.1177/1359105312459876 PMID:23104997

Richards, T., Montori, V. M., Godlee, F., Lapsley, P., & Paul, D. (2013). 'Let the patient revolution begin'. *British Medical Journal*, *346*(may14 1), 2614f. doi:10.1136/bmj.f2614

de Ridder, D., & Schreurs, K. (1996). Coping, social support and chronic disease: A research agenda. *Psychology Health and Medicine*, *1*(1), 71–82. doi:10.1080/13548509608400007

Royal College of General Practitioners. Enabling Patients to Access Electronic Health Records. Guidance for health professionals. London: RCGP; 2010 (www.rcgp.org.uk/clinical-and-research/practice-management-resources/health-informaticsgroup/~/

media/Files/CIRC/Health%20Informatics%20Report.ashx) (accessed November 2014)

Ryan, R. M., & Deci, E. L. (2000). 'Self-determination theory and the facilitation of intrinsic motivation, social development, and well-being'. *The American Psychologist*, *55*(1), 68–78. doi:10.1037/0003-066X.55.1.68 PMID:11392867

Schroeder, S. A. (2007). 'We can do better – improving the health of the American people'. *The New England Journal of Medicine*, *357*(12), 1221–1228www.nejm.org/doi/full/10.1056/. accessedMarch2014. doi:10.1056/NEJMsa073350 PMID:17881753

Shuler, J. A. (1996). Civic librarianship: Possible new role for depository libraries in the next century? *Journal of Government Information*, *23*(4), 415–419. doi:10.1016/1352-0237(96)00022-6

Smith, S. G., Curtis, L. M., Wardle, J., von Wagner, C., & Wolf, M. S. (2013). 'Skill set or mind set? Associations between health literacy, patient activation and health'. *PLoS ONE*, *8*(9), e74373www.ncbi.nlm.nih.gov/pmc/articles/PMC3762784/. accessedNovember2014. doi:10.1371/journal.pone.0074373 PMID:24023942

Snell, T., Wittenberg, R., Fernandez, J., Malley, J., Comas-Herrera, A., & King, D. (2011). Projections of Demand for Social Care and Disability Benefits for Younger Adults in England. Report of Research Conducted for the Commission on Funding of Care and Support. PSSRU Discussion paper 2800/3. London: Economics of Social and Health Care Research Unit. (www.pssru.ac.uk/pdf/DP2880-3.pdf) (accessed November 2014)

Staniszewska S, Bullock I. Can we help patients have a better experience? (2012)

Wanless, D. (2004). The Wanless report: Securing good health for the whole population. Norwich: HMSO; http://webarchive.nationalarchives.gov.uk/+/http:/www.hmtreasury.gov.uk/media/D/3/Wanless04_summary.pdf, accessed July 2013.

Stoves, J., Connolly, J., & Cheung, C. K. et al.. (2010). Electronic consultation as an alternative to hospital referral for patients with chronic kidney disease: A novel application for networked electronic health records to improve the accessibility and efficiency of healthcare. *Quality & Safety in Health Care*, *19*, e54. PMID:20554576

Stoves J, Wong A, Orlando A, Hipkiss V, Middleton J, Lampinen E, Coman T, Carlisle G, Green W, Connolly J (2014). Electronic patient record sharing between primary and secondary care to support renal pathways, British Journal of Renal Medicine, Vol. 19 No 2

The Care Record Guaranteed. (2011) (www.nigb.nhs.uk/pubs/nhscrg.pdf) (accessed November 2014)

The Patient Online. Road Map (2011) (http://www.rcgp.org.uk/patientonline) (accessed November 2014)

The Mid-Atlantic Renal Coalition (MARC). (http://www.esrdnet5.org/Home.aspx) (accessed December 2014)

The Renal Patient Support Group (RPSG). http://www.facebook.com/groups/RPSGroup/

The Renal Patient Support Group (RPSG) BlogSpot. http://shahidrpsg.blogspot.co.uk/

Timimi, F. (2012). The Use of Social Media in Healthcare, (http://newsblog.mayoclinic.org/2012/03/24/farris-timimi)

Welsh, N. H. S. Confederation (n.d.). From the Rockies to the Rhondda: Better patient care and better use of hospitals, What can Wales learn from Colorado? Cardiff: Welsh NHS Confederation. (Available at http://welshnhsconfed.ifanetsite.com/RockiesRhondda.htm) (accessed July 2013)

World Health Organization. (2005). Preventing chronic diseases: a vital statement. Switzerland: World Health Organization. (www.who.int/chp/chronic_disease_report/en/) (accessed March 2014)

Volandes, A. E., Ferguson, L. A., Davis, A. D., Hull, N. C., Green, M. J., Chang, Y., & Paasche-Orlow, M. K. et al. (2011). 'Assessing end-of-life preferences for advanced dementia in rural patients using an educational video: A randomized controlled trial'. *Journal of Palliative Medicine*, *14*(2), 169–177. doi:10.1089/jpm.2010.0299 PMID:21254815

Wolf, J. A., Niederhauser, V., Marshburn, D., & LaVela, S. (2014). "Defining Patient Experience," Patient Experience Journal: Vol. 1: Iss. 1, Article 3

Xie, B. (2009). Older adults' health information wants in the internet age: Implications for patient-provider relationships. *Journal of Health Communication*, *14*(6), 510–524. doi:10.1080/10810730903089614 PMID:19731124

Zautra, A. J. (1996). Investigations of the ongoing stressful situations among those with chronic illness. *American Journal of Community Psychology*, *24*(6), 697–717. doi:10.1007/BF02511031 PMID:9194327

This work was previously published in the International Journal of User-Driven Healthcare (IJUDH), 4(4); edited by Ashok Kumar Biswas, pages 17-33, copyright year 2014 by IGI Publishing (an imprint of IGI Global).

Chapter 10
Creating a Supportive Environment for Self-Management in Healthcare via Patient Electronic Tools

Sharazade Balouchi
Sewanee: The University of the South, USA

Ahmad Zbib
Heart and Stroke Foundation, Canada

Karim Keshavjee
InfoClin Inc, Canada & University of Victoria, Canada

Karim Vassanji
InfoClin Inc, Canada

Jastinder Toor
InfoClin Inc, Canada

ABSTRACT

Consumer electronic healthcare applications and tools, both Web-based and mobile apps, are increasingly available and used by citizens around the world. "eTools" denote the full range of electronic applications that consumers may use to assess, track, or treat their disease(s), including communicating with their healthcare provider. Consumer eTool use is prone to plateauing of use because it is one-sided (i.e., consumers use them without the assistance or advice of a healthcare provider). Patient eTools that allow patients to communicate with their healthcare providers, exchange data, and receive support and guidance between visits is a promising approach that could lead to more effective, sustained, and sustainable use of eTools. The key elements of a supportive environment for eTool use include 2-way data integration from patient home monitoring equipment to providers and from provider electronic medical records systems to patient eTools, mechanisms to support provider-patient communication between visits, the ability for providers to easily monitor incoming data from multiple patients, and for provider systems to leverage the team environment and delegate tasks to appropriate providers for education and follow-up. This is explored in this chapter.

DOI: 10.4018/978-1-5225-1928-7.ch010

INTRODUCTION

Patient-provider relationships rarely move beyond the confines of a doctor's office or hospital room. The typical patient-provider interaction is a time-honored tradition from the time of Hippocrates: a patient visits with his or her healthcare provider when experiencing symptoms or problems with his or her health. Based on this consultation and follow-up tests, the provider assesses the patient's condition and advises on the best method of treatment, which often includes prescribed medication, but also includes a variety of other modalities, such as physiotherapy, psychotherapy or non-pharmacological treatments. The patient proceeds by this method of treatment, or withdraws from it if he or she finds it ineffective or not feasible, until the next visit several months later. In between visits there is often no communication between the patient and the provider to discuss how the treatment is working. Although this approach does provide a great level of patient autonomy, it only works for low acuity diseases or when treatment regimes are relatively simple.

With the rapid growth in diagnostic and treatment modalities and preventive care approaches across a wide number of chronic diseases, it is increasingly difficult for patients to maintain their autonomy without additional supports. New technologies are trying to fill that gap, but may not provide the appropriate context and judgment patients need to maintain appropriate adherence to treatment recommendations over the long periods of time (sometimes decades) necessitated by today's preventive care protocols. For example, a patient with high cholesterol or high blood pressure may need to regularly monitor and treat his or her disease for 30, 40 or even 50 years to gain the benefits of stroke and heart attack prevention.

If medicine is to achieve economies of scale and capabilities, it is important that patients assume an active role in the management of their health because patients are more in tune with their own symptoms and healthcare providers are increasingly overworked. An approach that encourages patient involvement is self-management, which involves active collaboration between the patient and provider. Self-management is essential to long-term patient health, for it engages both the patient and provider to agree on the issues, establish goals, decide on priorities and agree on treatment plans (Schaefer et al 2009).

Electronic tools (eTools) are designed to assist patients with managing their diseases by identifying risk factors, monitoring symptoms, and facilitating communication with the patients' healthcare providers between visits (http://apps.nhs.uk/). eTools take many forms from personal health records to patient portals to mobile applications and social media. In particular, social media outlets and dedicated disease social networks have strong potential to enable the process of self-management since the effects and health outcomes from using social media appear positive (Merolli 2013).

A recent Pew Internet survey (2012) showed that over 70% of patients measure and track a health indicator for themselves or for a loved one. However, only 21% of patients use some form of technology to track their health; i.e., the remaining 49% track the metrics 'in their head'. This same rate appears in reports from the several years preceding 2012 as well, indicating a "plateaued" use of eTools in general. Plateaued use of specific health applications, as with many other apps, is quite common but poorly documented (Rudansky 2013). Nonetheless, it is an important metric for understanding the needs of users and providing tools that will work for them over an extended period of time. It also highlights the need for healthcare providers to reinforce the use of eTools, if they are to be effective in driving improved patient outcomes.

The marketplace distinguishes between two specific kinds of tools: *consumer* eTools – those applications that a person seeks out on his or her own to self-monitor health conditions – and *patient* eTools, which are designed for patients to use under the guidance of and through interaction with a healthcare provider. Consumer eTools do promote health awareness among patients but lack the patient-physician interaction necessary for long-term disease management. For example, consumer eTools are unlikely to integrate with the patient's electronic record maintained by their physician, thereby providing recommendations that may be at odds with what the patient's physician might recommend. Plateaued usage may be more likely in this setting because there is no reinforcing mechanism to encourage prolonged use. For this reason, this chapter focuses on how to create an environment where *patient* eTools can thrive. We analyze key barriers and enablers to incorporating them as part of a self-management program and make recommendations to healthcare providers on how to use patient eTools effectively. We believe that encouragement and accountability are two mechanisms that healthcare providers can use to support patients to continue using eTools for self-management and prevent plateauing of use. We also identify the clinical environment where eTools are most likely to succeed and examine the features that will make patient applications useful in the long run. Finally, we make recommendations to eTool developers on how to make their tools more effective for healthcare providers to use during their encounters with patients.

BACKGROUND AND LITERATURE REVIEW

Chronic diseases are the leading causes for 60% of deaths around the world, and the burden of chronic disease is predicted to rise over the next several decades. Self-management is critical in the case of chronic disease because lifestyle factors and medication adherence between healthcare provider visits are vital for the long-term health of patients. One definition of self-management is "the systematic provision of supportive interventions by healthcare staff to increase patients' skills and confidence in managing their health problems, including regular assessment of progress and problems, goal setting, and problem-solving support…the key feature of these interventions is the aim of increasing patients' ability to deal with day-to-day consequences of their disease to maintain a satisfactory quality of life" (Trappenburg 2012). In fact, the recently adopted definition of health includes self-management as a key component (Huber 2011).

Because more people are seeking out health information on the web and via their mobile devices, the role of healthcare providers in supplying quality advice is more important than ever. There are many advantages to patients using the Internet and social media to learn about healthcare. Social media platforms allow users to share stories of sickness and health, which function as important sources of encouragement and empowerment. Social support from peers is a significant catalyst for behavior change. Brandt et al (2013) found that consumers interacting on a smoking cessation blog shared their personal stories, provided emotional support to each other and provided congratulatory messages, which served as encouragement to continue down a difficult path.

Users can also recommend doctors and healthcare facilities to one another. Recent studies reveal a surprisingly large amount of trust in social media content posted by other patients; 46% trust content posted by other patients, 55% trust content posted by hospitals, 56% by nurses and 60% by physicians (Ottenhoff 2012). There is also a positive correlation between provider use of social media and the quality of care delivered to a patient (Beck 2002, Manary 2013). The current clinical trends favor patient self-management as the most efficient approach in healthcare for treating chronic disease (Wagner 2002, Coleman 2009). In addition to experiencing better health outcomes, patients that are actively engaged in managing their diseases incur lower healthcare costs (Hibbard 2013).

Internet-based interventions are effective ways of engaging individuals that fall outside the range of conventional care, such as marginalized individuals that do not have access to primary care or those who may be unwilling to seek out traditional care. Online health programs can also be kept up-to-date with the latest treatment strategies and can capture demographic and usage data in large volumes to improve program content and efficacy. In this way, electronic health (eHealth) interventions can overcome challenges that traditional care cannot.

Web-based interventions are inherently personalized because users can freely browse and interact with content that is most relevant to them. Customized web-based algorithms already exist and have been successfully implemented in other industries, such as online advertising, and eHealth programs can use similar technology to personalize user content. The eTool registration page can imitate the face-to-face clinical information gathering process by having users input health-related parameters that tailor the eTool's content for a program more fitted to the user's health needs.

Moreover, the web has the added benefit of discussion and support forums where users can interact with others experiencing similar challenges; some programs are even moderated by experts, which ensures that the quality of health information is accurate in addition to supportive.

There is evidence that internet-based intervention is effective in treating mental health and addiction problems because users that fear stigmatization or struggle to prioritize self-care benefit from the anonymity of web-based interventions and the accessibility of information. Although the evidence shows that counseling and tailored self-help methods are effective methods, these avenues are underused and must be more accessible and up-to-date.

A study conducted by researchers at Evolution Health assessed the most active social network participants on two web-based smoking intervention sites and found that while most users posted infrequently, those who did post made regular contributions that strongly drive social network traffic. The study also revealed that the majority of users that posted to discussion boards were recent quitters, who ceased smoking for less than one year. The two eHealth social networks compared were the publicly run Canadian Cancer Society's Smokers' HelplineOnline and the privately run StopSmokingCenter.net. However, it is not clear what demographics frequent posters share; gender, age, and past smoking/quitting habits did not reveal significant differences. The key to effective social networks is to maintain a group of regular posters who offer direct help information, but there is very little research that explains the correlation between frequent posters and disengaged users (van Mierlo, et al. 2012).

Another study assessed how users engage with online weight loss tools. The results show that clinical characteristics can provide some indication into how a user interacts with an online health program. For example, there may be a correlation between gender and weight loss treatment strategies. Whereas for women the psychological influence of food may be a stronger factor in engaging with a weight loss tool, other factors may be more influential for men seeking weight loss tools. However, there is still very little research into how user demographics impact engagement with online intervention tools (Binks M, et al. 2012).

Simply providing health information is not enough to engage patients to change their health behaviors (Burns 2012). Some patients may feel overwhelmed and unprepared to manage their own health while others simply require more in-depth information to adequately care for themselves. A customized approach to healthcare that incorporates different health beliefs, goals, and motivations would improve clinical outcomes, lower costs, and heighten patient satisfaction.

Five key constructs appear to play an important role in enhancing and mediating patient self-management and improving patient outcomes. These constructs are real-world constructs that can be supported by eTools or can be detracted by poorly designed eTools. These constructs are: 1) Patient activation, as measured by the Patient Activation Measure (PAM); 2) patient-physician communications and patient preferences for communication styles and approaches; 3) patient behavior change models and 4) health literacy and 5) interoperability of data from provider electronic medical records (EMRs) to eTools and from remote monitoring devices to EMRs. An additional construct may be important in some cases, but is considered out of scope for this chapter discussion, namely the impact of mild to moderate cognitive impairment on use of eTools (Archer 2014). The impact of cognitive impairment on patient's understanding of their disease, disease process and self-management is very poorly understood. Although some consider cognitive impairment to be a special case of low health literacy, further research on the impact of cognitive impairment on disease and self-management are required before incorporating design recommendations into the next generation of eTools.

Hibbard et al (2013) and others (Hibbard 2008, Rask 2009, Skolasky 2011, Mosen 2007) have shown that patient activation, as measured by the Patient Activation Measure (PAM), is correlated with: healthier behaviors such as, physical activity and a diet higher in fruits and vegetables; more appropriate use of the healthcare system, including seeking regular care and not delaying care; more consumer-like behaviors such as making a list of questions for the doctor and researching doctor qualifications; more activity in self-management such as logging disease parameters and attending specialist visits; and better control of their disease, such as better control of blood pressure, HbA1c and fewer hospitalizations.

More importantly, patient activation has been found to be modifiable. Interventions that lead to changes in patient activation are not yet well-understood, but changes in patient activation from a low level to a higher level are associated with better health outcomes. As our understanding of the factors that lead to activation increases, it is likely that interventions will become more effective at changing health outcomes through personal agency. Early work with use of web-based interventions shows promise of being able to increase patient activation even in the absence of tailoring messages to the stage of the patient's level of activation (Solomon 2012). However, the authors caution against assuming that a short-term intervention is likely to have long-term, sustainable effects on patient activation.

Much has been written about patient-provider communication (Lam 2013, Farin 2012, de Jongh 2012). Farin et al (2011, 2012) have developed the KOPRA tool which measures communication preferences of patients with chronic disease. The KOPRA tool measures patient's communication preference along four dimensions: 1) effective and open communications, 2) patient participation and orientation, 3) emotionally supportive communication and 4) communication about personal circumstances. Interestingly, patients with different diseases prioritize different dimensions.

Older patients have different preferences from those of young people (older people are more comfortable with directive communications with less patient participation), and preferences appear to change over time or at different stages of a disease. When patients are particularly sick, they much prefer a directive approach rather than an open approach. Farin et al (2012) have also developed a provider communication style assessment questionnaire for patients. The so-called KOVA tool is an adaptation of the KOPRA tool but assesses whether providers' communication behaviors are in line with preferences. These two tools are good ways of assessing the congruence between provider communication behaviors and patient preferences.

Lam (2013) and de Jongh (2012) assess patient preference for specific communication media. Whether patients prefer to communicate by email, text messaging, social media or telephone can depend on age or disease. The effectiveness of communication also depends on disease and medium. eTools can be designed to assess patients' communication preferences in different situations and at different times in their lives to make sure that communications between patients and providers are the most effective ones. Ensuring appropriate communications with patients can be daunting when there are so many dimensions required which change for different diseases, severities of disease and ages of patients. These are exactly the types of situations where technologies, properly designed, can excel.

There are many behavior change models that have been studied over the last few years, including Prochaska's (1992) venerable transtheoretical model (TTM) of change, motivational interviewing (MI) and the health risk intervention (HRI) model (Prochaska 2008). The transtheoretical model has the longest history of research and has over 150 publications devoted to it. The model posits that people are at different stages of change at various times in their lives. The model describes 5 stages: 1) Individuals in the precontemplation stage engage in risky behaviors, but are not considering changing their behaviors. They typically do not have any facts about the risks of their behaviors or have tried to make changes unsuccessfully and have regressed back into the precontemplation stage; 2) Contemplators are those who are considering making a change. They are usually stuck weighing the benefits and costs of changing and are not yet convinced that they should change; 3) Preparers are individuals who have a plan to make a change (e.g., quit smoking, lose weight, etc) because for them the benefits now outweigh the costs. Many have attempted a change in the past but have been unsuccessful. Although the Preparer has a plan, they may not have full commitment to the plan; 4) The Action stage is where the individual actually acts on their intent. They are doing what is required to make the change. If an individual has not sufficiently prepared for this stage, they are likely to revert back to their previous state; 5) Maintenance is the stage where the individual has successfully changed to a new set of behaviors for at least 6 months.

This model is well suited for development into eTools as the metrics are easily able to identify which stage a patient is in and can provide recommendations that are suited to the patient's stage. For example, while a patient who is in the Action stage may require encouragement and a reminder about the types of things that can lead to a relapse, a patient who is in the Precontemplation stage may need information about their disease and encouragement that behavior change is possible and sustainable. Chen et al (2012) report on a systematic review of eTools for smoking cessation. They concluded that eTools do have a small, but statistically significant impact on smoking cessation. Several other eTools for behavior change in a variety of health behaviors such as getting human papilloma virus vaccinations (Paiva 2014) and weight loss (Wee 2005) have been developed and tested.

A promising new area of behavior change is a method called adaptive elearning. As patients have increased access to technology and computers become more powerful, it is possible to create interactive tools that can assess a patient's knowledge and then provide them with the right information in the format that they like best and which is most effective at driving behavior change (Harris 2011). Although these authors reported poor results of this intervention that was found to be as costly as other current interventions, we speculate that costs are likely to come down and quality of the intervention is likely to go up over time. Adaptive elearning is likely here to stay.

Poor health literacy is well described as being associated with poor health and being disadvantaged when using the healthcare system. Patients with poor health literacy, which is estimated to be as high as 88% of patients over the age of 65, have a difficult time following treatment instructions, are more likely to make errors with their medications, have difficulty navigating the healthcare system, are more likely to be hospitalized and are more likely to incur higher costs (Health Literacy n.d).

eTools present a promising method to overcome poor health literacy. The ability to display pictures and graphs may help make numerical information more understandable. Showing patients pictures of their medications and displaying the time of day at which they are supposed to take them could be useful in communicating medication dosage information. Smith et al (2011) tried to automate a tool to improve the coherence of health text, building on a strong base of theoretical knowledge of how to write health related text in a manner that is easy to understand. Although they found that their approach was not scalable, it is only a matter of time before researchers crack the code on simplifying health text using automated algorithms.

Finally, eTools need to be able to get data from EMRs (Holbrook 2009) and share data with EMRs. Interoperability of data between healthcare provider systems and patient eTools is crucial for empowering patients to self-manage their diseases. Without interoperability, patients are blind in their use of eTools and their use is not sustainable.

Although the growing presence of sophisticated eTools that utilize complex notions of change in the realm of healthcare is engaging patients in the treatment of their own diseases and promoting health-consciousness, the drawbacks of a largely user-driven application are the lack of accountability, poor follow-up and lack of critical data that is usually in the hands of the provider. The literature shows that over the long-term users disengage from using these applications. This could be attributed to several factors including the feeling of discouragement due to a lack of improvement in one's condition, the lack of feedback and validation needed to course correct or encourage one to stay on track, a lack of accountability for change other than to oneself, or a variety of other personal reasons such as busy schedules and life events taking priority.

Despite these barriers, recent surveys confirm a strong willingness by both physicians and patients to engage in the use of electronic tools, if it can provide better quality care. (Ottenhoff 2013, McGowan 2012). However, this is where the literature's role ends as there is very little written about the role of eTools in: 1) enhancing communication between healthcare providers and patients on an on-going basis; after all, it is unrealistic to expect patients with complex chronic diseases to self-manage for the 3-6 months between provider visits without some support or guidance from their care team; 2) enhancing the ability of the provider to track and monitor patient progress in between visits; currently there is no payment model for this type of service, other than a capitation funding model which may not explicitly require it and the tools to manage multiple data streams are still relatively primitive; 3) increasing patient accountability because somebody is monitoring progress on an on-going basis (Demiris 2008, Rosser 2009, van Gemert-Pijnen 2011).

GETTING PAST THE PLATEAU IN ETOOL USE

The Problem

The current patient-provider rapport does not effectively support communication between patients and providers between doctor visits – where the bulk of treatment takes place. As a patient undertakes the prescribed method of treatment, he or she can encounter complications such as experiencing side effects from a new medication, failing to see improvement in his or her condition after an adequate period of use of medication, or getting mixed messages about the safety or efficacy of the medication from family, friends and the Internet. As a result, patients may decide to stop taking a medication or stop following a course of treatment. This means that until the next doctor's visit (usually several months later) a patient is not treating his or her disease, during which time a patient's condition can worsen. The result is that doctors become frustrated and patients become discouraged because there is no structure in place to enable effective communication between the two parties in between visits.

At present, patient-provider communication tends to take the form of checklisting for medical information, which fails to incorporate the patient's personal and daily social demands, which can significantly impact the success of patient self-care. Quantitative measures are poor motivators for patient health behavior change because they don't hold significant relevance for patients in their daily lives. Often, the demand of self-care competes with many other demands in an individual's life, and it is important that providers take these social demands into account when working with patients to develop an effective treatment plan so that care is more manageable. Patients become discouraged and are less likely to take action when they do not feel that they can change their condition in a significant way. Treatment plans that incorporate patients' social demands are more manageable. It is also important to relate quantitative health indicators to how a patient is feeling in terms of pain, tiredness, etc. rather than simply as a physical result. (Farvolden et al. 2009)

Even with the support of eTools, patients tend to lose interest in health applications over time. While many people are initially willing to use health applications, they eventually become unmotivated and disengaged, which hinders disease management.

Controversies

The issue of how much support providers can give patients and the source of this support is controversial. Some tools that support self-management are purely patient-driven, while others are largely physician-controlled (e.g. tethered PHRs). Although self-management is not a new concept, it has not been widely adopted by providers. However, the trend is changing and some healthcare practices are now more willing to participate than others. In order to reduce the barrier for adoption of self-management in the care process, the important issue of how to provide enough support through an eTool must be addressed so that patients can succeed without critically disrupting the clinical workflow process and without overburdening already busy healthcare practitioners.

Barriers

Most eTools on the market today fall into the consumer eTool category. They are one-sided because the patient can download them without a prescription or recommendation from a healthcare provider and use them to manage their health autonomously without the guidance of their physician, who has access to valuable information that may not be available to the patient. It is also easier to develop eTools that don't require integration with EMRs as there are currently no universal standards for seamless integration into EMRs. The information that a patient may be missing include lab results, physiological readings and examination findings, a listing of previous diagnoses, alternative treatments and other best practice knowledge. Ultimately, this can cause inconsistencies between what patients are doing and what physicians might recommend. There are currently few systems in place to facilitate the sharing of information between the patient and the provider when a patient opts to use a consumer eTool.

Even most patient eTools today do not use best practices in helping patients and providers have postive, empowering interactions. eTools lack the customization that can be provided by staging patients in level of activation and stage of change. By assessing the level of activation and the stage of change, eTools can better identify where patients are in the self-management continuum and provide more customized and more effective interventions. eTools also lack the sophistication of understanding patient communication preferences with regard to their disease, not just their communication channel preferences. Finally, eTools lack the ability to present material at the appropriate level of health literacy for each patient that uses the eTool. Without better interoperability and sensitivity to a wider range of patients and their heterogenous needs, eTools will continue to miss the mark with encouraging self-management.

On the provider side, a key barrier is a lack of training. Many believe that self-management is more time consuming, yet there is no clear evidence that engaging patients is more time consuming than the typical care approach and in fact, encouraging self-management may in fact lead to better compliance and therefore better patient outcomes. Therefore, temporary incentives for providers to adopt this method may be useful to overcome this misconception and barrier in the early stages of roll-out.

Providers also have few tools that allow them to manage data from multiple patients with multiple diseases; automated data collection from multiple eTools can easily overwhelm the current capacity of providers to manage incoming data. Lack of payment mechanisms to reimburse providers and lack of tools for reviewing, analyzing and responding to patient and remote device communications is yet another barrier preventing widespread adoption of these technologies.

Some critical barriers associated with adopting eTools into the primary care system include (Figure 1) concern for the privacy and security of patient personal information, lack of integration of eTools into the primary care workflow and lack of proof of their efficacy (Buijink 2012). Many information systems are not equipped to track patients throughout the care process. Furthermore, unlike the typical producer-consumer interaction that exists in a business transaction, the doctor-patient relationship involves greater risk because the stakes are so much higher. The threat of government regulation may also impede willingness to adopt and recommend eTools that may end up, for example, being withdrawn from the market because of impending regulatory requirements (FDA 2011).

Figure 1. Barriers and enablers of eTool use

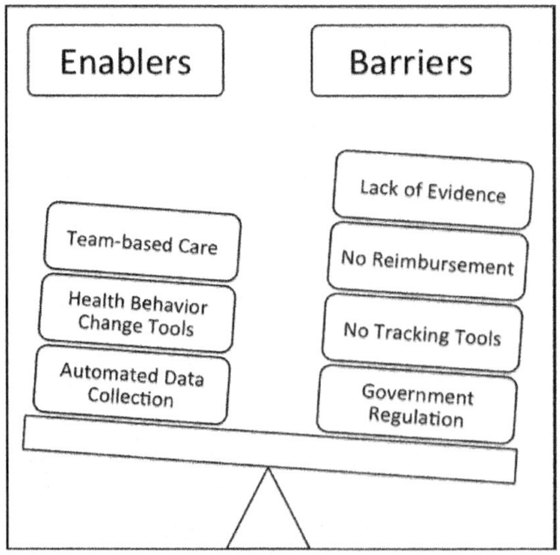

Enablers

Technological advances are facilitating the creation of more effective health tools. Automated data collection from a variety of devices is getting much easier and requires less effort from users, so patients are increasingly benefiting from applications without putting in very much work. Health behavior change tools and gamification of apps is another mechanism that keeps patients engaged with eTools longer. However, even gamified apps are soon abandoned if there are no strong external forces to help patients maintain use of their app for behavioral tracking and change over the long-term.

In addition to technological advances, other process and organizational enablers include team-based primary care, physician leadership within a culture of communication and quality improvement, support for patient self-management integrated into the primary care workflow, information technology support and an IT infrastructure that supports the use of eTools.

Although eTools are relatively new and it is still too early to be able to tell whether patients will use them for extended periods of time, patients do see their physicians for decades at a time and tend to be quite loyal to them. Basing a long-term intervention on known patterns of behavior (seeing a healthcare provider on a regular basis) is more likely to lead to success rather than relying on a relatively new technology to supplant existing relationships and ways of working.

Solutions and Recommendations

Based on interviews with key stakeholders (policy players, educational organizations and other organizations actively involved in designing, developing and deploying electronic channels of communication with healthcare providers), we identified several potential solutions.

An effective eTool will not only capture patient-collected data (e.g., home blood pressure readings, home blood sugar monitoring) but will also integrate with the provider's electronic medical record system (EMR) to collect relevant data for the management of the patient's condition (e.g., HbA1C for tracking diabetes, LDL for tracking high cholesterol, list of current medications, etc). The effective eTool will record a patient's healthcare goal, then track the patient's progress against that goal and send regular reports to providers so that they can support patients based on where they are in the treatment process.

Figure 2. Enabling environment for patient self-management and eTool use

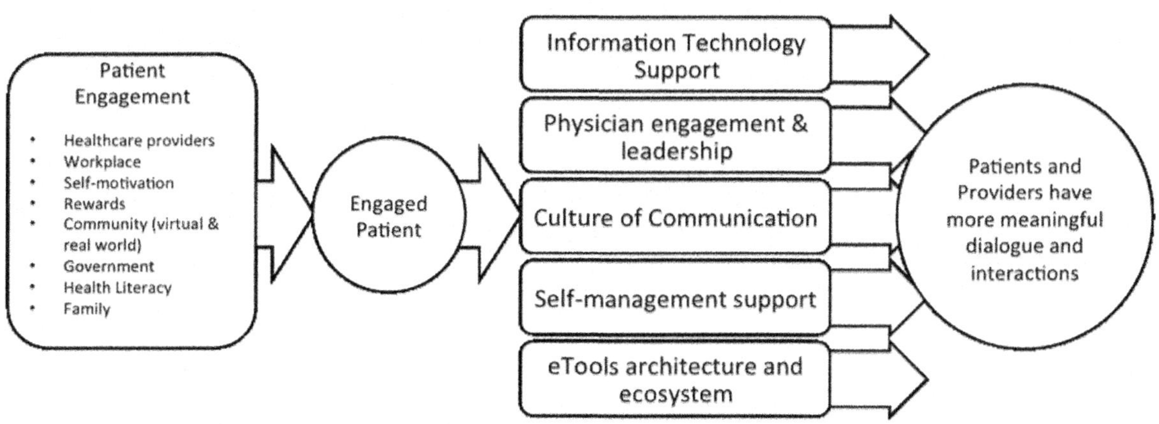

For example, an application might present a questionnaire shortly after a patient begins a new prescription. Through it, patients could voice concerns about side effects, new symptoms, and other treatment complications to their physicians in between visits. The application would send the questionnaire results to the provider, so they can gauge patient response to the treatment and provide feedback on how to proceed. eTools might also suggest questions for the patient to ask the provider.

Effective eTools also need to continue to use innovative best practices in enhancing patient self-management, including patient activation and patient behavior change. They also need to incorporate best practices in providing patients with communications in a manner that is congruent with their preferences and their expectations and in language that is easy to understand and implement.

Ultimately, patients benefit most from communicating with an advisor because technology alone cannot provide the accountability, encouragement and guidance that a human being can; therefore, healthcare management cannot be purely consumer-driven (Rock 2009, Rosser 2009). The self-management process must begin with a dialogue during which the provider recommends an eTool to the patient as a part of a self-management plan. Then, the provider requires some form of output or follow-up report from the eTool to serve as the focus for discussion at the next visit or as measure of efficacy in between visits. This focus on follow-up and on-going communication between visits creates the accountability that patients require to stay the course and continue using the app after the initial novelty has worn off. But before providers will adopt eTools, they must be effectively integrated into the primary care workflow.

The trend toward team-based care supports the integration of eTools into primary care workflows. The burden of follow-up need not fall on a single provider because different providers on the team can each address issues that are relevant to their domain; e.g., the team pharmacist can address medication issues while the dietician can address nutrition issues. If provider EMRs allowed providers to tag patient issues according to team member competencies, then the appropriate provider could follow-up with patients to help them address their issue. Providers should be able to escalate or 'refer' a patient to another provider, if necessary.

Furthermore, provider-side applications will need to allow the provider to quickly separate the signals from the noise that is likely to come from eTools, allowing them to focus on the medical events that are most important and ignore the thousands of normal findings that might be reported about patient physiological measurements or medication compliance.

Although providers keep asking for evidence of efficacy, the reality is that until there is better understanding of which workflows are effective and which ones are not, it is unlikely that we will be able to garner the evidence that eTools are effective in the way that pharmaceutical agents are shown to be effective. The mechanism of action for an eTool is completely different from that of a pharmaceutical agent, so it is unlikely that we will have randomized controlled trial level evidence for eTool efficacy and effectiveness in the near term. Other than interacting with the eTool itself, eTools by themselves do not have a plausible mechanism for changing patient behaviors on a sustainable basis. Rather, what we will see is that assisting patients in self-management is effective because of the education, knowledge and behavior change support that is provided to them. eTools will only be a mechanism to measure progress between visits and to ensure consistency, replicability and mass customization of the self-management process across many patients.

FUTURE RESEARCH DIRECTIONS

Health behavior change is a rapidly evolving field. The inclusion of patient activation and health behavior change principles into eTools is also gaining ground (Pal 2013). The gamification of consumer and patient eTools is one facet of this evolving area, which is fuelled by the increasing ubiquity of smartphones that allow for rapid design of useful applications (Primack 2012),

eTools are a promising technology, but still in their infancy. Some key areas requiring further research include: 1) Impact of gamification and health behavior change methods on short- and long-term adherence to eTool use (Primack 2012). The role of gamification and other health behavior modification methods in the overall self-management paradigm needs to be better understood. 2) A better understanding of the elements of self-management that are effective for specific diseases and why they might be more effective for those diseases (Savage 2011, Li 2011, Effing 2007). It may be difficult to program effective interventions into eTool applications without a sound theoretical underpinning for patient self-management and a robust empirical base for proving the efficacy of interventions. 3) A better understanding of the mechanisms by which social and information forces exerted by providers, families, friends and social media can support or detract from patient wellness behaviors and patient well-being. Patients are bombarded by information from a variety of sources, many of which can be conflicting (Carpenter 2013). How they navigate those social and informational forces can have a big impact on medication compliance and follow through.

More information on tailored interventions is necessary to identify which strategies are the best for a given situation, in order to provide a framework under which dynamic approaches can be followed. Further research that could present the dynamic range of self-management programs supported by evidence of positive outcomes would support the transition towards self-management practices in primary care. For example, which kind of self-management intervention works best for which kind of patients and chronic diseases would be helpful in deciding which approach to take.

Developing multimodal eTools will be essential, and getting the most relevant information to patients will be critical in keeping the tools engaging and meaningful.

CONCLUSION

Patient self-management demands effective communication between patients and providers. Further, it requires a supportive and enabling environment for patient education and support. Social media is a powerful tool in this process because it can support or detract from provider efforts through social reinforcement or by presenting conflicting information. This points out that providers do not work in a vacuum and that providers cannot shape or control all the forces that patients need to navigate when taking care of themselves. Providers can only guide and support patients on how to navigate those forces if they themselves are aware of them and have effective mechanisms to overcome them.

Stand-alone, specialized tools may be effective for short-term use, and encourage patients to engage in monitoring their own health. But for eTools to be effective in the long run, they must be complemented by patient-provider communication within a broader environment and culture that supports patient self-management and is information technology- and information management-enabled to take advantage of new and evolving eTools and best practices.

An effective self-management program must customize its approach to treatment because a one-size-fits-all attitude does not account for individual patient experiences, desires, and concerns. Since patients cannot always meet with a doctor to discuss health issues, health applications can provide temporary support to a patient in between doctor visits. But electronic tools must move beyond the limitations of consumer applications before healthcare providers will adopt them. Furthermore, incorporating eTools does not eliminate the role of healthcare providers in the treatment process but, rather, promotes collaboration between patients and providers to achieve the best treatment strategies. This means engaging patients in the care process. Healthcare providers are key motivators for patient progress, and, as such, they should require some tangible output from eTools to keep patients engaged and accountable for self-management.

REFERENCES

Archer, N., Keshavjee, K., Demers, C., & Lee, R. (2014). Online self-management interventions for chronically ill patients: Cognitive impairment and technology issues. *International Journal of Medical Informatics*, *83*(4), 264–272. doi:10.1016/j.ijmedinf.2014.01.005 PMID:24507762

Beck, R. S., Daughtridge, R., & Sloane, P. D. (2002). Physician-patient communication in the primary care office: A systematic review. *The Journal of the American Board of Family Practice*, *15*(1), 25–38. PMID:11841136

Binks, M., van Mierlo, T., & Edwards, C.L. (2012). Relationships of the Psychological Influence of Food and Barriers to Lifestyle Change to Weight and Utilization of Online Weight Loss Tools. *The Open Medical Informatics Journal*, (6), 9-14.

Bodenheimer, T., Wagner, E. H., & Grumbach, K. (2002). Improving primary care for patients with chronic illness. *Journal of the American Medical Association*, *288*(15), 1909–1914. doi:10.1001/jama.288.15.1909 PMID:12377092

Brandt, C. L., Dalum, P., Skov-Ettrup, L., & Tolstrup, J. S. (2013). After all–It doesn't kill you to quit smoking: An explorative analysis of the blog in a smoking cessation intervention. *Scandinavian Journal of Public Health*, *41*(7), 655–661. doi:10.1177/1403494813489602 PMID:23696257

Buijink, A. W., Visser, B. J., & Marshall, L. (2013). Medical apps for smartphones: Lack of evidence undermines quality and safety. *Evidence-Based Medicine*, *18*(3), 90–92. doi:10.1136/eb-2012-100885 PMID:22923708

Burns, J. (2012). The Next Frontier: Patient Engagement. *Managed Care*. Retrieved from http://www.managedcaremag.com/archives/1206/1206.engagement.html

Carpenter, D. M., Elstad, E. A., Blalock, S. J., & Devellis, R. F. (2014). Conflicting Medication Information: Prevalence, Sources, and Relationship to Medication Adherence. *Journal of Health Communication*, *19*(1), 67–81. doi:10.1080/10810730.2013.798380 PMID:24015878

Chen, Y. F., Madan, J., Welton, N., Yahaya, I., Aveyard, P., & Bauld, L. et al. (2012). Effectiveness and cost-effectiveness of computer and other electronic aids for smoking cessation: A systematic review and network meta-analysis. *Health Technology Assessment*, *16*(38). doi:10.3310/hta16380 PMID:23046909

Coleman, K., Austin, B. T., Brach, C., & Wagner, E. H. (2009). Evidence on the Chronic Care Model in the new millennium. *Health Affairs*, *28*(1), 75–85. doi:10.1377/hlthaff.28.1.75 PMID:19124857

de Jongh, T., Gurol-Urganci, I., Vodopivec-Jamsek, V., Car, J., & Atun, R. (2012). Mobile phone messaging for facilitating self-management of long-term illnesses. *Cochrane Database of Systematic Reviews*, *12*. doi:10.1002/14651858.CD007459.pub2 PMID:23235644

Demiris, G., Afrin, L. B., Speedie, S., Courtney, K. L., Sondhi, M., Vimarlund, V., & Lynch, C. (2008). Patient-centered applications: Use of information technology to promote disease management and wellness. *Journal of the American Medical Informatics Association*, *15*(1), 8–13. doi:10.1197/jamia.M2492 PMID:17947617

Effing, T., Monninkhof, E. M., van der Valk, P. D., van der Palen, J., van Herwaarden, C. L., & Partidge, M. R. et al. (2007). Self-management education for patients with chronic obstructive pulmonary disease. *Cochrane Database of Systematic Reviews*, *4*. doi:10.1002/14651858.CD002990.pub2 PMID:17943778

Farin, E., Gramm, L., & Kosiol, D. (2011). Development of a questionnaire to assess communication preferences of patients with chronic illness. *Patient Education and Counseling*, *82*(1), 81–88. doi:10.1016/j.pec.2010.02.011 PMID:20219317

Farin, E., Gramm, L., & Schmidt, E. (2012). Taking into account patients' communication preferences: Instrument development and results in chronic back pain patients. *Patient Education and Counseling*, *86*(1), 41–48. doi:10.1016/j.pec.2011.04.012 PMID:21570795

Farvolden, P., Cunningham, J. A., van Mierlo, T., & Selby, P. (2009). Using E-health programs to overcome barriers to the effective treatment of mental health and addiction problems. *Journal of Technology in Human Services*, *27*(1), 5–22. doi:10.1080/15228830802458889

Federal Drug Administration. (2011). *Draft Guidance for Industry and Food and Drug Administration Staff - Mobile Medical Applications.* Retrieved from http://x.co/1U9bc

Harris, J., Felix, L., Miners, A., Murray, E., Michie, S., & Ferguson, E. et al. (2011). Adaptive e-learning to improve dietary behavior: A systematic review and cost-effectiveness analysis. *Health Technology Assessment*, *15*(37), 1–160. PMID:22030014

Health Literacy. (n.d.). Retrieved from http://healthliteracy.ca/en/professionals-and-service-providers.html

Hibbard, J., & Cunningham, P. J. (2008). How engaged are consumers in their health and health care, and why does it matter? *Research Briefs*, *8*, 1–9. PMID:18946947

Hibbard, J. H., & Greene, J. (2013). What the evidence shows about patient activation: Better health outcomes and care experiences, fewer data on costs. *Health Affairs (Project Hope)*, *32*(2), 207–214. doi:10.1377/hlthaff.2012.1061 PMID:23381511

Holbrook, A., Pullenayegum, E., Thabane, L., Troyan, S., Foster, G., & Keshavjee, K. et al. (2011). Shared electronic vascular risk decision support in primary care: Computerization of Medical Practices for the Enhancement of Therapeutic Effectiveness (COMPETE III) randomized trial. *Archives of Internal Medicine*, *171*(19), 1736–1744. doi:10.1001/archinternmed.2011.471 PMID:22025430

Huber, M., Knottnerus, J. A., Green, L., Horst, H. V. D., Jadad, A. R., Kromhout, D., & Smid, H. (2011). How should we define health? *British Medical Journal*, *343*(6). doi:10.1136/bmj.d4163 PMID:21791490

Lam, R., Lin, V. S., Senelick, W. S., Tran, H. P., Moore, A. A., & Koretz, B. (2013). Older adult consumers' attitudes and preferences on electronic patient-physician messaging. *The American Journal of Managed Care*, *19*(10), eSP7–eSP11. PMID:24511886

Li, T., Wu, H. M., Wang, F., Huang, C. Q., Yang, M., Dong, B. R., & Liu, G. J. (2011). Education programmes for people with diabetic kidney disease. *Cochrane Database of Systematic Reviews*, *6*. doi:10.1002/14651858.CD007374.pub2 PMID:21678365

Manary, M. P., Boulding, W., Staelin, R., & Glickman, S. W. (2013). The patient experience and health outcomes. *The New England Journal of Medicine*, *368*(3), 201–203. doi:10.1056/NEJMp1211775 PMID:23268647

McCallum, S. (2012). Gamification and serious games for personalized health. *Studies in Health Technology and Informatics*, 85–96. doi:10.3233/978-1-61499-069-7-85 PMID:22942036

McGowan, B. S., Wasko, M., Vartabedian, B. S., Miller, R. S., Freiherr, D. D., & Abdolrasulnia, M. (2012). Understanding the factors that influence the adoption and meaningful use of social media by physicians to share medical information. *Journal of Medical Internet Research*, *14*(5), e117. doi:10.2196/jmir.2138 PMID:23006336

Merolli, M., Gray, K., & Martin-Sanchez, F. (2013). Health Outcomes And Related Effects Of Using Social Media In Chronic Disease Management: A Literature Review And Analysis Of Affordances. *Journal of Biomedical Informatics*, *46*(6), 957–969. doi:10.1016/j.jbi.2013.04.010 PMID:23702104

Mosen, D. M., Schmittdiel, J., Hibbard, J., Sobel, D., Remmers, C., & Bellows, J. (2007). Is patient activation associated with outcomes of care for adults with chronic conditions? *The Journal of Ambulatory Care Management*, *30*(1), 21–29. doi:10.1097/00004479-200701000-00005 PMID:17170635

Ottenhoff, M. (2012). Infographic: Rising Use of Social and Mobile in Healthcare. *The Spark Report*. Retrieved from http://x.co/1U9fJ

Paiva, A. L., Lipschitz, J. M., Fernandez, A. C., Redding, C. A., & Prochaska, J. O. (2014). Evaluation of the acceptability and feasibility of a computer-tailored intervention to increase human papillomavirus vaccination among young adult women. *Journal of American College Health*, *62*(1), 32–38. doi:10.1080/07448481.2013.843534 PMID:24313694

Pal, K., Eastwood, S. V., Michie, S., Farmer, A. J., Barnard, M. L., & Peacock, R. et al. (2013). Computer-based diabetes self-management interventions for adults with type 2 diabetes mellitus. *Cochrane Database of Systematic Reviews*, *3*. doi:10.1002/14651858.CD008776.pub2 PMID:23543567

Pew Internet and American Life Project. (2012). *CHCF Health Survey Aug 7-Sep 6, 2012*. Retrieved from http://www.pewinternet.org/Reports/2013/Tracking-for-Health/Summary-of-Findings.aspx

Primack, B. A., Carroll, M. V., McNamara, M., Klem, M. L., King, B., & Rich, M. et al. (2012). Role of video games in improving health-related outcomes: A systematic review. *American Journal of Preventive Medicine*, *42*(6), 630–638. doi:10.1016/j.amepre.2012.02.023 PMID:22608382

Prochaska, J. O., Butterworth, S., Redding, C. A., Burden, V., Perrin, N., & Leo, M. et al. (2008). Initial efficacy of MI, TTM tailoring and HRI's with multiple behaviors for employee health promotion. *Preventive Medicine*, *46*(3), 226–231. doi:10.1016/j.ypmed.2007.11.007 PMID:18155287

Prochaska, J. O., DiClemente, C. C., & Norcross, J. C. (1992). In search of how people change: Applications to addictive behaviors. *The American Psychologist*, *47*(9), 1102–1114. doi:10.1037/0003-066X.47.9.1102 PMID:1329589

Public Health Agency of Canada. (n.d.). Retrieved from http://www.phac-aspc.gc.ca/cd-mc/hl-ls/index-eng.php

Rask, K. J., Ziemer, D. C., Kohler, S. A., Hawley, J. N., Arinde, F. J., & Barnes, C. S. (2009). Patient activation is associated with healthy behaviors and ease in managing diabetes in an indigent population. *The Diabetes Educator*, *35*(4), 622–630. doi:10.1177/0145721709335004 PMID:19419972

Rock, D. (2009). Managing with the Brain in Mind. *Strategy+ Business, 56*, 1-11.

Rosser, B. A., Vowles, K. E., Keogh, E., Eccleston, C., & Mountain, G. A. (2009). Technologically assisted behavior change: A systematic review of studies of novel technologies for the management of chronic illness. *Journal of Telemedicine and Telecare*, *15*(7), 327–338. doi:10.1258/jtt.2009.090116 PMID:19815901

Rudansky, A. K. (2013, June 23). PayPal Founder's Fellowship Hatches Medication Reminder App. *Information Week Health Care.* Retrieved from http://x.co/1U6Xp

Savage, E., Beirne, P. V., Ni Chroinin, M., Duff, A., Fitzgerald, T., & Farrell, D. (2011). Self-management education for cystic fibrosis. *Cochrane Database of Systematic Reviews*, *7*. doi:10.1002/14651858.CD007641.pub2 PMID:21735415

Schaefer, J., Miller, D., Goldstein, M., & Simmons, L. (2009). *Partnering in Self-Management Support: A Toolkit for Clinicians*. Institute for Healthcare Improvement. Retrieved from http://www.ihi.org/resources/Pages/Tools/SelfManagementToolkitforClinicians.aspx

Skolasky, R. L., Green, A. F., Scharfstein, D., Boult, C., Reider, L., & Wegener, S. T. (2011). Psychometric properties of the patient activation measure among multimorbid older adults. *Health Services Research*, *46*(2), 457–478. doi:10.1111/j.1475-6773.2010.01210.x PMID:21091470

Smith, C. A., Hetzel, S., Dalrymple, P., & Keselman, A. (2011). Beyond readability: Investigating coherence of clinical text for consumers. *Journal of Medical Internet Research*, *13*(4), e104. doi:10.2196/jmir.1842 PMID:22138127

Solomon, M., Wagner, S. L., & Goes, J. (2012). Effects of a web-based intervention for adults with chronic conditions on patient activation: online randomized controlled trial. *Journal of Medical Internet Research*, *14*(1), e32. doi:10.2196/jmir.1924 PMID:22353433

Trappenburg, J., Jonkman, N., Jaarsma, T., van Os-Medendorp, H., Kort, H., & de Wit, N. et al. (2013). Self-management: one size does not fit all. *Patient Education and Counseling*, *92*(1), 134–137. doi:10.1016/j.pec.2013.02.009 PMID:23499381 van Gemert-Pijnen, J. E., Nijland, N., van Limburg, M., Ossebaard, H. C., Kelders, S. M., Eysenbach, G., & Seydel, E. R. (2011). A holistic framework to improve the uptake and impact of eHealth technologies. *Journal of Medical Internet Research, 13*(4), e111. doi:10.2196/jmir.1672 PMID:22155738

van Mierlo, T., Voci, S., Lee, S., Fournier, R., & Selby, P. (2012). Superusers in Social Networks for Smoking Cessation: Analysis of Demographic Characteristics and Posting Behavior from the Canadian Cancer Society's Smokers' Helpline Online and StopSmokingCenter.net. *Journal of Medical Internet Research, 14*(3), e66. doi:10.2196/jmir.1854 PMID:22732103

Wee, C. C., Davis, R. B., & Phillips, R. S. (2005). Stage of readiness to control weight and adopt weight control behaviors in primary care. *Journal of General Internal Medicine, 20*(5), 410–415. doi:10.1111/j.1525-1497.2005.0074.x PMID:15963162

ADDITIONAL READING

Berwick, D. (2010). *Connected for Health: using electronic health records to transform care delivery* (L. L. Liang, Ed.). Wiley.

KEY TERMS AND DEFINITIONS

Consumer: A person who uses goods and services voluntarily and of their own volition.

EMR: Software used by healthcare providers to document the care they provide. Usually used in real-time at the point of care.

eTool: A software application or website that is intended to help consumers or patients to monitor, track and/or treat a disease condition.

Gamification: Integration of game mechanics or game dynamics into software applications.

Patient: A person with a health condition who is in the care of a healthcare provider.

Team-Based Care: Interprofessional teams of healthcare providers who work together (virtually or in the real world) to provide care to patients in an integrated manner.

This work was previously published in Social Media and Mobile Technologies for Healthcare edited by Mowafa Househ, Elizabeth Borycki, and Andre Kushniruk, pages 109-125, copyright year 2014 by Medical Information Science Reference (an imprint of IGI Global).

Chapter 11
Informatics and Health Services: The Potential Benefits and Challenges of Electronic Health Records and Personal Electronic Health Records in Patient Care, Cost Control, and Health Research – An Overview

Nelson Ravka
York University, Canada

ABSTRACT

Personal electronic health records are seen as a key component to improved health care for patients, empowering motivated patients by giving them access to their own records resulting in increased self-care, shared decision making, and better clinical outcomes. Benefits through electronic record keeping would also accrue to health care providers through the availability and retrievability of data, reduced duplication of medical tests, more effective physician diagnosis and treatment, reduced incidence of prescription errors, and flagging inappropriate drug combinations. Utilizing information technology could also moderate the cost of health care services. Electronic health records would also improve clinical research through access to a large database of patient electronic records for research and determining best practices. Although potential benefits are considerable, many challenges to implementation must be addressed and resolved before this potential of improved health care provision and cost efficiency can be realized.

INTRODUCTION

Personal Health Records (PHRs) and Electronic Health Records (EHRs) are seen as key components to improving health care to patients as well as promoting wellness to the public at large (Tang, Ash, Bates, Overhage, & Sands, 2006). Electronic health records are digital depositories for clinician records and managed by clinicians or health institutions. Hayrinen et al. describe EHRs as repositories of patient data in digital form, stored and exchanged securely, and accessible by multiple authorized users that contain

DOI: 10.4018/978-1-5225-1928-7.ch011

retrospective, concurrent, and prospective information. Their primary purpose is to support continuing, efficient, and quality orientated health care (Hayrinen, Saranto, & Nykanen, 2008). An advisory panel to the U.S. government's Health Information Technology Adoption Initiative has listed the functions of EHRs as 1) having the ability to electronically collect and store data about patients, 2) having the ability to supply that information to health providers on demand, 3) having the ability to allow physicians to enter patient care orders on the computer, and 4) having the ability to provide health professionals with health care decision making support (Blumenthal & Glasor, 2007). Garde et al. describe EHRs as having the following necessary characteristics:

- **Patient-Centred:** The EHR relates to the patient, not an encounter with an institution.
- **Longitudinal:** A long-term record of patient care.
- **Comprehensive:** Record of care from all health care providers and institutions.
- **Prospective:** Plans, goals, orders, and evaluations are recorded (Garde, Knaup, Hovenga, & Heard, 2007).

Conceptually, PHRs are digital health information vehicles that can be managed by individuals (patients or surrogates) compared to EHRs that are managed by health providers or clinical institutions. Although there is no absolute consensus on what defines PHRs, a description suggested by the Markle Foundation's working group on policies for information sharing between doctors and patients is useful. It describes PHRs as: "an electronic application through which individuals can access, manage and share their health information...in a private, secure and confidential environment" (Markle Connecting for Health, 2004). The National Alliance for Health Information Technology further clarifies an idealized model of PHRs as "an electronic record of health-related information that conforms to a common interoperability standard allowing information to be drawn from multiple sources while being managed, shared and controlled by the individual" (Kahn, Aulakh, & Bosworth, 2009, p. 369).

There is a range of formats that PHRs can be classified. The simplest is a stand-alone patient-initiated application that is not linked with any other system. The patient enters their own health data using commercial applications. Google Health and Microsoft Health Vault are examples of companies that have introduced such systems. However there is a concern that patients would not keep records up to date in a stand-alone PHR (Tang et al., 2006). Consequently these PHRs could be unreliable instruments for conveying information to clinicians or health institutions. Tang, et al. suggest that although some information can be supplied by patients, clinicians must have access to their own past inputs to assist in decision making. They stated; "[T]he reliability of patient-entered data depends on the nature of the information per se, the patient's general and health literacy, and the specific motivations for recording the data." (Tang et al., 2006, p. 122) In a study conducted by Ira C. Denton, 1000 patients were offered their medical information in a stand-alone PHR system. Only 330 accepted. After 10 months, of those who responded to a survey, 37% continued to use the electronic record (Denton, 2001). According to Linda Reed, chief information officer, Atlantic Health; "[M]any people are more willing to keep their Facebook page updated than their medical records" (Page, 2010).

Acknowledging the limitations of stand-alone PHRs that depend on patient-only inputs, a more information reliable model would involve health records that are stored in the patient's EHR. Such a 'tethered' system of provider owned and maintained PHR would consist of a summary of clinically relevant health information that is made available to patients. These systems can include functionalities such as appointment requests and prescription renewals. There can also be an opportunity for patient input that can be uploaded and saved to the provider's EHR (Tang et al., 2006). A still more complex system involves the linking of different health care data sources in a seamless interoperative functionality to allow for the transfer of patient data from all sources to the provider's EHR and patient PHR (Tang et al., 2006). This most complex system consists of a portable, interoperable digital file in which selected, clinically relevant health data can be managed, secured and transferred. With this level of functionality, Steinbrook wrote in the New England Journal of Medicine:

Online repositories will allow patients to store, retrieve, manage, and share their health data—such as lists of medical problems, medical history, medications, allergies, immunizations, test results, insurance information, and doctors' visits over the internet (Steinbrook, 2008, p. 1653).

In a February 2005 symposium sponsored by the American College of Medical Informatics, participants concluded that PHRs that were linked to EHRs either through tethering or interconnectivity would provide much greater benefits than stand-alone PHRs (Tang et al., 2006). Tethered PHR adoption would be tied to the growth in EHR adoption (especially by primary care physicians who are the main source of patient data) and would have the additional role of advising and supporting patients in their health care and self-management (Archer, Fevrier, Lokker, McKibbon, & Straus, 2011).

BENEFITS OF PHRS AND EHRS

There is growing public interest for access to health records and a general belief that this access would be useful in allowing patients to assume more responsibility and decision-making for their own health-care (Tang & Lansky, 2005). This electronic modality would empower motivated patients by giving them access to their own records and allow them to manage and share their health information in a private, secure and confidential environment. Pagliari et al. list the functions of these PHRs that include:

- Access to providers' electronic clinical record which includes history, drugs and test results.
- Access to a personal health organizer (can include information on clinics, doctors, tests, dates, non-prescribed treatments and scanned documents).
- Access to self-management support such as care plans, graphing of symptoms, passive biofeedback, instructive or motivational feedback, decision aids and reminders.
- Enablement of secure patient-provider communication for booking appointments, reordering prescriptions, and seeking advice through patient-doctor e-mail.
- Easily accessed links to information concerning illness, treatments or self-care.
- Links to sources of support such as patient organizations or virtual peer networks.
- Improve or facilitate the capture of symptoms or health behaviour data by self-reporting or link to electronic monitoring devices. (Pagliari, Detmer, & Singleton, 2007)

Detmer et al. also include in PHR potential functionality the ability to review insurance eligibility and benefits, the processing of claims and payments and automated checking for drug interactions (Detmer, Raymond, Tang, & Bloomrosen, 2008).

The potential of PHRs accrues to both patients and providers. Pagliari et al. suggest that the potential functionalities of PHRs can provide patient empowerment through access to their personal data, health information and communication opportunities. They note that the potential exists for increased self-care, shared decision making and better clinical outcomes and that patient involvement can improve safety through flagging diagnostic and drug errors, recording non-prescribed medications or improving accessibility to test results or drug alerts (Pagliari, Detmer, & Singleton, 2007). Hayrinen et al. state that PHRs can:

...reduce geographic barriers to patient care and act as a point of record integration, particularly in fragmented health systems, thus improving continuity of care and efficiency. Although the number and quality of studies remains limited, existing research suggest improvements in communication and trust between patients and professionals, confidence in self-care, compliance in chronic disease, and accuracy of records. Patients particularly value online reordering of prescriptions, laboratory results, disease management plans, trend charts, drug lists and secure messaging (Hayrinen et al., 2008, p. 293).

Pagliari et al. summarize the benefits derived from the use of PHRs. Patient empowerment creates distinct benefits through better health and quality of life. Increased personal responsibility can drive health maintenance and self-care. Motivation to comply with treatment through increased participation in decision-making and acquisition of health knowledge can result from the use of PHRs. Quality of care improves with improved relationships with health care providers through better communication. Patients have more flexible access to services such as appointments, tests and electronic consulting. Patient safety is enhanced through reduced errors, quicker access to results and drug alerts. Patient care can be improved with knowledge of otherwise unreported health behaviours and drug use and potentially better collaboration between caregivers and health care providers (Pagliari et al., 2007).

Examples of the advantages of PHRs can be informative. Tang and Lee describe a common scenario:

Mary is 68 years old, has four chronic conditions, takes seven medications, and averages 12 visits per year to her six physicians. In between visits, she spends a lot of time on the telephone with them or their staff—making appointments, requesting prescription renewals and referrals, seeking test results, and asking questions that she forgot to bring up in person.... What if Mary could view her test results within hours after her blood was drawn? What if she could upload her home glucometer and blood-pressure readings so she could graph them and see how changes in her behaviour affect them? What if her health care team received copies of her readings and could recommend dose adjustments for her medications? And what if it all happened without an office visit (Tang & Lee, 2009, p. 1276)?

Wolter et al. illustrates another scenario of how a PHR can improve information sharing between health care providers:

A patient is visiting a cardiologist for the first time. The physician asks the patient what medications he is taking. This is not a simple question, and the patient has trouble recalling all the necessary information: which medications he takes, the dosage for each, how often he takes them, how long he has been taking them, and the prescribing physician for each. He is not entirely sure why he has been prescribed one of them (Wolter & Friedman, 2005, p. 28).

Demand is growing among the public for access to their health records (Detmer et al., 2008). A 2003 survey by the Markle Foundation found that 65% of respondents were interested in electronically accessing their own personal health records. 90% believed it was important to be able to track their symptoms or changes in health care on-line. 71% stated that PHRs would be helpful in clarifying doctors' instructions. 65% believed that it would help in preventing medical mistakes. 54% believed it would change the way they managed their own health. 60% thought it would improve care. When asked about specific features, 75% of respondents indicated PHRs would be useful to e-mail their doctor, 69% believed it would be useful to store immunization records, 65% would use it to transfer information to specialists, 63% would look up test results and 62% would track medication use. The survey found that those with chronic illnesses, frequent health care users and caregivers had the greatest interest in PHRs (Markle Connecting for Health, 2003). A second survey by the Markle Foundation in 2006 reconfirmed public interest (Markle Connecting for Health, 2006).

A case study by Chen et al. illustrates the benefits of PHRs to health care providers. Following the installation of an EHR system with PHR functionalities that included secure patient-provider messaging, the total office visit rate among Kaiser Permanente patients decreased by 26.2%. (Kaiser health care providers are salaried employees. Their salaries are not dependent on the number of patient visits.) Comparing before and after implementation of the EHR and PHR system, office visits decreased from 99.6% of all ambulatory care contacts to 66%. Scheduled telephone visits accounted for 30% of contacts post-installation and secure messaging accounted for 4%. Although marginal or unnecessary office visits were reduced, the new modalities of care allowed an increase in patient contacts of 8%. Additionally, benefits involved reduced direct costs to patients through reduced cost of travel and parking and reduced school or work time loss. Surveys showed that patients' overall satisfaction with the new system were at least as high as previously. They perceived that the interest taken in their care by their health care providers was as good after implementation of EHRs and PHRs (Chen, Garrido, Chock, Okawa, & Liang, 2009).

Pagliari et al. suggest that the potential benefit to health care providers goes beyond unnecessary consultations and corresponding reduced waiting lists. They see the possibility of lower costs through better health and reduced use of services and treatments. Finally, health care providers could benefit from reduced provider liability through increased safety and patient self-management of their own health issues (Pagliari et al., 2007).

However Dunn and Wynia question whether care providers are better off with the addition of patient information input through their PHRs. The line between empowering and overwhelming patients and doctors with data may create its own problems. They suggest:

[W]ith too much information, decisions may be inappropriately delayed. Information overload can occur and some information may be pushed out; usually, more recently acquired information is retained and used, even if it is not the most relevant. Information will also tend to be retained if it supports a preconceived notion. Mental fatigue or decision fatigue can occur from the labour of sifting through information, and fatigued decision makers might make fast, careless decisions or suffer from decision paralysis (Dunn & Wynia, 2010, p. 67).

Innovative design and functioning of PHRs could rescue the users from these issues. It is possible that large amount of information can be converted into a summary format that would also generate recommendations (Dunn et al., 2010). Development of such decision support functions would enhance the value of PHRs to health care providers, avoiding the potential of overwhelming information interfering with appropriate or timely decision making (Dunn et al., 2010).

Electronic health records provide the digital link to PHRs and the benefits to patients that can come of it. Benefits of electronic records would also accrue to health care providers. Menachem and Collum suggest potential advantages over paper-based record systems that include:

- Improved legibility, availability and retrievablity of records and data.
- Reduced likelihood of duplication or unnecessary medical tests.
- Shorter patient waiting lists.
- More effective physician diagnosis and treatment through real time access to current best practices.
- Reduced incidence of prescription errors.
- Improved management and monitoring of multiple prescriptions.
- Improved flagging of inappropriate drug combinations that can cause adverse drug reactions.
- Increased efficiency in the delivery of health services (Menachemi & Collum, 2011).

EHRs can also be beneficial in clinical research (Diamond, Mostashari, & Shirky, 2009). Compiling information from a large data base of patients' electronic records would allow for assessments of treatment choices and determining best practices, enhance clinical research processes, and determine the incremental benefits of new medicines as well as documenting the frequency and severity of adverse events (Lumpkin, 2007). EHRs can improve efficiency and contain costs through innovative designing and conducting of global clinical trials (EHR4CR, 2011).

The goals of the Electronic Health Records for Clinical Research project (EHR4CR) are examples of the potential of EHRs for clinical research. This EU research project jointly run be academics and industrial partners is intended to; "build, validate and deploy a Europe-wide innovative technological platform to re-use EHRs data for clinical research purposes" (EHR4CR, 2011). Its goals are to attract research and development investments in Europe, to increase access to innovative medicines and to improve health outcomes while accomplishing these objectives within applicable legal, ethical and privacy protections of patients. The initiative would seek to moderate the cost of clinical trials by more efficiently evaluating patient populations, improving protocol design and identifying suitable patients for clinical trials thus eliminating unnecessary repetitive re-entry of data, confirming reliability of data sources and rendering easier the detection and reporting of rare adverse events. The realization of these objectives would create significant efficiency gains, faster access to new drugs and improve health outcomes (EHR4CR, 2011).

There are difficult obstacles that interfere with these goals. They include patient privacy, autonomy and consent, and interoperability across institutions, countries and continents (Jensen, Jensen, & Brunak, 2012). West et al. note three requirements that would allow EHRs to be useful for clinical research:

1. The ability to assemble patient clinical information from all providers to assess care quality.
2. The standardizing of entry procedures for recording patient care to optimize text mining of information and facilitate the use of data for research and assessing care quality.
3. The means to avoid using patient identifiers in sections of EHRs related to clinical data to conform to privacy requirements (West et al., 2009).

The potential advantages conferred to clinical research from EHRs are exciting in its scope. However it will take time and research to develop the protocols and technical standards to realize this potential.

CHALLENGES TO THE USE OF PHRS AND EHRS

Interoperability

The promise of better health care through shared health care and clinical research that are the potential benefits of EHRs can only be realized if information can be distributed efficiently to authorized stakeholders (Taylor, Bower, Frederico, & Bigelow, 2005). Taylor et al. state that; "[E]ffective connectivity is required to avoid redundant tests; improve safety and coordination among providers; increase administrative efficiency; and improve consumers' compliance with prevention, disease management, and care guidelines" (Taylor, Bower, Frederico, & Bigelow, 2005). The Institute of Electrical and Electronics Engineers defines interoperability as the "ability of two or more components to exchange information and to use the information that has been exchanged" (Institute of Electrical & Electronics Engineers, 1990). If information technology does not allow for a systematic processing of information, clinicians will bear unnecessary costs and workload as well as compounding the chance of introducing data errors. Garde et al. state:

Captured data must be of high quality (i.e. correct and complete), high reliability and high flexibility. This requires a mixture of free text entries and highly structured and standardized data items and the use of integrity constraints and plausibility checks. Different information systems used by the various health care providers of shared care must be able to interoperate, so that one system can understand the context and meaning of information provided by another system" (Garde et al., 2007, p. 333).

Unfortunately, as Thomas Beale argues, many systems have proprietary software that makes them expensive to modify and extend (Garde et al., 2007). The key to the widespread use of EHRs is standardization (Garde et al., 2007). This is not an easy goal. With technological and scientific advancements, changes are constantly needed to increase the scope and application of EHRs as medical knowledge expands. Standardization must include the means to incorporate change (Garde et al., 2007). To be fully beneficial EHRs that currently differs not only from each proprietary system within jurisdictions but also from country to country must be harmonized (Begoyan, 2007).

Harmonization must address two areas of interoperability—functional and semantic (Garde et al.,2007. Functional interoperability involves the exchange of information between different EHR systems that is readable by humans (Begoyan, 2007). Semantic interoperability refers to the exchange of information between systems that is computer processable by the receiving system (Begoyan, 2007). Begoyan lists the requirements to achieve semantic interoperability as follows;

- The utilization of a standardized EHR Reference Model to define and coordinate the semantics of EHR information structures.
- Use of a standardized service interface to define and coordinate the semantics of interfaces between EHR and other services.
- Utilization of a standardized set of domain-specific concept models to address needs dealing with archetypes and templates for different domain concepts.
- Use of standardized terminologies to define the language that is used in archetypes (The first two prerequisites also apply to functional interoperability) (Begoyan, 2007, p. 3).

Begoyan identifies a number of national and international organizations responsible for developing standards for EHRs. They include ISO (International Organization for Standardization) whose activities are limited to the structure and function of the EHR and the systems that processes EHR; CEN (European Committee for Standardisation) that oversees the development of multi-disciplinary standards including the interoperability of EHRs; HL7 (Health Level Seven) that is involved in providing standards between different types of healthcare computer applications including incorporating clinical and administrative data; and DICOM (Digital Imaging and Communications in Medicine) that has developed the standard for medical image communication allowing an independent exchange between medical images and related information (Begoyan, 2007). At the time of his review, Begoyan suggested that HL7 version3; "can be the foundation of future health care environments" (Begoyan, 2007, p. 7). However until semantic interoperability is achieved, full EHR utilization will be hampered by incompatible EHR systems purchased by different users (Begoyan, 2007).

Taylor et al. contend that the low rate of EHR adoption and the lack of interoperability in systems not designed for sharing of health information is a major barrier to connectivity. They identify four market failures that perpetuate these barriers:

1. The disconnect between those that pay for the technology and those who benefit from it.
2. The lack of pressure to adopt a standards-based EHR system.
3. The lack of incentives to develop a standards-based system or share detailed electronic patient data with competitors.
4. The lack of widespread access to standardized patient care data that could improve general health care performance (Taylor et al., 2005).

Interoperability is the backbone to efficient use of health information technology (Taylor et al., 2005; Garde et al., 2007). It is also a formidable technical challenge to overcome (Hersh, 2004). Its importance for fulfilling the potential of EHRs is driving research in standardization that adequately addresses the harmonization issues of semantics and functionality (Begoyan, 2007).

Access and Literacy Challenges

The potential for PHR use can only be realized if the modality is accessible (Pirtle & Chandra, 2011). This requires a public that is computer competent, has access to the internet and has a degree of health literacy. It is estimated that 50% of U.S. adults would not comprehend the information that could be made available to them for the purpose of allowing them to make better health choices (Pirtle & Chandra, 2011). In the U.S. only 44% of low- income households have computers and only 34% have an internet connection (Beacom, 2010). Computer literacy and internet access are necessary conditions for on-line communications and accessing information. These criteria are least available to low income individuals. In addition, identified groups with low health literacy are populations over age sixty five, members of minorities or immigrant groups and those with chronic physical conditions (Kahn et al., 2009). Groups that are among the largest users of health care are the elderly and those with chronic conditions (Bodenheimer & Fernandez, 2005). As well, since poverty is a known determinate of ill health (McCally, et al., 1998) the poor can be included as disproportionate users of health-care (Wolter & Friedman, 2005; Wagstaff, 2002). If costs are not a barrier to accessing health care (as is the case in OECD countries with universal health care), then people of lower socio-economic status use more health care services than wealthier people (Asada & Kephart, 2007). It is likely that the largest users of health care resources are also the most health illiterate and the least likely to have computer or internet access. They would be excluded from the potential benefits of PHRs (Eyserbach, 2008).

This lack of access prevents disadvantaged groups from participating in social networking, denying them the ability to confer with peers and informing themselves of relevant information and what others are doing (Eyserbach, 2008). Thus the utilization of the power of the internet as a source of motivation and self-help is unavailable to the computer illiterate or those without access. These factors present a cautionary warning. Health maintenance and health recovery are multi-dimensional concepts that are related to many disciplines. Without addressing tangentially related issues, PHRs will be beneficial to a privileged part of the population and thus realize only a fraction of their potential.

Thus far those without computer or internet access have been excluded as candidates for PHR benefits (Pirtle & Chandra, 2011). However smart phones are becoming ubiquitous. This may be the future entry point to PHRs for disadvantaged groups who would otherwise not have access. Paglieri suggests; "[T]he emergence of mobile and wireless applications that allow remote submission of data to a shared record offer new possibilities and real time decision support" (Pagliari et al., 2007, p. 331). Much development work must be done to realize the potential of this way forward.

Denton has shown that many patients may not want to take the personal responsibility that PHRs allow (Denton, 2001). Therefore it may be a modality that is most suitable for certain motivated patients and caregivers (Tang et al., 2006). Paglieri et al. suggest that although surveys indicate that most people would like access to their health records, the most likely users and therefore the ones who would gain the most from PHRs would be those with long term conditions who have ongoing incentives to track their illness and treatments and patients experiencing periodic need for care that triggers an interest in information and communication (Pagliari et al., 2007). Caregivers and relatives of elderly parents or children in hospitals can benefit from PHRs by developing a partnership with health care providers through information sharing that could impact the patient's care (Pagliari et al., 2007).

Privacy and Security Challenges

Privacy and security are serious concerns for most people. The Personal Health Working Group of the Markle Foundation stated in 2003 that 91% of people reported that they were very concerned about the privacy and security of their personal health information (Kaelber, Jha, Johnston, Middleton, & Bates, 2008). Halanka et al. studied three functioning PHR systems that were clinic or institutional owned and maintained. A number of privacy and security challenges were common to all three systems. These include:

- Should the entire problem list be shared?
- Should the entire medication list and allergy list be shared?
- Should all laboratory and diagnostic test results be shared with the patient?
- Should clinical notes be shared with the patient?
- How should patients be authenticated to access the PHR?
- Should minors be able to have their own private PHR and should patients be able to share access to their PHRs via proxies?
- Should the PHR include secure clinician-patient messaging (Halamka, Mandl, & Tang, 2008)?

The authors noted that all three systems chose to share the entire problem list with patients and facilitated patient understanding by using full text descriptions of problems. One provided hyperlinks to provide explanatory information of diagnoses. All shared the entire medication list. All shared laboratory and diagnostic tests (where not restricted by jurisdictional laws) and established protocols so that disturbing information could first be conveyed by personal communication with a health care provider. All decided not to share clinical text notes. All implemented username and password protocols to ensure privacy. As to policy regarding PHRs and minors, each system determined their own unique policy. Although concerns existed about a lack of reimbursement involving secure messaging, all three provided the service. The authors noted that with careful attention to policy concerning privacy, security, data stewardship and personal control, PHRs can be successfully deployed (Halamka et al., 2008).

Further research is needed to develop a standard protocol for ensuring appropriate PHR privacy and security (Kaelber et al., 2008). Answers to questions such as who controls sharing of and access to a PHR of minors and non-competent patients and what would be an acceptable trade-off between verification of authenticity of a user and the interests of legitimate patient proxies must be debated and a policy consensus developed. A balance must be agreed on how much security is needed to allow easy patient access but difficult enough to prevent security breaches. Consideration must be given to the possibility of unintentially limiting PHR use if access is too difficult. Answers to what common procedures can be developed to allow access if passwords are forgotten or if the patient is incapacitated must be found. Kaelbe et al., referring to issues of privacy and security, ask what authentication methods would "ensure both privacy and security yet in doing so do not present a major barrier to access." (Kaelber et al., 2008, p. 731) How would the use of patient records for research be allowed while still protecting patient privacy? PHRs will only become commonplace when these privacy and security issues are resolved (Kaelber et al., 2008).

Adoption and Attitude Challenges for PHR Utilization

Use of PHRs will hinge on overcoming attitudinal and physical adoption barriers among patients and care providers (Kaelber et al., 2008). As previously noted, some limited research has shown interest among patients. However adoption has been low when access is available even when it was provided free of charge (Kaelber et al., 2008; Denton, 2001). The attitudes of physicians are even less well documented. Some studies show that providers are hesitant about adopting PHRs (Witry, Doucette, Daly, Levy, & Chrischilles, 2010). Physicians are concerned about any additional work that would be required that would not be compensated (Kaelber, Jha, Johnston, Middleton, & Bates, 2008). Witry et al. observed; "While providers believe PHRs have the potential to decrease errors and increase efficiency, they are concerned about how to integrate PHRs into patient appointments that are already too short" (Witry et al., 2010, p. 8). Archer et al., suggest a number of adoption issues among healthcare providers. These include; " new workflow demands and resistance to change, inadequate technology literacy, responsibility for ensuring the accuracy and integrity of health information across multiple interconnected data systems, and confidentiality and privacy risks" (Archer et al., 2011, p. 518). Physicians' limited view of PHR functions and benefits and their perception of barriers to its use may inhibit support for PHR use (Witry et al., 2010).

Cost many also be a barrier to PHR adoption (Tang et al., 2006). There is some data to indicate that motivated patients may be willing to pay $2-$5 per month (Archer et. Al., 2011). How would PHRs be subsidized? Archer and Fevrier-Thomas state:

[T]he diffusion of ePHRs to those who are genuinely motivated to adopt them will be a significant cost if done effectively. Until solid information can be collected and the future of such systems is decided, support for ePHRs will be a major public policy issue for healthcare systems administrators and funding agencies (Archer & Fevrier-Thomas, 2010).

The financial aspects of PHR and EHR integration in health care must be addressed and sufficient value to all participants must be apparent to justify their use (Tang et al., 2006).

THE BUSINESS CASE FOR PHRS AND EHRS

Adoption of PHRs will be affected by how much the various stakeholders would be willing to support it (Tang et al., 2006). There must be advantages in the PHR model that would make business sense to health care providers and patients. Walker and Carayon state that; "substantial evidence suggests that achieving the goal of higher-quality patient outcomes at decreased cost per outcome requires improved, patient-centered care processes" (Walker & Carayon, 2009, p. 475). The various providers and health care support services that must cooperate to supply the data and contribute to the functionality of the PHR must see where they will profit either through efficiency gains or remuneration for their involvement from their investment in time and software and hardware expenses (Tang et al., 2006). The introduction of provincial subsidies in Canada and allocation of funds towards healthcare information technology in the USA in the American Recovery and Reinvestment Act of 2009 (ARRA) are incentives to accelerate the use of EHRs that may hasten adoption in both countries (Blumenthal, 2009) (Webster, 2010).

The ARRA provided $17 billion as financial incentives to physicians and hospitals to adopt and use EHRs (Blumenthal, 2009). Blumenthal notes that; "[S]tarting in 2011, physicians can receive extra Medicare payments for the 'meaningful use' of a 'certified' EHR that can exchange data with other parts of the health care system" (Blumenthal, 2009, p. 1478). Meaningful use refers to the use of EHRs in a way that will improve quality and efficiency in the health care delivery system. Blumenthal states:

...if EHRs are to catalyze quality improvement and cost control, physicians and hospitals will have to use them effectively. This means taking advantage of embedded clinical decision supports that help physicians take better care of their patients (Blumenthal, 2009, p. 1479).

If PHRs are also to become widespread, patients will have to see significant value if they are to demand and support implementation. To some, empowerment in sharing in their health care with providers may prove to be sufficient incentive. Others may appreciate the communication functionalities of PHRs. Still others will value the savings in time and expenses by eliminating some physical visits to their health care providers (Kaelber & Pan, 2008). All these various advantages are intuitively self-serving and may only require education of the public that this new modality of care is available.

Enlisting the less motivated is more problematic. A study by Fosyth et al. showed that some patients did not want to understand their own medical information let alone contribute to its contents. They did not feel comfortable with even possessing their own medical records (Forsyth, Maddock, Iedema, & Lassere, 2010). A strategy for engaging these patients may revolve around convincing them of the merit of having these records available at medical appointments and emergency care visits. Those with limited English skills could appreciate the advantage of PHRs in reducing communication issues (Forsyth et al., 2010). (As previously noted, the problems of a lack of access to computers and computer illiteracy of disadvantaged groups are symptoms of larger social issues. The potential benefits of PHRs for these groups must be addressed through effective social policies that strive for equitable opportunity.)

A critical economic criterion for successful implementation involves the compensation to providers to enlist their cooperation in the communication functionality of PHRs (Blumenthal, 2009). Tethered PHR systems can allow for secure e-mail access between patient and physician as well as the facilitation of telephone appointments in lieu of office visits (Chen et al., 2009). Many current reimbursement models do not compensate physicians for these methods of communication (Blumenthal, 2009). In advance of determining changes in the payment to providers, research will be required to determine if these modalities of patient care are advantageous in:

1. Utilization of time.
2. Satisfaction by patients in their perception of care received.
3. Effectiveness of care and health outcomes compared to standard models of care (Yau, Williams, & Brown, 2011).

Answers to these questions through appropriate research would provide insight in the economic (as well as health) benefits that could drive the implementation of PHRs. Kaelber and Pan note that any cost savings and value to stakeholders including patients has yet to be demonstrated (Kaelber & Pan, 2008). Kaelber et al. state; "[I]n considering reimbursement reform, policymakers need additional information about the benefits of non-visit care to determine how best to compensate providers for it" (Kaelber et al., 2008, p. 733). These policy changes could affect one or more of the existing funding models of fee-for-service, salaried employment or capitation. As well, if PHR use can demonstrate improved health and health outcomes, a financial benefit can be accrued to the payer, which could provide an additional incentive to spread the system universally. Offering financial incentives to providers for utilizing EHR and PHR functionalities can be financed from the expected savings to the health care global budget.

PHR utilization in the fee-for-service funding model must address the new communication modalities. Currently, the fee-for-service funding model does not compensate providers for time spent in phone or e-mail communications with patients. If research confirms that the overall time needed to treat patients is reduced, the availability of extra time in the working day through substituting non-visit care for some office visits can allow an added flow of income from additional patients. This may balance a significant amount of the loss of income from reduced office visits. However, this theoretical scenario might not reflect any compelling reasons for providers to embrace the new modality. The time spent in voice or e-mail communications is still without compensation in the fee-for-service payment model. Working time is still expended without monetary reward. A new fee for voice or e-mail communications can reimburse providers for their time. If research also shows improved health and health outcomes using PHRs, a financial incentive involving increased fees to providers participating in the use of EHRs/PHRs may become a reasonable policy change. Any such policy changes must be based on health outcomes. Appropriate research and proof of concept demonstration initiatives must confirm whether the theoretical potential of PHRs is in fact translatable to actual improved health care, reduced appointments and reduced costs. A balance must be struck between additional fee payments and reduced global health care costs.

In payment models that involve salaried providers, there is less of a financial issue surrounding the utilization of PHRs. Providers will not be directly impacted monetarily if research shows improved health care outcomes with PHRs. Their working time and effort would not change if PHRs allow each provider to treat more patients. However salary levels may be altered to recognize the health care providers' role in improving health care efficiency. This salary adjustment may be a necessary incentive to reward providers for participating in the use of a more efficient and effective health care system.

Capitation models of provider compensation may be the most receptive of PHRs without requiring changes in the existing model. Capitation refers to a system of compensation to the provider that pays a fixed amount per patient per month without considering the amount of care or time each patient may require. If it can be shown that the use of PHRs can improve the health of patients and reduces the time required for each, there is an incentive for the provider to incorporate such a system into her practice. The outcome will be the same compensation while expending less time. Income can be maintained with less work or increased if more patients are added to the patient roster to fill the additional clinic time created through the use of PHRs.

If the use of PHRs can provide better health maintenance, improved health outcomes when care is needed and reduced use of resources, policy initiatives could be used to pursue the potential benefits of PHRs. A shift in funding amounts or funding methods to encourage providers to adopt the use of PHRs would further the goals of administrators in health care funding. Each compensation model would require some use of financial incentives to encourage the adoption of PHRs. However, the capitation model may be the method that provides the greatest natural incentive for adoption. Striving for efficiency is a characteristic of the capitation model and those working in that system would be the least resistant to utilize a tool that could improve efficiency. Their own financial interest in PHRs would be an incentive to encourage patients to utilize them. Government policy that encourages doctors to adopt a capitation remuneration model and include PHRs in their patient care strategy could be part of the effort to control health care costs.

Taylor et al. have attempted to monetize the potential benefits of incorporating Health Information Technology (HIT). Although referring specifically to the American system of health care, they estimate that $81 billion can be saved annually by using EHR systems. They estimate the cost of implementation for inpatient and outpatient systems of $7.6 billion per year during the adoption period. To attain these savings they note three requirements;

1. There must be widespread provider adoption of a standard-based EMR system.
2. There must be effective connectivity between providers and between providers and patients.
3. There must be intense efforts to improve quality and efficiency performance (Taylor et al., 2005).

Obstacles to attaining these benefits would be the cost of acquiring and implementing these systems, the uncertainty of financial benefits to providers, and the high initial physician time requirements to implement the system (Taylor et al., 2005).

Shekelle et al., examining five cost-benefit analyses involving the use of EHRs, reported that all predicted significant savings (Shekelle, Morton, & Keeler, 2006). Not all potential benefits are theoretical. The case study by Chen et al. examining the effects of Kaiser Permanente's utilization of EHRs and PHRs showed improvement in patient care efficiency through reduced office visits (Chen et al., 2009). This suggests cost benefits although the study did not examine per patient time savings accrued to providers through the introduction of health information technology. Documentation of actual financial benefits is largely unavailable. Chaudhry et al. concluded:

[P]ublished evidence of the information needed to make informed decisions about acquiring and implementing health information technology in community settings is nearly nonexistent. For example, potentially important evidence related to initial capital costs, effect on provider productivity, resources required for staff training (such as time and skills), and workflow redesign is difficult to locate in the peer-reviewed literature. Also lacking are key data on financial context, such as degree of capitation, which has been suggested as a model to be an important factor in defining the business case for electronic health record use (Chaudhry, et al., 2006, p. 748).

Chaudhry et al. showed evidence does exist that health information technologies do improve quality and efficiency. Examining the effects on health care in four benchmark research institutions following the installation of multifunctional health information technology systems that included decision support, they documented five effects:

1. More care was provided that was in adherence to guidelines and protocols.
2. Surveillance and monitoring for disease conditions and care delivery was improved.
3. Medication errors decreased.
4. Less patient care was required.
5. Utilization of time was inconclusive (Chaudhry, et al., 2006).

Oliver has reported on the improvement in the health record performance of the Veteran Health Administration (VHA) in the United States following the installation of an EHR system. He observed, "[T]he system increased the availability of patient-charts at the point of clinical encounter from 60% to 100% between 1995 and 2004. At least one in five medical tests in the US is repeated because of lost patient records, but lost records are no longer a problem in the VHA" (Oliver, 2008, p. 1213). Hurricane Katrina demonstrated the benefit of EHRs. Many New Orleans evacuees found themselves without their medical records. Brown et al. noted that; [T]he outcome was different for enrolled veterans. Their complete electronic clinical records were available from the rehosted VistA [VHA electronic records] system to authorized users with access to VA's secure network" (Brown, et al., 2007, p. S138).

The UK's Department of Health launched a project, the Whole System Demonstrator program, to determine whether ehealth would live up to the expectations claimed for it as part of a transformational delivery of health care. In their findings released December, 2011 the Department of Health stated:

....if used correctly telehealth can deliver a 15 percent reduction in A&E [ambulatory and elective] visits, a 20 percent reduction in emergency admissions, a 14 percent reduction in elective admissions, a 14 percent reduction in bed days and an 8 percent reduction in tariff costs. More strikingly they also demonstrate a 45 percent reduction in mortality rates" (KPMG International Cooperative, 2012, p. 13).

Further research is needed to quantify the cost savings of these effects within the global health care budget. Cost-benefit analyses projections are encouraging (Chaudhry, et al., 2006). The potential for savings through either reduced need for health care or more efficient provision of care is so compelling that agencies responsible for funding have embraced the technology as a method of controlling health care spending in an environment of aging societies, accelerating drug costs and increasingly sophisticated and costly health care (Blumenthal, 2009).

THE STATE OF RESEARCH ON PHRS

Too little is known about the actual benefits of PHRs. So little research has been initiated that Kaelber et al. warn; "....we believe the lack of evaluation and the current rudimentary understanding of how PHRs can specifically contribute to health care quality, safety, efficiency and patient satisfaction threatens the viability and sustainability of these systems" (Kaelber et al., 2008, p. 730). The authors note four areas of research opportunities for PHRs: function evaluation, adoption and attitudes, privacy and security and architecture. They suggest that currently function evaluation may be the most important area of research. This includes information collecting (retrieving from external sources), sharing, exchanging (two-way sharing), and self-management. These areas of functionality should be explored to assess their importance with respect to health care quality, safety, efficiency, cost, and patient and provider satisfaction (Kaelber et al., 2008).

Several issues regarding PHR privacy and security require investigation. Who controls sharing and access to a PHR of minors and non-competent patients requires further inquiry. Consensus must be found on acceptable trade-offs between verification of authenticity of a user and the interests of legitimate patient proxies. Research that would aid in establishing acceptable protocols is necessary to encourage widespread use of PHRs (Mandl et. al., 2001).

Research is needed to determine the model of PHR design of data collection, infrastructure and applications that will best support patient-centred health care. The issue of interoperability is a critical element of PHR functionality and standards for architecture compatibility must be explored (Kaelber & Pan, 2008).

Research to assess the business case for PHRs is critical to determine the viability of PHRs and whether the investments made in this field is warranted. Many current reimbursement models do not compensate providers for the new modalities of communication that PHRs provide (Kaelber & Pan, 2008). In advance of determining changes in the payment to providers, research must determine if these modalities of patient care are advantageous in utilization of time, satisfaction by patients in their perception of care received and effectiveness of care and health outcomes compared to standard models of care (Witry et. al., 2010). The research that would provide the necessary insight in the economic (as well as health) benefits will drive the progress in PHR implementation (Kaelber & Pan, 2008).

EHR AND PHR UTILIZATION: A WORLD VIEW

In 2011, a consortium of five of the largest health care providers in the U.S.—Kaiser Permanente, the Mayo Clinic, Geisinger, Intermountain Healthcare and Group Health, each with established EHR systems, committed to share patient records through an open source and make available the infrastructure to all health care providers in the U.S. to ensure general interoperability and connectivity. To further systemic integration of health care delivery, national content and exchange standards as set out by government would be followed to allow for interoperability with government systems (KPMG International Cooperative, 2012).

Oliver notes that the U.S. Veterans Health Administration provides an open source, public domain adaptable platform to allow any health care institution to access at no cost the EHR system that was developed for their own use (the Veterans Health Information Systems and Technology Architecture). The system engages all U.S. veterans and was developed over two decades developing from a hospital-based to a broader health-care system over that period. It provides stored information on medical charting, provider orders and patient progress notes (Oliver, 2008).

Denmark has an advanced IT system through "a public web-based portal that collects and distributes key healthcare information to citizens and healthcare professionals, and empowers patients to access the healthcare system more effectively" (KPMG International Cooperative, 2012, p. 11). The interface is adaptable to the needs of specific users. Patients have their own unique webpage that allows access to diagnosis and treatment information, booking of appointments, secure emails to health providers, ordering medications, monitoring self-compliance with medication and access to disease management systems (KPMG International Cooperative, 2012).

The United Kingdom embarked on a nation-wide EHR project in 2002. The program was intended to integrate patient records, prescription services, secure email communications and support archiving radiology images with the purpose of improving patient access to their health care providers and improve satisfaction with the service. However the project was delayed and scaled back in 2011, a result of insufficient clinical engagement, gaps in stakeholder expectations and problems with technology. The U.K. experience highlights the challenges in implementing EHRs. A critical component for successful implementation of the project involves the cooperation and collaboration between the various stakeholders. The differences in values, priorities and methodology between the political, clinical, academic, technical, and commercial players were a barrier to the ambitious initial expectations (KPMG International Cooperative, 2012).

The Australian state and territorial governments established a national authority to develop a system based on national standards for collecting, exchanging and securing health information. The intention from the outset was to attain full interoperability based on national standards. Engagement with all stakeholders was a strategic priority that fostered adoption and utilization (KPMG International Cooperative, 2012).

In 2011 Singapore began a coordination of information project of patient health care records that was available in providers' widely adopted individual EHR systems. The new National effort was to consolidate the information to form an integrated patient centred health care record that include diagnoses, allergies, immunizations, medications, treatment, referrals and care plans (KPMG International Cooperative, 2012).

The experience of the province of Ontario, Canada provides a cautionary tale. In 2002 the province of Ontario established the Smart Systems for Health Agency (SSHA) that was charged with overseeing the creation of a secure electronic network connecting the medical community. Between 2002 and 2008 approximately $1 billion was spent on this project (Office of the Auditor General of Ontario, 2009). In 2009 an audit by the Auditor General's office was released. It found that Ontario did not yet have an electronic record system that met the needs of health providers or the public. The report stated that the private IT network that was created remained underutilized because "there is insufficient health related information on it" (Office of the Auditor General of Ontario, 2009, p. 8). No thought had been given to how this private network would provide secure access to the public. The Auditor General criticized the endeavor for its lack of upfront strategic planning and overall lack of effective oversight as well as unrealistic timelines, inadequate integration of various components of the system, the inability of the end product to meet user requirements and the lack of cost-effective management.

MACRO AND MICRO FACTORS IN THE SUCCESSFUL IMPLEMENTATION OF EHR TECHNOLOGY

EHR and PHR models are exceedingly complicated to create and implement. Venkatramen et al., observed:

[W]hile there are hundreds of vendors currently serving the EMR systems market, there is limited data standardization across these systems. Further, these systems are so fine-tuned and built for a specific function that integration with other systems (for example, computerized patient order entry systems [CPOE}, automated drug dispensing systems [ADDS], and accounting/billing systems) becomes a nightmare (Venkatraman, Bala, Venkatesh, & Bates, 2008, p. 141).

Without proper protocols and planning the end result can be disappointing. Venkatraman et al. examined the VHA's IT systems and architecture and from this case study suggests six strategies to help in the development of EHR systems;

1. Develop a common operational database and application interface.
2. Use an interoperable system based on common standards and architecture to allow the seamless transfer of patient information.
3. Align clinical and administrative processes.
4. Develop a Web-based interface to allow access to patient data from any location.
5. Develop enterprise data warehouse and business intelligence systems as part of EHRs to allow for better clinical decisions and medical research.
6. Develop clinical decision support capabilities as part of EHR architecture (Venkatraman et al., 2008).

As important as the architecture and operational systems are to the successful use of EHRs, the actual process of implementation at the health provider's location is equally critical (Smith, 2003). Smith reported on the installation of an EHR system in a medical clinic. The ultimate success of the project was summarized by seven key factors;

- Clear definition of goals.
- Strong project leadership team to run the implementation.
- Project manager with sufficient, dedicated time.
- Strong physician leader to champion the project.
- Detailed analysis of work flow.
- High level of staff flexibility.
- Commitment to "plan for the worst; hope for the best" (Smith, 2003, p. 41).

Studer reviewed the literature examining the effect of organizational factors on successful EMR system implementation. A number of critical factors were identified:

1. Management support for the project and the communication of that support to the entire provider organization is essential.
2. A physician champion for the project must be identified.

3. Financial resources to purchase and implement the project and provide for ongoing maintenance must be budgeted. This must also include compensation for the reduction of productivity during and after implementation and financial incentives and rewards to members of the health provider team.
4. The organization must provide adequate initial and ongoing training for EHR system users and sufficient dedicated time must be scheduled for this training. This training must address any unrealistic expectations and emphasize the goals and benefits of the enterprise.
5. Ongoing and on-site technical support must be made available.
6. All members of the organization must have input in the design and implementation of the EHR system.
7. All physicians must be supportive of the goals, anticipated benefits and implementation process of the EHR system.
8. The system must be easy to learn and use and not interfere with the physician-patient interaction.
9. The system must have effective redundancy and backup safeguards (Studer, 2005).

It is only with sufficient planning and forethought that the implementation of a EHR system can be successfully achieved.

CONCLUSION

It is widely believed that the use of EHR's and PHR's will help provide better health care and do so more cost efficiently than present systems (Walker & Carayon, 2009). Witry et. al., state; "[D]evelopment of a national HIT [Health Information technology] infrastructure, including Electronic Medical Records (EMRs), Personal Health Records (PHRs), and medical record interoperability, has the potential to increase efficiency, decrease medical errors, and improve healthcare quality" (Witry et. al., 2010). At this point in the development and implementation of IT systems these beliefs are largely unproven (Kaelber & Pan, 2008). Little in the way of case studies has shown that the potential is indeed realizable. It is imperative that further research be undertaken in the various components of EHR and PHR systems development. This would include efforts to perfect the architecture and interoperability of electronic health record technology. Case studies must be completed to demonstrate that cost efficiency and health improvement are real benefits of EHRs and PHRs. Many stakeholders are invested in the belief that these systems will be transformative in the provision of health care and controlling health costs. It is critical for the widespread adoption of EHRs and PHRs to show that these assumptions are valid.

REFERENCES

Archer, N., Fevrier, U., Lokker, C., McKibbon, K., & Straus, S. (2011). Personal health records: A scoping review. *Journal of the American Medical Informatics Association, 18*, 515–522. doi:10.1136/amiajnl-2011-000105 PMID:21672914

Archer, N., & Fevrier-Thomas, U. (2010). An empirical study of Canadian consumer and physician perceptions of electronic personal health records. In *Proceedings of the Annual Conference, Administrative Sciences Association of Canada* (pp. 512-522). Regina, Canada: ASAC.

Asada, Y., & Kephart, G. (2007). Equity in health services use and intensity of use in Canada. *BMC Health Services Research*. doi:10.1186/1472-6963-7-41 PMID:17349059

Beacom, A. M. (2010). Communicating health information to disadvantaged populations. *Family & Community Health*, *33*(2), 152–162. doi:10.1097/FCH.0b013e3181d59344 PMID:20216358

Begoyan, A. (2007). An Overview of interoperability standards for electronic health records. *Integrated Design and Process Technology*, 1-8.

Berk, M., & Monkeit, A. (2001). The concentration of health care expenditures, revisited. *Health Affairs*, *20*(2), 9–18. doi:10.1377/hlthaff.20.2.9 PMID:11260963

Blumenthal, D. (2009). Stimulationg the adoption of health information technology. *The New England Journal of Medicine*, *260*, 1477–1479. doi:10.1056/NEJMp0901592

Blumenthal, D., & Glasor, J. (2007). Information technology comes to medicine. *The New England Journal of Medicine*, *356*(24), 2527–2534. doi:10.1056/NEJMhpr066212 PMID:17568035

Bodenheimer, T., & Fernandez, A. (2005). High and rising health care costs: Part 4: Can costs be controlled while preserving quality? *Annals of Internal Medicine*, *143*(1), 26–31. doi:10.7326/0003-4819-143-1-200507050-00007 PMID:15998752

Bourgeois, F., Taylor, P., Emans, S., Nigrin, D., & Mandl, K. (2008). Whose personal control? Creating private, personally controlled health records for pediatric and adolescent patients. *Journal of the American Medical Informatics Association*, *15*(6), 737–743. doi:10.1197/jamia.M2865 PMID:18755989

Brown, S., Fischetti, L., Graham, G., Bates, J., Lancaster, A., McDaniel, D.,... Kolodner, R. (2007). Use of electronic health records in disaster response: The experience of department of veterans affairs after hurricaine Katrina. *American Journal of Public Health, 97*(S1), S136-S141. doi:102105/AJPH 2006.10494B

Buckley, B., Murphy, A., & MacFarlane, A. (2011). Public attitudes to the use in research of personal health information from general practitioners' records: a survey of the Irish general public. *Journal of Medical Ethics*, *37*(1), 50–55. doi:10.1136/jme.2010.037903 PMID:21071570

Chaudhry, B., Wang, J., We, S., Maglione, M., Mojica, W., Roth, E., & Morton, S. (2006). Systematic review: Impact of health information technology on quality, efficiency, and costs of medical care. *Annals of Internal Medicine*, *144*, 742–752. doi:10.7326/0003-4819-144-10-200605160-00125 PMID:16702590

Chen, C., Garrido, T., Chock, D., Okawa, G., & Liang, L. (2009). The kaiser permanente electronic health record: Transforming and streamlining modalities of care. *Health Affairs*, *28*(2), 323–333. doi:10.1377/hlthaff.28.2.323 PMID:19275987

Coffield, R., DeLoss, G., & Mooty, G. (2008). The rise of the personal health record: panacea or pitfall of health information. *Health Law News. University of Houston. Health Law and Policy Institute*, *12*(10), 8–13.

Cushman, R., & Froomkin, A. (2010). Ethical, legal and social issues for personal health records and applications. *Journal of Biomedical Informatics*, *43*(5), S51–S55. doi:10.1016/j.jbi.2010.05.003 PMID:20937485

Denton, I. (2001). Will patients use electronic personal health records? Responses from a real-life experience. *Journal of Healthcare Information Management*, *15*(3), 251–259. PMID:11642143

Detmer, D., Raymond, B., Tang, P., & Bloomrosen, M. (2008). Integrated personal health records: transformative tools for consumer-centric care. *BMC Medical Informatics and Decision Making*, *8*(45). doi:10.1186/1472-6947-8-45 PMID:18837999

Diamond, C., Mostashari, F., & Shirky, C. (2009). Collecting and sharing data for population health: A new paradigm. *Health Affairs*, *28*(2), 454–466. doi:10.1377/hlthaff.28.2.454 PMID:19276005

Dunn, K., & Wynia, M. (2010). Dreams and nightmares:practical and ethical issues for patients and physicians using personal health records. *The Journal of Law, Medicine & Ethics*, *38*(1), 64–73. doi:10.1111/j.1748-720X.2010.00467.x PMID:20446985

EHR4CR. (2011). *EHR4CR executive summary*. EHR4CR.

Eyserbach, G. (2008). Medicine 2.0: Social networking, collaboration, participation, apomediation, and openness. *Journal of Medical Internet Research*, *10*(3), e22. doi:10.2196/jmir.1030 PMID:18725354

Follen, M., Castaneda, R., Mikelson, M., Johnson, D., Wilson, A., & Higuchi, K. (2007). Implementing health information technology to improve the process of health care delivery: A case study. *Disease Management*, *10*(4), 208–215. doi:10.1089/dis.2007.104706 PMID:17718659

Forsyth, R., Maddock, C., Iedema, R., & Lassere, M. (2010). Patient perceptions of carrying their own health information: Approaches towards responsibility and playing an active role in their own health--Implications for a patient-held health file. *Health Expectations*, *13*(4), 416–426. doi:10.1111/j.1369-7625.2010.00593.x PMID:20629768

Gans, D. (2005). Medical groups' adoption of electronic health records and information systems. *Health Affairs*, *24*(5), 1323–1333. doi:10.1377/hlthaff.24.5.1323 PMID:16162580

Garde, S., Knaup, P., Hovenga, E., & Heard, S. (2007). Towards semantic interoperability for electronic health records: Domain knowledge governance for open EHR archetypes. *Methods of Information in Medicine*, *46*(3), 332–343. PMID:17492120

Gaylin, D., Moiduddin, A., Mohamoud, S., Lundeen, K., & Kelly, J. (2011). Public attitudes about health information technology, and its relationship to health care quality, costs, and privacy. *Health Services Research*, *46*(3), 920–938. doi:10.1111/j.1475-6773.2010.01233.x PMID:21275986

Halamka, J., Mandl, K., & Tang, P. (2008). Early experiences with personal health records. *Journal of the American Medical Informatics Association, 15*(1), 1-7. doi: M256210.1197/jamia

Hayrinen, K., Saranto, K., & Nykanen, P. (2008). Definition, structure, content, use and impacts of electronic records: A review of the research literature. *International Journal of Medical Informatics*, *77*(5), 291–304. doi:10.1016/j.ijmedinf.2007.09.001 PMID:17951106

Hersh, W. (2004). Health care information technology: Progress and barriers. *Journal of the American Medical Association*, *292*(18), 2273–2274. doi:10.1001/jama.292.18.2273 PMID:15536117

Heubusch, K. (2008). IT standards for PHRs: Are PHRs ready for standards? Are standards ready for PHRs? *Journal of American Health Information Management Association*, *79*(6), 31–36. PMID:18604973

Hillestad, R., Bigelow, J., & Bower, A. (2005). Can electronic medical record systems transform health care? Potential health benefits, savings, and costs. *Health Affairs*, *24*, 1103–1117. doi:10.1377/hlthaff.24.5.1103 PMID:16162551

Honeyman, A., Cox, B., & Fisher, B. (2005). Potential impacts of patients access to their electronic records. *Informatics in Primary Care*, *13*, 55–60. PMID:15949176

Institute of Electrical & Electronics Engineers. (1990). *IEEE standard computer dictionary: A compilation of IEEE standard computer glossaries*. New York: IEEE.

Jensen, P., Jensen, L., & Brunak, S. (2012). Mining electronic health records: Towards better research applications and clinical care. *National Review*, *13*, 395–405. doi:10.1038/nrg3208 PMID:22549152

Kaelber, D., Jha, A., Johnston, D., Middleton, B., & Bates, D. (2008). A research agenda for personal health records. *Journal of the American Informatics Association, 15*(6), 729-736. doi:. M254710.1197/jamia

Kaelber, D., & Pan, E. (2008). The value of personal health record (PHR) systems. In *Proceedings of AMIA Annual Symposium* (pp. 343-347). AMIA.

Kahn, J., Aulakh, V., & Bosworth, A. (2009). What it takes: Characteristics of the ideal personal health record. *Health Affairs*, *28*(2), 369–376. doi:10.1377/hlthaff.28.2.369 PMID:19275992

Kharrazi, H., Chisholm, R., VanNasdale, D., & Thompson, B. (2012). Mobile personal health records: An evaluation of features and functionality. *International Journal of Medical Informatics*, *81*(9), 579–593. doi:10.1016/j.ijmedinf.2012.04.007 PMID:22809779

Kim, M., & Johnson, K. (2002). Personal health records: evaluation of functionality and utility. *Journal of the American Medical Informatics Association*, *9*(2), 171–180. doi:10.1197/jamia.M0978 PMID:11861632

Koppel, R., Metlay, J., & Cohen, A. (2005). Role of computerized physician order entry systems in facilitating medical errors. *Journal of the American Medical Association*, *293*, 1197–1203. doi:10.1001/jama.293.10.1197 PMID:15755942

KPMG International Cooperative. (2012). *Accelerating innovation: The power of the crowd*. KPMG.

Lee, R., & Garvin, T. (2003). Moving from information transfer to information exchange in health and health care. *Social Science & Medicine*, *56*, 449–464. doi:10.1016/S0277-9536(02)00045-X PMID:12570966

Liederman, E., & Morefield, C. (2003). Web messaging: a new tool for patient-physician communication. *Journal of the American Medical Informatics Association*, *10*, 260–270. doi:10.1197/jamia.M1259 PMID:12626378

Lumpkin, J. (2007). Archimedes: A bold step into the future. *Health Affairs*, *26*(2), w137–w139. doi:10.1377/hlthaff.26.2.w137 PMID:17259195

Maloney, F., & Wright, A. (2010). USB-based personal health records: an analysis of features and functionality. *International Journal of Medical Informatics*, *79*, 97–111. doi:10.1016/j.ijmedinf.2009.11.005 PMID:20053582

Mandl, K., Kohame, I., & Brandt, A. (1998). Electronic patient-physician communication: problems and promise. *Annals of Internal Medicine*, *129*, 495–500. doi:10.7326/0003-4819-129-6-199809150-00012 PMID:9735088

Mandl, K., Szolovits, P., & Kohane, I. (2001). Public standards and patients' control: how to keep electronic medical records accessible but private. *British Medical Journal*, *322*(7281), 283–287. doi:10.1136/bmj.322.7281.283 PMID:11157533

Markle Connecting for Health. (2003). *Americans want benefits of personal health records*. New York: Markle Foundation.

Markle Connecting for Health. (2004). *Connecting Americans to their healthcaare: Final report of the working group on policies for electronic information sharing between doctors and patients*. New York: Markle Foundation.

Markle Connecting for Health. (2006). *Survey finds Americans want electronic personal health information to improve own health care*. New York: Markle Foundation.

McCally, M., Haines, A., Fein, O., Addington, W., Lawrence, R., & Cassel, C. (1998). Poverty and ill health: Physicians can and should make a difference. *Annals of Internal Medicine*, *129*(9), 726–733. doi:10.7326/0003-4819-129-9-199811010-00009 PMID:9841606

McCray, A. (2005). Promoting health literacy. *Journal of the American Medical Informatics Association*, *12*, 153–163. PMID:15561782

Menachemi, N., & Collum, T. (2011). Benefits and drawbacks of electronic health record systems. *Risk Management and Healthcare Policy*, *4*, 47–55. doi:10.2147/RMHP.S12985 PMID:22312227

Middleton, B., Hammond, W., Brennan, P., & Cooper, G. (2005). Accelerating U.S. EHR adoption: How to get there from here: Recommendations based on the 2004 ACMI retreat. *Journal of the American Medical Informatics Association*, *12*, 13–19. doi:10.1197/jamia.M1669 PMID:15492028

Miller, R., West, C., Brown, T., Sim, I., & Ganchoff, C. (2005). The value of electronic health records in solo or small group practices. *Health Affairs*, *24*, 1127–1137. doi:10.1377/hlthaff.24.5.1127 PMID:16162555

Office of the Auditor General of Ontario. (2009). *Ontario's electronic health records initiative, special report*. Toronto, Canada: Office of the Auditor General of Ontario.

Oliver, A. (2008). Public-sector health-care reforms that work? A case study of the US veterans health administration. *Lancet*, *371*(9619), 1211–1213. doi:10.1016/S0140-6736(08)60528-0 PMID:18395583

Page, D. (2010, September). The two paths to PHRs. *Hospital and Health Networks Magazine*.

Pagliari, C., Detmer, D., & Singleton, P. (2007). Potential of electronic personal health records. *British Medical Journal*, *335*(7615), 330–333. doi:10.1136/bmj.39279.482963.AD PMID:17703042

Pirtle, B., & Chandra, A. (2011). An overview of consumer perceptions and acceptance as well as barriers and potential of electronic personal health records. *American Journal of Health Sciences*.

Poon, E., Blumenthal, D., Jaggi, T. H. M., Bates, D., & Kaushal, R. (2004). Overcoming bariers to adopting and impementing computerized physician order entry systems in U.S. Hospitals. *Health Affairs*, *23*(4), 184–190. doi:10.1377/hlthaff.23.4.184 PMID:15318579

Poon, E., Jha, A., Christino, M., Honour, M., Fernandopulle, R., Middleton, B., & Kaushal, R. (2006). Assessing the level of healthcare information technology adoption in the United States: A snapshot. *BMC Medical Informatics and Decision Making*, *6*(1). doi:10.1186/1472-6947-6-1 PMID:16396679

Powell, J., Fitton, R., & Fitton, C. (2006). Sharing electronic health records: the patient view. *Informatics in Primary Care*, *14*, 55–57. PMID:16848967

Pyper, C., Amery, J., Watson, M., & Crook, C. (2004). Patients' experiences when accessing their online electronic patient records in primary care. *The British Journal of General Practice*, *54*, 38–43. PMID:14965405

Shekelle, P., Morton, S., & Keeler, E. (2006). *Costs and benefits of health information technology*. Rockville, MD: Agency for Healthcare Research and Quality.

Smith, P. (2003). Implementing an EMR system: One clinic's experience. *Family Practice Management*, *10*(5), 37–42. PMID:12776405

Steinbrook, R. (2008). Personally controlled online health data--The next big thing in medical care. *The New England Journal of Medicine*, *358*(16), 1653–1656. doi:10.1056/NEJMp0801736 PMID:18420496

Studer, M. (2005). The effect of organizational factors on the effectiveness of EMR system implementation--What have we learned? *Electronic Healthcare*, *4*(2), 92–97.

Tang, P., Ash, J., Bates, D., Overhage, J., & Sands, D. (2006). Personal health records: Definitions, benefits, and strategies for overcomming barriers to adoption. *Journal of the American Medical Informatics Association*, *13*(2), 121–126. doi:10.1197/jamia.M2025 PMID:16357345

Tang, P., & Lansky, D. (2005). The missing link: Bridging the patient-provider health information gap. *Health Affairs*, *24*, 1290–1295. doi:10.1377/hlthaff.24.5.1290 PMID:16162575

Tang, P., & Lee, T. (2009). Your doctor's office or the internet? Two paths to personal health records. *The New England Journal of Medicine*, *360*(13), 1276–1278. doi:10.1056/NEJMp0810264 PMID:19321866

Taylor, R., Bower, A., Frederico, G., & Bigelow, J. (2005). Promoting health information technology: Is there a case for more-aggressive government action? *Health Affairs*, *24*(5), 1234–1245. doi:10.1377/hlthaff.24.5.1234 PMID:16162568

Venkatraman, S., Bala, H., Venkatesh, V., & Bates, J. (2008). Six strategies for electronic medical records systems. *Communications of the ACM*, *51*(11), 140–144. doi:10.1145/1400214.1400243

Waegemann, C. (2005). Closer to reality: Personal health records represent a step in the right direction for interoperability of healthcare IT systems and accessibility of patient data. *Health Management Technology*, *26*, 16–18. PMID:15932068

Wagstaff, A. (2002). Poverty and health sector inequalities. *Bulletin of the World Health Organization*, 97–105. PMID:11953787

Walker, J., & Carayon, P. (2009). From tasks to processes: The case for changing health information technology to improve health care. *Health Affairs*, *28*(2), 467–477. doi:10.1377/hlthaff.28.2.467 PMID:19276006

Wang, S., Middleton, B., & Prosser, L. (2003). A cost-benefit analysis of electyronic medical records in primary care. *The American Journal of Medicine*, *114*, 397–403. doi:10.1016/S0002-9343(03)00057-3 PMID:12714130

Webster, P. (2010). United States to compel physicians to make meaningful use' of electronic health records. *Canadian Medical Association Journal*, *182*(14), 1500–1502. doi:10.1503/cmaj.109-3361 PMID:20837690

Weitzman, E., Kaci, L., & Mandl, K. (2010). Sharing medical data for health research: The early personal health record experience. *Journal of Medical Internet Research*, *12*(2), e14. doi:10.2196/jmir.1356 PMID:20501431

Weitzman, E., Kelemen, S., Kaci, L., & Mandl, K. (2012). Willigness to share personal health record data for care improvement and public health: A survey of experienced personal health record users. *BMC Medical Informatics and Decision Making*, *12*(39). PMID:22616619

West, S., Blake, C., Liu, Z., McKoy, J., Oertel, M., & Carey, T. (2009). Reflections on the use of electronic health record data for clinical research. *Health Informatics Journal*, *15*(2), 106–121. doi:10.1177/1460458209102972 PMID:19474224

Witry, M., Doucette, W., Daly, J., Levy, B., & Chrischilles, E. (2010). Family physician perceptions of personal health records. *Perspectives in Health Information Management*, *7*(Winter), 1–12. PMID:20697465

Wolter, J., & Friedman, B. (2005). Health records for the people: Touting the benefits of the consumer-based personal health record. *Journal of American Health Information Management Association*, *76*(10), 28–32. PMID:16333941

Yamin, C., Emani, S., Williams, D., Lipsitz, S., Karson, A., Wald, J., & Bates, D. (2011). The digital divide in adoption and use of a personal health record. *Archives of Internal Medicine*, *171*(6), 568–574. doi:10.1001/archinternmed.2011.34 PMID:21444847

Yau, G., Williams, A., & Brown, J. (2011). Family physicians' perspectives on personal health records. *Canadian Family Physician Medecin de Famille Canadien*, *57*(5), e178–e184. PMID:21642732

ADDITIONAL READING

Bourgeois, F., Taylor, P., Emans, S., Nigrin, D., & Mandl, K. (2008). Whose personal control? Creating private, personally controlled health records for pediatric and adolescent patients. *Journal of the American Medical Informatics Association*, *15*(6), 737–743. doi:10.1197/jamia.M2865 PMID:18755989

Buckley, B., Murphy, A., & MacFarlane, A. (2011). Public attitudes to the use in research of personal health information from general practitioners' records: a survey of the Irish general public. *Journal of Medical Ethics*, *37*(1), 50–55. doi:10.1136/jme.2010.037903 PMID:21071570

Coffield, R., DeLoss, G., & Mooty, G. (2008). The rise of the personal health record: panacea or pitfall of health information. *Health Law News. University of Houston. Health Law and Policy Institute*, *12*(10), 8–13.

Cushman, R., & Froomkin, A. (2010). Ethical, legal and social issues for personal health records and applications. *Journal of Biomedical Informatics*, *43*(5), S51–S55. doi:10.1016/j.jbi.2010.05.003 PMID:20937485

Follen, M., Castaneda, R., Mikelson, M., Johnson, D., Wilson, A., & Higuchi, K. (2007). Implementing health information technology to improve the process of health care delivery: A case study. *Disease Management*, *10*(4), 208–215. doi:10.1089/dis.2007.104706 PMID:17718659

Gans, D. (2005). Medical groups' adoption of electronic health records and information systems. *Health Affairs*, *24*(5), 1323–1333. doi:10.1377/hlthaff.24.5.1323 PMID:16162580

Gaylin, D., Moiduddin, A., Mohamoud, S., Lundeen, K., & Kelly, J. (2011). Public attitudes about health information technology, and its relationship to health care quality, costs, and privacy. *Health Services Research*, *46*(3), 920–938. doi:10.1111/j.1475-6773.2010.01233.x PMID:21275986

Heubusch, K. (2008). IT standards for PHRs: are PHRs ready for standards? Are standards ready for PHRs? *Journal of American Health Information Management Association*, *79*(6), 31–36. PMID:18604973

Hillestad, R., Bigelow, J., & Bower, A. (2005). Can electronic medical record systems transform health care? Potential health benefits, savings, and costs. *Health Affairs*, *24*, 1103–1117. doi:10.1377/hlthaff.24.5.1103 PMID:16162551

Honeyman, A., Cox, B., & Fisher, B. (2005). Potential impacts of patients access to their electronic records. *Informatics in Primary Care*, *13*, 55–60. PMID:15949176

Kharrazi, H., Chisholm, R., VanNasdale, D., & Thompson, B. (2012). Mobile personal health records: An evaluation of features and functionality. *International Journal of Medical Informatics*, *81*(9), 579–593. doi:10.1016/j.ijmedinf.2012.04.007 PMID:22809779

Kim, M., & Johnson, K. (2002). Personal health records: evaluation of functionality and utility. *Journal of the American Medical Informatics Association*, *9*(2), 171–180. doi:10.1197/jamia.M0978 PMID:11861632

Koppel, R., Metlay, J., & Cohen, A. (2005). Role of computerized physician order entry systems in facilitating medical errors. *Journal of the American Medical Association*, *293*, 1197–1203. doi:10.1001/jama.293.10.1197 PMID:15755942

Lee, R., & Garvin, T. (2003). Moving from information transfer to information exchange in health and health care. *Social Science & Medicine*, *56*, 449–464. doi:10.1016/S0277-9536(02)00045-X PMID:12570966

Liederman, E., & Morefield, C. (2003). Web messaging: A new tool for patient-physician communication. *Journal of the American Medical Informatics Association*, *10*, 260–270. doi:10.1197/jamia.M1259 PMID:12626378

Maloney, F., & Wright, A. (2010). USB-based personal health records: an analysis of features and functionality. *International Journal of Medical Informatics*, *79*, 97–111. doi:10.1016/j.ijmedinf.2009.11.005 PMID:20053582

Mandl, K., Kohame, I., & Brandt, A. (1998). Electronic patient-physician communication: Problems and promise. *Annals of Internal Medicine*, *129*, 495–500. doi:10.7326/0003-4819-129-6-199809150-00012 PMID:9735088

Mandl, K., Szolovits, P., & Kohane, I. (2001). Public standards and patients' control: How to keep electronic medical records accessible but private. *British Medical Journal*, *322*(7281), 283–287. doi:10.1136/bmj.322.7281.283 PMID:11157533

McCray, A. (2005). Promoting health literacy. *Journal of the American Medical Informatics Association*, *12*, 153–163. PMID:15561782

Middleton, B., Hammond, W., Brennan, P., & Cooper, G. (2005). Accelerating U.S. EHR adoption: How to get there from here: Recommendations based on the 2004 ACMI retreat. *Journal of the American Medical Informatics Association*, *12*, 13–19. doi:10.1197/jamia.M1669 PMID:15492028

Miller, R., West, C., Brown, T., Sim, I., & Ganchoff, C. (2005). The value of electronic health records in solo or small group practices. *Health Affairs*, *24*, 1127–1137. doi:10.1377/hlthaff.24.5.1127 PMID:16162555

Poon, E., Blumenthal, D., Jaggi, T. H. M., Bates, D., & Kaushal, R. (2004). Overcoming bariers to adopting and impementing computerized physician order entry systems in U.S. hospitals. *Health Affairs*, *23*(4), 184–190. doi:10.1377/hlthaff.23.4.184 PMID:15318579

Pyper, C., Amery, J., Watson, M., & Crook, C. (2004). Patients' experiences when accessing their online electronic patient records in primary care. *The British Journal of General Practice*, *54*, 38–43. PMID:14965405

KEY TERMS AND DEFINITIONS

Architecture Compatibility: Refers to the ability of the software components of EHR systems to work effectively together.

Business Intelligence System: A decision support system that transfers raw data into meaningful and useful information for the purpose of better decision-making and data analysis.

Capitation: System of payment for providing health care services that specifies a constant monthly amount for each patient regardless of how much care is provided.

Electronic Health Records (EHRs): Depositories of patient files in digital form created, stored and managed by health care providers or health institutions.

Enterprise Data Warehouse: A central repository of data created by integrating data from multiple sources that can be used for decision support in clinical decision-making and data mining for medical research.

Fee-For-Service: System of payment for providing health care services that specifies a fixed amount for each service provided.

Functional Harmonization: The exchange of data between different ERS systems that is readable by humans.

Interoperability: The ability to exchange information in digital form between various information sources.

Interoperative PHR: PHR that derives its content from all sources that is automatically transferred to a provider's EHR and patient PHR.

Personal Health Records (PHRs): Digital health records of an individual managed by that individual.

Semantic Harmonization: Exchange of data between EHR systems that is computer processable by the receiving system.

Tethered PHR: PHR that derives its content from information compiled and stored by the patient's health provider or health institution in their EHR system and is made available to the patient.

This work was previously published in Research Perspectives on the Role of Informatics in Health Policy and Management edited by Christo El Morr, pages 89-114, copyright year 2014 by Medical Information Science Reference (an imprint of IGI Global).

Section 2
Medical Practice and Treatment

Chapter 12
The Perspectives of Medical Errors in the Health Care Industry

Kijpokin Kasemsap
Suan Sunandha Rajabhat University, Thailand

ABSTRACT

This chapter presents the overview of medical errors; drug prescription errors and prescribing; the overview of medical error disclosure; medical errors and telemedicine; medical errors and medical education; the overview of nursing medication errors; and the aspects of medical errors in the health care industry. Reducing medical errors, increasing patient safety, and improving the quality of health care are the major goals in the health care industry. Medical errors are caused by mistakes in drug prescription, dosing, and medical administration in inpatient and outpatient settings. Heath care-related guidelines, institutional safety practices, and modern health care technologies must be applied in hospitals, clinics, and medical offices to reduce the occurrence of medical errors. The chapter argues that understanding the perspectives of medical errors has the potential to enhance health care performance and reach strategic goals in the health care industry.

INTRODUCTION

Health care organizations face a wide range of internal and external factors that enable their ability to provide safe, quality, and reliable health care services (Pate & Swofford, 2016). Medical errors are one of the major threats for patient safety in all countries (Pazokian, Tafreshi, & Rassouli, 2014). Medical errors remain the most commonly occurring error in the health care area (Absulem & Hardin, 2011). The avoidable sources of medical errors include the failure to take a biopsy despite suspicious clinical findings, or incorrect clinicopathological correlations resulting in deleterious effects for the patient (Lehmann, Wesselmann, Weber, & Smentkowski, 2015). Clinicians involved in medical errors can experience significant distress (McLennan et al., 2015). The review and analysis of medical errors have emphasized their preventable potential for reoccurrence (Olaniyan, Ghaleb, Dhillon, & Robinson, 2015).

DOI: 10.4018/978-1-5225-1928-7.ch012

There is evidence that providers are reluctant to make the compensation for medical errors until a lawsuit is filed (Gawande, 2007). The rising health care costs, partially due to preventable medical errors, lead many hospitals to redouble their process improvement efforts (Gowen, McFadden, & Settaluri, 2012). The impact of digitization has important effect on teleexpertise, where a medical professional can remotely ask health care advices through the utilization of information and communication technology (ICT) toward providing medical treatment to a patient in remote environment (Doumbouya, Kamsu-Foguem, Kenfack, & Foguem, 2015). However, the outcome of such advice remotely obtained can lead to medical errors. It is important to determine whether the causes of the errors can be avoidable or not for the purposes of establishing the truth and assuring justice for the victims of medical errors (Doumbouya et al., 2015).

Providing effective health care service gains an increasing attention over the past few years (Chetouane & Ibraheem, 2016). There is an increasing need for the process improvement in health care systems regarding quality, safety, effectiveness, suitability, speed, efficiency, and uniformity (Institute of Medicine, 2001). Health care managers can make a major impact on safety culture development by promoting the patient safety-related strategies and fostering their employees' motivation to implement the health care improvement programs at the individual and departmental levels (Kagan & Barnoy, 2013). To improve patient safety, hospital managers should establish the reporting mechanisms at the national and international levels (Brady, Malone, & Fleming, 2009).

The chapter is based on a literature review of medical errors. The extensive literature of medical errors provides a contribution to practitioners and researchers by presenting the advanced issues of medical errors in order to minimize the medical errors in global health care.

BACKGROUND

For years, health care experts have recognized that medical errors exist and compromise health care quality (Vozikis, 2012). Errors are defined as any deviation from established standard operating procedures (Maskens et al., 2014). Studies of medical errors demonstrate that errors and adverse events are common in hospitals (Shah et al., 2009). Preventable error, malpractice, and complications can be considered as adverse events (Zientek, 2010). The adverse events rates and medical lawsuits are on the rise, whereas many medical errors are mostly due to negligence or malpractices which are preventable (Wong & Balasingam, 2013). Being able to understand health information and make decisions from that information is vital to patients' well-being (Kasemsap, 2017a).

Medical errors are the medical mistakes that can lead to serious consequences and even death of patients (Pazokian et al., 2014). Ammouri et al. (2015) indicated that patient safety is considered to be crucial to health care quality and is one of the major parameters monitored by all health care organizations around the world. Patient safety is a central issue of health care provision (Lehmann et al., 2015). Many quality improvement education programs have been introduced over the last decade with the purpose of enhancing patient safety (Gordon, Darbyshire, & Baker, 2012).

Patient safety remains a global challenge affecting many patients throughout the world (Schwappach, 2014). There are various approaches toward improving health care provision and patient safety in the health care industry (Lehmann et al., 2015). Critically ill patients need life saving treatments and are often exposed to medications requiring careful titration (Manias, Williams, & Liew, 2012). Improving patient safety hinges on the ability of health care providers to accurately identify, disclose, and report medical errors (Hobgood, Weiner, & Tamayo-Sarver, 2006). Learning and continuous improvement, hospital management support, supervisor expectations, communications about error, teamwork, and hospital handoffs are the major predictors of patient safety culture (Ammouri et al., 2015).

Medical interventions must account for differences in medical error identification, disclosure, and reporting by medicine provider type (Hobgood et al., 2006). Palmero et al. (2016) indicated that inexpensive and simple medication interventions can improve the intelligibility of prescriptions and reduce medication errors. Targeting the susceptible population groups and the dangerous aspects of the health care systems can be the effective approach to both medical error management and prevention (Olaniyan et al., 2015). In the digital society, there is a shift in the issue of designing and implementing health information system (Doumbouya et al., 2015).

Clinical practitioners play an essential role in the medical error reduction through providing accurate clinical information, procuring high-quality specimens, providing timely follow-up task on test results, effectively communicating on the potentially discrepant diagnoses, and advocating second opinions on the pathological diagnosis in specific situations (Raab & Grzybicki, 2010). Health professionals and patients must prepare themselves to take advantage of the established health care processes that improve the quality of health care service (Doumbouya et al., 2015). High self-efficacy and perceived effectiveness of the specific preventive actions considerably increase the likelihood of participation in medical error prevention (Schwappach & Wernli, 2010).

ADVANCED ISSUES OF MEDICAL ERRORS IN GLOBAL HEALTH CARE

This section provides the overview of medical errors; drug prescription errors and prescribing; the overview of medical error disclosure; medical errors and telemedicine; medical errors and medical education; the overview of nursing medication errors; and the aspects of medical errors in the health care industry.

Overview of Medical Errors

Medical errors are the consequence of multiple actions of the whole chain of organizational and individual interactions in which the individual does not have the intention of doing wrong (Garrouste-Orgeas, Flaatten, & Moreno, 2016). Medication errors can occur by patients and their health care providers in any stage of health care pathway (Gavgani, Oskouei, & Salehi, 2015). The ability to decrease medical errors depends on an understanding of the types and patterns of medical errors that occur in various settings (Henneman, Blank, Gattasso, Williamson, & Henneman, 2006). Clinical decisions based on the inaccurate sources of information can lead to medical errors, high treatment costs, and poor patient outcomes (Zaheer, 2015).

Since the 1970s, scientists have studied clinical decision making in order to improve its processes. Clinical decision making is called clinical reasoning, diagnostic reasoning, clinical judgment, and clinical inference (Ge et al., 2012). In scientific context, clinical decision making can be categorized into two modes (i.e., deductive mode and empirical mode). Clinical decision making is a critical aspect of clinical performance, having a high impact on quality and safety of care (Lucchiari & Pravettoni, 2012). Regarding deductive mode, when decisions are based on theoretical knowledge of diseases and the mechanisms of different treatments. Regarding empirical mode, when decisions are based on past experiences (Ge et al., 2012).

Different techniques are utilized in clinical decision-making process. The practical techniques include decision trees, Markov models, and simulation. Decision support systems play an important role in medical decision making (Azar & El-Metwally, 2013). Clinical reasoning is an important contributor to the quality of health care, but to achieve this quality of health care, the provided decisions in the clinical reasoning have to be safe. Goal Structuring Notation (GSN) is proposed to encourage communication among medical professionals and is more suitable for the analysis of medical errors (Doumbouya et al., 2015). Lawson and Daniel (2011) proposed a work in which they attempted to reduce and even eliminate diagnosis errors. The diagnosis errors encountered in health care systems are caused by cognitive errors.

Doumbouya et al. (2015) indicated that two categories of medical errors include process errors and knowledge errors. Process errors cover care system errors coordination, errors due to complementary examinations, such as drug prescription, results' management, errors related to medications, errors related to non-medications, and communication problems. Knowledge errors involve three concepts (i.e., errors in the execution of clinical tasks, errors in diagnosis, and wrong treatment decision with right diagnosis). Another area where medical errors have been explored is e-health cardiology (Gortzis & Nikiforidis, 2008). In e-health cardiology, two types of knowledge processes include knowledge tracing and knowledge cataloguing. Knowledge tracing demonstrates how a system executes and produces knowledge. Knowledge cataloguing classifies the knowledge that exists within the information system (Gortzis & Nikiforidis, 2008).

Based on knowledge processes, Gortzis and Nikiforidis (2008) proposed an important system (e.g., e-health cardiology environment) to minimize the medical errors in health care systems. Their approach is quite similar to teleexpertise since it allows collaboration among medical professionals. Gortzis and Nikiforidis (2008) achieved their goal by considering both knowledge tracing process and knowledge cataloguing process. Concerning knowledge tracing process that shows how the health care system executes and produces the knowledge, Gortzis and Nikiforidis (2008) demonstrated how the collected data is accepted or rejected. The collected data consists of a set of variables provided by the patients through portable devices. Each variable is related to the upper threshold and the lower threshold. The developed software performs the first filter by discarding data that is unrelated to the patients and then the data supposed to be valid can be systematically stored in the knowledge base.

Drug Prescription Errors and Prescribing

Prescribing is a complex task and a high-risk area of clinical practice (Brennan & Mattick, 2013). Celebi et al. (2010) indicated that prescribing correctly represents one of the most essential skills of a physician when it comes to patient safety. The prescribing errors that occur in hospitals are a source of health care concern (Tully, 2012). In 2007, the National Patient Safety Agency performed a study demonstrating that errors in prescribing led to nearly 12,000 adverse clinical incidents a year (Davies et al., 2011). Medical errors are common in health care settings, and the prescribing errors are the most common type (Harding, Britten, & Bristow, 2010). The tasks of prescribing, preparation, and administration of drugs are executed within a complex health care system (McDowell, Ferner, & Ferner, 2009). Ross et al. (2009) indicated that the prescribing errors account for a substantial proportion of medication errors and cause the significant medication problems.

Patients observe medical errors in the administration of drugs and they can be a valuable resource in the prevention of medical errors (Schwappach & Wernli, 2010). Drug prescription errors are a common and persistent problem in health care (Armitage, Newell, & Wright, 2010) and can be detrimental to patient care (Lewis et al., 2014). Electronic prescribing has a significant effect on the reduction of the prescribing errors (Shawahna et al., 2011). With the increasing number of adverse effects of drugs and the prescribing errors, the clinical pharmacologist plays an important role in introducing new drugs and in improving the effective use of current drugs (Williams, 2012).

Health professionals should establish the specific health care goals toward improving health literacy in strategic plans, programs, and educational initiatives (Kasemsap, 2017b). There is a need for more applied learning to develop the skill-based and applied aspects of drug prescribing toward improving the preparedness for drug prescription (Rothwell et al., 2012). National data regarding drug prescription is required in order to benchmark the independent nurses' prescribing practices in critical care (Carberry, Connelly, & Murphy, 2013). Insufficient knowledge is a significant factor in the nurses' drug administration errors (Hsaio et al., 2010).

Active failures are the unsafe acts committed by people who are in contact with the patient or system (Reason, 1990). Active failures take a wide variety of forms, such as slips, lapses, fumbles, mistakes, and procedural violations (Reason, 1990). Medical errors in drug prescription are frequently studied, but analyzing the data regarding drug administration is scarce (Niemann et al., 2015). Among all medication errors and adverse drug events, medication administration errors are common (Schwappach & Wernli, 2010). Medication administration errors are reported to occur in critical care settings, and can be associated with severe consequences (Mansour, James, & Edgley, 2012).

Overview of Medical Error Disclosure

Perception and satisfaction of patients with health care services are considered as the important parameters to evaluate the quality and competence of health care providers and the outcomes of their health care services in patients' health (Dias-Souza, 2016). The disclosure of medical error is useful in raising patient awareness, reducing their suffering, improving the quality of care, and limiting the consequences of the health care failure. Disclosing the medical errors to patients is an important part of patient care (Kaldjian et al., 2007). Kaldjian et al. (2006) indicated that four major domains of facilitating medical error disclosure include responsibility to patient, responsibility to self, responsibility to profession, and responsibility to community.

Effective risk management depends on establishing a reporting culture (Reason, 1997). The underreporting of medical administration errors is a threat to the quality of nursing care (Lin & Ma, 2009). The training and support of medical error disclosure can inform health care staff that the organization appreciates the honesty and integrity (Rathert & Phillips, 2010). Accreditation agencies (e.g., the Joint Commission on Accreditation of Healthcare Organization) encourage hospitals to voluntarily disclose information about medical errors (Rouse & Kaplan, 2008). The Joint Commission on Accreditation of Healthcare Organization has placed a great deal of emphasis on the patient safety-related strategies to reduce patient's identification errors (Koshy, 2005).

The disclosure of harmful errors to patients is recommended, but appears to be uncommon (White et al., 2011). Regarding medical error disclosure, the implementation of the anonymous reporting system with training is related to a statistically significant increase in the rate of reported medical errors (Taylor, Brownstein, Klein, & Strandjord, 2007). Nordén-Hägg et al. (2012) stated that introducing a web-based system for reporting the dispensing errors has a positive impact on the quantity of medical reports and completeness. Electronic reporting systems are the important components of the patient-safety movement, but are problematic, particularly in capturing information from physicians (Foster, Sidhu, Gadhia, & DeMusis, 2008).

Health care-related risk managers play a crucial role in promoting transparency in health care and enhancing patient safety (Gallagher et al., 2006). The organizational safety culture can encourage the medical error reporting by health care staff and can improve patient safety (Kagan & Barnoy, 2013). Shame and guilt are the subjective emotional responses that occur in response to the negative events (e.g., the making of medical mistakes and an experience of mistreatment), and are extensively studied in the field of psychology (Bynum & Goodie, 2014).

Sevdalis et al. (2010) stated that diagnostic errors present a particular challenge for medical error-related reporting systems because they involve clinical reasoning. Medical error reporting can be strengthened by human error theory, capturing a wide range of contributory medication factors to facilitate learning and encourage supportive medication actions (Armitage et al., 2010). Anoosheh et al. (2008) stated that medical outcomes that are identified from the process of practice error management should promote interventions designed to prevent future practice errors based on the contributory medication factors.

The reporting of near-miss medication events is significantly increased, suggesting that this is a beneficial format for gathering data on this type of medical error (Taylor et al., 2007). Guidance for nurses indicates that all medical errors and near misses should be immediately reported in order to facilitate the development of a learning culture (Haw, Stubbs, & Dickens, 2014). The supervisory discussion, the informal discussion, and near-miss reporting contain important information for improving clinical care (Rosenthal, Cornett, Sutcliffe, & Lewton, 2005). The registration of near misses prevents medical errors with serious consequences and thus improves the quality of care (Bosma, Veen, & Roukema, 2011).

Medical Errors and Telemedicine

Telemedicine is the use of telecommunication systems to deliver health care at a distance. Telemedicine can facilitate the efficient provision of health care services. Telemedicine bridges the challenges often encountered across different service levels including primary care, regional, and national care services, coordination between health care institutions, mobile medicine, medical and medical-social actors, promotion of virtual clustering, and new modalities for collaboration among medical partner organizations (Kamsu-Foguem & Foguem, 2014).

Elkin et al. (2013) described the usability-error ontology to handle medical errors in clinical contexts. The ontology can be employed to help improve the patients' treatment outcomes while ensuring the interoperability of the medical systems. In their ontology, the top level is categorized into two levels (i.e., cognitive errors and non-cognitive errors) since several medical errors are caused by human being. This work is interesting since it reveals the usability errors in the health information technology (health IT) or its interaction with users. However, the study of Elkin et al. (2013) does not explicitly discuss how medical professionals can collaborate with the important aspect in telemedicine.

Medical Errors and Medical Education

During the last decade, there has been a drive to improve the medical quality of patient care and prevent the occurrence of avoidable errors (Wong, Levinson, & Shojania, 2012). Accreditation standards and assessment methods, both during training and at end-of-training certification examinations, should explicitly target these medical competencies (Wong et al., 2012). Härkänen et al. (2015) indicated that observing real situations in clinical practice can provide undetected information regarding problems in the medication process. Although it is clear that the curriculum in medical schools should encompass quality and safety training to reduce patient safety in health care settings, many medical schools are slow to implement the reforms of medical education that are necessary to accomplish such a goal (DesHarnais & Nash, 2011).

Medical educators should increase exposure to exemplary responses to medical errors and help medical students learn from medical errors toward reducing medical errors in the future (Martinez & Lo, 2008). Training programs and managerial support, focusing on improving patient safety, need to be emphasized to prevent medical errors in the health care industry (Hwang & Hwang, 2011). Use of current health care equipment for medical procedures (e.g., central-line insertion and central-line care) is primarily dependent on the cognition of the health care staff (Bakdash & Drews, 2012). Deficiencies in the prescribing education and training are closely linked to the high frequency of medication errors (Sandilands et al., 2011). Methods for estimating the prevalence of physician dyscompetence include evaluating available data on medical errors, malpractice claims, disciplinary actions, quality control studies, medical record-related review studies, and physician's performance evaluation (Williams, 2006).

In medical education, medical trainees' perceptions and attitudes toward medical errors vary depending on whether the severity of outcome and whether the medical error is attributable to an individual or a team (Muller & Ornstein, 2007). Safe prescribing is a core competency in undergraduate medical education (Harding et al., 2010). The lack of preparedness of graduates for medical practice is related to a lack of exposure and preparation for clinical practice (Rothwell et al., 2012). Accepting responsibility for medical errors is recognized as prerequisite to medical education (Mazor, Fischer, Haley, Hatem, & Quirk, 2005).

The integration of simulation into the training of health care professionals provides the health care-related context for decision making and procedural skills in a high-fidelity environment, without having risk to patients (Gardner & Rich, 2014). Medical simulation can be applied in the training efforts to reduce medical errors concerning medical knowledge and patient care (Issenberg, Chung, & Devine, 2011). Medical simulation exhibits the causes of teamwork errors, latent errors, and error-producing conditions in emergency medical services (EMS) pediatric care (Lammers, Byrwa, & Fales, 2012). Woodfield et al. (2014) indicated that simulating cases and utilizing real drug charts are the effective methods for improving medical students' prescribing ability and confidence in medical emergencies.

Overview of Nursing Medication Errors

The nursing error relating to clinical management (NECM taxonomy) provides direction to clinicians and health care managers on various areas in clinical management that are most vulnerable to medical error (Tran & Johnson, 2010). Contributory medication factors to the nurse's medical errors include the reconciliation of medical errors, the types of drug distribution system, the quality of prescriptions, and the distractions during administration, excessive workloads, and nurse's medical knowledge (Brady et al., 2009).

Abdi et al. (2015) indicated that nurse managers can contribute to promoting a safety culture by encouraging staff to report medical errors, promoting learning from medical errors, and addressing inter-professional communication problems. When supported by their practice environments, nurses employ practices that can assist in interrupting medical errors before they reach the patients (Flynn, Liang, Dickson, Xie, & Suh, 2012). Nurses should carefully check medical administration in the high-alert situations toward reducing medical errors (Sheu, Wei, Chen, Yu, & Tang, 2009). Effective nursing handover is an opportunity for nurses to prevent medical errors by implementing more risk-aware handover strategies (Drach-Zahavy & Hadid, 2015).

Knowledge about nurses' error perception is crucial for establishing a sustainable risk management (Habermann, Foraita, & Cramer, 2013). There is a need to decrease the number and severity of medical administration errors, by increasing both nurse awareness and medical error reporting (Kelly & Wright, 2012). Identification of the conditions contributing to medication errors allows clinical nurses and administration systems to eliminate medical errors and to incorporate the changes that create a safer patient environment (Tang, Sheu, Yu, Wei, & Chen, 2007).

Aspects of Medical Errors in the Health Care Industry

Medication errors are a significant cause of morbidity and mortality in hospitalized patients (Brady et al., 2009). There is an increasing recognition that medical errors cause a global health problem, as many medical errors result in patient harm and increase costs to health care providers (Wheeler & Wheeler, 2005). Medical errors are affected by individual and work environment characteristics (Hwang & Hwang, 2011). Efforts to mitigate risk in the emergency department should include the diverse clinical specialties who work in this complex environment, with attention to those health conditions and potential errors with the highest risk (Brown, McCarthy, Kelen, & Levy, 2010).

The analysis of medical error patterns, contributory medication factors, and suggestions for error prevention can help reduce the frequency of medication events and improve patient care (Haw & Cahill, 2011). Medical errors have a serious effect on clinicians (McLennan et al., 2015). The implementation of the existing interventions at points within the system significantly offers the cost-effective approaches to improving medication safety in primary care (Olaniyan et al., 2015). Promoting the consistency between health care professionals as to what constitutes medication error contributes to the increased accuracy and compliance in the reporting of medical errors, thus creating effective health care policies toward reducing the occurrence of medical errors (Brady et al., 2009).

Measuring medical error typically results in the biased estimates of exposure-disease associations, the severity of the bias, and the nature of the bias concerning medical error patterns (Keogh & White, 2014). The quality function deployment matrix is used to translate the desired improvement in the malpractice costs into both medical decisions and diagnostic tests (Dror & Margol, 2015). The methods of Incident reporting (IR) and failure mode and effective analysis (FMEA) are widely used to detect and analyze the medical errors in health care settings (Daverio et al., 2015).

Computerized medication management systems are found to improve the medication safety (Redley & Botti, 2013). Standardized IT in the health care industry can reduce the preventable errors and increase patient safety (Koshy, 2005). Barcode labels, radio frequency identification tags (RFID), and palm vein-scanning technology are increasingly utilized in patient identification (Fastman & Kaplan, 2011). RFID solutions can be utilized to reduce the operating costs through decreasing labor costs, enhancing automation, improving the tracing procedure, and preventing the material loss (Kasemsap, 2015a). Concerning health care operations, RFID monitors the operating instruments and medical equipment during procedures to ensure all materials are accounted for (Kasemsap, 2017c).

Medical liability reform is viewed by many physician groups as a method of reducing medical malpractice litigation and lowering health care costs (Pegalis & Bal, 2012). Physicians cannot avoid the responsibilities and liabilities as a profession, when they provide the inappropriate advice to patients

(Nakayasu & Sato, 2012). The lack of cooperation among health care providers and the poor continuity of health care significantly contribute to medical errors (Kroll, Singleton, Collier, & Jones, 2008). Medication-ordering error rates are higher for the overnight and post-call physicians, particularly on the medical wards (Hendey, Barth, & Soliz, 2005).

Many medical errors are reported with the utilization of the paper-based tool than with the existing computerized error-reporting system (Kolovos, Bratton, & Levy, 2008). It can be more effective when the computerization of physicians' orders links to other computerized systems toward detecting and preventing the medical prescription errors (Shamliyan, Duval, Du, & Kane, 2008). Clinical decision support systems utilize IT to improve the quality of care by supporting the physician's decision-making process (Laing et al., 2015).

The medication errors found in many hospitals in Australia are the prescription-related ordering errors, dispensing, administration, and medication recording errors (Hodgkinson, Koch, Nay, & Nichols, 2006). Hodgkinson et al. (2006) stated that medical strategies to reduce medical errors include the establishment of computerized physician ordering entry systems combined with clinical decision support systems; individual medication supply systems when compared with other dispensing systems (e.g., ward stock approaches); the utilization of clinical pharmacists in the inpatient setting; and the checking of medication orders by nurses before dispensing medication.

Workload and lack of medical experience at the current ward are two important conditions that can lead to medical errors (Seki & Yamasaki, 2006). Health care organizations need to support clinicians in coping with the stress concerning medical errors (McLennan et al., 2015). In order to constitute a practical action to counteract the medical errors, it is necessary to consider major elements (e.g., human, technological, and organizational perspectives) that contribute to the occurrence of a critical medication event (Smorti, Cappelli, Zarantonello, Tani, & Gensini, 2014). Incorporating the apology into conversations between physicians and patients can address the needs of both parties and can play an important role in the effective resolution of disputes concerning the occurrence of medical errors (Robbennolt, 2009).

FUTURE RESEARCH DIRECTIONS

The classification of the extensive literature in the domains of medical errors will provide the potential opportunities for future research. Telemedicine is the utilization of medical information exchanged from one site to another via electronic communications to improve a patient's clinical health status. Telemedicine offers important benefits (e.g., improved access, cost efficiencies, improved quality, and patient demand). Telemedicine brings the health care value through its ability for the remote visits with patients, immediate access to health care professionals, real-time access to health data, and health monitoring capabilities (Kasemsap, 2017d).

Electronic health record (EHR) provides the ability to exchange complete health information about a patient in real time. EHR systems are very important in health care settings and have the potential to transform the health care system from a mostly paper-based industry to the one that utilizes the clinical data and other pieces of information to assist the health care providers in delivering the higher quality of care to their patients (Kasemsap, 2017e). Accurate, updated, and thorough information through EHR leads to a higher quality of care, from better diagnoses to reduced medication errors. The integration of health IT into primary care includes a wide variety of electronic methods that are used to manage information about people's health and health care, for both individual patients and groups of patients.

Effective health IT can lower costs, improve efficiency, and reduce medical error, while providing better patient care and service (Kasemsap, 2017f). An examination of linkages among telemedicine, EHR, health IT, TQM, and medical error reduction would seem to be viable for future research efforts.

Quality of performance is the numerical measurement of the performance of an organization or process assessed through measurement of physical products and statistical sampling of the output of processes (Kasemsap, 2014). In order to facilitate quality performance and achieve the effectiveness of the whole quality management system, researchers and managers should develop and maintain their organization's total quality management (TQM) practices related to quality performance in organization (Kasemsap, 2015b). Implementing Six Sigma within global operations offers a number of benefits, such as the improved customer loyalty, reduced cycle time, better time management, better employee motivation, improved strategic planning, and the reduced risk of defects (Kasemsap, 2016). Successful Lean health care efforts result in the measurable improvements in patient outcomes, such as improved quality, less harm due to preventable errors, better access, shorter waiting times, and better service (Kasemsap, 2017g). Recent developments in the robotic age have made robots and robotics more intelligent, affordable, and user-friendly in modern operations, ranging from manufacturing to health care (Kasemsap, 2017h). Reducing medical errors through the applications of TQM, Six Sigma, Lean health care, and robotics would be beneficial for future research directions.

CONCLUSION

This chapter explained the overview of medical errors; drug prescription errors and prescribing; the overview of medical error disclosure; medical errors and telemedicine; medical errors and medical education; the overview of nursing medication errors; and the aspects of medical errors in the health care industry. Reducing medical errors, increasing patient safety, and improving the quality of health care are the major goals in the health care industry. Medical errors are caused by mistakes in drug prescription, dosing, and medical administration in inpatient and outpatient settings. Heath care-related guidelines, institutional safety practices, and modern health care technologies must be applied in hospitals, clinics, and medical offices to reduce the occurrence of medical errors.

Health care organizations must clearly communicate with all health care providers that patient safety is their responsibility, and health care managers must define how the health care organizations deal with the unsafe practitioners toward reducing the medical errors. The perspective to effectively implement a safe medication-use process is the need for the well-defined, consistently applied, and highly standardized system process. The successful approach to the implementation of a safe medication-use process is the effective collaboration among health care leadership, health care providers, and patients. Health care organizations must provide the leadership, expectations, training, and structure to promote the coordinated functioning of caregivers and patients to enhance the quality of health care and reduce the medical errors.

Health care providers and health care organizations must adopt a proactive approach to the reduction of medical errors. The technologies and processes of health care systems must be continuously evaluated regarding the potential risks to patient safety. Understanding the perspectives of medical errors is necessary for health care organizations that seek to serve patients, increase health care performance, strengthen competitiveness, and achieve continuous success in the health care industry. Therefore, it is essential for health care organizations to understand their perspectives of medical errors and develop a strategic plan to regularly check their practical advancements toward minimizing the medical errors in the health care industry. Understanding the perspectives of medical errors has the potential to enhance health care performance and reach strategic goals in the health care industry.

REFERENCES

Abdi, Z., Delgoshaei, B., Ravaghi, H., Abbasi, M., & Heyrani, A. (2015). The culture of patient safety in an Iranian intensive care unit. *Journal of Nursing Management*, *23*(3), 333–345. doi:10.1111/jonm.12135 PMID:23902287

Absulem, S., & Hardin, H. (2011). Home health nurses' perceived care errors. *Rehabilitation Nursing*, *36*(3), 98–105. doi:10.1002/j.2048-7940.2011.tb00073.x PMID:21675394

Ammouri, A. A., Tailakh, A. K., Muliira, J. K., Geethakrishnan, R., & Al Kindi, S. N. (2015). Patient safety culture among nurses. *International Nursing Review*, *62*(1), 102–110. doi:10.1111/inr.12159 PMID:25495946

Anoosheh, M., Ahmadi, F., Faghihzadeh, S., & Vaismoradi, M. (2008). Causes and management of nursing practice errors: A questionnaire survey of hospital nurses in Iran. *International Nursing Review*, *55*(3), 288–295. doi:10.1111/j.1466-7657.2008.00623.x PMID:19522944

Armitage, G., Newell, R., & Wright, J. (2010). Improving the quality of drug error reporting. *Journal of Evaluation in Clinical Practice*, *16*(6), 1189–1197. doi:10.1111/j.1365-2753.2009.01293.x PMID:20807298

Azar, A. T., & El-Metwally, S. M. (2013). Decision tree classifiers for automated medical diagnosis. *Neural Computing & Applications*, *23*(7), 2387–2403. doi:10.1007/s00521-012-1196-7

Bakdash, J. Z., & Drews, F. A. (2012). Using knowledge in the world to improve patient safety: Designing affordances in health care equipment to specify a sequential "checklist". *Human Factors and Ergonomics in Manufacturing & Service Industries*, *22*(1), 7–20. doi:10.1002/hfm.20289

Bosma, E., Veen, E. J., & Roukema, J. A. (2011, November). Incidence, nature and impact of error in surgery. *British Journal of Surgery*, *98*(11), 1654–1659. PMID: 21706475 doi:10.1002/bjs.7594

Brady, A. M., Malone, A. M., & Fleming, S. (2009). A literature review of the individual and systems factors that contribute to medication errors in nursing practice. *Journal of Nursing Management*, *17*(6), 679–697. doi:10.1111/j.1365-2834.2009.00995.x PMID:19694912

Brennan, N., & Mattick, K. (2013). A systematic review of educational interventions to change behaviour of prescribers in hospital settings, with a particular emphasis on new prescribers. *British Journal of Clinical Pharmacology*, *75*(2), 359–372. doi:10.1111/j.1365-2125.2012.04397.x PMID:22831632

Brown, T. W., McCarthy, M. L., Kelen, G. D., & Levy, F. (2010). An epidemiologic study of closed emergency department malpractice claims in a national database of physician malpractice insurers. *Academic Emergency Medicine*, *17*(5), 553–560. doi:10.1111/j.1553-2712.2010.00729.x PMID:20536812

Bynum, W. E. IV, & Goodie, J. L. (2014). Shame, guilt, and the medical learner: Ignored connections and why we should care. *Medical Education*, *48*(11), 1045–1054. doi:10.1111/medu.12521 PMID:25307632

Carberry, M., Connelly, S., & Murphy, J. (2013). A prospective audit of a nurse independent prescribing within critical care. *Nursing in Critical Care, 18*(3), 135–141. doi:10.1111/j.1478-5153.2012.00534.x PMID:23577948

Celebi, N., Kirchhoff, K., Lammerding-Köppel, M., Riessen, R., & Weyrich, P. (2010). Medical clerkships do not reduce common prescription errors among medical students. *Naunyn-Schmiedeberg's Archives of Pharmacology, 382*(2), 171–176. doi:10.1007/s00210-010-0530-9 PMID:20535451

Chetouane, F., & Ibraheem, E. (2016). Surgery operations modeling and scheduling in healthcare systems. In P. Manolitzas, E. Grigoroudis, N. Matsatsinis, & D. Yannacopoulos (Eds.), *Effective methods for modern healthcare service quality and evaluation* (pp. 90–108). Hershey, PA: IGI Global. doi:10.4018/978-1-4666-9961-8.ch005

Daverio, M., Fino, G., Luca, B., Zaggia, C., Pettenazzo, A., Parpaiola, A., & Amigoni, A. et al. (2015). Failure mode and effective analysis ameliorate awareness of medical errors: A 4-year prospective observational study in critically ill children. *Paediatric Anaesthesia, 25*(12), 1227–1234. doi:10.1111/pan.12772 PMID:26432066

Davies, E. D., Schneider, F., Childs, S., Hucker, T., Krikos, D., Peh, J., & Cashman, J. et al. (2011). A prevalence study of errors in opioid prescribing in a large teaching hospital. *International Journal of Clinical Practice, 65*(9), 923–929. doi:10.1111/j.1742-1241.2011.02705.x PMID:21752165

DesHarnais, S. I., & Nash, D. B. (2011). Reforming way medical students and physicians are taught about quality and safety. *Mount Sinai Journal of Medicine: A Journal of Translational and Personalized Medicine, 78*(6), 834–841. doi:10.1002/msj.20302

Dias-Souza, M. V. (2016). Strategies for expanding access and improving the quality of pharmaceutical services. In P. Manolitzas, E. Grigoroudis, N. Matsatsinis, & D. Yannacopoulos (Eds.), *Effective methods for modern healthcare service quality and evaluation* (pp. 168–201). Hershey, PA: IGI Global. doi:10.4018/978-1-4666-9961-8.ch008

Doumbouya, M. B., Kamsu-Foguem, B., Kenfack, H., & Foguem, C. (2015). Argumentative reasoning and taxonomic analysis for the identification of medical errors. *Engineering Applications of Artificial Intelligence, 46*, 166–179. doi:10.1016/j.engappai.2015.08.009

Drach-Zahavy, A., & Hadid, N. (2015). Nursing handovers as resilient points of care: Linking handover strategies to treatment errors in the patient care in the following shift. *Journal of Advanced Nursing, 71*(5), 1135–1145. doi:10.1111/jan.12615 PMID:25641374

Dror, S., & Margol, D. (2015). Framework for analyzing malpractice cases to improve healthcare systems. *Quality and Reliability Engineering International, 31*(7), 1103–1113. doi:10.1002/qre.1851

Elkin, P. L., Beuscart-zephir, M. C., Pelayo, S., Patel, V., & Nøhr, C. (2013). The usability-error ontology. In M. Beuscart-Zéphir, M. Jaspers, C. Kuziemsky, C. Nøhr, & J. Aarts (Eds.), *Context sensitive health informatics: Human and sociotechnical approaches* (pp. 91–96). Amsterdam, The Netherlands: IOS Press.

Fastman, B. R., & Kaplan, H. S. (2011). Errors in transfusion medicine: Have we learned our lesson? *Mount Sinai Journal of Medicine: A Journal of Translational and Personalized Medicine, 78*(6), 854–864. doi:10.1002/msj.20296

Flynn, L., Liang, Y., Dickson, G. L., Xie, M., & Suh, D. C. (2012). Nurses' practice environments, error interception practices, and inpatient medication errors. *Journal of Nursing Scholarship*, *44*(2), 180–186. doi:10.1111/j.1547-5069.2012.01443.x PMID:22510244

Foster, P. N., Sidhu, R., Gadhia, D. A., & DeMusis, M. (2008). Leveraging computerized sign-out to increase error reporting and addressing patient safety in graduate medical education. *Journal of General Internal Medicine*, *23*(4), 481–484. doi:10.1007/s11606-007-0503-y PMID:18373149

Gallagher, T. H., Brundage, G., Summy, E. A., Bommarito, K. M., Ebers, A. G., Waterman, A. D., & Dunagan, C. et al. (2006). National survey: Risk managers' attitudes and experiences regarding patient safety and error disclosure. *Journal of Healthcare Risk Management*, *26*(3), 11–16. doi:10.1002/jhrm.5600260305

Gardner, A., & Rich, M. (2014). Error management training and simulation education. *The Clinical Teacher*, *11*(7), 537–540. doi:10.1111/tct.12217 PMID:25417983

Garrouste-Orgeas, M., Flaatten, H., & Moreno, R. (2016). Understanding medical errors and adverse events in ICU patients. *Intensive Care Medicine*, *42*(1), 107–109. doi:10.1007/s00134-015-3968-x PMID:26248952

Gavgani, V. Z., Oskouei, M. M., & Salehi, R. (2015). Patients' medication errors: How patients' inadequate information about their prosthetic heart valve diseases affects their healthcare. In *Healthcare administration: Concepts, methodologies, tools, and applications* (pp. 1081–1087). Hershey, PA: IGI Global. doi:10.4018/978-1-4666-6339-8.ch057

Gawande, A. (2007). *Better: A surgeon's notes on performance*. New York, NY: Metropolitan Books.

Ge, X., Rijo, R., Paige, R. F., Kelly, T. P., & McDermid, J. A. (2012). Introducing goal structuring notation to explain decisions in clinical practice. *Procedia Technology*, *5*, 686–695. doi:10.1016/j.protcy.2012.09.076

Gordon, M., Darbyshire, D., & Baker, P. (2012). Non-technical skills training to enhance patient safety: A systematic review. *Medical Education*, *46*(11), 1042–1054. doi:10.1111/j.1365-2923.2012.04343.x PMID:23078681

Gortzis, L. G., & Nikiforidis, G. (2008). Tracing and cataloguing knowledge in an e-health cardiology environment. *Journal of Biomedical Informatics*, *41*(2), 217–223. doi:10.1016/j.jbi.2007.09.001 PMID:17945541

Gowen, C. R. III, McFadden, K. L., & Settaluri, S. (2012). Contrasting continuous quality improvement, Six Sigma, and Lean management for enhanced outcomes in US hospitals. *American Journal of Business*, *27*(2), 133–153. doi:10.1108/19355181211274442

Habermann, M., Foraita, R., & Cramer, H. (2013). Categories of errors and error frequencies as identified by nurses: Results of a cross-sectional study in German nursing homes and hospitals. *Journal of Public Health*, *21*(1), 3–13. doi:10.1007/s10389-012-0531-x

Harding, S., Britten, N., & Bristow, D. (2010). The performance of junior doctors in applying clinical pharmacology knowledge and prescribing skills to standardized clinical cases. *British Journal of Clinical Pharmacology*, *69*(6), 598–606. doi:10.1111/j.1365-2125.2010.03645.x PMID:20565451

Härkänen, M., Ahonen, J., Kervinen, M., Turunen, H., & Vehviläinen-Julkunen, K. (2015). The factors associated with medication errors in adult medical and surgical inpatients: A direct observation approach with medication record reviews. *Scandinavian Journal of Caring Sciences*, *29*(2), 297–306. doi:10.1111/scs.12163 PMID:25213297

Haw, C., & Cahill, C. (2011). A computerized system for reporting medication events in psychiatry: The first two years of operation. *Journal of Psychiatric and Mental Health Nursing*, *18*(4), 308–315. doi:10.1111/j.1365-2850.2010.01664.x PMID:21418430

Haw, C., Stubbs, J., & Dickens, G. L. (2014). Barriers to the reporting of medication administration errors and near misses: An interview study of nurses at a psychiatric hospital. *Journal of Psychiatric and Mental Health Nursing*, *21*(9), 797–805. PMID:24646372

Hendey, G. W., Barth, B. E., & Soliz, T. (2005). Overnight and postcall errors in medication orders. *Academic Emergency Medicine*, *12*(7), 629–634. doi:10.1111/j.1553-2712.2005.tb00919.x PMID:15995095

Henneman, E. A., Blank, F. S. J., Gattasso, S., Williamson, K., & Henneman, P. L. (2006). Testing a classification model for emergency department errors. *Journal of Advanced Nursing*, *55*(1), 90–99. doi:10.1111/j.1365-2648.2006.03878.x PMID:16768743

Hobgood, C., Weiner, B., & Tamayo-Sarver, J. H. (2006). Medical error identification, disclosure, and reporting: Do emergency medicine provider groups differ? *Academic Emergency Medicine*, *13*(4), 443–451. doi:10.1111/j.1553-2712.2006.tb00324.x PMID:16531598

Hodgkinson, B., Koch, S., Nay, R., & Nichols, K. (2006). Strategies to reduce medication errors with reference to older adults. *International Journal of Evidence-Based Healthcare*, *4*(1), 2–41. PMID:21631752

Hsaio, G. Y., Chen, I. J., Yu, S., Wei, I. L., Fang, Y. Y., & Tang, F. I. (2010). Nurses' knowledge of high-alert medications: Instrument development and validation. *Journal of Advanced Nursing*, *66*(1), 177–190. doi:10.1111/j.1365-2648.2009.05164.x PMID:20423443

Hwang, J. I., & Hwang, E. J. (2011). Individual and work environment characteristics associated with error occurrences in Korean public hospitals. *Journal of Clinical Nursing*, *20*(21/22), 3256–3266. doi:10.1111/j.1365-2702.2011.03773.x PMID:21733027

Institute of Medicine. (2001). *Crossing in the quality chasm: A new health system for the 21st century*. Washington, DC: National Academies Press.

Issenberg, S. B., Chung, H. S., & Devine, L. A. (2011). Patient safety training simulations based on competency criteria of the Accreditation Council for Graduate Medical Education. *Mount Sinai Journal of Medicine: A Journal of Translational and Personalized Medicine*, *78*(6), 842–853. doi:10.1002/msj.20301

Kagan, I., & Barnoy, S. (2013). Organizational safety culture and medical error reporting by Israeli nurses. *Journal of Nursing Scholarship*, *45*(3), 273–280. PMID:23574516

Kaldjian, L. C., Jones, E. W., Rosenthal, G. E., Tripp-Reimer, T., & Hillis, S. L. (2006). An empirically derived taxonomy of factors affecting physicians' willingness to disclose medical errors. *Journal of General Internal Medicine*, *21*(9), 942–948. doi:10.1007/BF02743142 PMID:16918739

Kaldjian, L. C., Jones, E. W., Wu, B. J., Forman-Hoffman, V. L., Levi, B. H., & Rosenthal, G. E. (2007). Disclosing medical errors to patients: Attitudes and practices of physicians and trainees. *Journal of General Internal Medicine*, *22*(7), 988–996. doi:10.1007/s11606-007-0227-z PMID:17473944

Kamsu-Foguem, B., & Foguem, C. (2014). Telemedicine and mobile health with integrative medicine in developing countries. *Health Policy and Technology*, *3*(4), 264–271. doi:10.1016/j.hlpt.2014.08.008

Kasemsap, K. (2014). Unifying a framework of organizational culture, organizational climate, knowledge management, and job performance. In R. Perez-Castillo & M. Piattini (Eds.), *Uncovering essential software artifacts through business process archeology* (pp. 336–362). Hershey, PA: IGI Global. doi:10.4018/978-1-4666-4667-4.ch013

Kasemsap, K. (2015a). The role of radio frequency identification in modern libraries. In S. Thanuskodi (Ed.), *Handbook of research on inventive digital tools for collection management and development in modern libraries* (pp. 361–385). Hershey, PA: IGI Global. doi:10.4018/978-1-4666-8178-1.ch021

Kasemsap, K. (2015b). The role of total quality management practices on quality performance. In A. Moumtzoglou, A. Kastania, & S. Archondakis (Eds.), *Laboratory management information systems: Current requirements and future perspectives* (pp. 1–31). Hershey, PA: IGI Global. doi:10.4018/978-1-4666-6320-6.ch001

Kasemsap, K. (2016). Applying Lean Production and Six Sigma in global operations. In U. Akkucuk (Ed.), *Handbook of research on waste management techniques for sustainability* (pp. 44–74). Hershey, PA: IGI Global. doi:10.4018/978-1-4666-9723-2.ch003

Kasemsap, K. (2017a). The fundamentals of health literacy. In N. Wickramasinghe (Ed.), *Handbook of research on healthcare administration and management* (pp. 507–527). Hershey, PA: IGI Global. doi:10.4018/978-1-5225-0920-2.ch030

Kasemsap, K. (2017b). Promoting health literacy in global health care. In N. Wickramasinghe (Ed.), *Handbook of research on healthcare administration and management* (pp. 485–506). Hershey, PA: IGI Global. doi:10.4018/978-1-5225-0920-2.ch029

Kasemsap, K. (2017c). Radio frequency identification and mobile ad-hoc network: Theories and applications. In S. Bhattacharyya, N. Das, D. Bhattacharjee, & A. Mukherjee (Eds.), *Handbook of research on recent developments in intelligent communication application* (pp. 63–95). Hershey, PA: IGI Global. doi:10.4018/978-1-5225-1785-6.ch003

Kasemsap, K. (2017d). The importance of telemedicine in global health care. In N. Wickramasinghe (Ed.), *Handbook of research on healthcare administration and management* (pp. 157–177). Hershey, PA: IGI Global. doi:10.4018/978-1-5225-0920-2.ch010

Kasemsap, K. (2017e). Mastering electronic health record in global health care. In N. Wickramasinghe (Ed.), *Handbook of research on healthcare administration and management* (pp. 222–242). Hershey, PA: IGI Global. doi:10.4018/978-1-5225-0920-2.ch014

Kasemsap, K. (2017f). Analyzing the role of health information technology in global health care. In N. Wickramasinghe (Ed.), *Handbook of research on healthcare administration and management* (pp. 287–307). Hershey, PA: IGI Global. doi:10.4018/978-1-5225-0920-2.ch017

Kasemsap, K. (2017g). Lean thinking in global health care: Theory and applications. In N. Wickramasinghe (Ed.), *Handbook of research on healthcare administration and management* (pp. 120–141). Hershey, PA: IGI Global. doi:10.4018/978-1-5225-0920-2.ch008

Kasemsap, K. (2017h). Robotics: Theory and applications. In M. Moore (Ed.), *Cybersecurity breaches and issues surrounding online threat protection* (pp. 311–345). Hershey, PA: IGI Global. doi:10.4018/978-1-5225-1941-6.ch013

Kelly, J., & Wright, D. (2012). Medicine administration errors and their severity in secondary care older persons' ward: A multi-centre observational study. *Journal of Clinical Nursing*, *21*(13/14), 1806–1815. doi:10.1111/j.1365-2702.2011.03760.x PMID:21733025

Keogh, R. H., & White, I. R. (2014). A toolkit for measurement error correction, with a focus on nutritional epidemiology. *Statistics in Medicine*, *33*(12), 2137–2155. doi:10.1002/sim.6095 PMID:24497385

Kolovos, N. S., Bratton, S. L., & Levy, F. H. (2008). A novel error-reporting tool in pediatric intensive care. *Journal for Healthcare Quality*, *30*(3), 43–50. doi:10.1111/j.1945-1474.2008.tb01142.x PMID:18507240

Koshy, R. (2005). Navigating the information technology highway: Computer solutions to reduce errors and enhance patient safety. *Transfusion*, *45*(Suppl. 4), 189S–205S. doi:10.1111/j.1537-2995.2005.00619.x PMID:16181403

Kroll, L., Singleton, A., Collier, J., & Jones, I. R. (2008). Learning not to take it seriously: Junior doctors' accounts of error. *Medical Education*, *42*(10), 982–990. doi:10.1111/j.1365-2923.2008.03151.x PMID:18823517

Laing, G., Bruce, J., Skinner, D., Allorto, N., Aldous, C., Thomson, S., & Clarke, D. (2015). Using a hybrid electronic medical record system for the surveillance of adverse surgical events and human error in a developing world surgical service. *World Journal of Surgery*, *39*(1), 70–79. doi:10.1007/s00268-014-2766-x PMID:25167900

Lammers, R., Byrwa, M., & Fales, W. (2012). Root causes of errors in a simulated prehospital pediatric emergency. *Academic Emergency Medicine*, *19*(1), 37–47. doi:10.1111/j.1553-2712.2011.01252.x PMID:22251191

Lawson, A. E., & Daniel, E. S. (2011). Inferences of clinical diagnostic reasoning and diagnostic error. *Journal of Biomedical Informatics*, *44*(3), 402–412. doi:10.1016/j.jbi.2010.01.003 PMID:20093196

Lehmann, L., Wesselmann, U., Weber, B., & Smentkowski, U. (2015). Medical error analysis in dermatology according to the reports of the North Rhine Medical Association from 2004–2013. *JDDG: Journal der Deutschen Dermatologischen Gesellschaft*, *13*(9), 903–908. PMID:26882381

Lewis, P. J., Ashcroft, D. M., Dornan, T., Taylor, D., Wass, V., & Tully, M. P. (2014). Exploring the causes of junior doctors' prescribing mistakes: A qualitative study. *British Journal of Clinical Pharmacology*, *78*(2), 310–319. doi:10.1111/bcp.12332 PMID:24517271

Lin, Y. H., & Ma, S. M. (2009). Willingness of nurses to report medication administration errors in Southern Taiwan: A cross-sectional survey. *Worldviews on Evidence-Based Nursing*, *6*(4), 237–245. doi:10.1111/j.1741-6787.2009.00169.x PMID:19747183

Lucchiari, C., & Pravettoni, G. (2012). Cognitive balanced model: A conceptual scheme of diagnostic decision making. *Journal of Evaluation in Clinical Practice*, *18*(1), 82–88. doi:10.1111/j.1365-2753.2011.01771.x PMID:21999310

Manias, E., Williams, A., & Liew, D. (2012). Interventions to reduce medication errors in adult intensive care: A systematic review. *British Journal of Clinical Pharmacology*, *74*(3), 411–423. doi:10.1111/j.1365-2125.2012.04220.x PMID:22348303

Mansour, M., James, V., & Edgley, A. (2012). Investigating the safety of medication administration in adult critical care settings. *Nursing in Critical Care*, *17*(4), 189–197. doi:10.1111/j.1478-5153.2012.00500.x PMID:22698161

Martinez, W., & Lo, B. (2008). Medical students' experiences with medical errors: An analysis of medical student essays. *Medical Education*, *42*(7), 733–741. doi:10.1111/j.1365-2923.2008.03109.x PMID:18507766

Maskens, C., Downie, H., Wendt, A., Lima, A., Merkley, L., Lin, Y., & Callum, J. (2014). Hospital-based transfusion error tracking from 2005 to 2010: Identifying the key errors threatening patient transfusion safety. *Transfusion*, *54*(1), 66–73. doi:10.1111/trf.12240 PMID:23672511

Mazor, K. M., Fischer, M. A., Haley, H. L., Hatem, D., & Quirk, M. E. (2005). Teaching and medical errors: Primary care preceptors' views. *Medical Education*, *39*(10), 982–990. doi:10.1111/j.1365-2929.2005.02262.x PMID:16178824

McDowell, S. E., Ferner, H. S., & Ferner, R. E. (2009). The pathophysiology of medication errors: How and where they arise. *British Journal of Clinical Pharmacology*, *67*(6), 605–613. doi:10.1111/j.1365-2125.2009.03416.x PMID:19594527

McLennan, S. R., Engel-Glatter, S., Meyer, A. H., Schwappach, D. L. B., Scheidegger, D. H., & Elger, B. S. (2015). The impact of medical errors on Swiss anaesthesiologists: A cross-sectional survey. *Acta Anaesthesiologica Scandinavica*, *59*(8), 990–998. doi:10.1111/aas.12517 PMID:25952281

Muller, D., & Ornstein, K. (2007). Perceptions of and attitudes towards medical errors among medical trainees. *Medical Education*, *41*(7), 645–652. doi:10.1111/j.1365-2923.2007.02784.x PMID:17614884

Nakayasu, K., & Sato, C. (2012). Liability for telemedicine. *International Journal of E-Health and Medical Communications*, *3*(1), 1–21. doi:10.4018/jehmc.2012010101

Niemann, D., Bertsche, A., Meyrath, D., Koepf, E. D., Traiser, C., Seebald, K., & Bertsche, T. et al. (2015). A prospective three-step intervention study to prevent medication errors in drug handling in paediatric care. *Journal of Clinical Nursing*, *24*(1/2), 101–114. doi:10.1111/jocn.12592 PMID:24890332

Nordén-Hägg, A., Kettis-Lindblad, Å., Ring, L., & Kälvemark-Sporrong, S. (2012). Experiences of a nationwide web-based system: Reporting dispensing errors in Swedish pharmacies. *International Journal of Pharmacy Practice*, *20*(1), 25–32. doi:10.1111/j.2042-7174.2011.00159.x PMID:22236177

Olaniyan, J. O., Ghaleb, M., Dhillon, S., & Robinson, P. (2015). Safety of medication use in primary care. *International Journal of Pharmacy Practice*, *23*(1), 3–20. doi:10.1111/ijpp.12120 PMID:24954018

Palmero, D., Di Paolo, E. R., Beauport, L., Pannatier, A., & Tolsa, J. F. (2016). A bundle with a preformatted medical order sheet and an introductory course to reduce prescription errors in neonates. *European Journal of Pediatrics*, *175*(1), 113–119. doi:10.1007/s00431-015-2607-4 PMID:26272253

Pate, C. L., & Swofford, M. D. (2016). Organizational integration of decision analytic methods in healthcare settings. In P. Manolitzas, E. Grigoroudis, N. Matsatsinis, & D. Yannacopoulos (Eds.), *Effective methods for modern healthcare service quality and evaluation* (pp. 45–73). Hershey, PA: IGI Global. doi:10.4018/978-1-4666-9961-8.ch003

Pazokian, M., Tafreshi, M. Z., & Rassouli, M. (2014). Iranian nurses' perspectives on factors influencing medication errors. *International Nursing Review*, *61*(2), 246–254. doi:10.1111/inr.12086 PMID:24571495

Pegalis, S. E., & Bal, B. S. (2012). Closed medical negligence claims can drive patient safety and reduce litigation. *Clinical Orthopaedics and Related Research*, *470*(5), 1398–1404. doi:10.1007/s11999-012-2308-5 PMID:22419349

Raab, S. S., & Grzybicki, D. M. (2010). Quality in cancer diagnosis. *CA: a Cancer Journal for Clinicians*, *60*(3), 139–165. doi:10.3322/caac.20068 PMID:20444999

Rathert, C., & Phillips, W. (2010). Medical error disclosure training: Evidence for values-based ethical environments. *Journal of Business Ethics*, *97*(3), 491–503. doi:10.1007/s10551-010-0520-3

Reason, J. (1990). *Human error*. Cambridge, UK: Cambridge University Press. doi:10.1017/CBO9781139062367

Reason, J. (1997). *Managing the risks of organizational accidents*. Aldershot, UK: Ashgate.

Redley, B., & Botti, M. (2013). Reported medication errors after introducing an electronic medication management system. *Journal of Clinical Nursing*, *22*(3/4), 579–589. doi:10.1111/j.1365-2702.2012.04326.x PMID:22998067

Robbennolt, J. K. (2009). Apologies and medical error. *Clinical Orthopaedics and Related Research*, *467*(2), 376–382. doi:10.1007/s11999-008-0580-1 PMID:18972177

Rosenthal, M. M., Cornett, P. L., Sutcliffe, K. M., & Lewton, E. (2005). Beyond the medical record. *Journal of General Internal Medicine*, *20*(5), 404–409. doi:10.1111/j.1525-1497.2005.0098.x PMID:15963161

Ross, S., Bond, C., Rothnie, H., Thomas, S., & Macleod, M. J. (2009). What is the scale of prescribing errors committed by junior doctors? A systematic review. *British Journal of Clinical Pharmacology*, *67*(6), 629–640. doi:10.1111/j.1365-2125.2008.03330.x PMID:19094162

Rothwell, C., Burford, B., Morrison, J., Morrow, G., Allen, M., Davies, C., & Illing, J. et al. (2012). Junior doctors prescribing: Enhancing their learning in practice. *British Journal of Clinical Pharmacology*, *73*(2), 194–202. doi:10.1111/j.1365-2125.2011.04061.x PMID:21752067

Rouse, R. A., & Kaplan, J. B. (2008). Why do some hospital leaders "speak no evil" about their organizations' medical errors? *The Journal of Leadership Studies*, *2*(3), 6–16. doi:10.1002/jls.20070

Sandilands, E. A., Reid, K., Shaw, L., Bateman, D. N., Webb, D. J., Dhaun, N., & Kluth, D. C. (2011). Impact of a focussed teaching programme on practical prescribing skills among final year medical students. *British Journal of Clinical Pharmacology*, *71*(1), 29–33. doi:10.1111/j.1365-2125.2010.03808.x PMID:21143498

Schwappach, D. L. B. (2014). Risk factors for patient-reported medical errors in eleven countries. *Health Expectations*, *17*(3), 321–331. doi:10.1111/j.1369-7625.2011.00755.x PMID:22296575

Schwappach, D. L. B., & Wernli, M. (2010). Medication errors in chemotherapy: Incidence, types and involvement of patients in prevention. A review of the literature. *European Journal of Cancer Care*, *19*(3), 285–292. doi:10.1111/j.1365-2354.2009.01127.x PMID:19708929

Seki, Y., & Yamasaki, Y. (2006). Effects of working conditions on intravenous medication errors in a Japanese hospital. *Journal of Nursing Management*, *14*(2), 128–139. doi:10.1111/j.1365-2934.2006.00597.x PMID:16487424

Sevdalis, N., Jacklin, R., Arora, S., Vincent, C. A., & Thomson, R. G. (2010). Diagnostic error in a national incident reporting system in the UK. *Journal of Evaluation in Clinical Practice*, *16*(6), 1276–1281. doi:10.1111/j.1365-2753.2009.01328.x PMID:20727061

Shah, R. K., Lander, L., Forbes, P., Jenkins, K., Healy, G. B., & Roberson, D. W. (2009). Safety on an inpatient pediatric otolaryngology service: Many small errors, few adverse events. *The Laryngoscope*, *119*(5), 871–879. doi:10.1002/lary.20208 PMID:19358191

Shamliyan, T. A., Duval, S., Du, J., & Kane, R. L. (2008). Just what the doctor ordered. Review of the evidence of the impact of computerized physician order entry system on medication errors. *Health Services Research, 43*(1p1), 32–53.

Shawahna, R., Rahman, N. U., Ahmad, M., Debray, M., Yliperttula, M., & Declèves, X. (2011). Electronic prescribing reduces prescribing error in public hospitals. *Journal of Clinical Nursing*, *20*(21/22), 3233–3245. doi:10.1111/j.1365-2702.2011.03714.x PMID:21627699

Sheu, S. J., Wei, I. L., Chen, C. H., Yu, S., & Tang, F. I. (2009). Using snowball sampling method with nurses to understand medication administration errors. *Journal of Clinical Nursing*, *18*(4), 559–569. doi:10.1111/j.1365-2702.2007.02048.x PMID:18298506

Smorti, A., Cappelli, F., Zarantonello, R., Tani, F., & Gensini, G. F. (2014). Medical error and systems of signaling: Conceptual and linguistic definition. *Internal and Emergency Medicine*, *9*(6), 681–688. doi:10.1007/s11739-014-1108-1 PMID:25034521

Tang, F. I., Sheu, S. J., Yu, S., Wei, I. L., & Chen, C. H. (2007). Nurses relate the contributing factors involved in medication errors. *Journal of Clinical Nursing*, *16*(3), 447–457. doi:10.1111/j.1365-2702.2005.01540.x PMID:17335520

Taylor, J. A., Brownstein, D., Klein, E. J., & Strandjord, T. P. (2007). Evaluation of an anonymous system to report medical errors in pediatric inpatients. *Journal of Hospital Medicine*, *2*(4), 226–233. doi:10.1002/jhm.208 PMID:17683099

Tran, D. T., & Johnson, M. (2010). Classifying nursing errors in clinical management within an Australian hospital. *International Nursing Review*, *57*(4), 454–462. doi:10.1111/j.1466-7657.2010.00846.x PMID:21050197

Tully, M. P. (2012). Prescribing errors in hospital practice. *British Journal of Clinical Pharmacology*, *74*(4), 668–675. doi:10.1111/j.1365-2125.2012.04313.x PMID:22554316

Vozikis, A. (2012). Adverse events and medical errors in Greece: Knowledge creation and capture methods. In P. Ordóñez de Pablos & M. Lytras (Eds.), *Knowledge management and drivers of innovation in services industries* (pp. 95–101). Hershey, PA: IGI Global. doi:10.4018/978-1-4666-0948-8.ch009

Wheeler, S. J., & Wheeler, D. W. (2005). Medication errors in anaesthesia and critical care. *Anaesthesia*, *60*(3), 257–273. doi:10.1111/j.1365-2044.2004.04062.x PMID:15710011

White, A. A., Bell, S. K., Krauss, M. J., Garbutt, J., Dunagan, W. C., Fraser, V. J., & Gallagher, T. H. et al. (2011). How trainees would disclose medical errors: Educational implications for training programmes. *Medical Education*, *45*(4), 372–380. doi:10.1111/j.1365-2923.2010.03875.x PMID:21401685

Williams, B. W. (2006). The prevalence and special educational requirements of dyscompetent physicians. *The Journal of Continuing Education in the Health Professions*, *26*(3), 173–191. doi:10.1002/chp.68 PMID:16986149

Williams, D. (2012). Monitoring medicines use: The role of the clinical pharmacologist. *British Journal of Clinical Pharmacology*, *74*(4), 685–690. doi:10.1111/j.1365-2125.2012.04316.x PMID:22554404

Wong, B. M., Levinson, W., & Shojania, K. G. (2012). Quality improvement in medical education: Current state and future directions. *Medical Education*, *46*(1), 107–119. doi:10.1111/j.1365-2923.2011.04154.x PMID:22150202

Wong, R. S. Y., & Balasingam, U. (2013). Teaching medical law in medical education. *Journal of Academic Ethics*, *11*(2), 121–138. doi:10.1007/s10805-013-9184-9

Woodfield, G., O'Sullivan, M., Haddington, N., & Stanton, A. (2014). Using simulation for prescribing: An evaluation. *The Clinical Teacher*, *11*(1), 24–28. doi:10.1111/tct.12056 PMID:24405915

Zaheer, S. (2015). Implementation of evidence-based practice and the PARIHS framework. In *Healthcare administration: Concepts, methodologies, tools, and applications* (pp. 323–340). Hershey, PA: IGI Global. doi:10.4018/978-1-4666-6339-8.ch017

Zientek, D. M. (2010). Medical error, malpractice and complications: A moral geography. *HEC Forum*, *22*(2), 145–157. doi:10.1007/s10730-010-9130-9 PMID:20480208

ADDITIONAL READING

Al-Zahrani, W., & Sheikh, M. (2015). Detection of pre-analytical laboratory testing errors: Leads and lessons for patient safety. In M. Sheikh, A. Mahamoud, & M. Househ (Eds.), *Transforming public health in developing nations* (pp. 241–263). Hershey, PA: IGI Global. doi:10.4018/978-1-4666-8702-8.ch011

Buetow, S., Kiata, L., Liew, T., Kenealy, T., Dovey, S., & Elwyn, G. (2010). Approaches to reducing the most important patient errors in primary health-care: Patient and professional perspectives. *Health & Social Care in the Community*, *18*(3), 296–303. PMID:20141539

Caruba, T., Boussadi, A., Lenain, E., Korb-Savoldelli, V., Gillaizeau, F., Durieux, P., & Sabatier, B. (2015). A simulation study of the interception of prescribing errors by clinical pharmacists in an acute hospital setting. *Journal of Evaluation in Clinical Practice*, *21*(4), 673–680. doi:10.1111/jep.12363 PMID:25907983

Choo, J., Johnston, L., & Manias, E. (2014). Effectiveness of an electronic inpatient medication record in reducing medication errors in Singapore. *Nursing & Health Sciences*, *16*(2), 245–254. doi:10.1111/nhs.12078 PMID:23855683

Conte, D. (2013). Recognizing errors in medical literature. *Internal and Emergency Medicine*, *8*(2), 97–98. doi:10.1007/s11739-012-0887-5 PMID:23269531

Cottney, A., & Innes, J. (2015). Medication-administration errors in an urban mental health hospital: A direct observation study. *International Journal of Mental Health Nursing*, *24*(1), 65–74. doi:10.1111/inm.12096 PMID:25394525

Davis, R. E., Joshi, D., Patel, K., Briggs, M., & Vincent, C. A. (2013). The medical student as a patient: Attitudes towards involvement in the quality and safety of health care. *Journal of Evaluation in Clinical Practice*, *19*(5), 812–818. PMID:22620283

de Feijter, J. M., de Grave, W. S., Koopmans, R. P., & Scherpbier, A. J. J. A. (2013). Informal learning from error in hospitals: What do we learn, how do we learn and how can informal learning be enhanced? A narrative review. *Advances in Health Sciences Education: Theory and Practice*, *18*(4), 787–805. doi:10.1007/s10459-012-9400-1 PMID:22948951

Dumitrescu, A., & Ryan, C. A. (2014). Addressing the taboo of medical error through IGBOs: I got burnt once! *European Journal of Pediatrics*, *173*(4), 503–508. doi:10.1007/s00431-013-2168-3 PMID:24240665

Fyhr, A., & Akselsson, R. (2012). Characteristics of medication errors with parenteral cytotoxic drugs. *European Journal of Cancer Care*, *21*(5), 606–613. doi:10.1111/j.1365-2354.2012.01331.x PMID:22335508

Groszkruger, D. (2014). Diagnostic error: Untapped potential for improving patient safety? *Journal of Healthcare Risk Management*, *34*(1), 38–43. doi:10.1002/jhrm.21149 PMID:25070255

Huckels-Baumgart, S., & Manser, T. (2014). Identifying medication error chains from critical incident reports: A new analytic approach. *Journal of Clinical Pharmacology*, *54*(10), 1188–1197. doi:10.1002/jcph.319 PMID:24782100

Ison, M. G., Holl, J. L., & Ladner, D. (2012). Preventable errors in organ transplantation: An emerging patient safety issue? *American Journal of Transplantation*, *12*(9), 2307–2312. doi:10.1111/j.1600-6143.2012.04139.x PMID:22703471

Kalbfleisch, J. D., & Wolfe, R. A. (2013). On monitoring outcomes of medical providers. *Statistics in Biosciences*, *5*(2), 286–302. doi:10.1007/s12561-013-9093-x

Khalili, H., Farsaei, S., Rezaee, H., & Dashti-Khavidaki, S. (2011). Role of clinical pharmacists' interventions in detection and prevention of medication errors in a medical ward. *International Journal of Clinical Pharmacology, Therapy and Toxicology*, *33*(2), 281–284. PMID:21394569

Kooienga, S., & Stewart, V. T. (2011). Putting a face on medical errors: A patient perspective. *Journal for Healthcare Quality*, *33*(4), 37–41. doi:10.1111/j.1945-1474.2010.00121.x PMID:21733023

Lawton, R., Carruthers, S., Gardner, P., Wright, J., & McEachan, R. R. C. (2012). Identifying the latent failures underpinning medication administration errors: An exploratory study. *Health Services Research*, *47*(4), 1437–1459. doi:10.1111/j.1475-6773.2012.01390.x PMID:22375850

Leroy, P. (2011). Medical errors: The importance of the bullet's blunt end. *European Journal of Pediatrics*, *170*(2), 251–252. doi:10.1007/s00431-010-1283-7 PMID:20809247

Manias, E., Kinney, S., Cranswick, N., & Williams, A. (2014). Medication errors in hospitalised children. *Journal of Paediatrics and Child Health*, *50*(1), 71–77. doi:10.1111/jpc.12412 PMID:24397451

Menon, S., Singh, H., Meyer, A. N. D., Belmont, E., & Sittig, D. F. (2014). Electronic health record–related safety concerns: A cross-sectional survey. *Journal of Healthcare Risk Management*, *34*(1), 14–26. doi:10.1002/jhrm.21146 PMID:25070253

Palmieri, P. A., Peterson, L. T., & Noeding, M. N. (2015). Health information technology: Anticipating, recognizing, and preventing disruptions in complex adaptive healthcare systems. In *Healthcare administration: Concepts, methodologies, tools, and applications* (pp. 1–22). Hershey, PA: IGI Global. doi:10.4018/978-1-4666-6339-8.ch001

Seidling, H. M., Lampert, A., Lohmann, K., Schiele, J. T., Send, A. J. F., Witticke, D., & Haefeli, W. E. (2013). Safeguarding the process of drug administration with an emphasis on electronic support tools. *British Journal of Clinical Pharmacology*, *76*(Suppl. 1), 25–36. doi:10.1111/bcp.12191 PMID:24007450

Siklósi, B., Novák, A., & Prószéky, G. (2016). Context-aware correction of spelling errors in Hungarian medical documents. *Computer Speech & Language*, *35*, 219–233. doi:10.1016/j.csl.2014.09.001

Tallentire, V. R., & Smith, S. E. (2012). Medical error: Time to get real? *Medical Education*, *46*(7), 632–634. doi:10.1111/j.1365-2923.2012.04292.x PMID:22691143

Thomas, L., Cordonnier-Jourdin, C., Benhamou-Jantelet, G., Diviné, C., & Le Louët, H. (2011). Medication errors management process in hospital: A 6-month pilot study. *Fundamental & Clinical Pharmacology*, *25*(6), 768–775. doi:10.1111/j.1472-8206.2010.00907.x PMID:21210845

Varjavand, N., Nair, S., & Gracely, E. (2012). A call to address the curricular provision of emotional support in the event of medical errors and adverse events. *Medical Education*, *46*(12), 1149–1151. doi:10.1111/medu.12074 PMID:23171256

Zhang, Q., Li, Y., Li, J., Mao, X., Zhang, L., Ying, Q., & Zhang, M. et al. (2012). Patients for patient safety in China: A cross sectional study. *Journal of Evidence-Based Medicine*, *5*(1), 6–11. doi:10.1111/j.1756-5391.2012.01164.x PMID:23528115

KEY TERMS AND DEFINITIONS

Health Care: The act of taking preventative or necessary medical procedures to improve a person's well-being.

Information: The data that is specific and organized for a purpose.

Information Technology: The set of tools, processes, and equipment employed to collect, process, and present the information.

Medication: The set of drugs, used to improve a particular condition or illness.

Medicine: A substance, especially in the form of a liquid or a pill, that is a treatment for illness or injury.

Patient: A person who is receiving medical care.

Physician: A medical doctor, especially one who has the health care skill.

Prescription: A piece of paper on which a physician writes the details of drugs that patient requires.

This work was previously published in Impact of Medical Errors and Malpractice on Health Economics, Quality, and Patient Safety edited by Marina Riga, pages 113-143, copyright year 2017 by Medical Information Science Reference (an imprint of IGI Global).

Chapter 13
Waiting for Health Care Services

Stefan Janzek-Hawlat
Vienna University of Technology, Austria

Hilda Tellioğlu
Vienna University of Technology, Austria

ABSTRACT

Waiting for health care services have impact on people from several perspectives. First of all, seen from patients' point of view, due to psychologically and physically burden short waiting times are an indication of quality. Second, seen from health care systems' point of view, short waiting times can be a competitive advantage for health care providers. Finally, short-waiting times can contribute to a more effective system applied in health care. In this chapter, the impact of waiting times of patients are analyzed on all three levels based on quantitative and qualitative study carried out by the authors as well as on the foregoing literature review. The situation of patients and their requirements are shown, strategies to reduce waiting times are presented by also considering the role of information and communication technologies, and several relevant questions raised are answered.

INTRODUCTION

A new kind of patient has entered the healthcare sector (Carpman, Grant, & Simmons, 1986; Marberry, 2006; Marsh, 1993), an active one who wants to participate directly in healthcare decisions and is therefore increasingly responsible for his or her own health (Wallner, 2013). At the same time, this new patient demands service quality and person-centred care that causes a paradigm shift in the understanding of healthcare and in the definition and perception of services provided for it. One of the impacts is to move the focus of healthcare in many western societies from a paternalistic approach to a shared decision making process, in which the needs of the patient are central (Emanuel & Emanuel, 1992; Gillon, 1994). In such a setting patient-participation and informed consent are fundamental rights (Kizer, 2001). Another impact is creating a more patient-friendly environment in hospitals and at resident physicians (Mangold, Peintinger, & Kopetzki, 2010).

DOI: 10.4018/978-1-5225-1928-7.ch013

Increasing requirements to service quality and focusing on person-centred services have also impact on the healthcare sector as any other business sector. In healthcare patients – in this context they are the consumers – demand the right to safety, to information, to choose among alternatives, and the right to be heard (Kennedy, 1962). However, healthcare is different than the other business areas; it is a highly complex field. It is not always easy for consumers to contract or consent, sometimes because of their current health condition (e.g., in case of mentally ill patients or patients in a coma), sometimes because of the complexity of the medical situation and related diagnosis or treatment procedures.

Nevertheless, patients' autonomy has become more important in the last few decades. The US-Institute of Medicine, for example, states patient-centeredness as one of the six aims for increasing general healthcare quality provided (Adams, Greiner, & Corrigan, 2004). The World Health Organization World Alliance for Patient Safety (2005) highlights the determinant of including patients and their family into the healthcare decisions (Pittet, Allegranzi, Storr, & Donaldson, 2005). Increasing patient participation in processes and health-related decision-making as well as the changing role of patients to consumers can improve the quality of care and through this the healthcare system in general (Longtin et al., 2010; Lancet, 2005). In the "Vienna Recommendations on Health Promoting Hospitals" from 1997, the WHO, sub-organisations, and their member states announced official documents that confirmed the same statement and furthermore claimed that it would also improve the efficiency of healthcare systems (World Health Organization [WHO], 1997; Committee on Patient Safety and Quality Improvement, 2005; General Medical Council [GMC], 2013; Nursing & Midwifery Council [NMC], 2015; Brink-Muinen et al., 2006). About 15 years after "Vienna Recommendations", the Austrian government has included "patient empowerment" in the on-going healthcare reform (Grazie & Wimmer-Puchinger, 2014). One of its ten targets is to increase health literacy by improving the involvement of the citizens in their own health issues.

Due to the demographic changes in Europe, the frequency of the use of healthcare services increases (Statistik Austria, 2015a, 2015b). Putting the needs of patients in the centre, Austria shows good numbers in the quality and quantity of healthcare services provided. On the one hand, 7.7 hospital beds and 4.75 doctors per 1,000 inhabitants as well as a life expectancy of 80 years paint a favourable picture of a high quality healthcare system in Austria[1] (Mundi Index, 2012). Looking at the number of healthy life years (60 years)[2] and the health expenditure of 10.8% of the GDP (Gross Domestic Product)[3], the Austrian healthcare system is in the midfield of the European Union (WHO, 2015). But, there is further place for improvement. Several surveys show the most potential for improvement lies in the waiting times in hospitals and at resident doctors: The main problem is still the waiting for meeting a physician and a "two-tier healthcare system"[4]. The question is how to reduce the waiting times, how to focus on health instead of illness, and how to strengthen the patient-centred approach (Deloitte, 2011).

So far, waiting for healthcare services have got only little public attention in Austria. There is almost no data available. A questionnaire published in 2009 showed that the average waiting time at general practitioners (GP) is 34 minutes and at specialists 28 minutes (Fischer, 2009). The question whether electronic appointment systems lower waiting times of patients was not studied. This chapter aims to evaluate and analyse waiting process and waiting environment on an organisational and structural level, and tries to find solutions to decrease waiting times as they have negative impact on citizens (Bailey, 1952), support infections (Eck, DeBaun, & Pugliese, 2001), and are a financial burden for patients, clinics, and the Austrian healthcare and economy system in general (Fleischer, 2011).

In this chapter, findings of a study done at the Vienna University of Technology are presented (Janzek-Hawlat, 2015). Besides showing the reasons and the duration of waiting times, the main part focuses on the study of ICT based tools, which are able to reduce waiting times by increasing patient engagement and participation. This paper aims to answer the following research questions:

- What are the reasons for waiting in outpatient clinics and at hospitals?
- How long is the average waiting time for patients at general practitioners and at hospital ambulances?
- How are waiting times perceived by patients?
- Are there any convincible improvements to decrease the burden of waiting and make waiting more comfortable for patients?
- Are there differences in waiting times at healthcare institutions with and without electronic appointment systems?
- How can ICT based solutions help decrease waiting times by increasing patient participation?

Waiting for healthcare services has effects on different levels. First of all, from the patients' point of view (Bailey, 1952; Eck et al., 2001), short waiting times are an indication of quality and are able to reduce the psychologically and physically burden which likely occur due long waiting times (Arneill & Devlin, 2002). Second, seen from a healthcare system's point of view, short waiting times can be a competitive advantage for healthcare providers. Finally, short-waiting times can contribute to a more effective and efficient system applied in healthcare (Fleisher, 2013). To sum up, in this chapter the impact of waiting for healthcare services is analysed on all these three levels based on our quantitative and qualitative study and the literature review. The situation of the patients and their requirements are shown, strategies to reduce waiting times are presented, and the questions listed above are answered and discussed.

The next section summarises the relevant state of the art literature related to waiting for healthcare services. After introducing the methodology applied for this research work, results are presented, structured in four areas: the origin of waiting, waiting times per se, perception of waiting, solutions for reducing waiting times. The chapter is finalised with a conclusion including future work.

WAITING IN HEALTH CARE

In the healthcare sector, there are in general two kinds of waiting. First, patients wait in waiting rooms of doctors' offices or hospital ambulances to meet the physician. Second, there is waiting for appointments, diagnostic procedures like MRT, surgeries, or transplantation of organs. Both issues are important and currently important topics of public discussions (Laschet, 2014; Staeck, 2014; Lammers, 2014), but only the first will be the subject of interest in this chapter.

Long waiting and queues in healthcare services are associated with several negative impacts. First, waiting is usually associated with being non-productive. Second, due to the unpredictability of waiting times, waiting often delays one's follow-up activities, which might be business or spare-time related. Third, waiting cause stress, frustration, and anger to the people waiting (Wijayasinghe, 2013). Furthermore, while waiting in waiting rooms of healthcare facilities patients might be infected by others also waiting in the same area (Eck et al., 2001). This leads to the paradox situation that long waiting can decrease the patients' health condition.

When patients wait for healthcare services they decrease the idle time of physicians. Professionals' time has been found 37.5 times more valuable than patients' time (Bailey, 1952). A peculiarity of waiting for healthcare is that the patient can change the service provider only under considerable expense. The patient has in general no access to information about waiting times in other healthcare providing institutions. Especially in hospitals and clinics, it can be psychologically difficult to change the physician, once a patient is already in treatment. Even the change of a family doctor is associated with effort because, for instance, the new GP might not have access to necessary previous healthcare data.

There are several studies on waiting for healthcare services. Norman and Bailey took a closer look on waiting times and appointment systems at outpatient clinics based on data from the Nuffield Provincial Hospital (Bailey, 1952). Due to the use of mathematical models, they examined a series of 50 hypothetical clinics, each with 25 patients. They found out that the best appointment interval is between 5 and 5.5 minutes as the average waiting time and the consultant's time wasted is about 7 to 8 minutes. However, they also showed that the increase of patient's waiting time clearly decreases the consultant's average wasted time. For instance, when patients wait about 17 minutes, the consultant's wasted idle time is reduced between 1 to 2 minutes. Furthermore, they showed that the waiting times of patients have a positive skew. Within the mentioned study 30% of the patients were waiting up to 5 minutes, 25% between 5 and 10 minutes, 15% between 10 and 15 minutes, 12% had no waiting times, and the rest more than 15 minutes. They concluded that a suitable appointment system decreases waiting times without increasing the idle time of physicians. The best situation is when appointments at regular intervals are equal to the average consultation time, and the arrival of the physician is at the same time as the second patient. Miceli and Wolosin (2004) found out that longer waiting times correlate negatively with satisfaction with healthcare services. But they also showed that good communication and a strong relationship between the healthcare provider and the patient is able to reduce those negative effects. So, transparency and being aware of waiting times including their origin are important for patients' satisfaction. Becker and Douglass categorise the waiting process in an ambulatory waiting room into three steps (Becker & Douglass, 2008): 1) time for pre-process which is the arrival time of the patient till the patient is taken into the exam room; 2) time for in-process that is the time between entering and leaving the exam room; and 3) time for post-process that is the remaining time from leaving the exam room till exiting the building. In this chapter slightly different categories are used: 1) waiting for the administrative work at the administrative desk; 2) waiting in waiting area; and 3) time for in-process.

There has only been little research about the correlation of real waiting times, perceived waiting times, and attractiveness of the waiting area. De Man et al. (2005) showed that the perceived waiting time correlates with the perception of the quality of service in nuclear medicine. The perceived waiting time was higher than the actual waiting time. The time inside the exam room was found too short. If patients are given information about the reasons for their waiting the difference between perceived and actual waiting time decreases. Arneill and Devlin (2002) confirmed de Man's results and they detected a relationship between the quality of care, perceived waiting times, anxiety, staff-patient interaction, and attractiveness of the physical setting for patients in an out-patient facility. Based on a study in emergency care departments (Becker & Douglass, 2008) patients tend to overestimate shorter waiting times and underestimate longer waiting times. 23% of the patients thought that they waited 0-5 minutes. In fact, only 15% of them waited 0-5 minutes. 11% of the patients thought they waited over 30 minutes. Actually, 25% of them waited over 30 minutes. Furthermore, they found out that in more attractive environments patients experienced a larger difference between actual and perceived times.

Taylor states two kinds of psychological and physiological responses to waiting can be observed: 1) uncertainty including annoyance, irritability, stress; and 2) anger (Taylor, 1994). Entertainment programs such as providing TV or magazines, outdoor views, refreshments as well as giving patients a choice what they can do while waiting could dramatically reduce those negative implications (Haggard & Hosking, 2003).

Becker and Douglass (2008) found a strong significant correlation between the level of anxiety and the attractiveness of a clinic. A well-designed environment is able to reduce stress and psychological harm of waiting patients. Arneill and Devlin (2002) emphasised how the design of outpatient waiting rooms influences the perception of the quality of healthcare services. More comfortable designed waiting areas are associated with greater perception of provided healthcare (Devlin, 2008; Marberry, 2006). Furthermore, healthcare staff can also perform better after small design changes of their work environment (Becker & Poe, 1980). So, there is a relation between the design of the environment, performance and attitude of healthcare staff, and patients' satisfaction with the healthcare services. This paper takes up this issue and asks the patients how the environment could be changed to make the waiting more comfortable. However, this question includes only comparable small changes like a water dispenser or more magazines. It does not include general redesigns of buildings, as this would often be impossible.

The result of more than 7,000 questionnaires filled in by German physicians to study the adherence to schedules of patients (Hartmannbund, 2014) was that in 1 in 10 appointments at GPs and in 1 in 7 appointments at specialist patients did not show up at all.

This chapter takes up those points within a questionnaire by asking the waiting patients how the waiting process in a certain institution is perceived (possible answers are "long", "ok", and "short"), and how one feels while waiting (possible answers are "comfortable", "neutral", and "uncomfortable"). This distinction enables to search for a correlation between those two factors. We study waiting times of an emergency hospital ambulance for follow-up examination and treatment. The focus lies on the waiting inside the waiting room and the administrative desk. We chose a hospital for our study because hospitals are places where the healthcare chain can be followed. It is the "the chain of operations that need to be performed to produce a particular health service" (Vissers & Beech, 2005). Defining such an effective healthcare chain enables the creation of strategic management tools to allocate resources to increase operational effectiveness and linking organisational objectives with operational processes to increase patients' satisfaction (Armistead, 1999).

METHODOLOGY

There are two research traditions, which differ in regard to the approach, data, aim, and usage (Erzberger, 1998). The objective tradition (1) on the one hand aims to verify correlations. Following a positivistic, quantitative, and rational approach, it tries to check hypothesis for explorative empirical science. The subjective tradition (2) on the other hand aims to find new correlations. It follows an interpretative and qualitative approach using qualitative data to generate hypothesis. Both research traditions have their place in the scientific community and also in the research presented in this chapter.

Figure 1 points out that we used mixed method research approach in our study. On the one hand, each step depends on one or more previous steps (Przyborski & Wohlrab-Sahr, 2010; Gläser & Laudel, 2009; Mayring, 2002; Girtler, 2001). On the other, we combined quantitative data with qualitative to

Figure 1. Mixed method research approach shows the process flow with activities and results of our methodology

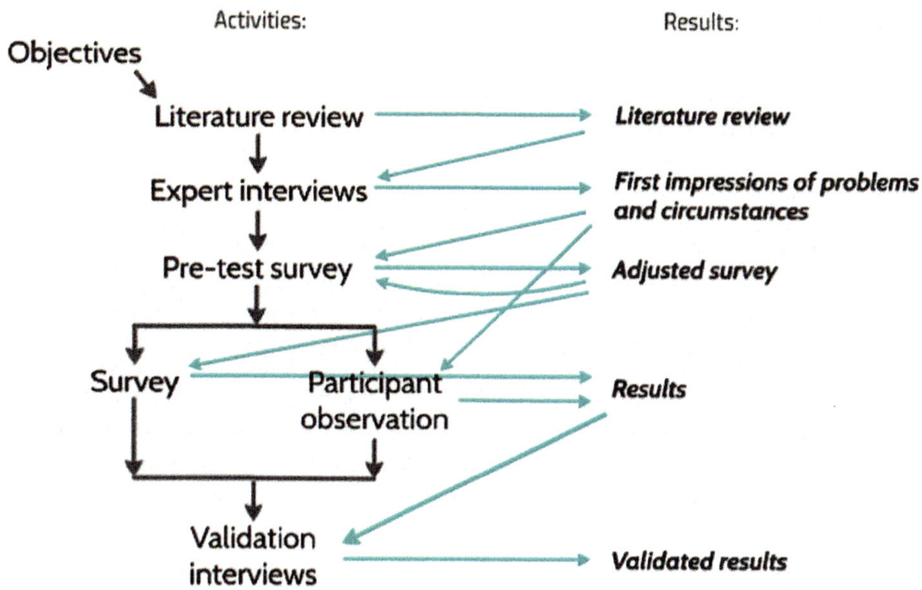

first setup the quantitative data inquiry parameters and then to explain the quantitative data gathered by putting it into context.

Within the first step of our methodology, the objectives were defined. Then the literature was used firstly to get an insight into the study area and secondly to define a proper methodology. Based on the results from the literature review, semi-structured, guideline-based, problem-centred expert interviews (Strauss, 1998) were conducted to get detailed insight and knowledge concerning the topic of waiting at the chosen physicians and the hospital ambulances. Based on the expert interviews, the questionnaire for the patients was designed. Before handing out, it was pre-tested several times till the questions were comprehensible and understandable. After the pre-tests, the questionnaire was handed out to the patients at the waiting rooms of a hospital ambulance and several GP offices. Parallel to and shortly after the survey phase, participant observation took place to examine the processes, which lead to waiting times, the environment of the waiting areas, and how the patients acted during the waiting time. Finally, the results were discussed with and validated through a subset of the resident physicians included in the study. The data was presented and physicians were given the opportunity to comment and reflect. The method was again a semi-structured, guideline-based, problem-centred expert interview.

We captured the quantitative data at two different kinds of environments (Janzek-Hawlat, 2015): at 4 GPs offices and at a hospital ambulance. In a first expert interview with the GPs the study was introduced and explained, the procedure was clarified, and the questions were asked. The semi-structured open interview was recorded, a participant observation was scheduled and questionnaires at the GP's waiting room were set up. In total there were 63 questionnaires filled in at GPs' offices. The head of the occupational medicine at the hospital was the expert interviewed. We spent a whole day for observation at the hospital's ambulance for follow-up care. This particular ambulance was chosen because the patients were normally not severely injured, had usually time and the ability to fill out the questionnaire that was given. In sum, there were 60 questionnaires filled in at the hospital.

In the following section, we present our empirical material and our findings. First, we show some relevant quantitative data. Second, we put the empirical data into context by using the evidence from the qualitative inquiry and discussing it. We derive results and discussion points based on our study.

SOME FIGURES FROM OUR STUDY

Our study showed that the majority of the patients at the hospital ambulance had an appointment between 9 a.m. and 9:29 a.m. *Figure 2* shows the distribution of appointments made in our study. This example also shows that the scheduling process (with or without an appointment system) must be truly integrated in the workflow of a healthcare provider. Otherwise it causes additional waiting time for its patients.

There is no significant difference between waiting times at the administrative desk at the hospital ambulance and at resident physicians. While the majority of the patients were waiting less than six minutes in all these environments, some patients wait more than 11 minutes. In all the observed offices there was only one person working at the administrative desk. Questions like extension of long-term medications or the writing of sick notes might increase the waiting time at administrative desks. Some patients suggested providing an additional desk for administrative services. On the other hand, physicians in our study said that they couldn't afford to employ additional administrative persons. They calculate these additional costs in terms of patients: "Another employee is not affordable. One hour *(of an administration staff)* costs around 10-20 patients. Hiring another employee would make it necessary to have more patients, what decreases the time I have for each patient."

Patients at the hospital ambulance for follow-up care normally get an appointment calculated by the computer. The computer system is supposed to assign an appointment every 15 minutes. This allocation is not displayed in the system. Patients' appointments were at 8:00 (5 times out of 47 surveys), 9:00 (12 times out of 47 surveys) or 10:00 (6 times out of 47 surveys). Some patients even got an appointment at 9:20, which would be impossible according to the computer system. So either the right appointment time does not reach the patient due to false communication or the system is flawed. 60% of patients at the hospital ambulance for follow-up care waited between 60 and 120 minutes (see *Figure 3*). 8% were waiting less than 30 minutes, 20% waited more than 120 minutes. The median was 90 minutes.

The median waiting time at resident physicians with an electronic appointment system was 17 minutes, at physicians without any electronic appointment system 64 minutes. Waiting times at physicians using appointment systems are clearly lower than at physicians not using one. However, both numbers

Figure 2. Distribution of the appointments at the hospital ambulance within our study

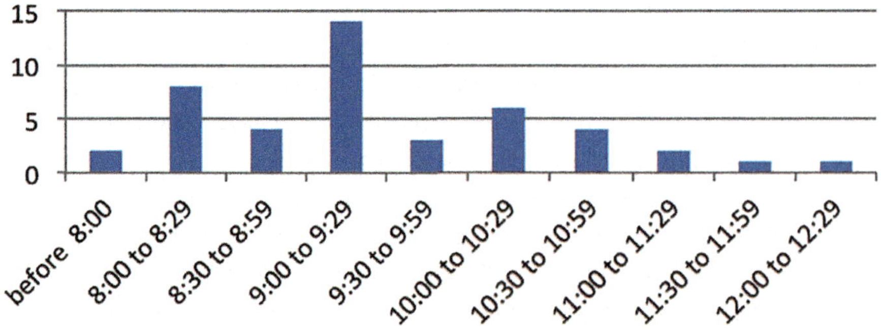

Figure 3. Distribution of the waiting times at the hospital ambulance studied

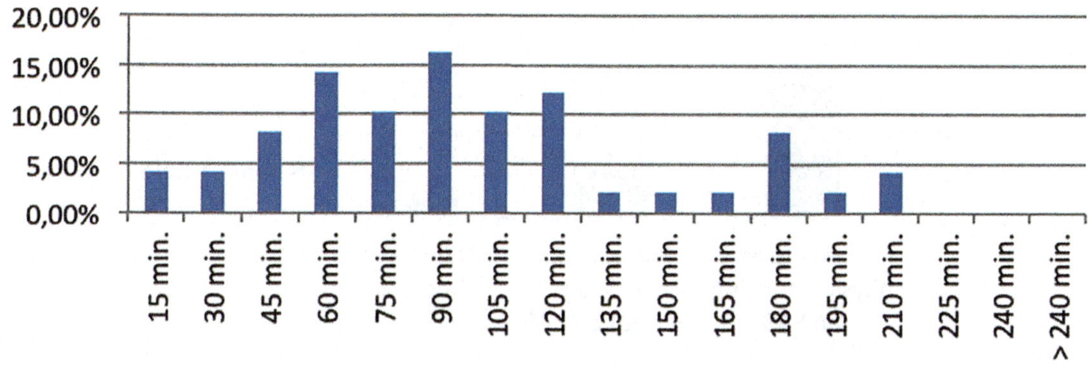

are clearly lower than waiting times at the hospital. *Figure 4* shows the distribution of waiting times for hospital ambulance patients and patients at resident physicians studied.

Within the study the question asked to the patients was: "How do you perceive the waiting time?" The results show a clear tendency (see *Figure 5*). The shorter the waiting time, the more comfortable the patients feel, which is obvious. While 66.7% of the patients at the physicians using an electronic appointment system (EAS) feel comfortable, only 25% of the patients at physicians without an EAS and 10.2% of the patients at the hospital feel comfortable in their waiting environment.

DISCUSSION

This section contains results and findings from the analysis of the collected qualitative and quantitative data supplemented by key results from the related work. Before presenting patient participation tools which target the reduction of waiting times, the issue of waiting will be described and discussed from different point of views including the reasons for waiting times and their average length. The section is structured by the questions asked in the introduction of the chapter.

Figure 4. Distribution of waiting times for hospital ambulance patients and patients at resident physicians studied

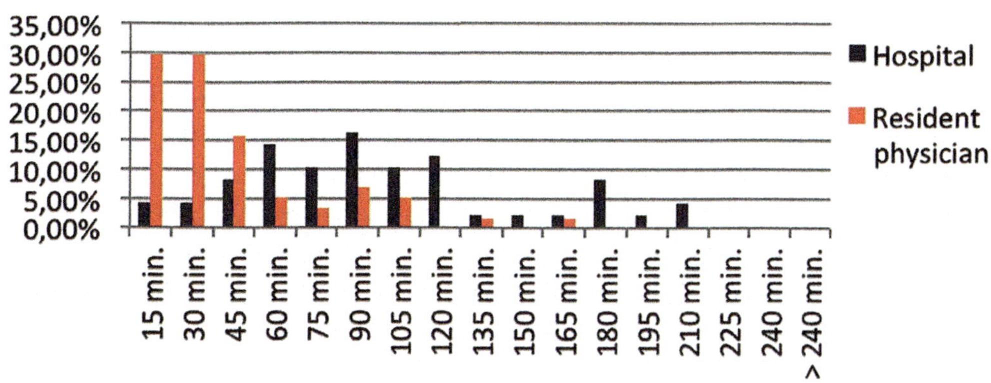

Figure 5. Perception of the waiting time by patients in the study (EAS=Electronic Appointment System)

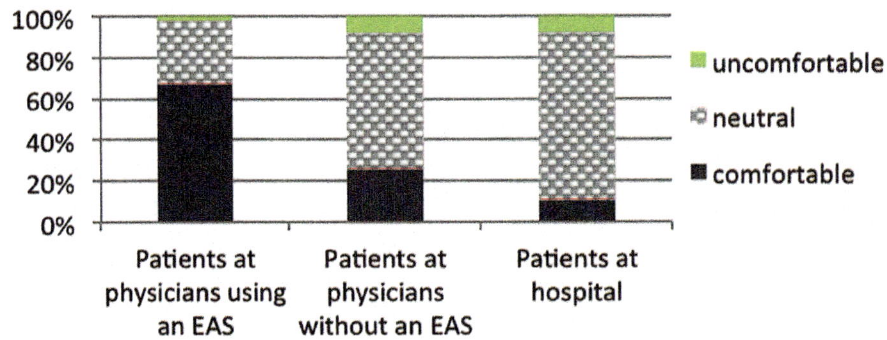

The Origin for Waiting in Health Care

One approach to detect the causes of waiting in healthcare is process-oriented modelling of the healthcare flows. Modelling the physician-patient-interaction as well as the business processes of the doctor's office and the hospital ambulance makes possible to identify waiting situations. In this research the processes are not modelled because of the complexity of generalising for different healthcare providers: Some physicians claim that "there is no medical process" and that it is "difficult to standardise a medical process". The process starting from the first contact with the patients and ending with their diagnoses and treatment are found very inhomogeneous especially if the office organisation of a GP or specialist is considered. A process from one medical institution cannot be compared to the process of another one. Designing such a process would lead to an either very complex or inaccurate outcome. Also the research literature confirms that a standardisation of medical processes is hard to achieve. A study concludes that the incalculable medical everyday life, e.g., that a call from another institution concerning a patient during the office hours can lead to longer waiting times (Wijayasinghe, 2013), or an emergency patient arrives and the whole waiting list must be rearranged (Chan, 2013).

Patients normally call before visiting the physicians' office. During these calls patients are asked to state the medical issues, so a certain suitable time slot can be reserved for them. That is not always doable with all patients. Some patients might be able to express themselves others might not. This kind of problems is related to health literacy. Health literacy is a function of the interaction between individuals in health context, which they are opposed to. This applies to the patient, physician but also to the administrative personnel such as the receptionists or nurses. A lack of health literacy concerns especially the lower social classes (Nielsen-Bohlman, Panzer, & Kindig, 2004). However, the improvement of scheduling systems is one of the main claims of the patients studied.

One cannot imagine running a healthcare institution without using an electronic appointment system. However, there are some shortcomings in the application of such systems: If a system is not flexible enough to vary the duration of the time slot reserved for a patient later on and this patient does not appear at the right time, gaps in the schedule occur. If the next patient is not available, the time until s/he arrives is wasted time. A survey from the Hartmannbund (2014) in Germany states that one in seven patients misses an appointment at resident specialist and one in ten patients misses an appointment at GPs. The problem becomes bigger if a patient comes later than the appointment. This causes even longer waiting times (Hartmannbund, 2014). At the hospital of this study, the majority of patients (45 out of 60) had an appointment and 24.4% of them came late (11 out of 45). These numbers show that coming late to an appointment is quite often the case. For that reason and to prevent idle time, physicians overbook their appointment schedule as they expect – based on their own experiences – a certain amount of patients to come late or not to show up. So, they might reserve shorter time slots for the patients, so that the gap is not that big or that the next patient is already waiting and can be treated first, if another patient comes late. Norman and Bailey showed that long waiting times decrease the consultants' average time wasted (Bailey, 1952). Such systems fail when more patients come on schedule than estimated. This could then lead to the situation that the schedule falls apart and patients have to wait although having an appointment. Consequently, patients feel that appointments are not working well and start disregarding them.

Waiting Time Per Se

Waiting times captured in this study are comparable to the results from other studies (Dansky & Miles, 1997; Becker & Douglass, 2008). Within their survey in an emergency care department, Dansky and Miles (1997) found out that patients waited on average 55 minutes in the waiting area before entering the exam room. Becker and Douglass (2008) included different kinds of waiting times into their study such as total time in clinic, time spent with doctor, and time spent in the examination room. The average total time in the clinic was 63 minutes, the total waiting time was 48 minutes, and the time spent with a physician was 13 minutes.

Only one third of the participants of our survey perceived the waiting time at the hospital ambulance as "long". Almost two thirds thought the waiting time was "ok". This perception of waiting times is similar to the perception of waiting times at the GPs without an electronic appointment system. However, the waiting at the hospital triggered most often "neutral" (more than 80%) sensations. This indicates that people are used to long waiting times at hospitals and that is why they are neutral to their occurrence.

To overcome the physical and psychological burden of waiting (Taylor, 1994), hospitals often offer some kind of entertainment program such as TV or magazines in the waiting area. However, two fundamental issues are not provided to the patient: First, information about the waiting time or their position in the waiting line. Second, giving people the opportunity to leave the waiting room for some time, as they have to wait in front of the exam rooms so they do not miss their call (Haggard & Hosking, 2003). More than 60% of the patients of the hospital (37 out of 60) would have liked to know how much longer they had to wait. Forwarding this information to the patients would boost the perceived involvement of the patient into the administrative processes. It would not only enable a better understanding for long waiting times, but also dissolve the stress and tension of patients, as they are not able to estimate the time till they can see a doctor.

To increase the attractiveness and consequently decrease the anxiety of patients (Becker & Douglass, 2008) the following improvements were suggested by the patients: They would like to have more magazines and medical journals to read and to have more space in the waiting area. But the most important thing for them was to know how long they have to wait. To comply with this request, it would be necessary to show the waiting queue on the available screens in the waiting area. Then patients would know the approximate waiting time. This would reduce stress and tenseness of patients drastically as they could, e.g., go to the restrooms without having the feeling that they might miss their call.

It is interesting to see that physicians without electronic appointment systems (EAS) estimate the time that patients wait for them quite well, while physicians with an EAS overestimate this time. 50% of the patients of physicians without an EAS state that the duration of the waiting was "ok", but 41.7% considered they were waiting too "long". In contrast, 51.4% of the patients of physicians with an EAS regarded the time they waited for the physician as "ok" and 48.6% said that they waited a "short" time. The majority of patients at physicians without an EAS felt "neutral" concerning waiting. This result is similar to the hospital results, where most of the patients had also a "neutral" feeling towards waiting. Again, the results differ from the results of physicians with an EAS. There, two thirds of the patients considered waiting as "comfortable".

Improvements required by patients for waiting areas at the resident physicians are similar to the improvements required in the hospital setting. Here patients would like to have more magazines and more medical journals as well. They also would like to have a drink dispenser. It is interesting to see that some patients request more space than others. The need to know how much longer they have to wait is not as high as in the hospital, but was addressed by some patients explicitly. Due to a smaller and more individual system at the resident physicians compared to the hospital, it is not easy to display and explain the queue mechanisms. However, small improvements like a drink dispenser or magazines are acceptable for the resident physicians. The validation interviews showed that physicians are under certain conditions willing to apply the suggested improvements, e.g., provide water or more magazines. On the contrary, costly improvements such as drink dispenser or displaying waiting times are not accepted due to financial reasons.

Perception of Waiting

The impact of waiting on patients and physicians is completely different. Patients are affected directly as they lose the waiting time immediately. Physicians are affected in a different way. First of all, they feel the pressure of patients waiting and therefore they may reduce the treatment time per single patient. Furthermore, they face the anger and impatience once the long waiting patient is treated (Becker & Douglass, 2008). Second, the longer the waiting queue, the larger the waiting room has to be. Third, the probably biggest effect for physicians is that they have a bad reputation on online platforms about rating physicians and their services.

Our study showed that the median waiting time at resident physicians using an EAS has been lower than any other. Patients at physicians with an EAS perceive waiting times as shorter and more pleasant. Long waiting times in combination with an EAS increase patients' dissatisfaction drastically. Patients at the hospital ambulance in this study had to wait much longer and felt much less comfortable in the provided waiting environment.

Solutions for Reducing Waiting Times

The question regarding Electronic Appointment Systems (EASs) was to find out whether they have positive or negative impact on waiting times. Resident physicians have two ways of organising their office: to use an EAS, reserve time slots, and process patients within the reserved time; or to call one patient after the other and give them as much time as they need. The results of our study show that waiting times are lower at physicians with an EAS. The average waiting time is between 10 and 20 minutes at physicians with an EAS and 23.5 and 77.5 minutes at physicians without an EAS.

Our findings show that there are some problems for administrative staff if a physician introduces an EAS to the office. This occurs because the work type and workload of administrative staff changes through the EAS. A lot of administrative work is shifted from the physician to the administrative personnel when using an EAS.

The survey included several questions concerning the general acceptance of the tools suggested in the literature. Besides the implementation of ICT based tools, the possibility of changes within the intra-institutional processes, which are developed in cooperation with physicians and administrative personnel, are evaluated.

A topic, which has been of much debate lately in literature but also in the public, is the emergence of online doctors. Within such a setting, a patient sits at home in front of the computer connected to the doctor via camera and microphone. On the one hand, this tool enables the patient to wait at home in a familiar surrounding which makes the waiting time much more comfortable. On the other hand, it gives the physicians independence from space. Online medical consulting provides patients the possibility to choose time and place of the consultation. Patients are able to communicate with their physicians from home or from another convenient place. This topic has been of much debate in the literature lately because there have already been several providers, which offer online consultations.

The acceptance of online doctors within our study is miscellaneous. About two thirds of the waiting patients participating in the survey at one resident physician's office can imagine visiting their doctor online. The majority of the patients at the other resident physician's office cannot imagine visiting their doctor online. To find out the reasons for this, further studies are necessary. Patients at the hospital, who had to wait much longer than patients at resident physicians, were torn. 47.4% can imagine visiting their doctor online, 52.6% cannot. Those results correspond to the results from a study in Germany, where up to 44% of patients can imagine visiting a doctor online (Techniker Krankenkasse [TK], 2014). It is interesting to see that the higher the education level of patients, the more they are willing to see their physician online.

Remarkably, the question of visiting an online doctor is not related to waiting. People who are waiting longer do not tend to visit doctors online. It is rather depending on the way the physician works and maybe also depending on demographic factors like age or being a digital native or not. The results clearly show the importance of the Internet in the healthcare sector and correspond with the results from a study by Google (2012), which says that the Internet (meaning mainly the hospitals' websites) is the most frequented resource prior to a healthcare consumption. The fact that more than 60% of the patients visit two or more hospital websites before visiting a healthcare institution shows how important the online presence of healthcare institutions is.

Another idea for reducing waiting time by using ICT solutions is publishing waiting times online to enable patients to choose either when to visit a certain healthcare facility or to choose one out of several reachable healthcare facilities (Chan, 2013). There have been several attempts to publish waiting times online in different countries. Several hospital departments use the platform *twitter* and other social media platforms to publish waiting times. *Figure 6* shows on the left side an example of the Progress West Hospital in St. Louis Missouri (USA), which tweets the waiting times of the emergency department. Public hospitals in Vancouver (Canada) chose another way. They founded a platform where the waiting times from all emergency departments are published centrally, shown on the right side of *Figure 6*. Based on this information, patients have the possibility to choose where to go. It is then their choice.

Publishing waiting times online has two positive effects (Dansky & Miles, 1997; Miceli & Wolosin, 2004; De Man et al., 2005): First, by giving patient information about internal processes and the reasons how long they will wait, which increases acceptance of waiting times. Second, publishing waiting times online has the power to equalise the distribution of patients and healthcare facilities over time and place. The willingness of the patients to look at published waiting times has also been one of the subjects of the questionnaire in our study. The majority of the patients (79,3% of the patients at the hospital, 58,7%

Figure 6. Online published waiting times of the Progress West Emergency Department in Missouri, USA [accessed 10.11.2014] (left); Canadian online platform showing waiting times online [accessed 06.07.2015 17:32] (right).

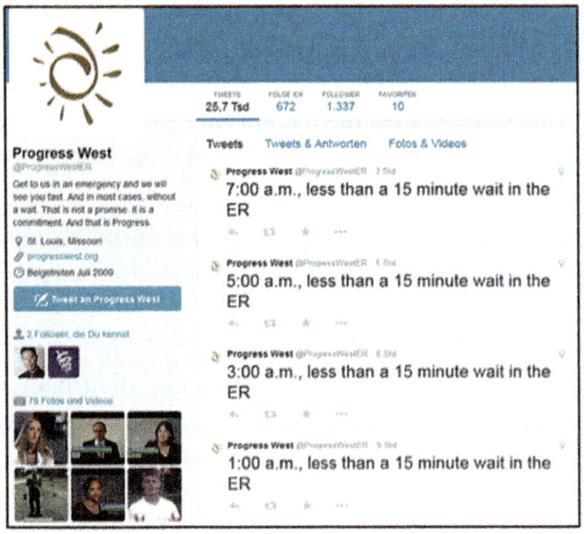
25,7 Tsd
672
1.337
10
Progress West
Tweets
Tweets & Antworten
Fotos & Videos
7:00 a.m., less than a 15 minute wait in the ER
5:00 a.m., less than a 15 minute wait in the ER
3:00 a.m., less than a 15 minute wait in the ER
1:00 a.m., less than a 15 minute wait in the ER

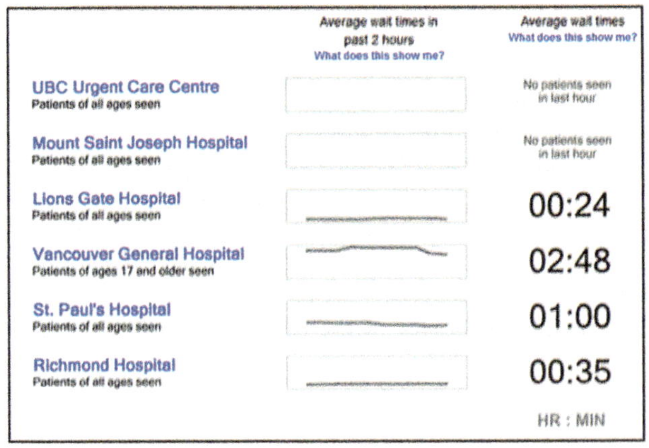

of the patients at resident physicians) who took part in the study are in favour of seeing waiting times online. Furthermore, 83% of the patients at hospitals and 73,8% of the patients at resident physicians, who would like to see waiting times online, would also plan their visit according to this information.

CONCLUSION

The question of whether patients want to participate in healthcare processes at all is an ambiguous one. Several studies have been done on this question and the results are diverse (Guadagnoli & Ward, 1998; Levinson, Kao, Kuby, & Thisted, 2005; Strull, Lo, & Charles, 1984; Little et al., 2001; Say, Murtagh, & Thomson, 2006; Mandell, Poses, Kazis, & Duefield, 2000). Naturally the willingness for participation is highly dependent on the subject (Longtin et al., 2010). Decisions, which are less or not dependent on medical knowledge or expertise, should involve patients more than issues which are highly complex, especially in medical terms (Little et al., 2001). Waiting is a good example. Patients could be included in dealing with the problems of waiting for healthcare and finding out ways to overcome these problems. No special medical knowledge is necessary to be involved in this challenge and it has in fact impact to everyone.

In this chapter after studying waiting times for patients and physicians at hospitals and outpatient clinics the impact of waiting is analysed on three levels based on our quantitative and qualitative study and literature review: from patients' point of view, from healthcare providers' point of view, and from the healthcare system's point of view. The situation of the patients and their requirements are shown, strategies to reduce times, especially for waiting for the administrative work at the administrative desk, for waiting in waiting area and for waiting for in-process, are presented, and the questions listed in the introduction of the chapter are answered.

One of the main results is that waiting times depend very much on the fact whether the doctor has an electronic appointment system (EAS) or not. The study shows that waiting times can be decreased substantially by using an EAS. While patients visiting doctors not using an EAS had to wait 64 minutes in median, the median was only 17 minutes at doctors with an EAS. However, there is of course room for improvement concerning the allocation of the time slots for each patient at an EAS. Some patients find it very hard to describe what kind of medical condition they want to discuss with the doctor on the telephone while making the appointment. One of the reasons for that is the lack of health literacy.

Another finding is that the majority of patients are willing to use ICT based tools, which are supposed to decrease waiting times. Patients are willing to visit their doctor online or plan the hospital or doctors' visit according to published waiting times of certain healthcare institutions. The implementation of such tools would not only decrease waiting times, they would also increase patient empowerment and the involvement in healthcare service consumption, which again could increase health literacy. Better health literacy would then lead to a better communication between healthcare providers and consumers. Appointments could then be planned easier or more efficiently, which would in then increase the patients' flow.

The question on what kind of patients is more likely to use ICT tools, for instance, for reducing waiting times still remains. Factors such as age or socioeconomic levels obviously influence patients' participation remarkably and should therefore be considered in future work to identify technological or organisational ways to reduce waiting for patients in healthcare sector (Levinson et al., 2005; Say et al., 2006; Gaston & Mitchell, 2005; McKinstry, 2000; Rosen, Anell, & Hjortsberg, 2001; Cassileth, Zupkis, Sutton-Smith, & March, 1980; Rothenbacher, Lutz, & Porzsolt, 1997).

The most obvious reason for waiting for healthcare services is that there are too many patients and too few doctors or hospitals (Blake, 2006). Hiring more physicians at a hospital by increasing the quantity of the healthcare provided, shifting work from physicians to other healthcare staff, or distributing patients better over existing healthcare providers might help solving this problem. These issues have a political, financial, and economic dimension that cannot be dealt with in this chapter. As a next step the EASs and other (online) information systems need to be designed and adapted that help provide patients the above-mentioned functionality like showing the reasons for waiting or how much time left to meet the doctor or get the treatment. These need to be evaluated again "in the wild" to improve the circumstances that cause waiting times and so to reduce waiting for patients.

REFERENCES

Adams, K., Greiner, A. C., & Corrigan, J. M. (2004). *1st Annual Crossing the Quality Chasm Summit: A Focus on Communities*. Washington, DC: National Academies Press.

Armistead, C. (1999). Knowledge management and process performance. *Journal of Knowledge Management*, *3*(2), 143–157. doi:10.1108/13673279910275602

Arneill, A. B., & Devlin, A. S. (2002). Perceived Quality of Care: The Influence of the Waiting Room Environment. *Journal of Environmental Psychology*, *22*(4), 345–360. doi:10.1006/jevp.2002.0274

Bailey, N. T. (1952). A Study of Queues and Appointment Systems in Hospital Out-Patient Departments, with Special Reference to Waiting-Times. *Journal of the Royal Statistical Society. Series B. Methodological*, *14*(2), 185–199.

Becker, F., & Douglass, S. (2008). The ecology of the patient visit: Physical attractiveness, waiting times, and perceived quality of care. *The Journal of Ambulatory Care Management*, *31*(2), 128–141. doi:10.1097/01.JAC.0000314703.34795.44 PMID:18360174

Becker, F., & Poe, D. B. Jr. (1980). The effects of user-generated design modifications in a general hospital. *Journal of Nonverbal Behavior*, *4*(4), 195–218. doi:10.1007/BF00986197

Blake, H. (2006). *Waiting Line Models,* Retrieved from http://www.csus.edu/indiv/b/blakeh/mgmt/documents/OPM101SupplC.pdf

Brink-Muinen, V. D., Van Dulmen, S. M., De Haes, H. C., Visser, A. P., Schellevis, F. G., & Bensing, J. M. (2006). Has patients' involvement in the decision-making process changed over time? *Health Expectations*, *9*(4), 333–342. doi:10.1111/j.1369-7625.2006.00413.x PMID:17083560

Carpman, J. R., Grant, M. A., & Simmons, D. A. (1986). *Design that cares: planning health facilities for patients and visitors*. Chicago: American Hospital Pub.

Cassileth, B. R., Zupkis, R. V., Sutton-Smith, K., & March, V. (1980). Information and participation preferences among cancer patients. *Annals of Internal Medicine*, *92*(6), 832–836. doi:10.7326/0003-4819-92-6-832 PMID:7387025

Chan, K. (2013). *Going to the ER? Real-time hospital emergency wait times now online*. Retrieved from http://www.vancitybuzz.com/2013/04/hospital-emergency-room-wait-times-online/

Committee on Patient Safety and Quality Improvement. (2005). ACOG Committee Opinion No. 320: Partnering with patients to improve safety. *Obstetrics and Gynecology*, *106*(5), 1123–1128. doi:10.1097/00006250-200511000-00057 PMID:16260544

Dansky, K. H., & Miles, J. (1997). Patient satisfaction with ambulatory healthcare services: Waiting time and filling time. *Hospital & Health Services Administration*, *42*(2), 165–177. PMID:10167452

De Man, S., Vlerick, P., Gemmel, P., De Bondt, P., Matthys, D., & Dierckx, R. (2005). Impact of waiting on the perception of service quality in nuclear medicine. *Nuclear Medicine Communications*, *26*(6), 541–547. doi:10.1097/00006231-200506000-00010 PMID:15891598

Deloitte. (2011). *Umfrage 2011 zum Gesundheitswesen in der Schweiz. Wichtigste Ergebnisse, strategische Auswirkungen*.

Devlin, A. S. (2008). Judging a Book by Its Cover: Medical Building Facades and Judgments of Care. *Environment and Behavior*, *40*(3), 307–329. doi:10.1177/0013916507302242

Eck, E. K., DeBaun, B., & Pugliese, G. (2001). *The Contagious Patient: Identifying, Containing, and Treating Appropriately.* Retrieved http://www.infectioncontroltoday.com/articles/2001/12/the-contagious-patient.aspx

Emanuel, E. J., & Emanuel, L. L. (1992). Four models of the physician-patient relationship. *Journal of the American Medical Association*, *267*(16), 2221–2227. doi:10.1001/jama.1992.03480160079038 PMID:1556799

Erzberger, C. (1998). *Zahlen und Wörter: Die Verbindung quantitativer und qualitativer Daten und Methoden im Forschungsprozeß*. Dt. Studien-Verlag.

Fischer, T. (2009). *Die ärztliche Versorgung im niedergelassenen Bereich aus dem Blickwinkel der Patienten: Schlaglichter auf ein vernachlässigtes Gebiet der Gesundheitspolitik.*

Fleisher, J. (2013). Hospitals Duel Over Wait Times. *The Wall Street Journal.*

Gaston, C. M., & Mitchell, G. (2005). Information giving and decision-making in patients with advanced cancer: A systematic review. *Social Science & Medicine*, *61*(10), 2252–2264. doi:10.1016/j.socscimed.2005.04.015 PMID:15922501

General Medical Council. (2013). *Good Medical Practice.* Retrieved from http://www.gmc-uk.org/guidance/news_consultation/20477.asp

Gillon, R. (1994). Medical ethics: Four principles plus attention to scope. *BMJ (Clinical Research Ed.)*, *309*(6948), 184–188. doi:10.1136/bmj.309.6948.184 PMID:8044100

Girtler, R. (2001). *Methoden der Feldforschung.* Stuttgart: UTB GmbH. (in German)

Gläser, J., & Laudel, G. (2009). *Experteninterviews und qualitative Inhaltsanalyse: als Instrumente rekonstruierender Untersuchungen.* Wiesbaden: VS Verlag für Sozialwissenschaften.

Google (2012). *The Digital Journey to Wellness: Hospital Selection Infographic.*

Grazie, D., & Wimmer-Puchinger, B. (2014). Rahmen-Gesundheitsziel 3 - Gesundheitskompetenz der Bevölkerung stärken, Bericht der Arbeitsgruppe. Bundesministerium für Gesundheit, Editor (in German).

Guadagnoli, E., & Ward, P. (1998). Patient participation in decision-making. *Social Science & Medicine*, *47*(3), 329–339. doi:10.1016/S0277-9536(98)00059-8 PMID:9681902

Haggard, L., & Hosking, S. (2003). *Healing the Hospital Environment: Design, Management and Maintenance of Healthcare Premises.* London: Taylor & Francis.

Hartmannbund. (2014). *Umfrage „Termintreue" – Datenbasis.* Retrieved from http://www.hartmannbund.de/uploads/Landesverb%C3%A4nde/Niedersachsen/2014-07-09_Handout-Presse.PDF (in German).

Janzek-Hawlat, S. (2015). *Impact of waiting times in health care* [Master Thesis]. Faculty of Informatics, Vienna University of Technology.

Kennedy, J. F. (1962). *Special message to Congress on protecting consumer interest.* Presidential Papers. President's Office Files.

Kizer, K. W. (2001). Establishing healthcare performance standards in an era of consumerism. *The New England Journal of Medicine*, *286*(10), 1213–1217. PMID:11559267

Lammers, W. M. (2014). *So lässt sich die Wartezeit in der Praxis reduzieren.* ÄrzteZeitung. (in German)

Lancet, T. The Lancet. (2005). Will consumerism lead to better health? *Lancet*, *366*(9483), 343. doi:10.1016/S0140-6736(05)66999-1 PMID:16060053

Laschet, H. (2014). *Kommentar zur Wartezeit-Umfrage: Säumige Patienten?* ÄrzteZeitung. (in German)

Levinson, W., Kao, A., Kuby, A., & Thisted, R. A. (2005). Not all patients want to participate in decision making. A national study of public preferences. *Journal of General Internal Medicine*, *20*(6), 531–535. doi:10.1111/j.1525-1497.2005.04101.x PMID:15987329

Little, P., Everitt, H., Williamson, I., Warner, G., Moore, M., Gould, C., & Payne, S. et al. (2001). Preferences of patients for patient centred approach to consultation in primary care: Observational study. *BMJ (Clinical Research Ed.)*, *322*(7284), 468–540. doi:10.1136/bmj.322.7284.468 PMID:11222423

Longtin, Y., Sax, H., Leape, L. L., Sheridan, S. E., Donaldson, L., & Pittet, D. (2010). Patient Participation: Current Knowledge and Applicability to Patient Safety. *Mayo Clinic Proceedings*, *85*(1), 53–62. doi:10.4065/mcp.2009.0248 PMID:20042562

Mangold, M., Peintinger, M, & Kopetzki, C. (2010). Behandlungsablehnung trotz vitaler Indikation. RdM - Recht der Medizin 2010/4. (in German)

Mansell, D., Poses, R. M., Kazis, L., & Duefield, C. A. (2000). Clinical factors that influence patients' desire for participation in decisions about illness. *Archives of Internal Medicine*, *160*(19), 2991–2996. doi:10.1001/archinte.160.19.2991 PMID:11041908

Marberry, S. O. (2006). *Improving Healthcare with Better Building Design*. Chicago, IL: Health Administration Press.

Marsh, G. E. Jr. (1993). Hospital Interior Architecture: Creating Healing Environments for Special Patient Populations. *The New England Journal of Medicine*, *328*(12), 894–895. doi:10.1056/NEJM199303253281224

Mayring, P. (2002). *Einführung in die qualitative Sozialforschung*. Weinheim: Beltz. (in German)

McKinstry, B. (2000). Do patients wish to be involved in decision making in the consultation? A cross sectional survey with video vignettes. *BMJ (Clinical Research Ed.)*, *321*(7265), 867–871. doi:10.1136/bmj.321.7265.867 PMID:11021866

Miceli, J., & Wolosin, R. J. (2004). *You're running late - now what? Patient satisfaction, wait time and physician behavior.* Orlando, Florida: World organization of national colleges, academies and academic associations of General Practitioners/Family Physicians.

Mundi Index. (2012). *Land Vergleich > Krankenhausbetten pro Einwohner*. Retrieved from http://www.indexmundi.com/g/r.aspx?v=2227&l=de

Nielsen-Bohlman, L., Panzer, A. M., & Kindig, D. A. (2004). *Health literacy: A prescription to end confusion*. Washington, D.C.: National Academies Press.

Nursing & Midwifery Council. (2015). *The code - Professional standards of practice and behaviour for nurses and midwives*. Retrieved from http://www.nmc.org.uk/standards/code/

Pittet, D., Allegranzi, B., Storr, J., & Donaldson, L. (2005). 'Clean Care is Safer Care': The Global Patient Safety Challenge 2005–2006. *International Journal of Infectious Diseases*, *10*(6), 419–424. doi:10.1016/j.ijid.2006.06.001 PMID:16914344

Przyborski, A., & Wohlrab-Sahr, M. (2010). *Qualitative Sozialforschung: Ein Arbeitsbuch*. München: Oldenbourg Wissenschaftsverlag. (in German)

Rosen, P., Anell, A., & Hjortsberg, C. (2001). Patient views on choice and participation in primary health care. *Health Policy (Amsterdam)*, *55*(2), 121–128. doi:10.1016/S0168-8510(00)00122-6 PMID:11163651

Rothenbacher, D., Lutz, M. P., & Porzsolt, F. (1997). Treatment decisions in palliative cancer care: Patients' preferences for involvement and doctors' knowledge about it. *European Journal of Cancer, 33*(8), 1184–1189. doi:10.1016/S0959-8049(97)00034-8 PMID:9301440

Say, R., Murtagh, M., & Thomson, R. (2006). Patients' preference for involvement in medical decision making: A narrative review. *Patient Education and Counseling, 60*(2), 102–114. doi:10.1016/j.pec.2005.02.003 PMID:16442453

Staeck, F. (2014). *Wartezeiten-Debatte: Regierung gegen Vergleich von PKV mit GKV*. ÄrzteZeitung. (in German)

Statistik Austria. (2015a). *Demographie*. Retrieved from http://www.statistik.at/web_de/statistiken/soziales/gender-statistik/demographie/

Statistik Austria. (2015b). *Stationäre Aufenthalte*. Retrieved from http://www.statistik.at/web_de/statistiken/gesundheit/stationaere_aufenthalte/index.html

Strauss, A. L. (1998). *Grundlagen qualitativer Sozialforschung: Datenanalyse und Theoriebildung in der empirischen soziologischen Forschung*. Fink. (in German)

Strull, W. M., Lo, B., & Charles, G. (1984). Do patients want to participate in medical decision making? *Journal of the American Medical Association, 252*(21), 2990–2994. doi:10.1001/jama.1984.03350210038026 PMID:6502860

Taylor, S. J. (1994). Waiting for Service: The Relationship between Delays and Evaluations of Service. *Journal of Marketing, 58*(2), 56–69. doi:10.2307/1252269

Techniker Krankenkasse. (2014). *TK-Meinungspuls Gesundheit 2014*. Retrieved from http://www.tk.de/tk/themen/meinungspuls-gesundheit-oktober-2014/meinungspuls-gesundheit-oktober-2014-studienband/660168

Vissers, J., & Beech, R. (2005). *Health operations management: Patient flow logistics in health care. Routledge health management series*. London, NY: Routledge.

Wallner, J. (2013). Rechtsethischer Anspruch und faktische Grenzen von Patientenaufklärung und Informed Consent. [in German]. *Zeitschrift für Gesundheitspolitik, 2013*(4).

Wijayasinghe, D. S. (2013). *I arrive on time but end up waiting to see my doctor. Why?* The Globe and Mail.

World Health Organization. (1997). The Vienna Recommendations on Health Promoting Hospitals.

World Health Organization. (2015). *Health expenditure, total (% of GDP)*. Retrieved from http://www.who.int/gho/health_financing/total_expenditure/en/

KEY TERMS AND DEFINITIONS

Electronic Appointment System: A piece of software to book appointments online, here for healthcare institutions.

Health Literacy: Ability to read, understand, describe and use healthcare information that is needed for health decisions or treatment.

Mixed Method Research Approach: Research approach applying mixed (qualitative and quantitative) methods in which each step depends on one or more previous steps.

Outpatient Clinics: A clinic, department or ward of a hospital that provides diagnosis and care for patients not staying overnight.

Qualitative Research: Exploratory research for understanding reasons of phenomena inquired quantitatively.

Waiting Time: The time patients have to wait for a physician or for appointments, diagnostic procedures in hospitals or at resident doctors.

ENDNOTES

1 http://www.indexmundi.com/g/r.aspx?v=2227&l=de
2 http://epp.eurostat.ec.europa.eu/statistics_explained/index.php/Healthy_life_years_statistics/de
3 http://www.statistik.at/web_de/presse/073804
4 https://www.gesundheit.gv.at/Portal.Node/ghp/public/content/gesundheitsbarometer.html

This work was previously published in Transformative Healthcare Practice through Patient Engagement edited by Guendalina Graffigna, pages 276-301, copyright year 2017 by Medical Information Science Reference (an imprint of IGI Global).

APPENDIX

Interview Guideline at the Resident Physician and Hospital

Part A

A1: What are the main patient processes?
A2: What are the reasons for waiting times?
 A2.1: Are there inner organisational reasons?
 A2.2: Are there external reasons?
A3: How long is the average waiting time?
A4: Are there any possibilities to decrease waiting times?
 A4.1: Are there inner organisational possibilities to decrease waiting times?
 A4.2: Are there possibilities outside the organisation to decrease waiting times?
 A4.3: Are there IT-based solutions, which could decrease waiting times?
A5: Are you using an appointment system?
 A5.1: What is the percentage of your patients using your appointment system?
 A5.2: What is the percentage of your patients who could use your appointment system?
 A5.3: Are appointment systems in general decreasing waiting times?

Part B

B1: How is the office/hospital equipped?
 B1.1: At the reception
 B1.2: In the waiting area
B2: Are there any entertainment facilities within the waiting area?

Questionnaire for Patients Waiting in the Hospital Waiting Area or Resident Physician

Part A: "Waiting"

A1: At what time did you arrive in the waiting area?
A2: How long was the waiting time at the administrative desk?
A3: Do you have an appointment?
 Yes I no
 A3.1: If yes, at what time?
A4: How do you sense the length of the waiting time here normally?
 Long I ok I short
A5: How do you sense the waiting in the waiting area?
 Pleasant I neutral I unpleasant
A6: What would it need to make the waiting time more pleasant (multiple answers)?

Books and magazines | more media entertainment | more space | increase cleanness | new design of the waiting area | water dispenser | more informative literature | I would like to know how much longer I have to wait | others…

A7: Are you coming alone or in company?
Partner | friend | child/children | other … | I'm here alone

A7.1: If you are coming in company, what would this person do if he or she wouldn't be here?
Working | free time | homework | others…

A7.2: If you are coming with a child, is there enough entertainment provided for the child?
Yes | no

A8: What would you do if you wouldn't be here?
Working | free time | homework | cure at home | other…

Part B: Decrease Waiting Time

B1: Could you imagine visiting your doctor online?
Yes | no

B2: Would you like to see waiting times online?
Yes | no

B2.1: Would you plan your visit according to the online waiting times?
Yes | no

B3: Do you prefer a strict appointment system?
Yes | no

B4: Do you have other suggestions to decrease the waiting time?

Part C: Demographics

C1: Please state your age

C2: What is your sex?

Chapter 14
The Past, the Present, and the Future:
Examining the Role of the "Social" in Transforming Personal Healthcare Management of Chronic Disease

Elizabeth Cummings
University of Tasmania, Australia

Leonie Ellis
University of Tasmania, Australia

Paul Turner
University of Tasmania, Australia

ABSTRACT

This chapter examines how the rapid diffusion of social media and Mobile Web is impacting personal healthcare management amongst those living with chronic disease. Despite a recent increase in research in this area (Moorhead, et al., 2013), evaluating the "social" still poses challenges to conventional notions of the "Internet empowered" patient and the best ways to support the management of chronic disease (Østbye, et al., 2005). The chapter argues that there is a need for advancing conceptual thinking on how health and IT are now interacting at the level of individual patients/citizens and how this is continuing to transform health professional-patient interactions (Glasgow, et al., 2008). By drawing on examples of e-health research, the chapter illustrates how notions of the "social" and "technology" have evolved over time from medically centred e-health through to patient-centred e-health. The chapter considers how this evolution may lead to a future focus on community-centred personal healthcare of chronic disease supported by "social" e-health tools, applications, and services that continue to blur the more conventional boundaries between health professionals, patients, and their social networks.

DOI: 10.4018/978-1-5225-1928-7.ch014

INTRODUCTION

The term social media covers a wide array of technologies, applications and services including social networking sites like Facebook, media-sharing platforms like YouTube, BitTorrent and Flickr, and an array of user content including Wikis, Blogs and micro-blogging services like Twitter. Despite some continuing definitional ambiguity in the literature, there is general agreement that social media involves interaction on-line around the generation, communication and exchange of user-generated content (Kaplan & Haenlein, 2010; Kietzmann et al, 2011). Simultaneously growth in the use of mobile devices (mobiles, tablets, laptops etc.) and mobile networks to access content on the internet has also expanded rapidly particularly during the last five years (Kelly, 2013). While this trend is uneven globally, it is noticeable that some of the most rapid adopters of 'mobile web' are countries with rapidly developing economies including Brazil, Russia, India and China (BRICs). These countries are also increasingly aware of the need to address the changing healthcare challenges arising within their increasingly affluent populations (Bhaumik, 2013). The diversity of analysis on growth social media uptake is evident with graphs and tables presenting data according to social media types, user timelines, size, duration and by companies or industries. As an example Figure 1 presents social media penetration by country as at March 2013.

Combined, the near exponential growth in the adoption and use of social media and mobile web (Qualman, 2013) has, perhaps not surprisingly, led to the their deployment by a range of healthcare stakeholders including governments and public & private sector healthcare provider organisations; healthcare

Figure 1. Social media penetration (source@wearesocialsg)

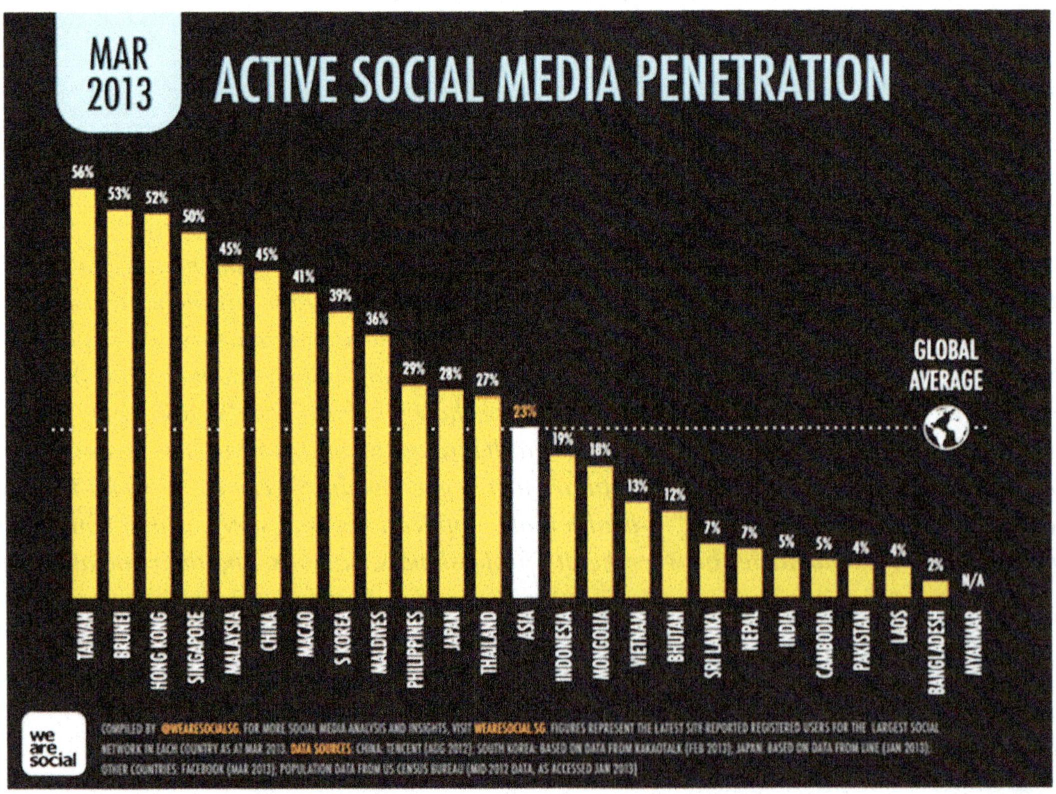

professionals and researchers; and patients/citizens (Thackeray et al, 2008; Moen et al, 2009; Colineau & Paris, 2010). Noticeably, the primary aims and objectives for using these 'social' technologies have varied considerably across the different stakeholders and have also changed over time. Governments and healthcare provider organisations have tended to have a strong focus on health information dissemination that has more recently given rise to trends that use social technologies for broader community engagement and awareness raising. Clinicians initially tended to focus on their own professional networks and on keeping their expertise up-to-date, but more recently some have been reaching out to their patients through these technologies to extend their services e.g. <www.ozdocsonline.com.au>.

For patients these social technologies primarily emerged as a way of either complementing or *by-passing* conventional sources of health related information. These technologies continue to be used to seek/share health information/advice, personal experiences and knowledge of medications/medical services, and to offer support and/or track personal healthcare (Househ, 2013). More recently there have been a number of other trends related to patient use of these social technologies. One major trend has been the emergence of private sector providers entering the social media market to support patients on-line health activities, for example, <www.patientslikeme.com> (Ellis, Showell, Turner, 2013). Another has been evidence of negative impacts on health arising from misinformation (Syed-Abdul et al, 2013) and/or reinforcement of negative behaviours (Hanson et al, 2013) as a result of 'social' networking.

The focus of this chapter is to examine how these different trends are impacting on personal health care management amongst an increasingly significant group of healthcare users – those living with chronic disease. More specifically, the chapter aims to examine how these different trends challenge conventional thinking about those living with chronic disease and the best ways to support their personal healthcare management (Kuijpers et al, 2013; Østbye et al, 2005). In this context, by drawing on examples of e-health research into management/self-management of chronic disease, the chapter illustrates how notions of the 'social' and 'technology' are being transformed by social media and mobile web.

The chapter argues that there is a need for advancing conceptual thinking on how health and ICTs (e-health) are now interacting at the level of individual patients/citizens and how these changes require improved sophistication in approaches to the management of chronic disease by health professionals and health informatics specialists. Critically, the chapter argues that the challenge for the future is how best to ensure that social media benefits for personal healthcare management outweigh the potential dangers for patients/citizens in terms of privacy breaches, data misuse, exploitation and/or misinformation (Adams, 2010; Corea et al, 2010).

BACKGROUND

This section provides background on how approaches to both the management of chronic disease and the use of e-health in supporting this management have changed over time. To contextualise these changes it is useful to briefly consider current and future predicted pressures on the health care environment as the result of the increase in chronic and complex conditions, ageing populations and the sustained increase in life expectancy exhibited in most countries around the world.

In one sense, current and predicted pressures on health care budgets, systems and resources are the direct result of the successful delivery of healthcare services that has occurred in most advanced economies since post-World-War 2. Developments in medicines, clinical practices, health technologies and increasing social affluence have all contributed significantly to a reduction in infectious diseases and injury as the major causes of premature death or disability. Simultaneously with these changes however, has been the emergence of increases in the prevalence of risk factors leading to chronic disease (Wagner et al., 2001). As increasing numbers of citizens' live longer, increasing numbers also live with complex chronic conditions or disability. In many developed countries this trend has been compounded by a reduction in the overall birth rate such that for at least another twenty years the ratio of aged citizens living with one or more chronic disease relative to the population as a whole will continue to rise. These factors have combined to make finding cost effective and efficient solutions to the management of chronic disease a priority. They have also put considerable pressure on the health budgets of most developed countries with the percentage of GDP spend on health continuing to rise in ways predicted to be unsustainable in the near future.

As an example, Australia is trying to address its rapidly ageing population by approaches that promote healthy ageing as part of strategies to support the maintenance of high quality healthcare services into the future. Current estimates are that between 2010 and 2050 the number of people between the ages of 65 and 84 will more than double, and the number of very old (85 years and over) will more than quadruple. In Australia, chronic conditions already contribute to more than 80% of the total health burden and contribute significantly to decreased quality of life for many patients/citizens and their carers. Based on the national health survey for 2007-08, an estimated 75% of Australians already had a long-term condition. It is also known that the number of long-term conditions that people report increases with age such that 50% of those aged 65 years or older are likely to have five or more long-term conditions (AIHW, 2010).

Chronic conditions are ongoing in nature and are rarely, if ever, completely cured (AIHW, 2012). Given the variety of chronic diseases/conditions it can be difficult to provide a single definition however it is clear that most chronic conditions exhibit the following characteristics:

- They have complex and multiple causes;
- They usually have a gradual onset, although they can have sudden onset and acute stages;
- They occur across the life cycle, although they become more prevalent with older age;
- They can compromise quality of life by causing physical and/or mental impairment or disability;
- They are long term and persistent, leading to a gradual deterioration of health; and
- They tend initially not to be immediately life threatening, but they are the most common and leading cause of premature mortality.

The increasing costs and the increasing incidence of chronic conditions have placed emphasis on ensuring the patient journey is proactive, planned, coordinated, and efficient (Coleman et al., 2009). It has also led to awareness that existing models of chronic disease management were not sustainable and that alternatives needed to be examined.

CHRONIC DISEASE MANAGEMENT AND CHRONIC DISEASE SELF-MANAGEMENT

Traditional approaches to chronic disease management rely on a health care model that positions the clinician-patient relationship as one in which the clinician is the sole source of expertise and decision making authority (Charles, Gafni, & Whelan, 1997). With the growth in the incidence of chronic disease, it has now been recognized that this approach is both unsustainable and inappropriate (Wagner et al, 1996; <www.improvingchroniccare.org>).

As a result, a number of more integrated and collaborative approaches have emerged that aim to variously support improved continuity of care, use of evidence based practices and direct involvement of patients and their carers. These include collaborative management (Von Korff, Gruman, Schaefer, Curry, & Wagner, 1997), patient empowerment (Funnell et al., 1991), shared decision making (Charles, Gafni, & Whelan, 1997), the partnership model (Holman & Lorig, 2000), and the chronic care model (Wagner, 1998; Wagner et al., 2001). Following Wagner et al, the chronic care model provides a general framework for these approaches and highlights that for successful self-management interventions there are a number of essential elements including: Collaborative problem definition; Targeting, goal setting and planning; Self-management training and support services; and Active and sustained follow-up.

These elements aim to ensure the development of self-management initiatives that enable patient's to define their problems in conjunction with their health professionals. This includes identifying the issues that are of greatest importance to the patient and clinician as the basis for the setting of realistic goals and the development of personalised care plans. To enhance the probability of success it is important that any processes are guided by the patient's readiness to change and the development of their self-efficacy skills. Ensuring that patients are provided with instruction about disease management, behavioural support, and physical activity and that they also have the emotional demands of living with a chronic condition addressed appear to be also be very important success factors (Coleman, 2009; IoM, 2012)

While these approaches vary in emphasis, all share a common perspective that clinicians, patients and their carers should share information and where possible make choices together (Barrett, 2005). Of course, underlying this focus on collaboration is the assumption that patients have the right to take part in all health decisions (Charles, Gafni, & Whelan, 1997), and that they are capable, with appropriate support, of making valuable contributions to these decisions (Wagner et al., 2001). This assumption has been criticized because of the fact that many patients living with chronic conditions may be unwilling or unable to take on these new responsibilities and that furthermore, even if they do, that the result will necessarily be improved quality of care (Cummings & Turner, 2010).

There is however a growing body of evidence reporting positive outcomes from attempts to 'empower' some patients and engage in more integrated care practices in relation to chronic disease (Coleman et al, 2009). But it is also clear that these outcomes are not evenly spread amongst those living with chronic conditions and that other socio-economic and educational factors are important in contributing to the capacity of patients to achieve positive health outcomes (Showell & Turner, 2013). This stated, for many patients the opportunity to engage in self-management is a positive development. Self-management being defined here as simply the active participation of patients/citizens in the own personal health care management. Clearly self-management does not mean patients managing their conditions in isolation. It requires an effective partnership between patient, carer and health service provider. Working together to ensure that essential care requirements are available when needed and that the various people involved in the care are informed and work together to ensure the best possible outcomes for patients (Harvey, Battersby, & Misan, 2003).

Evidence highlights that many patients engaged in self-management make better use of health care professionals' time and particularly where they have developed effective self-management skills (Barlow, Turner, & Wright, 2000; Lorig et al., 1999). Systematic reviews indicate clear clinical benefits for patients with conditions such as diabetes and hypertension through self-management programmes.

However, such reviews are limited by the heterogeneity of interventions and outcomes (Chodosh et al., 2005; Warsi, LaValley, Wang, Avorn, & Solomon, 2003; Warsi, Wang, LaValley, & Avorn, 2004). The increased ability to self-manage conditions and prevent or mitigate deterioration are linked to improving patient control of their condition (Cummings, 2008). However, this requires a more patient centred system based upon a deep understanding of both the patient and their perceptions of health care (Simborg, 2010).

As will be discussed below in relation to the use of technology this implies that what works for one patient may not work for another and this does create difficulties for health care systems that tend towards 'one-size fits all' approaches as they attempt to move towards patient centred care (Novak et al., 2013)

E-HEALTH AND CHRONIC DISEASE SELF-MANAGEMENT

As highlighted in the previous section of this chapter there is already a considerable body of health research in the areas of chronic disease management, self-management, active ageing, and independent living (Lorig et al., 2006, Jessup et al., 2006, Camarinha-Matos and Afsarmanesh, 2011).

Much of this work has utilised information and communication technologies (ICTs) to support interventions (Lorig et al, 2006, Cummings et al, 2010; Kuijpers et al, 2013). Many of these technology supported health interventions have been critiqued for their overly simplistic assumptions about the relationships between information provision and improved health outcomes (Cummings & Turner, 2010). In parallel with these types of disease specific technology supported health interventions, there has also been research focused on broader lifestyle change and wellness management amongst those with chronic diseases. However, as indicated previously, a major challenge how to ensure the sustainability of these lifestyle changes, which is an area of research that continues to receive limited attention (Freyne et al, 2011).

From a technological perspective, it is evident that there are significant differences amongst older people in the adoption and use of ICT. In Australia, where internet access and the penetration of computing technology is relatively high, a number of studies have confirmed that lack of internet access or computing technology continues to be correlated with a range of factors including low incomes, living in rural areas, low educational levels and old age (Fox, 2011, Gilhooly et al. 2009). To avoid accentuating this e-health divide, increased digital inclusion and use of assistive technologies can deliver benefits for the elder and those with chronic conditions such as increased independence and social participation (Gilhooly et al., 2009). However, there is also significant potential for the further isolation of already marginalised groups as more and more social, political and commercial services are transferred onto the Internet and those without ICT skills or access are further marginalized through a digital divide (Gilhooly et al., 2009; Niehaves and Plattfaut, 2010).

Following Niehaves and Plattfaut (2010), the single most important predictor of whether older people used ICT was their expectation of the benefits that ICT could bring them. Other factors identified as barriers to the adoption of ICT by older people include lack of interest, feeling too old, fear of new technology (fear of breaking it), lack of resources and access, lack of IT skills and experience, cost and concerns about security and privacy (Olphert et al., 2005; Charness & Boot, 2009). These factors are compounded by age-related decline as loss of vision, dexterity and motor skills make it more difficult for older or disabled people to use technologies (Olphert et al., 2005). Most of these impairments are directly correlated with chronic conditions.

Another dimension of these barriers relates to differences in people's health literacy. Following, Pearce-Brown et al. (2009) and Jordan et al. (2008) it has become evident that health literacy and the capacity to self-management are correlated. Personal capacity to seek, access, understand and use health information and services directly influences participation in treatment decisions. People with lower health literacy are those most likely to have chronic conditions and in turn they are the least able to manage those conditions (Hawkins et al. 2010; Pearce-Brown et al. 2009). Improved self-management may help compensate for lower levels of health literacy and improve health-related behaviours (Hibbard et al. 2007). However, currently there is little evidence on the costs of poor health literacy and the cost-effectiveness of interventions to improve health literacy (Eichler et al. 2009).

Clearly it is highly complex and challenging to genuinely understand individual patient's capacities and experiences in interacting with these technologies per se, as well as how they may contribute to improved self-management (Cummings and Turner, 2010). In recognition of this complexity, more recent approaches to the use of e-health to support chronic disease self-management have become more patient-centred and attempted to involve patients directly in the design of the solutions (Roehrer et al, 2013).

Two of the author's on this chapter have been directly involved in the design, implementation and evaluation of e-Health systems to support chronic disease self-management programs with a range of patient cohorts living with one or more chronic conditions including COPD and CF (Cummings, Chau, & Turner, 2009; Cummings et al., 2010; Cummings & Turner, 2007, 2008; Cummings & Turner, 2010; Roehrer, Cummings, Beggs et al., 2013; Roehrer, Cummings, Ellis, & Turner, 2011; Roehrer, Cummings, Turner et al., 2013). Below is a brief summary of some of this research work relating to one major project.

The Pathways Home project sought to support daily self-monitoring and recording of symptoms by patients suffering from two chronic respiratory conditions: chronic obstructive pulmonary disease (COPD), and cystic fibrosis (CF). The main purpose was to test the hypothesis that by assisting patients in the processes of identification, and comprehension about their condition they can initiate early action in relation to changes in their condition and so decrease the severity of exacerbations and slow their decline. The project was premised on the view that where possible patients should play a central role in decisions about their own health and that providing evidence-based knowledge to patients would enhance their ability to participate in self-management of their condition.

The COPD arm aimed to assist older people with COPD to achieve self-management skills, mediated through the development of self-efficacy for patient-identified health behaviours. The project supported self-management through self-monitoring and recording of symptoms (preferably in an electronic format) with a graphical longitudinal feedback report provided to participants and their mentors. Evaluation of this project appeared to indicate that the use of the online patient diary impedes or limits the development of self-efficacy for self-management in people suffering from moderate to severe COPD but that other social benefits can be achieved as the participants become more housebound by their condition (Cummings, 2008; Cummings et al, 2010).

The CF arm of the Pathways project was an investigation to see if an ICT tool, in this case a mobile phone application, could be developed for the use of daily symptom monitoring. The study hoped to discover if individuals with CF would use the tool and if the use of the ICT tool made a difference to the self-management behaviours and quality of life for individuals with CF. This was undertaken by was the support of mentoring activity through ICT, feedback from participants also indicated that further research was needed (Cummings et al., 2011). Pathways Home demonstrated that mentoring assisted with developing self-efficacy for self-management behaviours, but the pilot study was too small to make definitive conclusions on the ICT arm (Cummings et al., 2011).

The Pathways Home CF project was then extended to explore the effect of its implementation for a group of adolescents and older children with CF based in Queensland. The aim of this project was to examine task-specific self-efficacy and self-monitoring and the project was designed to improve self-management behaviours and quality of life amongst CF patients (Roehrer et al., 2013). The project ran for six months, with a further six months of follow up. Data collection involved both quantitative and qualitative assessments collected at commencement, 3, 6 and 6 months post completion. Again this consisted of an electronic diary and participants were able to view a summary of their feedback to monitor changes in their symptoms. The project mentors were also able to review their patients remotely. The outcomes of this project provided sufficient positive response from the qualitative data and usage statistics to indicate that further investigation with a broader scope encompassing a more sophisticated suite of products to support the CF community may be beneficial. Useful information was also obtained on aspects of self- monitoring that were not viewed favourably by these younger CF patients such as the need to enter diary data on a daily basis, which not surprisingly was not an attractive option for young adolescents (Roehrer et al., 2013).

This resulted in the development of a final project, the myCF project, which utilised web based resources that could also be accessed via mobile devices. This project had three proposed outcomes: development of a web based information portal which contained expert reviewed health information sheets and links to other relevant sites; Increasing the availability of community support from peers and other families through a secure online chat room; and introduction of a health mentor system of trained health professionals to encourage the development of self-monitoring and increase self-awareness about their condition.

What the above examples highlight is the complexity of using e-health to sustainably support chronic disease self-management in a manner that produces benefits recognized by both the patients and the health professionals (Kuijpers et al, 2013). A major conceptual challenge is addressing the implicit info-centrism that emerges within these types of intervention i.e. the prioritization of the importance of information provision per se. The implicit assumption that axiomatically through the provision of additional information patients will achieve better outcomes ignores the psychosocial, attitudinal and contextual factors that are important for good healthcare and the capacity to self-manage.

Figure 2. Timeline and relationship between projects

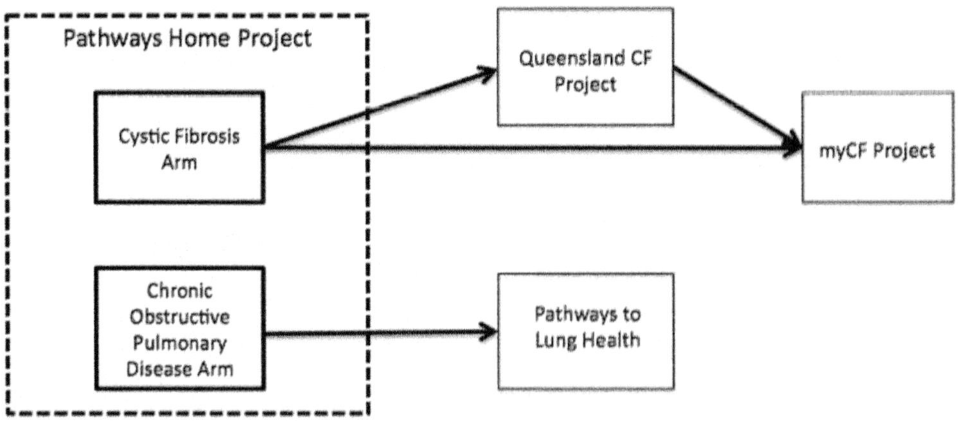

It is in this context that the emergence of social media and mobile web are transforming personal health care management of chronic disease and challenging some key assumptions that are embedded in health systems and health informatics approaches to support self-management.

CHRONIC DISEASE AND THE 'SOCIAL'

The above discussion has highlighted the complexity of supporting personal health care management of chronic disease. This situation has become even more complex as increasing numbers of patients and their carers adopt social media and mobile web in relation to their health.

This chapter argues that the impact of this 'social' use of information and communication technologies in personal healthcare management amongst many of those living with chronic conditions is further transforming conventional health professional – patient interactions, attitudes and expectations. In particular, it is evident that:

- Patient to Patient interactions through social media and mobile web are changing the nature and flow of information available on living with chronic conditions in ways that have the potential to both complement or *clash* with information provided by health care professionals;
- Exposure to social media platforms is changing patients' expectations, experiences and preferences for how information should be presented. Most of these contrast markedly with conventional approaches to the design and deployment of e-Health being deployed by health professionals;
- The dramatic adoption and diffusion of social media and mobile web across the population of those living with chronic conditions has already started to challenge many of the assumptions held by health professionals and health informatics specialists about who their service users are, what they need and want and how services should be provided, as more patients access alternative and more readily available information, peer-support and advice through social media and mobile web.

It is argued that these changes require advancement in conceptual thinking on how health care systems and health informatics solutions can be used to optimize the benefits of for individual patients/citizens engage in personal health care management of chronic disease. More critically, looking to the future, health professionals and health informatics specialists need to ensure that social media benefits for personal healthcare management outweigh the potential dangers for patients/citizens in terms of privacy breaches, data misuse, exploitation and/or misinformation (Adams, 2010; Corea et al, 2010).

In trying to understand how social media and mobile web are transforming the nature of health communications it is useful to consider the Keitzmann et al (2011) framework that describes seven major building blocks in terms of form and function exhibited by different social media. These building blocks have been summarized by Moorehead et al (2013) as follows:

- **Identity:** The nature and extent users reveal themselves on-line;
- **Conversations:** The nature and extent users communicate with each other;
- **Sharing:** The nature and extent users exchange, distribute, and receive information and content;
- **Presence:** The nature and extent users are aware of each other's availability on-line;

- **Relationships:** The nature and extent users socially relate to one another;
- **Reputation:** The nature and extent users are aware of and understand the social standing and trustworthiness of information, content and other users;
- **Groups:** The nature and extent users are aligned, structured and/or form identifiable communities.

What this framework highlights is how social media and the mobile web are changing the nature of spatial and temporal interactions between health content and patients. As Fox (2011) reports while health professionals remain the most important source of information increasing numbers of 'highly-engaged patients and caregivers' are playing an active role in sharing with others what they are learning through social media. Fox (2011) latest results indicate that of the 74% of USA adults who use the internet surveyed:

- 80% looked on-line for information concerning any of 15 health topics such as a specific disease or treatment.
- 34% read someone else's commentary or experience about health or medical issues on an online news group, website, or blog.
- 18% have gone online to find others who might have health concerns similar to theirs.
- 62% use social media platforms: and of these,
    - 23% of social network site users followed their friends' personal health experiences or updates on the site;
    - 17% of social network site users have used social networking sites to remember or memorialize other people who suffered from a certain health condition.

Significantly, while younger users still dominate social media platforms, increasing numbers of older and lower income users are using these platforms to find health related information (Chou et al, 2009; Kontos et al, 2010). This simultaneously challenges conventional thinking on the e-health divide and also raises concerns about the types of information these users are obtaining, its reliability and trustworthiness as well as the types of behavior interactions through these 'social' channels create? To date, these questions have remained under-explored. Indeed, as the most recent review of research into social media in health highlights, despite considerable optimism about the benefits of social media in healthcare the quality of evidence validating its impact remains low. This is especially the case in relation to the impact of social media amongst specific patient groups for example, those living with chronic disease (Moorhead et al, 2013).

DISCUSSION

This chapter has highlighted the reality that social media and the mobile web are now being adopted and used by increasing numbers of patients including those living with chronic conditions. This continuing trend and its impacts pose several questions for how health professionals and health informaticians should best respond given that major concerns are beginning to emerge about the quality and reliability of health information available through these 'social' channels, the potential for breaches of patient privacy and confidentiality and the dangers of inaccurate, misleading or harmful information being consumed by vulnerable user groups such as those living with chronic conditions (Adams, 2010a; Adams, 2010b).

For health professionals the first step in responding to the 'social' is to acknowledge that it is happening! Thereafter, exploring ways that social media can be leveraged to enhance health communications with patients and improve the quality and reliability of information and advice accessed will be important. Critically, health professionals must recognise that evidence that their patients are accessing social media for health information does not imply that these patients have necessarily high levels of health literacy (Jordan et al, 2010). Indeed, there is some evidence to suggest that using social channels to find health information is precisely because many patients find health information provided through conventional health service channels to be unhelpful or unusable. It is important for health professionals to recognise that without attempts to reach out to patients using these social channels there is a real danger that 'untethered social media use' may accentuate rather than mitigate existing health care challenges and inequalities amongst patients/citizens in terms of healthcare services (Simborg, 2010).

For health informaticians it is evident that the rapid adoption and use of social media and mobile web by patients is both simultaneously an opportunity and a challenge. For those living with chronic conditions the diversity of impairments and co-morbidities make it extremely challenging to ensure systems, applications and services are appropriate, user-friendly and useful for all users. However, that increasing numbers of patients are now on-line, presents greater opportunities to build applications and services to engage directly with them as part of the design, implementation and evaluation of 'social' health services. Indeed, it can be argued that the growth in use of social media for health amongst patients reveals an unmet appetite to engage on-line that is not being met by conventional healthcare channels. Certainly the emergence of private sector providers in this space supports this perspective (Ellis et al, 2013).

While it is important to avoid simply replacing patient dependency on health professionals for patient dependency on e-health systems, applications or services, there may be an opportunity to support and facilitate greater community-centred applications and services that leverage patients 'social' appetites. These types of applications and services open up the possibility of developing ways to mitigate the dangers of information overload and/or of patients receiving conflicting advice that may inhibit their ability to engage in self-management. In these more community-centred models social media and mobile web become platforms to complement other channels and as mechanisms to provide emotional, psycho-social and peer support amongst patients moderated by a range of health professionals working collaboratively (Frost et al, 2008). These emerging models do however suggest the need for a fundamental shift in thinking by health professionals in relation to their use of e-health and support of chronic disease self-management (Cummings & Turner, 2010; Kuijpers et al, 2013).

More broadly this community-centred approach leveraging social media platforms connects with a large body of published research that approaches self-management by investigating mechanisms to support positive lifestyle changes amongst a diverse range of users (Webb et al, 2010). While much of this research is focused on interventions with specific diseases, mechanisms to support prevention through wellness management have started to emerge as an important area of investigation. These types of intervention are focused on modifying problematic behaviours and/or promoting healthy lifestyles tailored to individual's context (Portnoy et al, 2007). While some of these investigations have critiqued the value of 'stages of change' models (Trans-theoretical models) for guiding interventions (Adams & White, 2005), most view the deployment of personalised interactive information services as useful tools to support these types of lifestyle change interventions (Yardley et al, 2010). Although it is acknowledged that user studies still point to significant challenges in how best to design these services and evaluate their impact across different types of users and contexts of use.

In attempting to enhance personal health care management amongst those living with chronic disease another challenge continues to be how to ensure sustainability of self-management and lifestyle changes and to reduce subsequent behaviour regression or reversal (Demiris et al, 2008). In this context, patients' adoption and use of social media opens up the possibility of finding new ways to personalise health systems, applications and services. More specifically, community-centred models leveraging peer communication and support may generate new ways of:

- Making health interventions 'sticky' in terms of maintaining interest in use amongst different types of users and in terms of being able to adapt to changing user needs in personal health care management (Baghaei et al, 2011);
- Making interventions persuasive in terms of enhancing sustainability of initiated health and lifestyle changes over time (Torning & Oinas-kukkonen, 2009).

Looking to the future this chapter suggests that responding to the growth of social media for health may lead to more community-centred personal e-health. In this vision, the community is dynamically formed in multiple different ways – patients communicating with and advising each other, patients and health professionals working in partnerships, and patients, carers, families and healthcare professionals communicating in a more fluid and integrated manner to form genuinely supportive communities (local or virtual) to aid patients to self-manage their conditions and live longer independently in their respective communities.

FUTURE RESEARCH DIRECTIONS

There are multiple opportunities for future research in the area of social media use in relation to transforming personal health care management of chronic disease. Whilst to date most of the research the authors have undertaken has been exploratory, and the results mixed, it is understood that there is a need to develop more explanatory research and undertake robust evaluation. Certainly longitudinal studies will be of use to determine whether the use and engagement with social media and mobile web changes patient behaviours in a sustained manner. These will require larger sample sizes than have previously been used and so a mixed methodological approach may be appropriate.

There is also further evidence required into how differentials in health literacy, cultural and linguistic diversity, gender, age, level of educational attainment and socio-economic affluence interact with the use of social media and patient's abilities to gain or sustain positive changes in their self-management behaviours.

Finally, different countries have different health care systems and also data protection standards. An investigation of the risks and issues that may arise through the on-line sharing of health information across jurisdictions would be beneficial. This could then be used to develop methods of providing education to users regarding methods of assessing risks and maintaining their privacy and confidentiality when using on-line social media for health care.

CONCLUSION

This chapter has examined the emerging impact of the increasing adoption of social media and mobile web on personal health care management amongst those living with chronic diseases and conditions. It has highlighted that to engage in this examination is challenging and complex as is the result of the diversity of factors and types of users, applications and health systems involved. The chapter has argued that one impact of the increasing adoption and use of social media and mobile web is to challenge many current notions about who and how patients are engaging with management of their own health. This has included insights how some patients are complementing and/or by-passing health professionals to obtain peer support, advice and insight from other patients. While from one perspective these changes appear to support the idea of 'internet empowered patients', it was also highlighted that many users of social media for health may have limited health literacy and may be obtaining health information that is inaccurate, misleading or even harmful from their peers. It was also highlighted that in the internet space many users may be inexperienced in terms of understanding how their on-line behaviours may jeopardise their privacy and confidentiality.

This chapter has also considered how this complexity also poses challenges for healthcare systems and health informatics solutions. It has tried to examine these impacts and to explore what types of tailored/personalised information technology solutions might complement/leverage these social media and mobile web trends. One suggested approach is a move towards more community-centred solutions that leverage peer communications and the 'social' to more meaningfully tailor solutions to the attributes and lifestyles of those living with chronic disease. The future is certainly developing rapidly and we need to recognise the changing landscape that is transforming patients – health professional interactions, attitudes and expectations around the personal management of chronic disease.

It is anticipated that this chapter has contributed to advancing conceptual thinking on how health and IT are now interacting at the level of individual patients/citizens as a result of the emergence of social media and mobile web. It is hoped that the case has been made for the need for improved sophistication in the approaches to the management of chronic disease being developed by health professionals and health informatics specialists. Critically, the chapter has pointed out that the challenge for the future is how best to ensure that the benefits of social media benefits for personal healthcare management outweigh the potential dangers for patients/citizens in terms of privacy breaches, data misuse, exploitation and/or misinformation (Adams, 2010; Corea et al, 2010).

REFERENCES

Adams, S. A. (2010a). Blog-based applications and health information: Two case studies that illustrate important questions for Consumer Health Informatics (CHI) research. *International Journal of Medical Informatics*, *79*(6), e89–e96. doi:10.1016/j.ijmedinf.2008.06.009 PMID:18701344

Adams, S. A. (2010b). Revisiting the on-line health information reliability debate in the wake of web 2.0: an inter-disciplinary literature and website review. *International Journal of Medical Informatics*, *79*(6), 391–400. doi:10.1016/j.ijmedinf.2010.01.006 PMID:20188623

Andersen, N. B., & Söderqvist, T. (2012). *Social Media and Public Health Research* (Working Paper/Technical Report). Faculty of Science, University of Copenhagen.

Australian Institute of Health and Welfare (AIHW). (2010). *Australia's health 2010. Australia's health series no. 12. Cat. no. AUS 122*. Canberra, Australia: AIHW.

Australian Institute of Health and Welfare (AIHW). (2012). *Risk factors contributing to chronic disease chronic disease, Cat. no. PHE 157*. Canberra, Australia: AIHW.

Baghaei, N., Kimani, S., Freyne, J., Brindal, E., Berkovsky, S., & Smith, G. (2011). Engaging Families in Lifestyle Changes through Social Networking. *International Journal of Human-Computer Interaction, 27*(10), 971–990. doi:10.1080/10447318.2011.555315

Bhaumik, S. (2013). BRICS nations agree to collaborate on research and public health challenges. *BMJ (Clinical Research Ed.), 346*, f369. PMID:23335476

Camarinha-Matos, L. M., & Afsarmanesh, H. (2011). *Collaborative Ecosystems in Ageing Support*. Paper presented at PRO-VE'11. São Paulo, Brazil.

Charness, N., & Boot, W. R. (2009). Aging and information technology use: Potential and barriers. *Current Directions in Psychological Science, 18*(5), 253–258. doi:10.1111/j.1467-8721.2009.01647.x

Chou, W., Hunt, Y., Beckjord, E., Moser, R., & Hesse, B. (2009). Social media use in the United States: implications for health communication. *Journal of Medical Internet Research, 11*(4), 48. doi:10.2196/jmir.1249 PMID:19945947

Coleman, K., Austin, B. T., Brach, C., & Wagner, E. H. (2009). Evidence on the Chronic Care Model in the new millennium. *Health Affairs, 28*(1), 75–85. doi:10.1377/hlthaff.28.1.75 PMID:19124857

Colineau, N., & Paris, C. (2010). Talking about your health to strangers: Understanding the use of online social networks by patients. *New Review of Hypermedia and Multimedia, 16*(1-2), 141–160. doi:10.1080/13614568.2010.496131

Correa, T., Willard Hinsley, A., & de Zúñiga, H. G. (2010). Who interacts on the Web? The intersection of users' personality and social media use. *Computers in Human Behavior, 26*(2), 247–253. doi:10.1016/j.chb.2009.09.003

Cummings, E. (2008). *An investigation of the influence of an online patient diary on the health outcomes and experiences of people with chronic obstructive pulmonary disease (COPD) participating in a mentored self-management clinical controlled trial*. (PhD Thesis). University of Tasmania, Hobart, Australia.

Cummings, E., Chau, S., & Turner, P. (2009). Assessing a Patient-Centered E-Health Approach to Chronic Disease Self-Management. In E. V. Wilson (Ed.), *Patient-Centered E-Health*. Hershey, PA: Medical Information Science Reference.

Cummings, E., Robinson, A., Courtney-Pratt, H., Cameron-Tucker, H., Wood-Baker, R., & Walters, E. et al. (2010). Pathways Home: Comparing Voluntary IT and Non-IT Users Participating in a Mentored Self-Management Project. *Studies in Health Technology and Informatics, 160*, 23–27. PMID:20841643

Cummings, E., & Turner, P. (2007). Considerations for deploying web and mobile technologies to support the building of patient self-efficacy and self-management of chronic illness. In L. Al-Hakim (Ed.), *Web Mobile-Based Applications for Healthcare Management*. Hershey, PA: Idea Group, Inc. doi:10.4018/978-1-59140-658-7.ch011

Cummings, E., & Turner, P. (2008). Considerations for Deploying Web and Mobile Technologies to Support the Building of Patient Self-Efficacy and Self-Management of Chronic Illness. In S. Clarke (Ed.), *End-User Computing: Concepts, Methodologies, Tools, and Applications* (Vol. 2, pp. 1053–1064). Hershey, PA: Information Science Reference. doi:10.4018/978-1-59904-945-8.ch076

Cummings, E., & Turner, P. (2010). Patients at the Centre: Methodological Considerations for Evaluating Evidence from Health Interventions Involving Patients use of Web-Based Information Systems. *The Open Medical Informatics Journal*, *4*, 188–194. PMID:21594007

Demiris, G., Afrinb, L., Speedie, S., Courtney, K. L., Sondhie, M., & Vimarlund, V. et al. (2008). Patient-Centered Applications: Use of Information Technology to promote Disease management and Wellness. *Journal of the American Medical Informatics Association*, *15*(1), 8–13. PMID:17947617

Dickerson, S. S., Reinhart, A., Boemhke, M., & Akhu-Zaheya, L. (2011). Cancer as a Problem to Be Solved: Internet Use and Provider Communication by Men With Cancer. *Computers, Informatics, Nursing*, *29*(7), 388–395. doi:10.1097/NCN.0b013e3181f9ddb1 PMID:20975535

Eichler, K., Wieser, S., & Brügger, U. (2009). The costs of limited health literacy: A systematic review. *International Journal of Public Health*, *54*(5), 313–324. doi:10.1007/s00038-009-0058-2 PMID:19644651

Ellis, L., Showell, C., & Turner, P. (2013). Social Media and patient self management: Not all sites are created equal. In *Proceedings of Information Technology and Communications in Health (ITCH) Conference*. IOS Press.

Fox, S. (2011). *The Social Life of Health Information*. Retrieved from http://www.pewinternet.org/Reports/2011/Social-Life-of-Health-Info.aspx

Freyne, J., Berkovsky, S., Baghaei, N., Kimani, S., & Smith, G. (2011). Personalised Techniques For Lifestyle Change. In *Proceedings of the 13th International Conference on Artificial Intelligence in Medicine in Europe*. Bled, Slovenia: AIME.

Gilhooly, M. L., Gilhooly, K. J., & Jones, R. B. (2009). Quality of life: conceptual challenges in exploring the role of ICT in active ageing. In Information and Communication Technologies for Active Ageing – Opportunities and Challenges for the European Union. IOS Press.

Glasgow, N. J., Jeon, Y.-H., Kraus, S. G., & Pearce-Brown, C. L. (2008). Chronic disease self-management support: The way forward for Australia. *Med J*, *189*(10), 14.

Hanson, C. L., Cannon, B., Burton, S., & Giraud-Carrier, C. (2013). An Exploration of Social Circles and Prescription Drug Abuse Through Twitter. *Journal of Medical Internet Research*, *15*(9), e189. doi:10.2196/jmir.2741 PMID:24014109

Hawkins, A. O., Kantayya, V. S., & Sharkey-Asner, C. (2010). Health literacy: A potential barrier in caring for underserved populations. *Disease-a-Month*, *56*(12), 734–740. doi:10.1016/j.disamonth.2010.10.006 PMID:21168579

Hibbard, J., Mahoney, E., Stock, R., & Tusler, M. (2007). Self-management and health care utilization: Do increases in patient activation result in improved self-management behaviors? *Health Services Research*, *42*(4), 1443–1463. doi:10.1111/j.1475-6773.2006.00669.x PMID:17610432

Hopgood, A. A. (2005). The State of Aritificial Intelligence. *Advanced in Computers, 65*, 1–75. doi:10.1016/S0065-2458(05)65001-2

Househ, M. (2013). The Use of Social Media in HealthCare: Organisational, Clinical and Patient Perspectives. In *Proceedings of Information Technology and Communications in Health (ITCH) Conference*. IOS Press.

Huber, J., Ihrig, A., & Peters, T. et al. (2011). Decision-making in localized prostate cancer: Lessons learned from an online support group. *BJU International, 107*(10), 1570–1575. doi:10.1111/j.1464-410X.2010.09859.x PMID:21105988

Institute of Medicine (IoM). (2012). *Living well with chronic illness: A call for public health action*. Washington, DC: The National Academies Press.

International Telecommunications Union (ITU). (n.d.). *ICT data and statistics*. Retrieved from http://www.itu.int/ITU-D/ict/statistics/

Jessup, M., Courtney-Pratt, H., Robinson, A., Cameron-Tucker, H., Walters, H., & Wood-Baker, R. et al. (2006). Cementing Pathways Home: Enhancing quality of life for people with chronic obstructive pulmonary disease (COPD). *Ageing International, 31*, 232–240. doi:10.1007/BF02915231

Jones, J., Hook, S., Park, S., & Scott, L. (2011). Privacy, security and interoperability of mobile health applications. In *Proceedings of the 6th international conference on universal access in human-computer interaction*. Orlando, FL: Springer-Verlag.

Jordan, J. E., Briggs, A., Brand, C., & Osborne, R. H. (2008). Enhancing patient engagement in chronic disease self management support initiatives in Australia: The need for an integrated approach. *The Medical Journal of Australia, 189*(10). PMID:19143585

Jordan, J. E., Buchbinderb, R., & Osbourne, R. H. (2010). Conceptualising health literacy from the patient perspective. *Patient Education and Counseling, 79*(1), 36–42. doi:10.1016/j.pec.2009.10.001 PMID:19896320

Kaplan, A. M., & Haenlein, M. (2010). Users of the world, unite! The challenges and opportunities of social media. *Business Horizons, 53*(1), 59–68. doi:10.1016/j.bushor.2009.09.003

Kelly, N. (2013, June 6). 7 Trends in Global Internet Growth You Can't Afford to Ignore. *Huffington Post*. Retrieved from http://www.huffingtonpost.com/nataly-kelly/seven-trends-in-global-in_b_3382907.html

Kietzmann, J. H., Hermkens, K., McCarthy, I. P., & Silvestre, B. S. (2011). Social media? Get serious! Understanding the functional building blocks of social media. *Business Horizons, 54*(3), 241–251. doi:10.1016/j.bushor.2011.01.005

Kontos, E. Z., Emmons, K. M., Puleo, E., & Viswanath, K. (2010). Communication inequalities and public health implications of adult social networking site use in the United States. *Journal of Health Communication, 15*(Suppl 3), 216–235. doi:10.1080/10810730.2010.522689 PMID:21154095

Korda, H., & Itani, Z. (2013). Harnessing Social Media for Health Promotion and Behavior Change. *Health Promotion Practice, 14*(1), 15–23. doi:10.1177/1524839911405850 PMID:21558472

Kuijpers, W., Groen, W. G., Aaronson, N. K., & Van Harten, W. (2013). A Systematic Review of Web-Based Interventions for Patient Empowerment and Physical Activity in Chronic Diseases: Relevance for Cancer Survivors. *Journal of Medical Internet Research, 15*(2), e37. doi:10.2196/jmir.2281 PMID:23425685

Lorig, K., Ritter, P., Laurent, D., & Plant, K. (2006). Internet-Based Chronic Disease Self-Management: A Randomized Trial. *Medical Care, 44*, 964–971. doi:10.1097/01.mlr.0000233678.80203.c1 PMID:17063127

Moen, A., Smørdal, O., & Sem, I. (2009). Web-based resources for peer support-opportunities and challenges. *Studies in Health Technology and Informatics, 150*, 302–306. PMID:19745318

Moorhead, S. A., Hzlett, D. E., Harrison, L., Carroll, J. K., Irwin, A., & Hoving, C. (2013). New Dimension of Health Care: Systematic Review of the Uses, Benefits, and Limitations of Social Media for Health Communication. *Journal of Medical Internet Research, 15*(4), e85. doi:10.2196/jmir.1933 PMID:23615206

Neiger, B. L., Thackeray, R., Van Wagenen, S. A., Hanson, C. L., West, J. H., Barnes, M. D., & Fagen, M. C. (2012). Use of Social Media in Health Promotion Purposes, Key Performance Indicators, and Evaluation Metrics. *Health Promotion Practice, 13*(2), 159–164. doi:10.1177/1524839911433467 PMID:22382491

Niehaves, B., & Plattfaut, R. (2010). *T-Government for the Citizens: Digital Divide and Internet Technology Acceptance among the Elderly*. Paper presented at the T-Gov Workshop. London, UK.

Olphert, C. W., Damodaran, L., & May, A. J. (2005). *Towards digital inclusion – Engaging older people in the 'digital world'*. Paper presented at the Accessible Design in the Digital World Conference. Dundee, UK.

Østbye, T., Yarnall, K. S. H., Krause, K. M., Pollak, K., Gradison, M., & Lloyd Michener, J. (2005). Is There Time for Management of Patients With Chronic Diseases in Primary Care? *Annals of Family Medicine, 3*(3), 209–214. doi:10.1370/afm.310 PMID:15928223

Pearce-Brown, C., Glasgow, N., Jeon, H., Jenkins, S., & Douglas, K. (2009). *Health literacy and self management in COPD: The same, different or misunderstood?* Paper presented at the PHC Research Conference. New York, NY.

Portnoy, D. B., Scott-Sheldon, L. A., Johnson, B. T., & Carey, M. P. (2008). Computer-delivered interventions for health promotion and behavioural risk reduction: A meta-analysis of 75 randomized controlled trials, 1988 – 2007. *Preventive Medicine, 47*, 3–16. doi:10.1016/j.ypmed.2008.02.014 PMID:18403003

Qualman, E. (2013). *Socialnomics: How Social Media Transforms the way we live and do business* (2nd ed.). John Wiley & Sons.

Roehrer, E., Cummings, E., Beggs, S., Turner, P., Hauser, J., & Micallef, N. et al. (2013). Pilot evaluation of web enabled symptom monitoring in cystic fibrosis. *Informatics for Health & Social Care*. doi: 10.3109/17538157.2013.812646 PMID:23957685

Roehrer, E., Cummings, E., Ellis, L., & Turner, P. (2011). The role of user-centred design within online community development. *Studies in Health Technology and Informatics, 164*, 256–260. PMID:21335720

Roehrer, E., Cummings, E., Turner, P., Hauser, J., Cameron-Tucker, H., & Beggs, S. et al. (2013). Supporting cystic fibrosis with ICT. *Studies in Health Technology and Informatics, 183*, 137–141. PMID:23388270

Schwarzer, R. (1999). Self-regulatory Processes in the Adoption and Maintenance of Health Behaviours. *J Health Psychol March, 4* (2), 115-127.

Showell, C., & Turner, P. (2013). The PLU problem: are we designing personal ehealth for People Like Us? In *Proceedings of Information Technology and Communications in Health (ITCH) Conference*. IOS Press.

Simborg, D. (2010). Consumer empowerment versus consumer populism in healthcare IT. *Journal of the American Medical Informatics Association, 17*, 370–372. doi:10.1136/jamia.2010.003392 PMID:20595301

Syed-Abdul, S., Fernandez-Luque, L., Jian, W.-S., Li, Y.-C., Crain, S., & Hsu, M. et al. (2013). Misleading Health-Related Information Promoted Through Video-Based Social Media: Anorexia on YouTube. *Journal of Medical Internet Research, 15*(2), e30. doi:10.2196/jmir.2237 PMID:23406655

Thackeray, R., Neiger, B. L., Hanson, C. L., & McKenzie, J. F. (2008). Enhancing promotional strategies within social marketing programs: Use of web 2.0 social media. *Health Promotion Practice, 9*(4), 338–343. doi:10.1177/1524839908325335 PMID:18936268

Torning, K., & Oinas-Kukkonen, H. (2009). Persuasive system design: State of the art and future directions. In *Proceedings of the 4th International Conference on Persuasive Technology*. New York: ACM.

Wagner, E. H., Austin, B. T., Davis, C., Hindmarsh, M., Schaefer, J., & Bonomi, A. (2001). Improving chronic illness care: translating evidence into action. *Health Affairs, 20*(6), 64–78. doi:10.1377/hlthaff.20.6.64 PMID:11816692

Wagner, E. H., Austin, B. T., & Von Korff, M. (1996). Improving outcomes in chronic illness. *Managed Care Quarterly, 4*(2), 12–25. PMID:10157259

Webb, T. L., Joseph, J., Yardley, L., & Michie, S. (2010). Using the Internet to promote Health Behaviour Change: A systematic review and meta analysis of the impact of theoretical basis, use of behaviour change techniques, and mode of delivery on efficacy. *Journal of Medical Internet Research, 12*(1). doi:10.2196/jmir.1376 PMID:20164043

Yardley, L., Morrison, L. G., Andreou, P., Joseph, J., & Little, P. (2010). Understanding reactions to an Internet delivered healthcare intervention: Accommodating user preferences for information provision. *BMC Medical Informatics and Decision Making*, (1): 52. doi:10.1186/1472-6947-10-52 PMID:20849599

KEY TERMS AND DEFINITIONS

Info-Centrism: This refers to prevalence of thinking that prioritises the role of information over other factors. This type of thinking presumes that the provision of information axiomatically is the answer to any problem addressed.

This work was previously published in Social Media and Mobile Technologies for Healthcare edited by Mowafa Househ, Elizabeth Borycki, and Andre Kushniruk, pages 76-93, copyright year 2014 by Medical Information Science Reference (an imprint of IGI Global).

Section 3
Patient Care

Chapter 15
Best Practices to Promote Patient and Donor Engagement to Care in Living Donor Transplant

Emanuela Saita
Catholic University of the Sacred Heart, Italy

Enrico Minetti
Careggi University Hospital, Italy

Susanna Zanini
Niguarda Ca' Granda Hospital, Italy

Chiara Acquati
University of Houston, USA

ABSTRACT

Increasing evidence has demonstrated that patients' involvement promotes better health care outcomes and cost-effectiveness of services. However, limited literature is available about the experience of living donor kidney transplantation and best practices to promote patients and donors' engagement. Aim of the present chapter is to review the literature about patient engagement in the context of chronic kidney disease, and to introduce an innovative protocol developed to promote potential donors and recipients' participation and adherence to care at the Niguarda Ca' Granda Hospital in Milan (Italy). Results are critical to reflect on the identification of best practices for patients' engagement in the context of chronic kidney disease. Through a better understanding of the emotional and affective dynamics and the relational implications that may influence the elaboration of the information given by health care providers, it will be possible to develop evidence-informed interventions.

INTRODUCTION

Increasing evidence has demonstrated that patients' involvement in decision making about their treatment and care promotes better health care outcomes, higher satisfaction with care and cost-effectiveness of services (Majani & Cavallini, 2010; Stockie, 2012; Berwick, 2010; Ocloo & Fulop, 2012; Hibbard & Greene, 2013; Provenzi, Borgatti, Menozzi, & Montirosso, 2015). With increasing demand for a more

DOI: 10.4018/978-1-5225-1928-7.ch015

active role of patients in the management of their health (Crawford et al., 2002; Davis, Schoenbaum, & Audet, 2005; Bellardita et al., 2012; Barello, Graffigna, Savarese, & Bosio, 2014a; Barello, Graffigna, Vegni, & Bosio, 2014b; Menichetti, Libreri, Lozza, & Graffigna, 2014; Graffigna, Barello, & Riva, 2013; Barello & Graffigna, 2015), patient engagement (PE) is more and more considered as a key factor in the improvement of health behaviors and outcomes in the context of chronic diseases (Graffigna, Barello, Libreri, & Bosio, 2014). However, limited literature is available about the experience of living donor kidney transplantation and best practices to promote patients and donors' activation and engagement (Boulware et al., 2013).

Until sixty years ago kidney insufficiency was a lethal disease. Nowadays the scenario has changed, although this illness is still a life-threatening disease in some underdeveloped areas where dialysis is not provided by the healthcare system. Despite its severity, symptoms of the progressive loss of renal function are often absent and the patient does not perceive to be "ill" or the individual is simply not aware of the seriousness of the condition. It has been noticed that the body of the patient suffering from renal insufficiency often adjusts to the disease and its evolution over time, with the consequence that indications from the medical team about changes in diet or medications are difficult to be negotiated (Polaschek, 2003). It therefore follows that a discrepancy exists between the recommendations of the medical team and the subjective experience of the patient, who often becomes non-compliant if the changes in care and treatments are not well-communicated (Kugler, Vlaminck, Haverich, & Maes 2005; Schell, Green, Tulsky, & Arnold, 2013). It follows that behavioral changes and best adherence to therapies are achieved only if patients internalize the need for self-change (McCarley, 2009).

The provision of information to the patient is critical since the moment of diagnosis for two main reasons. First, an effective communication with the patient is essential to address concerns and questions about the medical treatment (in particular, the surgery). Second, as the individual will need to take several medications and undergo numerous medical examinations, it is important that the process is clearly explained and understood in its complexity. Hence, information is key to engage patients evaluated as clinically and psychologically eligible for a transplant (Saita, Zanini, & Fenaroli, 2012).

The practice of living-donor kidney transplantation has significantly increased in the recent past and it represents an effective way to address the growing demand for organs (Fehrman-Ekholm, Duner, Brink, Tyden, & Elinder, 2001). Furthermore, it ensures a shorter waiting period and fewer complications. Within the context of chronic kidney disease, living-donation has registered a growing interest among individuals with this illness, their relatives and friends. As family members and close ones have started to consider themselves potential donors, greater demand for information has occurred and an increased number of health care professionals are now involved in explaining practices and evaluating potential kidney donors and recipients (LaPointe Rudow et al., 2015).

In the midst of this complexity, the present chapter has two objectives: (1) to review the literature about patient engagement in the context of chronic kidney disease and (2) to present an innovative protocol developed at the Niguarda Ca' Granda Hospital in Milan (Italy) to promote patients and relatives' participation and adherence to care.

BACKGROUND

Chronic kidney disease has been defined as a "reduced glomerular filtration rate, increased urinary albumin excretion, or both" (Jha et al., 2013; p. 260) and represents an increasingly concerning public health issues. Data from the Global Burden Disease study (2010) indicate that in an interval of 20 years, from 1990 to 2010, chronic kidney disease became the 18th cause of deaths worldwide, with an increment second only to HIV and AIDS (Lozano et al., 2013). Most recent data indicate that more than 70 million people worldwide are affected by the disease (Braun, Sood, Hogue, Lieberman, & Copley-Merriman, 2012; Levey et al., 2009), and this number is expected to grow in the near future (Diamantidis & Becker, 2014). End-stage kidney disease (ESKD) requires life-saving dialysis or kidney transplantation. Worldwide, the number of patients receiving renal replacement therapy (RRT) is estimated to be more than 1.4 million with an increase in incidence of 8% annually (Schieppati & Remuzzi, 2005).

Complications from chronic kidney disease include cardiovascular mortality, increased mortality at all stages, kidney disease progression, acute kidney injury, cognitive decline, anemia and bone disorders. (Jha et al., 2013; Go, Chertow, Fan, McCulloch, & Hsu, 2004). Several strategies to reduce these complications and to assist patients' management of the disease are available. However, adherence to the recommended treatments, diet and lifestyle changes is challenging, as it is expected that the patient and his support network are able to understand, implement and maintain over time kidney-related self-care strategies (Tout, Davis, Velasquez, Banerjee, & Powe, 2013; Dageforde & Cavanaugh, 2013; Bear & Stokie, 2014). This limited adherence to self-management behaviors like managing medications, dietary recommendations and co-morbid conditions next to renal replacement therapies is confirmed extensively by the literature, as non-adherence among patients on dialysis ranges from 25% to 86%. (Kluger et al., 2005; Denhaerynck et al., 2007; Gerbino et al., 2011).

The patient suffering from kidney disease is therefore expected not only to make significant changes in his lifestyle, but also to develop communication skills necessary to improve the quality of the interaction with the health care system (Dageforde & Cavanaugh, 2013; Berkman, Sheridan, Donahue, Halpern, & Crotty, 2011). The Institute of Medicine defines health literacy as "the degree to which individuals can obtain, process, understand and communicate about health-related information needed to make informed health decisions" (cited in Berkman, Davis, & McCormack, 2010; Institute of Medicine, 2012). It has been identified as a critical competence to master, as low health literacy is associated with limited prevention, more hospital stays and higher mortality (Berkman et al., 2011). Studies consistently indicate that limited health literacy among kidney disease patients is associated with greater risk of mortality, higher blood pressure, more missed dialysis treatments and more frequent ER visits (Boulware, Carson, Troll, Powe, & Cooper, 2009; Wright, Wallston, Elasy, Ikizler, & Cavanaugh, 2011; Kleinpeter, 2003; Pollock & Jaffrey, 2007; Cavanaugh et al., 2010; Foster et al., 2011; Grubbs, Gregorich, Perez-Stable, & Hsu, 2009; Green et al., 2011; Adeseun, Bonney, & Rosas, 2012; Osborn, Cavanaugh, Wallston, White, & Rothman, 2009; Green et al., 2013).

Berkman and colleagues report that in the last decade more than forty health literacy interventions have been published (Berkman et al., 2011) with the objective to improve the effectiveness of information delivered and increase opportunities for shared decision-making. Despite the availability of educational materials (Bear & Stockie, 2014; Dageforde & Cavanaugh, 2013), approximately one-third of patients with advanced chronic kidney disease and end-stage renal disease still report low health literacy about their illness (Fraser et al., 2013; Fadem et al., 2011; Young, 2013; Finkelstein et al., 2008; Pierratos, 2013; Schell, 2012; Green et al., 2011) and education tools are not routinely implemented as part of clinical protocols (Bear & Stockie, 2014).

However, findings from a recent report confirms that patients are interested in research that targets improved communication with their providers, the selection of dialysis modality, next to the management of emotional and physical symptoms (Manns et al., 2014).

Among the available treatments, kidney transplantation is an option for patients with advanced chronic kidney disease and end-stage renal disease when a patient is considered medically and psychologically eligible. The evaluation process that precedes the approval requires an intense level of patient engagement. Despite this, the literature about kidney transplant is limited (Devraj & Gordon, 2009). Furthermore, it is now well accepted that support from significant others plays a critical role to a successful kidney transplant, as caregivers are expected to facilitate self-care and promote effective health decisions. Difficulties with the administration of medicine, errors in the dosage of medications and poor health outcomes are some of the problems associated with limited literacy of caregivers (Yin, Dreyer, Foltin, van Schaick, & Mendelsohn, 2007; Lau et al., 2010).

Therefore, the attention of the multidisciplinary healthcare team should be placed on the development of programs and educational materials aimed at increasing patients and caregivers' engagement and adherence to treatment protocols. In the case of kidney transplant from living donor, this is extremely challenging given the relationship between donors and recipients, as well as the impact on their respective quality of life. Despite this, a review of the literature conducted by the authors has revealed a gap about protocols to promote patients and donors' engagement. Although a few centers have started to develop some experiences (see this link https://www.youtube.com/watch?v=fvdL8_WNxLA for the protocol used by the Azienda ospedaliero-universitaria in Novara), protocols from both the Italian and the international context and -more importantly- evidence of their efficacy/effectiveness have not been published yet. Hence, the present contribution aims to fill this gap by introducing the Informative Groups on Kidney Transplantation from Living Donor.

MAIN FOCUS OF THE CHAPTER

Issues, Controversies, Problems

Since 1979, one hundred eighty-six kidney transplants have been successfully completed at the Nephrology Unit of the Ca' Granda Niguarda Hospital. The first transplant from a blood-related donor took place in 1979, while the first transplant from a living donor not blood related was completed in 1987. Within the Unit, in 2002 the Clinical Psychology Service has received the mandate to conduct psychological assessments of living donor transplant candidates. This process is aimed at identifying possible psychological risks for the donor and the recipient, and to report about the psychological well-being of candidates as requested by the Italian public administration. The first assessment is conducted through meetings with potential donors and recipients, as mandated by the guidelines of Italian Society of Nephrology, the National Centre for Transplants, and the law number 458 of June 26th, 1967. However, this strategy soon appeared to be insufficient and incomplete because of the limited information and feedback provided by participants.

An initial reflection on the experience led the investigators to identify key topics to assess. In particular, motivation and self-determination of the possible donor next to psychosocial characteristics of the recipient were rated as crucial, since personality traits like psychoticism, limited adherence to treatment and ability to deal with stress have been associated to higher chance of rejection (Calia, Ferrarese, Zecchini, & Orlandelli, 2006; Lovera et al., 2000; Fisher, 2003; Rupolo & Poznanzki, 1999). The difficulty to follow indication from the healthcare team, both at the present time and earlier, represents another core aspect to investigate. Predictors of non-adherence among kidney recipients have been identified in four categories: socio-economic and cultural variables (occupation and dimension of social network), psychological and psychiatric characteristics (thought process, anxiety disorders, mood disorders, substance abuse), pre-transplant non adherence (for the renal disease or other associated illnesses), and the health literacy of the patient (information about illness, treatments, risks factors, etc). This last category is of particular interest for psychologists, as it gives the professional the opportunity to guide the patient in a process of knowledge and management of the illness that prevents complications and promote quality of life. To reduce non-adherence to the transplantation protocol, the first step was then to develop a program to increase patients' engagement.

Despite it is generally accepted that engagement reduces drop-outs and complications, to date procedures that involve the team as a whole do not exists. This is the reason to offer the readers a description of the protocol implemented in the last years at the Ca' Granda Niguarda Hospital, where this program precedes the medical evaluation. In particular, this protocol is truly multidisciplinary, as doctors, nurses and psychologists contribute to the selection of contents and to its implementation. Finally, the program has been inspired by a first standardization of the psychological assessment of patients and donors candidates and it represents an active strategy of engagement.

DESCRIPTION OF THE PROTOCOLS

Step One: The Development of the SICADR (Fact Sheet for the Potential Kidney Donor)

A central component of the new protocol is the SICADR - Scheda Informativa per il Candidato Alla Donazione di Rene/*Fact Sheet for the Potential Kidney Donor* (Minetti, Zanini, & Saita. 2011) which summarizes the essential information in simple sentences with the best balance of scientific precision and comprehensibility. This informative sheet, initially implemented in 2004 (Lennerling & Nyberg, 2004; Minetti, Zanini, & Civati, 2004), has multiple purposes. First, it was introduced to standardize the information given by different health care professionals. Second, it contributed to limit the amount of missing information in the patient-doctor meeting. Similarly, it assisted balancing pros and cons to promote awareness and self-determination in the decision-making process about care and treatment. Finally, it promoted a mutual feedback between the individual and the health care professional to improve the quality of the informative exchange.

This form is designed to meet the informational needs of the donor, with the goal to involve the individual from the beginning of the transplant experience. It has been reported in the literature that potential donors sometimes show a tendency to not listen and remember only part of the information given during the consultation with the medical team; especially details about potential risks associated with the removal of a kidney (Saita & Zanini, 2011). This behavior seems to reflect defensive tendencies from the anxiety associated with the surgery and the following impact on the quality of life of the potential donor. Hence, it is crucial to provide the donor with multiple opportunities to review significant information during the decision process, as highlighted by all the guidelines for living donor transplants.

The SICADR has been introduced as a routine step of the evaluation: it is provided during a meeting with the psychologist after the potential donor has already met with the physician. Copies are also made available to the primary care physician of the potential donor, to the Third Party Committee and the judge. The SICADR has been consistently reviewed over time and a final version (available in English – see

Appendix 1) has been prepared in 2009 using the data from follow-up calls with donors. Its efficacy has also been evaluated in following studies and results have been presented at the Technical-Scientific Meeting of the Nord Italian Transplant network and at the 2010 ELPAT International Congress (Minetti et al., 2004; Minetti, Zanini, & Saita, 2011).

However, the clinical experience has highlighted that informational support, although necessary, it is not sufficient to promote donors and recipients' engagement because of the role intra-psychical and relational factors have in this process. Given the limited literature available about this topic, the research team has then decided to engage in a qualitative study to better understand the emotional and affective dynamics that may contribute to a different processing of the information provided by the healthcare team. The project was aimed at exploring representations and meanings associated with the living donor transplant experience. Two were the objectives of the study: first, to examine how organ donation and transplant were experienced by potential donors and recipients, trying to identify which aspects contribute to the difficulties of making the decision. Second, authors wanted to explore the effects organ donation has on the family dynamics, with the long term goal to confirm the hypothesis that the organ donation can only take place in families where giving and receiving are characterized by authenticity and positive exchange. This qualitative research was conducted through the methodology of the focus group, which involves that a group of people are asked questions about perceptions, beliefs and attitudes about a certain topic. It is a method extremely used in social sciences, especially when the investigator is trying to collect preliminary knowledge (Krueger, 1994).

Focus groups were conducted by two researchers with extensive knowledge of renal disease and the meetings were aimed at examining three different areas: the individuals' representations of what organ donation is and the meanings associated with the word; the motivations for organ donation; and the information needed to make the decision (both for donors and recipients). Each focus group meeting was audiotaped and transcribed by the researchers. Participants, 12 potential donors and recipients, completed informed consent form before the beginning of the study. Transcripts of the meetings were then analyzed with T-LAB (Lancia, 2004; Lancia 2012), a statistical software aimed at analyzing, comparing and graphically representing contents. Results indicate that the kidney transplant from a living donor can be placed within a relational dynamic: the motivation to give and to receive are both influenced by the relationship between the donor and the recipient. The level of intimacy and closeness between donor and recipient emerges as the most relevant factor in the decision making process: the higher the bond between them, the higher the desire to donate (Saita et al., 2012).

Step Two: GITREV Groups (Informative Groups on Kidney Transplantation from Living Donor)

From these initial results, the authors have developed informative groups about kidney transplant from living donor dedicated to potential recipients and donors treated at the Ca' Granda Niguarda Hospital. Called GITREV (Gruppi Informativi sul Trapianto di Rene da Vivente/ *Informative Groups on Kidney Transplantation from Living Donor*), they represent a multidisciplinary strategy to increase the level of participants' engagement.

While it is known from the literature that the first level of patient engagement is direct patient care (Carman et al., 2013), in which subjects get information about a condition and answer questions about treatment preferences, this is not enough in living-donor kidney transplantation. In the selection of living donors, guiding ethical principles are important (the absence of coercion or monetary reward, autonomy, beneficence, and no maleficence) and a psychological assessment is required. Furthermore, deciding for living-kidney transplantation requires an ongoing discussion with the patient and the family because of the numerous psychological implications which affect both the kidney donor and the recipient. As a consequence, past donors and recipients were invited to be part of the meeting along with the multidisciplinary team. The GITREV groups represent an essential step of the educational journey of patients and potential donors, as they are not limited to the provision of information but they recognize the ability of the individual to make informed decisions about health issues (Rossi Ferrario et al., 2009).

The GITREV meetings are organized in two moments. At first a nephrologist, a surgeon, a nurse, and a psychologist present information about kidney transplantation (the same information included in SICADR) according to the criteria of gradual disclosure, choosing non-technical language, and using images to support the description of the procedures involved. Some time for questions is included to address issues and needs of participants. In the second part of the meeting, a small group approach is used. Under the guidance of two facilitators trained in group work and with expertise in kidney transplantation's psychosocial issues, potential donors and recipients discuss about the information received. The goal is to promote free expression of emotions, worries and concerns from the participants, without fear of negative evaluation by the health care providers. The use of a peer to peer approach, for both donors and recipients, helps to provide understanding of the transplantation procedure and to improve their health and well-being. In addition to surgical information, the candidate to transplantation may learn something about a real experience and receive informal knowledge from other donors or recipients. Furthermore, a group setting is useful to facilitate discussion and to collect information about the adequacy of candidates (possible coercion, expectations, aspirations, hopes, and the quality of the relationships) and to explore the real motivation (Saita & Zanini, 2011; Saita et al., 2012).

THE EVALUATION OF GITREV

The Efficacy of GITREV Groups: Preliminary Findings

A comprehensive evaluation of the efficacy of the GITREV groups is currently underway, and preliminary findings are presented here. To date, data have been collected and analyzed about the first three GITREV groups. Two perspectives have been considered: the experiences of the members of the healthcare team leading these groups and those of potential donors and recipients. Between 4 to 6 team members have been involved in the evaluation of each group, for a total of 14 professionals. Semi-structured interviews were conducted by psychologists about topics like: satisfaction of the healthcare team members, satisfaction of the participants and feedback about the experience. The interviews were audiotaped, transcribed and analyzed with the textual analysis software ATLAS.ti (Chiarolanza & De Gregorio, 2007).

For every area investigated codes have been created, with a procedure similar to the one used by the Grounded Theory methodology (Glaser & Strauss, 1967). The goal was to identify theoretical models underlying the data by examining the relationship between codes. From codes, categories have been created and narrative themes have been investigated in the texts. The analysis of the participation of potential donors and recipients has been conducted focusing on the questions subjects asked to members of the team and group leaders during the informative and discussion session. Questions from 25 participants (12 potential recipients: 9 men and 3 women, and 13 potential donors: 11 women and 2 men) have been analyzed with the T-LAB software (Lancia, 2004). This software allows researchers to conduct a number of statistical analysis to gain a more detailed understanding of the text compared to the paper-pencil strategy. Using this software, a text (in this case the transcripts from the three GITREV group sessions) is prepared for analysis through a series of steps, which include text segmentation, automatic lemmatization and key-term selection. Subsequently, researchers are given the choice to conduct three main types of analysis: co-occurrence analysis, thematic analysis, and comparative analysis. In the present work, a Thematic Analysis of Elementary Contexts has been conducted, with the goal to extract thematic clusters from the transcripts of the meetings. Separate analyses have been conducted on the two moments of the GITREV groups: during and after the informative session, and during the group discussion.

Participants' and Team Members' Experience of the GITREV Groups

Seven codes (major themes) have been identified from the researchers, using the same words used by the participants as suggested by the literature (Tarozzi, 2008). Connections between codes have been established through similarities and juxtaposition, to create two categories.

The first category, called "*exhaustive contents*" refers to the comprehensiveness of the information provided and the possibility to deepen and to examine more in detail questions or concerns of potential donors and recipients. Both members of the healthcare team and participants highlighted this as the key characteristic of the group experience. The second category, called "*participation*" refers to the satisfaction reported from health care professionals and participants about the way the GITREV groups have been conducted. They all positively commented on the fact that communication was not univocal (from the "expert" to the audience) but bi-directional. Furthermore, participants particularly enjoyed the closeness experienced with the other members of the group, the opportunity to get to know better other potential donors and recipients, and to share the emotional aspects associated with the disease. It is very interesting to comment about reported concerns and positive consequences of the transplant, which were similar among potential donors and recipients. Donors were concerned about the change in the quality of life of the patient moving from dialysis to transplant and the following treatment regime, while recipients reported worries about the risks of nephrectomy for donors. Both, however, anticipate reciprocal positive changes for their relationship. For example, among married couple's partners expected a positive change due to the end of dialysis and to an increased physical well-being of the patient. Among dyads composed by a parent and a son or a daughter, the identified improvement was the higher quality of life of the patient, while among siblings the act of organ donation represented a way to strengthen their affective bond.

Throughout a series of following analysis the core category has emerged. Using the words of a members of the healthcare team, it has been named "*As Virgil for Dante*" to illustrate how the informative groups were perceived as a guide and support in a challenging moment of their lives. Like Virgil in the Divine Comedy has walked with Dante in the afterlife, guiding him through Hell, Purgatory and Paradise, so the groups have assisted potential donors and recipients walking through the different challenges of the transplant experience. This core category has been placed in relation with the others, in order to describe how members of the healthcare team have perceived and experienced from an intra-psychic point of view the participation in the GITREV groups (see Figure 1).

Figure 1. Professionals: Core category and its relations with the other categories

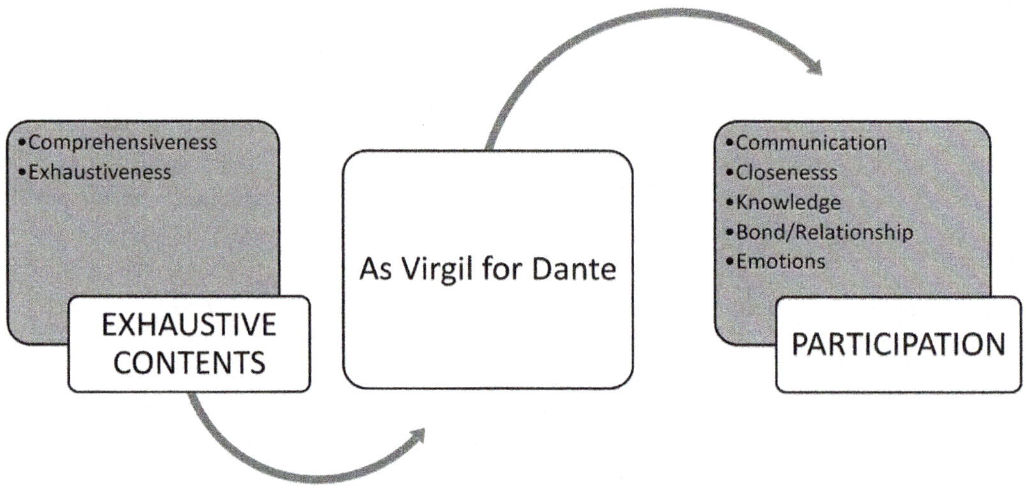

Potential Donors and Recipients' Experience on the GITREV

It is, however, the analysis of the questions asked by potential donors and recipients that is essential to describe the aspect of participation. Among the questions asked at the end of the first part of the GIT-REV, which account for 15% of the total (see Figure 2), four thematic clusters emerge (see Figure 3). The first one refers to *medical aspects* like pain management, or the efficacy of anti-rejection therapy and accounts for 24.23% of the variance. The second cluster, accounting for 28.39% of the variance, is organized around information that pertains to *nursing*. In the third cluster (29.06% of variance), lemmas refer to *psychological issues* like the risks for depressive disorders associated to a failed transplant. Finally, the fourth cluster, which accounts for 18.32% of the variance, is organized around *legal implications* of organ donation like healthcare coverage for the donor (see Figure 3).

Figure 2. Potential donors and recipients: percentages of questions in first part (1) and in the second part (2) of the GITREV

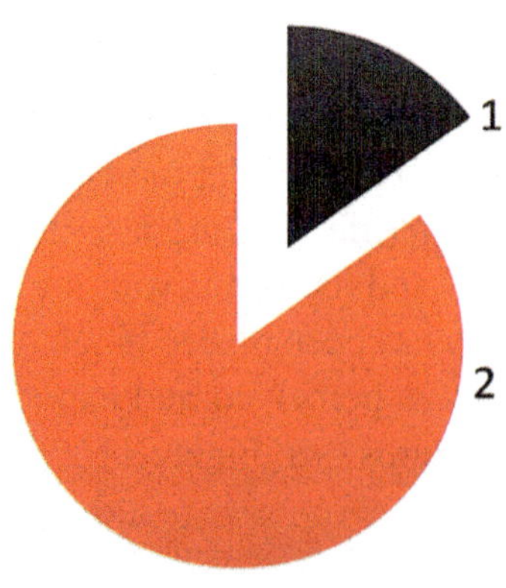

Figure 3. Thematic cluster in the first part of the GITREV

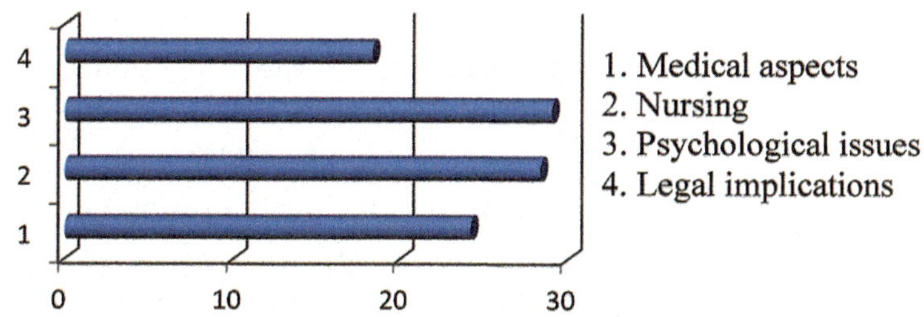

Questions asked during the group discussion, in the second half of the GITREV meeting, represent 85% of the questions asked during the whole session. Five are the thematic clusters identified through the analysis, which can be summarized in two macro areas: *information* and *emotions*. Among the macro area of information, one cluster pertains to confirm the information given by the healthcare team in the first part (20.23% of variance). A second cluster, which explains 19.07% of the variance, refers only to the need of information and clarification about post-operative pain and its management (for example, about the intensity of post-operative pain, and the dosage of anti-pain medication)

Focusing on the macro area of emotions, one cluster (accounting for 26.25% of variance) refers to the expressions of fear that both donors and recipients communicated to the team about aspects that couldn't be controlled like the survival of the donor during the surgical procedure. Hope and joy were part of another cluster explaining 24.27% of variance, while the relationship between donor and recipient is addressed in the third one (which accounts for 10.18%). From the way the questions are organized in the two moments of the group meeting, it is possible to affirm that the opportunity to meet and exchange perspectives and questions with peers promotes the active engagement of potential donors and recipients. In a similar way, participation and discussion contribute to higher satisfaction also among members of the healthcare team (see Figure 4).

SOLUTIONS AND RECOMMENDATIONS

The study has strong implications for clinical practice and patient engagement. First of all, the experience presented in this chapter is unique within the field of patient engagement in the context of chronic kidney disease. While previous studies have been limited to motivational interviewing in nursing and

Figure 4. Thematic cluster in the second part of the GITREV

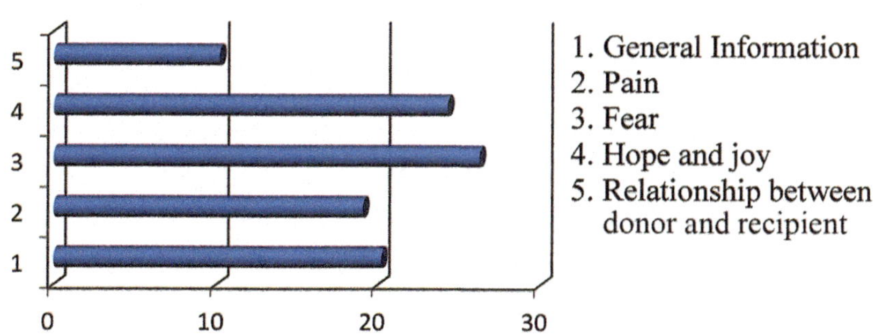

patient navigation programs (McCarley, 2009; Jolly et al., 2015), the GITREV contributes to foster patient engagement as a "process-like and multidimensional experience" (Graffigna et al., 2014, p. 1). Similarly, our findings are in line with previous studies identifying a positive relationship between engagement and quality of life (Barello & Graffigna, 2014).

From this initial analysis it is possible to appreciate how the GITREV group experience represents a setting where a tapestry of communication occurs: the medical description of the transplant process provided by the medical team is intertwined with questions and concerns of potential donors and recipients. Similarly, cognitive aspects intersect with the emotional dimensions of fear and hope. These last themes have been addressed only in a limited way by the literature. However, they tend to strongly emerge in the moment there is the opportunity for an open confrontation and a bi-directional communication between the healthcare team and potential organ donors and recipients. As health professionals explain the protocol and its side-effects to patients and their caregivers, so they are also in a position to ask questions and -more importantly- to voice their concerns and emotions.

In particular, this type of analysis has allowed the researchers to investigate the psychological implications of the introduction of a model of patient engagement as well as to evaluate attitudes towards transplantation. Results of the present work are therefore critical to reflect on the identification of best practices for patients' engagement and adherence to care in the context of chronic kidney disease. Through a better understanding of the emotional and affective dynamics and the relational implications that may influence the elaboration of the information given by health care providers, it will be possible to develop evidence-informed intervention with this population. Specifically, from our experience, donors are interested in knowing what could be the benefits for the recipients, while recipients' focus of attention is to understand risks for donors. It is therefore possible to affirm that both donors and recipients expect mutual and dyadic benefits.

We have mentioned earlier that this work was inspired by the desire to address barriers to effective communication between the team and potential organ donors and recipients as they occur in the clinical practice. One of the most delicate moment of the renal disease is the passage from conservative treatments to the dialysis or transplant. This passage is discussed with the patient by considering pros and cons of the different treatment options, giving priority to the patient's and his/her family's quality of life. In the case a living donor is available, a transplant can be completed before the dialysis (preemptive transplant). The transplant represents the best therapy for chronic renal insufficiency for the right candidate, and it is considered as life-extending because of its ability to improve the individual's quality of life and postpone death. A study has in fact demonstrated that Italian patients in dialysis show lower quality of life than transplanted patients (Mazzoni, Laghi, & Cicognani, 2013).

It is however well-known the limited availability of organs and, when an organ from a dead donor is not available, family members often offer themselves as potential donors. In case of blood-relatives, they are encouraged because of higher immunological compatibility and the lower risk of organ rejection, while for non-blood related potential donors it is often the desire to improve the health of their loved ones. Living organ donation is a topic that is creating increasing attention among patients and their relatives with the subsequent need for more information (Minetti et al, 2004). This information should be not only exhaustive, but also easy to understand for the patient in order to not compromise the success of the transplant.

FUTURE RESEARCH DIRECTIONS

The present contribution presents some limitations and it cannot be considered exemplificative of all the informative protocols about kidney transplant. On the contrary, it has been the absence of shared procedures both in the International and in the Italian context that has supported the description of the protocol implemented at the Ca' Granda Niguarda Hospital and its preliminary evaluation. Subjects, methodologies and statistical analyses have been inspired by an ethical dimension, aimed at listening to the needs of the individual with chronic kidney disease and the desire to help potential donors. In the future, this humanistic perspective should be supported by a stronger scientific rigor, in line with the directions of evidence-based medicine. However, the process leading to kidney transplant from living donor -because of its intrinsic complexity- requires analyses and strategies of study flexible and adjustable for the clinical practice. An integrative approach is necessary to assess situations and personal characteristics that poorly fit with the transplant but also to activate resources from the family and social context of the patient.

This type of transplant offers the opportunity to give without the certainty of a restitution: the aim of organ donation is then placed within the relationship between individuals and family members (Cigoli, 2006). Donation is characterized by positive connotations, and it is perceived as an idealistic and altruistic act because it requires to overcome a natural and genetically strong instinct to self-conservation, which is manifested through the care for one's integrity and safety (Saita, 2012). Given these considerations, chronic kidney disease can be considered a *we-disease* (Bodenmann, 2005; Kayser, Watson, & Andrade, 2007), an illness that affects both members of the dyad and their relationship. By assuming this perspective, it is within the relationship that it is possible to find a cure characterized by taking care of the patient, the close one and their relationship (Saita et al., 2012).

CONCLUSION

In this chapter we wanted to offer an initial reflection about some clinical practices influenced by the problems experienced by healthcare professionals working with patients with chronic kidney disease. These practices have promoted new spaces of communication among disciplines. The hope is that this first experience will contribute to increased confrontation between Medicine and Psychology with the long term goal to a more effective work with the patient, as suggested by some recent contributions (Saba, Saita & Novelli, 2011).

Summarizing, this chapter has originated from a serious clinical problem: patients and caregivers' engagement and adherence to transplant's protocol procedures and requirements, next to the efficacy of these protocols. These issues are at the core of the transplantation practice, because the success of the surgery is influenced by the adherence of the patient to the treatment and by the engagement of both potential donors and recipients. It is necessary to move from the idea that donors and recipients simply have to obey to prescribed guidelines, and to introduce the idea of a true partnership between them and the healthcare team.

Starting from issues and problems experienced by the members of the healthcare team, the protocol presented in the chapter has been developed. In its current form, the GITREV represents a multidisciplinary educational intervention that involves medical, nursing and psychological information. Informative aspects about the illness and its treatment are mixed with more expressive contents, like the possibility to share in a group setting emotional aspects and to take an active role. In this sense the GITREV promotes that ability of the members of the healthcare team to manage the diversity of situations that arise when health consumers are engaged in clinical decision making described by Barello and Graffigna (2015). This practice is coherent with the literature (Majani & Cavallini, 2010), which highlights how adherence in kidney transplant from a living donor requires higher active engagement from the patient, the donor and the family members who are expected to become involved in the preparation for the transplant.

As described before, in order to create the current protocol numerous steps have been taken and several instruments have been used. However, over time their limitations in the ability to address issues and concerns raised by patients and their relatives have emerged. Through an ongoing reflection, it has been possible to review and make adjustments to a previous clinical practice unable to address the complexity of the living donor transplant. As a consequence, a new dialogue between disciplines has started, and new strategies have emerged.

Chronic kidney disease therefore requires a constant exchange between Medicine, Psychology and Social Sciences. They all contribute to the promotion of care for patients and their relatives, as Medicine is focused on the promotion of prevention and care, Psychology assists understanding emotions and meanings associated to health and illness, and Social Sciences take in consideration the context and the multiple systems people are part of. Finally, the methodology adopted to improve patient engagement involves patient, family and health care providers in an active partnership aimed at ensuring the best quality of care. For this reason the protocol presented can be easily adapted into routine practice.

REFERENCES

Adeseun, G. A., Bonney, C. C., & Rosas, S. E. (2012). Health literacy associated with blood pressure but not other cardiovascular disease risk factors among dialysis patients. *American Journal of Hypertension*, *25*(3), 348–353. doi:10.1038/ajh.2011.252 PMID:22237154

Barello, S., & Graffigna, G. (2014). Engaging patients to recover life projectuality: An Italian cross-disease framework. [Epubaheadofprint]. *Quality of Life Research: An International Journal of Quality of Life Aspects of Treatment, Care and Rehabilitation*. doi:10.1007/s11136-014- 0846-x PMID:25373927

Barello, S., & Graffigna, G. (2015). Engagement-sensitive decision making: training doctors to sustain patient engagement in medical consultations. In G. Graffigna, S. Barello, & S. Triberti (Eds.), *Patient Engagement: A Consumer-Centered Model to Innovate Healthcare* (pp. 78–93). Berlin: De Gruyter Open. doi:10.1515/9783110452440-008

Barello, S., Graffigna, G., Savarese, M., & Bosio, A. C. (2014a). Engaging patients in health management: Towards a preliminary theoretical conceptualization. *Psicologia Della Salute*, *3*(3), 11–33. doi:10.3280/PDS2014-003002

Barello, S., Graffigna, G., Vegni, E., & Bosio, A. C. (2014b). The challenges of conceptualizing patient engagement in health care: A lexicographic literature review. *Journal of Participatory Medicine*, *6*, e9.

Bear, R. A., & Stockie, S. (2014). Patient engagement and patient-centred care in the management of advanced chronic kidney disease and chronic kidney failure. *Canadian Journal of Kidney Health and Disease*, *1*(1), 24. Published online21October2014. doi:10.1186/s40697-014-0024-7 PMID:25780613

Bellardita, L., Graffigna, G., Donegani, S., Villani, D., Villa, S., Tresoldi, V., & Valdagni, R. (2012). Patient's choice of observational strategy for early-stage prostate cancer. *Neuropsycholological Trends*, *12*, 107–116. doi:10.7358/neur-2012-012-bell

Berkman, N. D., Davis, T. C., & McCormack, L. (2010). Health literacy: What is it? *Journal of Health Communication*, *15*(sup2Suppl. 2), 9–19. doi:10.1080/10810730.2010.499985 PMID:20845189

Berkman, N. D., Sheridan, S. L., Donahue, K. E., Halpern, D. J., & Crotty, K. (2011). Low health literacy and health outcomes: An updated systematic review. *Annals of Internal Medicine*, *155*(2), 97–107. doi:10.7326/0003-4819-155-2-201107190-00005 PMID:21768583

Berwick, D. M. (2010). *What patient-centered care should mean*. Retrieved from http://patientprivacy-rights.org/wp-content/uploads/2010/02/What-Patient-Centered-Should-Mean.pdf

Bodenmann, G. (2005). Dyadic coping and its significance for marital functioning. In T. A. Revenson, K. Kayser, & G. Bodenmann (Eds.), *Couples coping with stress: Emerging perspectives on dyadic coping* (pp. 35–50). Washington, DC: American Psychological Association. doi:10.1037/11031-002

Boulware, L. E., Carson, K. A., Troll, M. U., Powe, N. R., & Cooper, L. A. (2009). Perceived susceptibility to chronic kidney disease among high-risk patients seen in primary care practices. *Journal of General Internal Medicine*, *24*(10), 1123–1129. doi:10.1007/s11606-009-1086-6 PMID:19711135

Boulware, L. E., Hill-Briggs, F., Kraus, E. S., Melancon, J. K., Falcone, B., Ephraim, P. L., & Powe, N. R. et al. (2013). Effectiveness of educational and social worker interventions to activate patients' discussion and pursuit of preemptive living donor kidney transplantation: A randomized controlled trial. *American Journal of Kidney Diseases*, *61*(3), 476–486. doi:10.1053/j.ajkd.2012.08.039 PMID:23089512

Braun, L., Sood, V., Hogue, S., Lieberman, B., & Copley-Merriman, C. (2012). High burden and unmet patient needs in chronic kidney disease. *International Journal of Nephrology and Renovascular Disease*, *5*, 151–163. doi:10.2147/IJNRD.S37766 PMID:23293534

Calia, R., Ferrarese, D., Zecchini, J., & Orlandelli, E. (2006). *Vissuti Psicosociali nel Trapianto di rene: Pazienti in lista di attesa, nel post-trapianto e nel ri-trapianto* [Psychosocial Experiences in Kidney Transplant: Patients waiting for transplant, post-transplant and re-transplant]. Roma: Accademia Lancisiana.

Carman, K. L., Dardess, P., Maurer, M., Sofaer, S., Adams, K., Bechtel, C., & Sweeney, J. (2013). Patient And Family Engagement: A Framework For Understanding The Elements And Developing Interventions And Policies. *Health Affairs*, *32*(2), 223–231. doi:10.1377/hlthaff.2012.1133 PMID:23381514

Cavanaugh, K. L., Wingard, R. M., Hakim, R. M., Eden, S., Shintani, A., Wallston, K. A., & Ikizier, T. A. et al. (2010). Low health literacy associates with increased mortality in ESRD. *Journal of the American Society of Nephrology*, *21*(11), 1979–1985. doi:10.1681/ASN.2009111163 PMID:20671215

Chiarolanza, C., & De Gregorio, E. (2007). *Lavorare con ATLAS.ti. Come analizzare i processi psico-sociali* [*Working with ATLAS.ti. How to Analyze Psychosocial Processes*]. Roma: Carocci.

Cigoli, V. (2006). *L'albero della discendenza. Clinica dei corpi familiari* [*The Descendents' Tree. A Clinical Approach to Family Bodies*]. Milano: Franco Angeli.

Crawford, M. J., Rutter, D., Manley, C., Weaver, T., & Bhui, K. (2002). Systematic review of involving patients in the planning and development of healthcare. *BMJ (Clinical Research Ed.)*, *325*(7375), 1263. doi:10.1136/bmj.325.7375.1263 PMID:12458240

Dageforde, L. A., & Cavanaugh, K. L. (2013). Health Literacy: Emerging Evidence and Applications in Kidney Disease Care. *Advances in Chronic Kidney Disease*, *20*(4), 311–319. doi:10.1053/j.ackd.2013.04.005 PMID:23809283

Davis, K., Schoenbaum, S. C., & Audet, A. M. (2005). A 2020 vision of patient-centered primary care. *Journal of General Internal Medicine*, *20*(10), 953–957. doi:10.1111/j.1525-1497.2005.0178.x PMID:16191145

Denhaerynck, K., Manhaeve, D., Dobbels, F., Garzoni, D., Nolte, C., & De Geest, S. (2007). Prevalence and consequences of nonadherence to hemodialysis regimens. *American Journal of Critical Care*, *16*(3), 222–235. PMID:17460313

Devraj, R., & Gordon, E. J. (2009). Health literacy and kidney disease: Toward a new line of research. *American Journal of Kidney Diseases*, *53*(5), 884–889. doi:10.1053/j.ajkd.2008.12.028 PMID:19324481

Diamantidis, C. J., & Becker, S. (2014). Health information technology (IT) to improve the care of patients with chronic kidney disease (CKD). *BMC Nephrology*, *15*(7). Available at http://www.biomedcentral.com/1471-2369/15/7. doi:10.1186/1471-2369-15-7 PMID:24405907

Fadem, S. Z., Walker, D. R., Abbott, G., Friedman, A. L., Goldman, R., Sexton, S., & Peters, T. G. et al. (2011). Satisfaction with renal replacement therapy and education: The American Association of Kidney Patients Survey. *Clinical Journal of the American Society of Nephrology; CJASN*, *6*(3), 605–612. doi:10.2215/CJN.06970810 PMID:21330485

Fehrman-Ekholm, I., Dunér, F., Brink, B., Tydén, G., & Elinder, C. G. (2001). No Evidence of Accelerated Loss of Kidney Function in Living Kidney Donors: Results from a cross-cultural follow-up. *Transplantation*, *72*(3), 444–449. doi:10.1097/00007890-200108150-00015 PMID:11502974

Finkelstein, F. O., Story, K., Firanek, C., Barre, P., Takano, T., Soroka, S., & Mendelssohn, D. et al. (2008). Perceived knowledge among patients cared for by Nephrologists about chronic kidney disease and ESRD therapies. *Kidney International*, *74*(9), 1178–1184. doi:10.1038/ki.2008.376 PMID:18668024

Fisher, M. S. Sr. (2003). Psychosocial evaluation interview protocol for living related and living unrelated kidney donors. *Social Work in Health Care*, *38*(1), 39–61. doi:10.1300/J010v38n01_03 PMID:14984248

Foster, M., Brice, J. H., Shofer, F., Principe, S., DeWalt, D., Falk, R., & Ferris, M. (2011). Personal disaster preparedness of dialysis patients in North Carolina. *Clinical Journal of the American Society of Nephrology; CJASN*, *6*(10), 2478–2484. doi:10.2215/CJN.03590411 PMID:21852660

Fraser, S. D., Roderick, P. J., Casey, M., Taal, M. W., Yuen, H. M., & Nutbeam, D. (2013). Prevalence and associations of limited health literacy in chronic kidney disease: A systematic review. *Nephrology, Dialysis, Transplantation*, *28*(1), 129–137. doi:10.1093/ndt/gfs371 PMID:23222414

Gerbino, G., Dimonte, V., Albasi, C., Lasorsa, C., Vitale, C., & Marangella, M. (2011). Adesione Alla Terapia Del Paziente In Emodialisi [Adherence to Care for the Patient in Dyalisis]. *Giornale Italiano di Nefrologia*, *28*(4), 416–424. PMID:21809311

Glaser, B., & Strauss, A. (1967). *The Discovery of Grounded Theory: Strategies for Qualitative Research*. New York: Aldine.

Go, A. S., Chertow, G. M., Fan, D., McCulloch, C. E., & Hsu, C. Y. (2004). Chronic kidney disease and the risks of death, cardiovascular events, and hospitalization. *The New England Journal of Medicine*, *351*(13), 1296–1305. doi:10.1056/NEJMoa041031 PMID:15385656

Graffigna, G., Barello, S., Libreri, C., & Bosio, C. A. (2014). How to engage type-2 diabetic patients in their own health management: Implications for clinical practice. *BMC Public Health*, *14*(1), 648. doi:10.1186/1471-2458-14-648 PMID:24966036

Graffigna, G., Barello, S., & Riva, G. (2013). Technologies for patient engagement. *Health Affairs*, *32*(6), 1172–1172. doi:10.1377/hlthaff.2013.0279 PMID:23733998

Green, J. A., Mor, M. K., Schields, A. M., Sevick, M. A., Palevsky, P. M., Fine, M. J., & Weisbord, S. D. et al. (2011). Prevalence and demographic and clinical associations of health literacy in patients on maintenance hemodialysis. *Clinical Journal of the American Society of Nephrology; CJASN*, *6*(6), 1354–1360. doi:10.2215/CJN.09761110 PMID:21551025

Green, J. A., Mor, M. K., Shields, A. M., Sevick, M. A., Arnold, R. M., Palevsky, P. M., & Weisbord, S. D. et al. (2013). Associations of health literacy with dialysis adherence and health resource utilization in patients receiving maintenance hemodialysis. *American Journal of Kidney Diseases*, *62*(1), 73–80. doi:10.1053/j.ajkd.2012.12.014 PMID:23352380

Grubbs, V., Gregorich, S. E., Perez-Stable, E. J., & Hsu, C. Y. (2009). Health literacy and access to kidney transplantation. *Clinical Journal of the American Society of Nephrology; CJASN*, *4*(1), 195–200. doi:10.2215/CJN.03290708 PMID:19056617

Hibbard, J., & Greene, J. (2013). What the evidence shows about patient activation: Better health outcomes and care experiences; fewer data on costs. *Health Affairs*, *32*(2), 207–214. doi:10.1377/hlthaff.2012.1061 PMID:23381511

Institute of Medicine. (2012). *How Can Health Care Organizations Become More Health Literate? Workshop Summary*. Washington, DC: National Academies Press.

Jha, V., Garcia-Garcia, G., Iseki, K., Li, Z., Naicker, S., Plattner, B., & Yang, C. W. et al. (2013). Chronic kidney disease: Global dimension and perspectives. *Lancet*, *382*(9888), 260–272. http://www.ncbi.nlm.nih.gov/pubmed/23727169. doi:10.1016/S0140-6736(13)60687-X PMID:23727169

Jolly, S. E., Navaneethan, S. D., Schold, J. D., Arrigain, S., Koning, V., Burrucker, Y. K., & Nally, J. V. et al. (2015). Development of a chronic kidney disease patient navigator program. *BMC Nephrology*, *16*(1), 69. doi:10.1186/s12882-015-0060-2 PMID:26024966

Kayser, K., Watson, E., & Andrade, J. T. (2007). Cancer as a we-disease: Examining the process of coping from a relational perspective. *Families, Systems & Health*, *25*(4), 404–418. doi:10.1037/1091-7527.25.4.404

Kleinpeter, M. A. (2003). Health literacy affects peritoneal dialysis performance and outcomes. *Advances in Peritoneal Dialysis. Conference on Peritoneal Dialysis*, *19*, 115–119. PMID:14763046

Krueger, R. A. (1994). *Focus groups. A practical Guide for Applied Research*. Thousand Oaks, CA: Sage Publications.

Kugler, C., Vlaminck, H., Haverich, A., & Maes, B. (2005). Nonadherence with diet and fluid restrictions among adults having hemodialysis. *Journal of Nursing Scholarship*, *37*(1), 25–29. doi:10.1111/j.1547-5069.2005.00009.x PMID:15813583

Lancia, F. (2004). *Strumenti per l'analisi dei testi. Introduzione all'uso di T-LAB* [*Instruments for Textual Analysis. An Introduction to the Use of T-LAB*]. Milano: Franco Angeli.

Lancia, F. (2012). T-LAB 8.0 – User's Manual. Available at http://tlab.it/it/bibliography.php

LaPointe Rudow, D., Hays, R., Baliga, P., Cohen, DJ, Cooper, M., & Danovitch, G, M.,... & Rodrigue, J. R. (2015). Consensus conference on best practices in live kidney donation: Recommendations to optimize education, access, and care. *American Journal of Transplantation*, *15*(4), 914–922. doi:10.1111/ajt.13173 PMID:25648884

Lau, D. T., Berman, R., Halpern, L., Pickard, A. S., Schrauf, R., & Witt, W. (2010). Exploring factors that influence informal caregiving in medication management for home hospice patients. *Journal of Palliative Medicine*, *13*(9), 1085–1090. doi:10.1089/jpm.2010.0082 PMID:20836633

Lennerling, A., & Nyberg, G. (2004). Written information for potential living kidney donors. *Transplant International*, *17*(8), 449–452. doi:10.1111/j.1432-2277.2004.tb00468.x PMID:15322746

Levey, A. S., Schoolwerth, A. C., Burrows, N. R., Williams, D. E., Stith, K. R., & McClellan, W. (2009). Comprehensive public health strategies for preventing the development, progression, and complications of CKD: Report of an expert panel convened by the Centers for Disease Control and Prevention. *American Journal of Kidney Diseases*, *53*(3), 522–535. doi:10.1053/j.ajkd.2008.11.019 PMID:19231739

Lovera, G., Basile, A., Bertolotti, M., Comazzi, A. M., Clerici, C. A., Gandione, M., & Ponton, P. et al. (2000). L'assistenza psicologica nei trapianti d'organo. [Psychological Care in Organ Transplants]. *Annali dell'Istituto Superiore di Sanita*, *36*(2), 225–246. PMID:11213654

Lozano, R., Naghavi, M., Foreman, K., Lim, S., Shibuya, K., Aboyans, V., & AlMazroa, M. A. et al. (2013). Global and regional mortality from 235 causes of death for 20 age groups in 1990 and 2010: A systematic analysis for the Global Burden of Disease Study. *Lancet*, *380*(9859), 2095–2128. doi:10.1016/S0140-6736(12)61728-0 PMID:23245604

Majani, G., & Cavallini, L. (2010). Il ruolo del paziente nella gestione di una terapia a lungo termine. Dalla compliance all'adherence. [Patient's role in the management of a long term treatment. From compliance to adherence]. *Giornale Italiano di Nefrologia*, *27*(3), 316–318. PMID:20540027

Manns, B., Hemmelgarn, B., Lillie, E., Crowe, S., Cyr, A., Gladish, M., & Laupacis, A. et al. (2014). Setting research priorities for patients on or nearing dialysis. *Clinical Journal of the American Society of Nephrology; CJASN*, *9*(10), 1813–1821. doi:10.2215/CJN.01610214 PMID:24832095

Mazzoni, D., Laghi, M., & Cicognani, E. (2013). Qualità della vita e fattori psicosociali nei pazienti con insufficienza renale [Quality of life and psychosocial factors in patients with Renal Insufficiency]. *Psicologia della Salute*, *3*, 5–27. doi:10.3280/PDS2013-003001

McCarley, P. (2009). Patient empowerment and motivational interviewing: Engaging patients to self-manage their own care. *Nephrology Nursing Journal*, *36*(4), 409–413. PMID:19715108

Menichetti, J., Libreri, C., Lozza, E., & Graffigna, G. (2014). Giving patients a starring role in their own care: A bibliometric analysis of the on-going literature debate. [Epubaheadofprint]. *Health Expectations*, n/a. doi:10.1111/hex.12299 PMID:25369557

Minetti, E., Zanini, S., & Civati, G. (2004). *Scheda informativa per il potenziale donatore vivente di rene* [[*Fact Sheet for the Potential Kidney Donor]*]. Ancona: Riunione Scientifica Nord Italia Transplant Program.

Minetti, E., Zanini, S., & Saita, E. (2011). Evaluation of Effectiveness of Information for the Candidate to Kidney Donation. In W. Weimar, M. Bos, & J. van Buschbach (Eds.), Organ Transplantation: Ethical, Legal and Psychological Aspects (pp. 322-328), Vol II, Pabst Science Publisher.

Ocloo, J. E., & Fulop, N. J. (2012). Developing a 'Critical' approach to patient and public involvement in patient safety in the NHS: Learning lessons from other parts of the public sector? *Health Expectations*, *15*(4), 424–432. doi:10.1111/j.1369-7625.2011.00695.x PMID:21711471

Osborn, C. Y., Cavanaugh, K., Wallston, K. A., White, R. O., & Rothman, R. L. (2009). Diabetes numeracy: An overlooked factor in understanding racial disparities in glycemic control. *Diabetes Care*, *32*(9), 1614–1619. doi:10.2337/dc09-0425 PMID:19401443

Pierratos, A. (2013). Patient Education in Chronic Kidney Disease and Dialysis. *Seminars in Dialysis*, *26*(2), 135–137. doi:10.1111/sdi.12081 PMID:23520986

Polaschek, N. (2003). Negotiated care: A model for nursing work in the renal setting. *Journal of Advanced Nursing*, *42*(4), 355–363. doi:10.1046/j.1365-2648.2003.02627.x PMID:12752880

Pollock, J. B., & Jaffery, J. B. (2007). Knowledge of phosphorus compared with other nutrients in maintenance dialysis patients. *Journal of Renal Nutrition*, *17*(5), 323–328. doi:10.1053/j.jrn.2007.05.009 PMID:17720101

Provenzi, L., Borgatti, R., Menozzi, G., & Montirosso, R. (2015). A dynamic system analysis of dyadic flexibility and stability across the Face-to-Face Still-Face procedure: Application of the State Space Grid. *Infant Behavior and Development*, *38*, 1–10. doi:10.1016/j.infbeh.2014.10.001 PMID:25463152

Rossi Ferrario, S., Zotti, A. M., Pasetti, C., Comazzi, F., Giorgi, I., Negri, M., & Omarini, P. et al. (2009). Communicating medical information: A little lesson from italian patients. *Giornale Italiano di Medicina del Lavoro Ed Ergonomia*, *31*(3Suppl B), b12–b16. PMID:20518222

Rupolo, G., & Poznanzki, C. (1999). *Psicologia e psichiatria del trapianto d'organi* [*Psychology and Psychiatry on Organ Tranplants*]. Milano: Masson.

Saba, G. W., Saita, E., & Novelli, M. (2011). Pearls Toolbox: l'equipaggiamento psicologico per il medico [Pearls Toolbox: Psychological tools for the medical doctor]. In E. Saita (a cura di) Pensare alla salute e alla malattia [Thinking of Health and Illness] (pp. 53-67). Milano: EDUcatt.

Saita, E. (2012). Il corpo condiviso. La motivazione a donare parti di sé. [The Shared Body. The motivation to donate a part of him/herSelf]. *Ricerche di Psicologia*, *4*, 639–641.

Saita, E., & Zanini, S. (2011). Donare un rene: le determinanti di una scelta. (Donating a Kidney: determinants of the choice). In G. Castelnuovo, R. Menici, & M. Fedi (Eds.), *La donazione in Italia. Situazione e prospettive della donazione di sangue, organi, tessuti, cellule e midollo osseo* [Donation in Italy. Current Status and Prospectives in Blood, Organs, Tissues, Cells and Bone-Marrow]. (pp. 195–205). Milano: Springer-Verlag.

Saita, E., Zanini, S., & Fenaroli, V. (2012). Il trapianto di rene da vivente: Le motivazioni a donare e a ricevere un rene. [Kidney Transplant from Living Donor: Motivations to Give and Receive a Kidney]. *Ricerche di Psicologia*, *4*, 693–711. doi:10.3280/RIP2012-004008

Schell, J. O., Green, J. A., Tulsky, J. A., & Arnold, R. M. (2013). Communication Skills Training for Dialysis Decision-Making and End-of-Life Care in Nephrology. *Clinical Journal of American Society of Nephrology*, *8*(4), 675–680. doi:10.2215/CJN.05220512 PMID:23143502

Schell, J. O., Patel, U. D., Steinhauser, K. E., Ammarell, N., & Tulsky, J. A. (2012). Discussion of kidney disease trajectory by elderly patients and Nephrologists: A qualitative study. *American Journal of Kidney Diseases*, *59*(4), 495–503. doi:10.1053/j.ajkd.2011.11.023 PMID:22221483

Schieppati, A., & Remuzzi, G. (2005). Chronic renal disease as a public health problem: Epidemiology, social, and economic implications. *Kidney International*, *68*(Suppl. 98), S7–S10. doi:10.1111/j.1523-1755.2005.09801.x PMID:16108976

Stockie, S. (2012). *Making patient-centred care a reality for Ontario Hospitals* [Unpublished MBA Thesis]. York University, Toronto.

Tarozzi, M. (2008). *Che cos'è la grounded theory* [*What Grounded Theory is*]. Roma: Carocci.

Tout, D. S., Davis, E., Velasquez, A., Banerjee, T., & Powe, N. R. (2013). Assessment of Printed Patient-Educational Materials for Chronic Kidney Disease. *American Journal of Nephrology*, *38*(3), 184–194. doi:10.1159/000354314 PMID:23970127

Wright, J. A., Wallston, K. A., Elasy, T. A., Ikizler, T. A., & Cavanaugh, K. L. (2011). Development and results of a kidney disease knowledge survey given to patients with CKD. *American Journal of Kidney Diseases*, *57*(3), 387–395. doi:10.1053/j.ajkd.2010.09.018 PMID:21168943

Yin, H. S., Dreyer, B. P., Foltin, G., van Schaick, L., & Mendelsohn, A. L. (2007). Association of low caregiver health literacy with reported use of non-standardized dosing instruments and lack of knowledge of weight-based dosing. *Ambulatory Pediatrics*, *7*(4), 292–298. doi:10.1016/j.ambp.2007.04.004 PMID:17660100

Young, B. A. (2013). Health Literacy in Nephrology: Why is it Important? *American Journal of Kidney Diseases*, *62*(1), 3–6. doi:10.1053/j.ajkd.2013.04.003 PMID:23773837

KEY TERMS AND DEFINITIONS

SICADR: Scheda Informativa per i Candidati alla Donazione di Rene.
GITREV: Gruppo Informativo Trapianto di Rene tra Viventi.

This work was previously published in Transformative Healthcare Practice through Patient Engagement edited by Guendalina Graffigna, pages 1-28, copyright year 2017 by Medical Information Science Reference (an imprint of IGI Global).

APPENDIX

SICADR: Fact Sheet for the Potential Kidney Donor

Information for Potential Kidney Donors

During the presentation of the process of evaluating your suitability to donate a kidney, the nephrologist and clinical psychologist described many aspects in order to help you make a free and informed decision concerning the donation.

We here summarise the key points and ask you to indicate whether you have clearly understood the information received.

1. Living donor kidney transplant represents an alternative to cadaveric donor kidney transplant and to dialysis.
   I understand [ ] *yes* [ ] *no*
2. The evaluation of the suitability of a donor is intended to minimise the following risks:
   - The risk of an unwilling donation.
   - The risk of the operation.
   - The risk of diseases affecting the remaining kidney.
   - The risk of the failure of the kidney transplantation.
   - The risk of transmitting a disease to the recipient.

     Minimising these risks does not mean excluding them with absolute certainty.
     I understand [ ] *yes* [ ] *no*
3. The evaluation process provides an opportunity of discovering any diseases and initiating possible treatments.
   I understand [ ] *yes* [ ] *no*
4. The decision as to which surgical technique is used to harvest the kidney (traditional or video-laparascopic) is made by the surgeon on the basis of the specific characteristics of the donor. The average duration of hospitalisation is seven days.
   I understand [ ] *yes* [ ] *no*
5. The complications depend on the surgical procedure; they tend to be higher with the video laparascopic technique. It is essential that, before the operation, donors give their consent to receive transfusions in the case of intra- or postoperative haemorrhaging.
   I understand [ ] *yes* [ ] *no*
6. A transplanted kidney has an average life of about 15 years. A kidney transplant does not constitute a complete recovery since the recipient will need pharmacologic therapy to prevent rejection for all the kidney life.
   I understand [ ] *yes* [ ] *no*
7. The results of kidney transplantation from a living donor (a relative or otherwise) are better than those of transplantation from a cadaveric donor.
   I understand [ ] *yes* [ ] *no*

8. While convalescing, donors cannot undertake any strenuous physical activities for a period of about two months. Subsequently, all physical activities can be resumed without any limitation. Check-up examinations at our Centre are foreseen one, three, six and twelve months after the operation, and are subsequently recommended every year.
   I understand [ ] *yes* [ ] *no*
9. The evaluation of the suitability of a donor involves many resources, and can therefore only be started if the donor is convinced that he/she really intends to make the donation.
   I understand [ ] *yes* [ ] *no*
10. Donors can freely interrupt the process at any time before the operation.
   I understand [ ] *yes* [ ] *no*
11. Years after having made a donation, donors describe the experience positively regardless of its outcome.
   I understand [ ] *yes* [ ] *no*
12. The donation of a kidney must be totally voluntary and so no form of payment is allowed; donors must feel free of any responsibility towards the recipient if the process of donation is interrupted for any reason.
   I understand [ ] *yes* [ ] *no*

Date................................ Signature...................................

This information sheet was jointly drawn up by:

Struttura Complessa di Nefrologia, Struttura Semplice Dipartimentale
Dialisi e Terapia del Trapianto Renale Servizio di Psicologia Clinica
Responsabile: Dott. Enrico Minetti Referente per la SC di Nefrologia: Dr.ssa Susanna Zanini, Ambulatorio Trapianti Tel. 02.6444.2670 Ambulatorio Tel. 02.6444.2306
Version 2.0 6/2009.
Azienda Ospedaliera
Ospedale Niguarda Ca' Granda
Piazza Ospedale Maggiore, 3 - 20162 Milano
Tel. 02/6444.2521 – Fax: 02/6444.2909

Chapter 16
A Need for Greater Collaboration:
Initiatives to Improve Transitions of Care

Mariette Sourial
Palm Beach Atlantic University, USA

Angelica Constanzo
University of Kansas Hospital, USA

Jo Ann M. Bamdas
Florida Atlantic University, USA

Marina E. Ishak
Palm Beach Atlantic University, USA

ABSTRACT

Patient safety concerns have risen to such levels that multiple organizations and initiatives have been created to reduce hospital readmissions and medication errors in the United States healthcare system. Interprofessional education and collaborative practice (IPECP) has become a center of focus in healthcare education and the competency-based programs help health providers function more effectively as a team, train new university and college healthcare students to become ready for collaborative practice, and assist in making new policies and practices to improve today's healthcare system. This chapter provides a comprehensive overview of healthcare initiatives created to help lower hospital readmission rates and polypharmacy errors. These projects, programs, and initiatives optimize patient care while minimizing costs. With pharmacists, physicians, nurses, social workers, and other professionals and caregivers build better teams with improved communication and understanding each other's roles and responsibilities, the global healthcare system will overcome the numerous challenges.

INTRODUCTION

A Patient's Story

TP is a 78-year old African American female who presented to the hospital complaining of shortness of breath. Her shortness of breath in addition to throbbing headaches began a few days ago and worsened today, for which she was admitted. Her past medical history is significant for hypertension, reduced ejec-

DOI: 10.4018/978-1-5225-1928-7.ch016

tion fraction heart failure, non-valvular atrial fibrillation, and hypothyroidism. Patient denies smoking or using illicit drug. She reported compliant with her medications and was taking the following, which were written on a piece of a paper: lisinopril 10 mg by mouth daily, carvedilol 6.25 mg by mouth twice daily, furosemide 80 mg by mouth twice daily, diltiazem hydrochloride 120 mg by mouth once daily, rivaroxaban 15 mg by mouth daily, and levothyroxine 75 mcg by mouth every morning. Her pulse upon admission varied from 151 to 92 and her blood pressure between 144/76 mmHg to 160/91 mmHg. Her serum creatinine was 1.9 and her blood urea nitrogen was 35 (her baseline was a serum creatinine of 1.7). Other pertinent labs were within normal limits. ECG showed atrial fibrillation with rapid ventricular response. Upon hospitalization, some of her medication regimens were changed – carvedilol was increased to 12.5 mg by mouth twice daily, lisinopril was decreased to 5 mg by mouth once daily, and furosemide 80 mg by mouth once daily was switched to bumetanide 1 mg by mouth once daily. The discharge instructions were provided by the healthcare team, yet the patient could not recall the discussion. She was confused with regard to the complexity of her medical conditions and the changes in her medication regimen, which were necessary for her post-discharge home care.

Two days later, the patient was readmitted to the hospital with similar symptoms. Upon further discussion, it appears that the patient was confused in her medication regimens and was taking her medications inappropriately. Luckily, she had brought with her the medication bottles, and was referred to the clinical pharmacist for medication reconciliation. The patient was taking carvedilol 12.5 mg by mouth twice daily along with her original regimen of 6.25 mg by mouth twice daily, for a total of 18.75 mg by mouth twice daily. We also discovered that the rivaroxaban 15 mg required prior authorization, but she was going off a physician sample that had a few pills left. Her diltiazem bottle was found to be emptied and dated since last month. When asked, the patient claimed it did not have refills and she had not had been able to visit her cardiologist yet.

Problem

TP's story powerfully reminds the importance of safe and effective transitions of care. She left the healthcare setting without being fully able to care for her conditions due to the lack of appropriate education based on her level of understanding and to gaps in communication between the healthcare providers. In order to be proactive in her own care, TP could have used a notebook to write down important information for discussion with her healthcare providers.

Predominantly, communication gaps are one of the major causes of ineffective transitions of care. Healthcare providers may not communicate information completely between the members of the team, to the patient, or their caregivers. Various risk factors that may contribute to such communication breakdowns include different expectations between senders and receivers, a culture that lacks teamwork and respect, a culture that does not promote a successful hand-off, inadequate time, and lack of standardized procedures (The Joint Commission, Joint Commission Center for Transforming Healthcare, & Joint Commission Resources, n.d.).

Secondly, a patient's level of understanding of the provided education is another major challenge in transitions of care. The patient's understanding can affect the way their health is managed. Sometimes, patients and caregivers receive conflicting information about their health, are excluded from the decision making, and are confused in their medication regimens, as seen in this patient. TP had multiple comorbid conditions and was taking multiple medications with various dosing regimens, placing her at risk for medication errors. Patients and caregivers sometimes are also excluded from the decisions making. Furthermore, unclear instructions related to timely follow-up may pose an obstacle to the patient's health (The Joint Commission et al., n.d.).

Solution

This story provides several examples of many real world polypharmacy problems occurring daily. This unfortunate readmission could have been prevented with a proper and accurate medication history as well as improved communication among health professionals. A healthcare team including a physician, nurse, pharmacist, and others as appropriate also should include the patient in their decision making. Furthermore, the team should collaborate with effective communication techniques from the moment the patient enters into their care. Each member of a healthcare team needs to be held accountable for ensuring that the patient's healthcare needs are coordinated and met across the different settings. While the healthcare team is accountable for the care of the patient, the patient also has the responsibility of taking care of their own health. Each of the various professionals are entrusted with a unique body of knowledge that they use in practice. For example, pharmacists in TP's case should have looked at her medication therapy and should have ensured that the prescribed medications indicated for her medical conditions were safe, effective, affordable, and that TP could adhere to the regimen.

Other topics of concern needing solutions for this patient center on patient education, on the patient's voice in decision making, and on discharge planning. Appropriate patient education given at the level of TP's understanding should have been done for her medications and medical conditions. A great need exists for the healthcare team to empower and hear the patient's voice and place them at the core of any health decision making. Moreover, proper discharge planning is needed with steps taken to ensure that the patient has sufficient knowledge and understanding of their medical condition and care plan as well as access to contact information and follow up. These areas of concern addressed are just a few that can lead to many preventable readmissions; this stresses the need for better coordination of care with all team members participating across settings to save costs as well as improve the quality and safety of patient care.

Implications

It is important to understand the term care transition or transitions of care. According to the American Society of Health System Pharmacists (ASHP, 2016), a resource for pharmacists, student pharmacists, and others, the term care transitions:

... is the movement of a patient from one setting of care to another. In concert with physicians, nurses, and others who contribute to the overall medical care of patients, pharmacists optimize medication therapy that translates into improved outcomes, reduced readmissions, and the overall goal of improved quality of life for patients.

According to Coleman and Boult (2003), the American Geriatrics Society published a position statement defining transitional care as a "set of actions designed to ensure the coordination and continuity of healthcare as patients transfer between different locations or different levels of care within the same location" (p. 556).

In a study by Jencks, Williams, and Coleman (2009), almost one fifth of the Medicare patients who had been discharged from a hospital were rehospitalized within 30 days. During transitions of care patients become vulnerable, especially to medication-related errors. In a study conducted by Foster, Murff, Peterson, Gandhi, and Bates (2003), nearly one out of five patients experienced an adverse drug event post discharge, ranging from abnormal laboratory findings to permanent disabilities (pp. 164-165). During hospitalization, drugs may be added or discontinued from a patient's medication regimen or dosing may be altered. A systematic review by Tam et al. (2005) revealed that 10-67% of patients had at least one error in their prescription medication histories (p. 511). Patients with complex medical conditions often find themselves cared for in many different healthcare settings and/or see different practitioners. Despite collaborative care teams, communication can be less than ideal. In an acute care setting, hospitalists often focus on the critical diagnosis while deferring chronic disease management to the patient's primary care provider. Several studies discussed later explore the use a transitional care pharmacist and demonstrate the benefit of pharmacist involvement in the continuum of care process. Incorporating accurate medication reconciliation into hospital practice improves transitions of care, yet chart reviews reveal that over half of all hospital medication errors occur at the interfaces of care (Rozich & Resar, 2001). To address deficiencies, cooperative systems should be put in place between different settings and professionals.

PATIENT PROTECTION AND AFFORDABLE CARE ACT

Under the Patient Protection and Affordable Care Act (2010), new financial incentives and penalties have been implemented to optimize the healthcare system and improve patient outcomes. One important initiative through the Centers for Medicare & Medicaid Services (CMS, 2016b) has been Medicare's Hospital Readmissions Reduction Program (HRRP), which began in October 2012. This program penalizes hospitals with excess unplanned 30-day readmissions for *initial* hospitalization. The penalties apply due to specific health conditions such as pneumonia, heart attacks, heart failure, chronic obstructive pulmonary disease, and hip/knee replacement regardless of whether the patient was readmitted to the same or another hospital as well as regardless of the reason for the readmission. The reduction in Medicare payments for Inpatient Prospective Payment System (IPPS) hospitals has been increasing each year, with a 1% reduction in 2013, 2% in 2014, and 3% in 2015 (CMS, 2016b). Thus, the main focus of several hospitals has been to lower those readmission rates. In turn, new opportunities have been created for collaboration among healthcare providers and even at the education level among students of various healthcare disciplines. Hospitals work at improving their discharge processes such as creating patient-friendly educational health videos, printing patient-tailored brochures, and incorporating transitional care initiatives to follow-up post-discharge either through phone calls or with a visit.

INNOVATIVE COMMUNITY TRANSITIONS OF CARE INITIATIVES

Several innovative initiatives designed by hospitals, as well as through colleges and universities, help increase patient safety and decrease readmission rates. Some include improving the medication reconciliation process, enhancing patient health education, improving patient discharge communication, coordinating care with the patient's providers, and reducing medical complications during the hospital stay. Many care coordination and transitions of care initiatives have emerged to address the challenges that have risen by the HRRP. These initiatives such as Project RED (Re-Engineered Discharge) (Project RED, 2014), and others such as Avoid Readmission through Collaboration (ARC, 2013b), Project BOOST (Better Outcomes for Older adults through Safe Transitions) (Society of Hospital Medicine, 2015), Script Your Future (Script Your Future, 2016), and Pharm2Pharm (University of Hawai'i at Hilo, 2012) have proven to be successful in overcoming some of those challenges and are discussed in this chapter. These are by no means a comprehensive list as there are other numerous successful initiatives currently available. With a continued push to collaborate, healthcare organizations should continue to seek collaborative partnerships and invest in sustaining them. Furthermore, to prepare health professional students for collaborative partnership in practice, many academic institutions are investing in interprofessional education as means to set the standard for such team-based practice and patient safety.

In the next few sections, collaborative opportunities are explored and discussed. In addition, proven transitional care initiatives designed specifically to address the challenges in the HRRP are highlighted in order to benefit the institutions, providers, and, ultimately, patients.

DISCUSSION

Interprofessional Collaboration

As the healthcare system has evolved, providers' integration has occurred through the formation of interdisciplinary teams. Institutions have been adopting new models in order to increase efficiency and improve patient outcomes (McDaniel & Robertson, 1995). These healthcare professionals share the same primary goal of serving patients. While each provider has their own set of duties and primary focus, their overall commitment to healthcare allows for collaborative work to ensure optimum patient care. An interprofessional team includes a physician, nurse, pharmacist, social worker, and others as appropriate. This interactive team communicates, collaborates, and coordinates a patient's care plan. The team begins this at admission and continues it throughout the entire inpatient stay, then focuses on a successful transition to outpatient (The Joint Commission et al., n.d.).

The health care team should be interprofessional and include a physician, a nurse, and a pharmacist, among other providers. An overview of the roles, responsibilities, education, and brief overview of these team members are discussed next.

Physician

The primary leader in an interprofessional team is the physician. The educational background of a physician is built on the foundation of medical school. Medical school consists of a total of four years: two being didactic, where students learn in the classroom setting, and two experiential, where they go on rotations in different focused medical settings. Post-graduation and upon licensure, physicians earn the title of Medical Doctor (MD) or Doctor of Osteopathic Medicine (DO). These physicians must undergo multiple post graduate years (PGY) of residency training where they practice, but also focus on sharpening their skills before completing final training. If a physician wants to specialize in a specific field of medicine, additional training is necessary. Physicians are considered a team leader as their primary role focuses on diagnosing. After determining a diagnosis, it is the responsibility of the physician to prescribe and coordinate the patient's overall healthcare plan with other providers on the team. Other duties a physician may have on a collaborative team includes providing referrals to other specialized practitioners who are specific to the patient's needs (The University of Texas at Austin, n.d.).

Over the past decade, there has been an increase in the amount of patients needing medical attention. This rise in the number of patients have outnumbered the amount of physicians available to attend to them.

Physician Assistants (PAs)

Physician assistants (PAs) can play a prominent role in healthcare when physicians are scarce. PAs undergo similar training as physicians; however, instead of a total of a 4-year program, it is a total of three years. The first two years are devoted to didactic coursework and the remaining year to clinical experience with participation in rotations in different settings. After completion of a PA program, PAs are not required to undertake a residency and can immediately start working (American Academy of Physician Assistants, 2006). While medical doctors can practice independently, PAs cannot. Each must share the responsibility of the patient with a supervising physician to provide optimum patient care. The responsibility of the PA includes diagnosing, interpreting and ordering labs, and prescribing. When a PA prescribes a medication, they are acting on behalf of the supervising physician. However, some variation of prescribing controlled substances may differ among states.

Physician's duties sometimes can become overwhelming due to an influx of patients or lack of time. One potential solution to this problem includes incorporating PAs on an interdisciplinary team where more patients can be seen and treated, thereby maximizing time and resources that are given to each patient. Although physicians and PAs provide the initial provider encounter for the patient, nurses have the most direct contact with the patient.

Nurse

In addition, nurses play a crucial role of a healthcare team as they ensure patient needs and communicate requests to other members of the healthcare team. Nurses are able to capture this component as their educational background allows for it. Nurses typically undergo a 3- to 4-year program that is divided into didactic and clinical experience (American Association of Colleges of Nursing [AACN], 2016). Upon completion of the program, nurses earn the title of being a registered nurse (RN). The roles and responsibilities of nurses depend on the designation of the nurse (Registered Nurse, Nurse Practitioner, and others). Some nurses may desire to expand their duties and go through more schooling to become an advanced registered nurse practitioner (ARNP) or doctor of nurse practitioner (DNP). ARNPs and DNPs have extended responsibilities because of being able to diagnose and prescribe medications; however, some differences exist between states regarding the ability to prescribe controlled substances. All types of nurses, however, are able to practice in different settings including, but not limited to hospitals, nursing homes, and clinics. Nurses monitor vitals, labs, and symptoms of the patient that may require immediate attention. Ever since Medicare started penalizing institutions for readmissions, hospitals have reset their focus on reducing readmissions rates. Nurses can play a pivotal role in avoiding this penalty by engaging in the patient's discharge process. Nurses collect discharge information, receive reconciled medications, and review the discharge plan with the patient; they also are commonly the ones leading the discharge when a patient is ready to leave the hospital. Because of how accessible nurses are, they are able to collaborate with the patient's family and the healthcare team to ensure the line of communication is clear to all.

Another study by Balaban, Weissman, Samuel, and Woolhandler (2008) examined nurses taking initiative for the patient's discharge care plan. A comprehensive discharge form was filled out by the physician and given to the nurse to review with the patient. This form included new medications to be taken and addressed communication issues that commonly occur during care transitions. After discharge, a follow up phone call was set up by the nurse to assess the patient's status, review the discharge form, and answer any concerns the patient may have had (Balaban et al., 2008)

Pharmacist

Another primary member of the healthcare team is the pharmacist. Pharmacists go to pharmacy school, which consists of a total of four years, similar to physicians. A traditional program typically consists of three years of didactic coursework and one year of experiential practice. Upon licensure pharmacists earn the title of Doctor of Pharmacy (PharmD). After completion of the PharmD degree, pharmacists have the option of doing a residency. The roles and responsibilities of the pharmacist vary by the setting of which they work. Overall, pharmacists serve as the medication experts on the healthcare team and their duties include ensuring that the patient's medications are appropriate for their indication, effective, and safe as well as cost-effective. Pharmacists ensure the correct medication is given with the appropriate dose for the right indication; also each can adjust doses as necessary. In addition, these doctors monitor for drug and disease interactions and potential allergic reactions. They also can order specific labs to ensure therapeutic levels of drugs are met. Pharmacists are trained heavily in the area of pharmacokinetics and understand factors that affect the medications in regards to absorption, distribution, and elimination, and how medications are affected throughout these parameters (General Pharmaceutical Council, 2016).

Pharmacists play an integral role in ensuring that patients receive therapeutic amounts of their medications and contribute in various transitions of care models due to their vast knowledge in pharmacotherapy and ability to manage medication regimens while optimizing patient care and reducing healthcare costs. Pharmacists have been reported to have reduced readmission rates by 86% through the integration of their services on a team (Zillich et al., 2014). A prospective pilot study by Sebaaly et al. (2015) viewed the number and severity of medication errors identified by a pharmacist prior to patient discharge. Medication errors encompassed omission of medications; extra medications; and inappropriate medications based on age, weight, antibiotic susceptibilities, wrong dose, frequency, or dosage form. A total of 84 errors were identified in a group of 67 patients, with the highest medication error being in chronic disease management. This was translated to a total of $42,300 in cost avoidance simply by allowing a pharmacist to perform a detailed comprehensive medication review (CMR). This detailed CMR allowed the pharmacist to be able to determine the reason for discrepancies in the admission and discharge medication orders (Sebaaly et al., 2015). Another study by Kilcup, Schultz, Carlson, and Wilson (2003) studied the rate of hospital readmission and financial savings with pharmacist intervention. By implementing post-discharge medication reconciliation, pharmacists could follow up with patients regarding medication management after transitioning out of the hospital. By utilizing a pharmacist, four readmissions were prevented per 100 patients. This equates to a financial saving of $35,478 per 100 patients after considering the cost of readmission and cost of labor of a clinical pharmacist (Kilcup et al., 2003). Integrating pharmacists on an interprofessional team has proven to reduce the cost of healthcare and readmission rates, while improving patient outcomes.

It is important to leverage the skills of each member of the interprofessional team and maximize their roles and responsibilities. This is one of the many reasons why the members of an interprofessional team need to know each other's roles and responsibilities. Many other healthcare professionals such as social workers, physical therapists, nutritionists, and certified diabetic educators contribute meaningfully to the care of patients. Through collaborative efforts between the healthcare professionals and the patients as well as their caretakers, the patient's care experience can be improved, the populations' health also can be improved, and healthcare expenditures can decrease, all of which are the critical objectives of what is known as the "Triple Aim" by the Institute for Healthcare Improvement (IHI, 2016).

Interprofessional Education (IPE) and Collaborative Practice (CP)

Interprofessional collaboration has been shown to be essential in optimizing patient care and patient safety while improving healthcare costs. Many academic institutions have incorporated interprofessional education as a foundational component of their curricula. The Interprofessional Education Collaborative (2016) has created four core competencies for interprofessional education, which includes shared ethics and values, roles and responsibilities, and communication as well as teams and teamwork. As healthcare continues to evolve, there are new opportunities constantly for health providers to work together with the same ultimate goal in mind – better patient care.

Patient safety and transitions of care have been significant aspects of IPECP competency concerns for many professional organizations and initiatives including the AACN (2016a), American Association of Colleges of Osteopathic Medicine (AACOM, 2016), American Association of Colleges of Pharmacy (AACP, 2016), American Dental Education Association (ADEA, 2016), Association of American Medical Colleges (AAMC, 2016), Association of Schools of Public Health (ASPH, 2016), and Agency for Healthcare Research and Quality (ARHQ, 2016). ARHQ has been proactive, particularly for many team-based learning opportunities at basic, master, and advanced levels of training educators and leaders to make patient safety a priority with the TeamSTEPPS® Strategies and Tools to Enhance Performance and Patient Safety (ARHQ, 2016). Interprofessional Education (IPE) also has become an area of focus for the AACP, with several groups, including these authors from the AACP Interprofessional Education Task Force, working on developing resources to promote and support IPE planning and development. In a review by Buring et al. (2009), there is fundamental information and background on the definition of IPE, evidence to support IPE and its need, student competencies and objectives for IPE, barriers to implementation of IPE, and elements critical for successfully implementing IPE.

The field of IPECP has been around for approximately 40 years (Brandt, 2015). Interprofessional education has been initiated, developed, and instituted around the world fueled by calls from the World Health Organization's (WHO, 2010) "Framework for Action on Interprofessional Education and Collaborative Practice." Like the United States and Canada, international efforts have been ongoing in Europe equally as long. Arguably, the largest influence in Europe is the professional organization, the Centre for the Advancement of Interprofessional Education (CAIPE, 2016) in the United Kingdom, which grows in advocacy and advancement every year. Also, the European Interprofessional Education Network (EIPEN, n.d.) was "one of the first interprofessional education networks to be formed." Furthermore, EIPEN (n.d.) has stated, "Initially... EIPEN... was led by the UK Higher Education Academy, a group of universities and CAIPE obtained European funding to set up a network in approximately 2007." Throughout the years, EIPEN has undergone change such as expansion and development of conferences around the world. CAIPE and EIPEN, along with major initiatives from professional organizations in

Canada such as the Canadian Interprofessional Education Health Collaborative (CIHC, 2016), have propelled the movement forward. The growth of interprofessional education and collaborative practice is evidenced by both a National Center for Interprofessional Education and Practice (2015) that was founded in 2012 and funded by several agencies including the Josiah Macy Jr. Foundation, Robert Wood Johnson Foundation, and Gordon and Betty More Foundation. In addition, two new journals were created in 2015; namely, the *Journal of Interprofessional Education and Practice* and the *Journal of Research in Interprofessional Practice and Education.* In the last year or two only one major journal has focused on interprofessional education and/or collaborative practice; namely, the *Journal of Interprofessional Care*, which is available to a researcher when becoming an annual CAIPE member.

In the United States, several key milestones for IPE and IPECP stemmed from a major report, "Educating for the Health Team" by the Institute of Medicine (IOM, 1972). In 1999, the Institute of Medicine created another report "To Err is Human: Building a Safer Health System," and then in 2001 created the Crossing the Quality Chasm. Other organizations such as AHRQ created efforts on retraining to building interprofessional (IP) teamwork and team-based care through TeamSTEPPS training face-to-face and with masters and advanced training face-to-face and online. Finally, the American Recovery and Reinvestment Act (ARRA) of 2009 and the Patient Protection and Affordable Care Act (2010) have placed emphasis on medical home, population health, improved primary care outcomes, and more.

Universities throughout the United States have been creating and instituting IPE/IPCP programs for a number of years. Two of the most prominent and experienced initiatives developed over time are the University of Washington's (UW, 2016) Center for Health Science Interprofessional Education, Research, and Practice and the University of Minnesota (2015) where the National Center for Interprofessional Practice and Education is housed. The Center was founded by Dr. Pam Mitchell, who is the current director for the Center for Health Sciences Interprofessional Education. Dedicated individuals like Dr. Pam Mitchell and dedicated professional organizations fuel the IPECP movement forward, including those initiated and growing in Florida.

Several large Florida universities built IPECP programs, courses, and certificates while some smaller universities have instituted interprofessional education programs as well. One of the first universities in Florida to create an interprofessional education program across their university was University of Florida (Davidson & Waddell, 2005). These programs provide students in pre-professional programs and professional programs with the competencies needed to prepare future clinicians to move into various health professions. In 2011, FAU created an Interprofessional Education program for medical, nursing, and social work students and faculty to begin training and developing future practitioners for the healthcare system (Jacomino et al., 2015).

Palm Beach Atlantic University (PBAU), a private university, created an IPE program with faculty from the Colleges of Nursing and Pharmacy after shadowing FAU's program and leadership. After consulting with FAU's Office of Interprofessional Education director, PBAU's School of Pharmacy students and faculty were invited by FAU's director to participate in FAU's IPE development session on healthcare policy and quality, which focused on the readmission rate and care transition problems. The students were prepared for the problems of care transition and readmission and then instructed to create a care transition plan together. In the 2014-2015 academic year 16 pharmacy students attended the March IPE session, along with faculty who served as team facilitators. For the 2015-2016 academic year, PBAU was invited back to FAU's care transition and reducing hospital readmission discussions for the third Interprofessional Education Development Session (IPEDS) series in February. The first session had 12 students and three faculty members participating. PBAU's Dr. Mariette Sourial wrote to FAU's Dr.

Jo Ann Bamdas that she felt "we planted seeds in the session that would be fruitful by the time the students went into practice. We believe that students learned new ways of thinking that made them realize the value of each discipline present" (email communication, February 17, 2016). Having pharmacy students on the team added a layer of team building that benefited both private and public university students and faculty. Since FAU does not have a school of pharmacy and PBAU does not have a medical school or school of social work, new knowledge was shared and transferred into practice that would not have been accomplished without collaborating across institutional borders.

The intent of the public university's final workshop session in a series of three was to discuss the Patient Protection and Affordable Care Act (2010) and the challenge to hospitals for a patient's readmission within 30 days of release. Each academic year, FAU serves approximately 250 medicine, nursing, and social work students, who work in teams of 3-5. The program includes a welcome and introduction to a panel of the session's committee members from each of the colleges/schools. After an introduction into the problem of care transition and readmission, students are asked to create a care transition plan directed at a local hospital. Next the panel members listen to the students' recommendations. At the conclusion of volunteering the transition plans, panel members ask students to debrief.

Because students consistently ask to participate in real-world situations rather than simulated exercises or didactic lessons from PowerPoint presentations, Palm Beach Atlantic University and Florida Atlantic University have tried to create opportunities to learn from community partners. Also, in the past two years, FAU has partnered with a local hospital whose interprofessional staff, led by the nursing department, joined the university faculty members to listen to students' plans and give feedback in real-world terms. The hospital leadership team models for students the process for an interprofessional team collaborating. The pharmacist, physician, social worker/cases manager, and nurse from the hospital include an introduction of each other's education, roles and responsibilities, and communication as they work collaboratively in a team.

In the current year's 2015-2016 collaboration between the two universities, both PBAU and FAU have decided to continue partnering and IPECP expansion, which will benefit university, students, faculty, and staff. In that vein, the goal has been to cross the public versus private university system divide. One major change currently is underway: Mariette Sourial has been invited to join the committee that plans the third workshop for students and faculty on transitions of care. This change also adds the voice of pharmacy to the original IPE working group team when viewing real case studies from the local hospital volunteering to participate. After two years working with one local hospital, this year the universities will work with another hospital in the community to view how the leadership collaborates for transitions of care and counteracts readmission rates. The development of the universities' partnership no doubt will include several hospitals in the future since students, faculty, administrators, and hospital leaders want to prepare and be prepared for improving the healthcare system. Hospitals and universities can form initiatives for working together so that each can learn together as a team.

TRANSITIONS OF CARE INITIATIVES THROUGH INTERPROFESSIONAL COLLABORATION

Currently, many initiatives exist to increase the awareness of healthcare collaboration as the patient transitions from one care setting to another and to emphasize the Triple Aim (IHI, 2016). According to the IHI (2016), the Triple Aim approach strives to optimize health system performance, and consists of "three critical objectives: (a) improving the patient experience of care (including quality and satisfaction), (b) improving the health of populations, and (c) reducing the per capita cost of health care."

By implementing transition of care models, readmission rates can be greatly decreased as well. Integrating interprofessional collaborative practice in these initiatives ensures optimum patient care and patient safety. Many initiatives have emerged, which focus on improving transitions of care through collaborative efforts. The ARC (2013b) initiative, based in California, focuses on reducing readmission rates after discharge. In 2013, ARC helped reduce over 6,400 readmissions in a 3-year period. This initiative not only reduced readmission, but helped save healthcare over $62 million. ARC works by enlisting a number of hospitals that participate in the ARC Action Network. This network allows participating hospitals to submit their readmission information through the ARC website where five measures are entered. These five ARC measures include:

1. Percent of 30-day readmissions.
2. Percent of 90-day readmissions.
3. Responses to HCAHPS patient survey question #23: "During this hospital stay, staff took my preferences and those of my family or caregiver into account in deciding what my healthcare needs would be when I left."
4. Responses to HCAHPS patient survey question #24: "When I left the hospital, I had a good understanding of the things I was responsible for in managing my health."
5. Responses to HCAHPS patient survey question # 25: "When I left the hospital, I clearly understood the purpose for taking each of my medications." (ARC, 2013a)

Additionally, other hospitals may add other unique measures that their hospital uses to oversee readmissions. In this database, hospitals can view their own readmission information and collaborative care over a period of time and compare their information to others to see others performing in comparison.

Another transitions of care initiative is Project RED (2104), developed by a research group at Boston University Medical Center. This initiative focuses on revamping the workflow in a transition of care setting in order to improve patient safety, while reducing readmission rates. At the time of discharge, the nurse discharging the patient is the main caregiver responsible for their transition out of the hospital. The charge nurse must oversee 11 components that are to be reviewed with the patient. These include:

1. Educating the patient about his/her diagnosis.
2. Making follow up appointments and any post-discharge testing for follow-up and post-discharge testing.
3. Discussing any tests or studies that have been completed in the hospital.
4. Organizing post-discharge services.
5. Confirming their medication plan.
6. Reconciling the discharge plan with standard of care guidelines.
7. Reviewing what to do should a problem arise.
8. Expediting discharge summary to physicians.
9. Assessing the degree of understanding of patient through the "teach-back" method.
10. Giving the patient a written discharge plan at the time of discharge.
11. Providing reinforcement via telephone two to three days after discharge. (Project RED, 2014).

This initiative aims for optimum care and strives to reduce healthcare costs. It has been reported through a study that Project RED has saved up to $412 per patient, equivalent to a 33.9% reduction in overall costs (Brian et al., 2009, p. 184).

Another initiative, Project BOOST (Better Outcomes for Older adults through Safe Transitions) is led by the Society of Hospital Medicine (SHM, 2015). Their mission seeks to improve the care of patients when transitioning from inpatient to outpatient. The primary focus of this initiative includes identifying high risk patients prone to re-hospitalization, reducing potential adverse events, reducing 30-day readmission rates, improving HCAHPS measures associated with discharge, and improving communication and work flow among healthcare providers.

The board members on Project BOOST's consist of medical doctors along with representatives from AHRQ, Blue Cross and Blue Shield Association, CMS, Centers for Disease Control and Prevention (CDC), IHI, The Joint Commission, Kaiser Permanente, and many more. These mentors assist in providing evidence-based clinical interventions for hospitals to integrate into their systems.

Project BOOST encompasses a comprehensive intervention tool that was developed by experts practicing evidence-based medicine. It also provides a variety of management tools including the teach-back training method for interdisciplinary teams to implement with patients and other providers. To ensure continuity in care while minimizing gaps in miscommunication, BOOST allows sites to communicate with and learn from each other via the BOOST Listserv and BOOST Community site. Hospitals may choose to use any or all of these resources. Much of this information can be accessed on the BOOST Data Center, which is an online resource that allows different sites to store and benchmark data and to generate reports. In 2012 almost 4,000 sites had adapted the project BOOST toolkit, with reports of a 21% reduction in 30-day all cause readmission rates after implementation of BOOST. BOOST not only improves readmission rates, but also specifically caters to patients to have an increased level of medical service through collaboration (Society of Hospital Medicine, 2015).

Collaboration among Pharmacists

The ASHP (2010) 2015 initiative empowers pharmacists to be the medication experts during transitions of care (Goal 1, objective 1.6). Pharmacists are well suited to identify and resolve medication-related problems related to transitional care, activities that are core fundamentals to pharmaceutical care. Their roles ultimately can lead to identifying and resolving medication-related errors, decreasing adverse drug events upon discharge, and reducing unnecessary emergency room visits. Pharmacists are trained to evaluate a patient's drug therapy to ensure it is indicated, safe, and effective, and that the patient can adhere to it. Through patient interactions, pharmacists also can see whether the patient is able to use the medications as intended. For example, upon interviewing a patient, the pharmacist may discover that a particular patient was on an insulin regimen at home, which was not included in the medication list at the hospital. If, upon discharge, a different insulin regimen was prescribed, it could lead to the patient taking both regimens and being place at risk of having a hypoglycemic event, which could lead to a readmission. Therefore, if a pharmacist is involved in discharge counseling, this could be addressed and an adverse drug event could have been prevented. Furthermore, The Joint Commission's (2016) National Patient Safety Goals in Ambulatory Healthcare stresses the importance of medication reconciliation and the role of communicating effectively the medications to the next provider. Pharmacy organizations such as these have strived to put together in place a system to help with safer practices and to engage the patients in healthcare decisions (The Joint Commission, 2016).

As an integral function, medication management needs to be seen at all interfaces of change as patients' transition from one care setting to another. Adverse drug events are a major cause of avoidable hospital readmissions and lack of medication adherence has been a lead cause of post-discharge adverse events.

The University of Hawaii at Hilo (2012) created an innovative project focused on pharmacist-to-pharmacist collaboration, known as "Pharm2Pharm." The model is geared toward transitions of care and care coordination and aims at improving patient safety while reducing medication-related hospitalizations and emergency room visits, especially in rural communities. It involves the collaboration between hospital pharmacists and community pharmacists to close the medication-related gaps as patients transition from the hospital to the community setting. This establishment of hospital and community pharmacists' teamwork is a great exemplary model for other institutions to follow as well (University of Hawai'I at Hilo, 2012).

Another study conducted by Calvert et al. (2012), titled "PILOT-EBM: Patient Focused Intervention to Improve Long-term Adherence to Evidence Based Medications," evaluated the effectiveness of a program to help patients with heart disease stay on their medications. The lead coordinator was the inpatient pharmacist for medication management, who was involved in a collaborative effort with the community pharmacist identified by the patient. The inpatient pharmacist addressed patient and caregiver barriers to adherence identified by the care team. These adherence barriers then were discussed by the inpatient pharmacist with the community pharmacist and information was sent to the primary care. The community monitored refill records and communicated discrepancies to the patient's care team (Calvert et al., 2012).

Collaboration with Patients and Caregivers

A pharmacist integrated into a patient's healthcare team has the potential to improve patient's health and to increase their healthcare delivery. This integration also promotes collaboration between other healthcare providers, professionals, patients, and their caregivers (CDC, 2013). It is not every day that caregivers are considered to play an active role in the chain to achieving adequate healthcare. Yet, caregivers generally are the main ingredient to a patient's healthcare. They usually take over the transition of patient care, so why are they not engaged as partners of care during this vital transition for patients? Discharge processes vary between institutions; yet, how often do these processes involve patients and their caregivers? Practical ways to achieve patient and caregiver engagement include asking questions about their care, using the "teach-back" method (restating the information learned), and sharing beliefs and concerns with the healthcare team. Oftentimes, it is the goal to educate the patient on their health. While that is true, there have been discussions about the need to start looking at the big picture to see the entire line of transition (American Pharmacists Association [APhA], 2014).

Several major questions often asked within the health field include: Who is ultimately responsible for managing a patient's healthcare? Is the patient only responsible? Does the physician or pharmacist make sure any information is relayed to the patient? Is the family member of the patient the responsible caregiver? No one exact answer exists to these questions. It is a joint effort of all those involved in the care of patient to make sure the best care is provided (Interprofessional Education Collaborative, 2016). Patient self-management of their healthcare success requires collaboration to promote and achieve better transitions of care. Successful self-management can prevent costly readmissions, improve healthcare outcomes, and enhance patient satisfaction and experiences with their healthcare (Naylor & Keating, 2008).

Transitions of care remains a critical area of concern that healthcare providers and institutions continually focus their efforts to maximize results. During transitions of care, healthcare information, accountability, responsibility, and authority are transferred to the patient (Schulz et al., 1997). Unfortunately, sometimes the transitions of these three major components do not occur as smoothly as anticipated and follow up to care or confusion potentially can occur. The Joint Commission et al. (n.d.) implemented a 3-year initiative to define ways in which to achieve effective transition of patients between different healthcare settings in order to provide safe and quality care for patients regardless of the setting. Today, with a growing awareness of the importance of transition of care, several tools to facilitate seamless care continue to be developed. Various tools readily available to patients, providers, and caregivers can assist and smooth out the processes associated with the transition of care.

TOOLS AND PROGRAMS FOR HEALTH PROVIDERS

While several tools currently are under development, many resources and tools now assist and ensure effective transitions of care. One organization, AHRQ (2007), has developed a toolkit, which is focused on assessing a patient's health literacy in order to ease communication between patients and providers to improve health outcomes.

In addition to AHRQ's toolkit, several tests have been developed for healthcare providers to assist in assessing the health literacy of their patients and their caregivers. One test, the Rapid Estimate of Adult Literacy in Medicine Short Form (REALM-SF), is a 7-item recognition assessment that provides some indication of the person's health literacy. Another test, the Short Assessment of Health Literacy Spanish and English (SAHL-S&E) is longer and is comprised of an 18-item assessment of a patient's health literacy (AHRQ, 2007).

Also, other implemented programs help health professionals and patients during care transitions. In collaboration, two major pharmaceutical organizations, the ASHP and APhA developed a program called the Medication Management in Care Transitions (MMCT). This program assists in the transitions of care by pharmacists and in collaboration with patients and their caregivers (ASHP & APha, n.d.).

Another program that emerged through the Affordable Care Act by the Centers for Medicare & Medicaid Services is called the Community-based Care Transitions Program (CCTP). This program examines and identifies ways to improve patient care transitions in hopes of reducing readmissions for Medicare patients/beneficiaries (CMS, 2016a).

A national campaign, Script Your Future, led by the National Consumers League, helps patients take an active role in their healthcare by encouraging medication adherence to promote a healthier life (Script Your Future, 2016). This campaign aims to help people manage chronic and debilitating disease states such as diabetes, chronic obstructive pulmonary disease (COPD), asthma, and hypertension by supporting the importance of taking medications as prescribed and directed by their physician. Patients not taking their medications as prescribed or directed put their health and, more importantly, their future at risk. Healthcare costs rise daily in today's society. The United States spends more on healthcare than most other countries (Anderson, 2005). One way to contain healthcare costs includes adhering to the prescribed medication regimen, which, in turn, can prevent a readmission.

The Script Your Future (2016) campaign includes a website that allows patients and their caregivers to create a personal pledge to take medications as prescribed to help reinforce its importance. Some other tools available on their website include text reminders, Script Your Future wallet cards in languages such as Spanish and English, an adherence estimator, and a pocket size medication list have available at all times and to bring to doctor visits. Recently, the campaign has begun providing pharmacy students and faculty around the country with a unique opportunity to participate in a competition held nationally. The competition encourages teams to develop ideas and initiatives for raising awareness about the importance of medication adherence in the transitions of care of patients (Script Your Future, 2014).

The City of New York Health and Mental Hygiene in conjunction with the Fund for Public Health in New York (FPHNY) developed an initiative, the Medication Adherence Project (Starr & Sacks, 2010), for patients with several chronic and debilitating disease states, reinforcing effective communication by pharmacists and all healthcare providers. A major barrier to successful patient care identified by the MAP Initiative was lack of medication adherence. To overcome the barrier, MAP provides tools and resources to achieve optimal patient results in outcomes in this specific patient population. MAP created several objectives to facilitate the transition of care process and adherence barrier. The tools and resources available by the MAP initiative are targeted for everyone on the healthcare team. A 2-part guide assists in increasing effective communication. The first part is the guide, which contains medication adherence basics for providers, tools, and icebreakers to facilitate the training. The second part of the guide consists of the actual trainer curriculum, which serves as a guide to create MAP training sessions for anyone on the healthcare team (Starr & Sacks, 2010).

HEALTH LITERACY

One major influence of adherence to a prescribed regimen is the patient's health literacy. Limited literacy has been associated with poor health status, poor outcomes, and a barrier to successful transition of care. Individuals with limited literacy also tend to have higher incidences of illness and hospitalizations compared to individuals with higher literacy and reading skills. The National Adult Literacy Survey found that roughly 44 million Americans, or about one quarter of the adult population, are considered by definition to be illiterate (National Center for Education Statistics [NCES], n.d.). Many of the health brochures, health information, and education information printed for patients traditionally have been written at a 10th grade reading level or above (NCES, n.d.). Often, providers supply information to educate the patient and assist in understanding their disease states or next steps, but actually the patient may not comprehend what it means. AHRQ (2007) has developed resources including four tools to assist in measuring health literacy in our patient population.

Health literacy evaluation occurs in several ways including education level, reading level, barriers in language, and more. Oftentimes healthcare professionals may engage the patient they want to educate and assist; however, sometimes the person responsible for administering the patient's medication or daily activities does not understand what they are being told or are not informed at all; as a result, issues such as medication adherence and proper patient therapy are affected. Patients who may have difficulty in obtaining, processing, and understanding basic health information and services can have a health coach help them navigate through the health system or can designate a caregiver who can build relationships with the patient's healthcare providers. Health providers also should be cognizant of the patient's and caregiver's health literacy level and tailor the information they provide in a manner that they can understand and use. For example, the use of pictures to illustrate how to take a medication is a great way to help visualize the drug regimen. The American Medical Association has recognized that limited patient literacy is an actual barrier to effective treatment for patients (Parker, 2000).

PATIENT ENGAGEMENT

Patients need to play a more active role in their health. They are the central hub for all their health information and services. It not only is important for them to become involved in decision making, but also to be their own health advocate. One example of how to achieve this is through the use of the "teach-back" method, where patients and/or caregivers are asked to demonstrate their understanding of the instructions by explaining back in their own words what they have been informed. Patient's goals and preferences need to be accounted for during the decision making as they may directly influence the medication regimen. In an IOM report entitled "To Err is Human," patients with low level of involvement in their care become a major obstacle as well as the lack of awareness of the patient's voice during decision making (Kohn, Corrigan, & Donaldson, 2000). Achieving therapeutic goals are not necessarily the goals of the individual patient. Every patient should understand the information being received, which includes the diagnosis and the degree of uncertainty of their medical problems, the risks and benefits of the treatments options, the expected recovery time, and the healthcare providers and the costs involved. Patients should be empowered to share their beliefs and concerns with their healthcare providers. Whenever a new medication is prescribed, patients should ask their provider: "What am I taking?" "What am I taking this for?" "When should I take it?" "Are there any side effects?" "Are there any special instructions?" "What if I miss a dose?" The patients also should be aware of any past medications used and discontinued as well as any allergies and what happened to them when they had an allergic reaction. Through informed consent, each patient should become involved with their healthcare providers in making decisions about their healthcare and be the 'champions' in their own care, a movement led by the World Health Organization (WHO, 2016) called Patients for Patient Safety.

CONCLUSION

Everyone either may be a caregiver at some point in their lives or may need one during their lifetime. Sometimes caregiving can occur gradually, while other times it may happen rapidly. Studies have shown that most caregivers are not as prepared for their role as they would like to be. Caregiver participation has shown improvement in outcomes for patients, especially those with physical, mental, and cognitive disorders. Also, participation contributes to greater patient satisfaction and improves the patient's continuity of care. Caregivers are just as vital in the line of communication as patients when it comes to providing effective care. Caregiver education is needed to achieve goals, obtain desired results, and ensure effective patient transition when caregivers are involved. Proper education and incorporation of caregivers into the healthcare of an individual is not only convenient but necessary (Pinquart & Sorensen, 2003).

Many other great organization and initiatives are taking place now. As healthcare systems begin to adjust their practices to help reduce readmissions and overall healthcare costs as well as to improve patient care and safety, a much greater need exists for the healthcare professional to be accountable, collaborate as a team, and engage patients and their caregivers. Healthcare in the United States still is fragmented despite all these national efforts; however, there is progress being made in coming together and achieving the "Triple Aim" to improve the patient experience of care, including quality and satisfaction; to improve the health of populations; and to reduce the per capita cost of healthcare.

FUTURE TRENDS

Healthcare professional organizations have identified several topics of great concern for an interprofessional healthcare team's competencies. Some of the concerns discussed in this chapter are situations involving a growing aging population and chronic disease management, along with many patient safety issues such as polypharmacy and miscommunication. But healthcare reforms and focusing on better care, better health, and lower costs as well as transitions of care and the likelihood of 30-day readmission rates will be a continuing concern in the future. In addition to highlighting some gaps in healthcare, this chapter also has pointed to solutions to create a seamless healthcare system between provider, educator, patient, and caregiver. Experts in other disciplines have pointed to other trends in the healthcare system of which all interprofessional team members need to be cognizant. One profession investigated by Stanton and Lammon (2008) showed "predicted changes in [nurse] case management" (p. 161). Three of these trends included: "transitions of care, informatics in healthcare …, and the impact of an aging population …" (Stanton & Lammon, 2008, pp. 163-164).

As one gazes into the future, one may predict several opportunities and problems that will continue to be with us such as the growth of technology in healthcare. With the new informatics, telehealth, mobile health, and digital health market growing seemingly every day, knowledge, skill, and imagination will increase benefits to those who have access. But some tools may create challenges and barriers that conflict with each other. In fact, in some ways one may not think about the ramifications of some unforeseen medical dilemmas. As technology develops, particularly online courses, and training programs emerge, pharmacists, nurses, social workers, literally everyone, will need to be able to work together to benefit all stakeholders. With the advent of technology making healthcare systems seemingly easier to use, complications certainly will emerge. These conflicts and obstacles will continue affecting transitions of care and readmission rates for hospitals as well as for educators.

With the challenges at hand today, one also can gaze into the future to predict the effect of childhood chronic disease as well as physical and mental health problems. Arguably those most at risk are youth with a number of cognitive and physical disabilities. Other challenges will continue, such as access and equitable arrangements for those living in rural areas versus those in affluent areas, and will have a major impact on policy and politics. In addition, the population growth of aging Baby Boomers needing additional medical care professionals and those individuals ready to retire from the healthcare professions will invariably cause concern for transitions of care and the need for interprofessional teams to work together to solve problems.

Finally, the future of education and training will continue being affected deeply by the push for an interprofessional education and collaborative practice framework and its competencies in institutions and in the workforce. Simply put, healthcare professionals and educators cannot continue working in isolation, with silo mentalities, or within hierarchical structures and systems. As described in the *Business Dictionary*, silo mentalities are:

a mind-set present in some companies when certain departments or sectors do not wish to share information with others in the same company. This type of mentality will reduce the efficiency of the overall operation, reduce morale, and may contribute to the demise of a productive company culture. ("Silo mentality," 2016)

But many chances to improve group and team communication abound. Creating initiatives at the local and state level will bring healthcare professionals together. Workforce development state and educational initiatives such as the recent State University System of Florida's "Think Florida" (n.d.) will call on universities to reflect on the partnerships between student's knowledge, skill, and attitudes, along with workforce development. The process by which healthcare and education systems communicate and collaborate as a team will move the country forward.

This chapter has highlighted the need for patients to have a strong interprofessional team where everyone understands each other's role and responsibility and collaborates. This chapter also has captured the need for patients to take ownership of their health, the need to understand the comprehensive growth of communication and collaboration in the healthcare system today, and the need to move into the future.

REFERENCES

Agency for Healthcare Research and Quality. (2007). *Health literacy measurement tools (revised)*. Retrieved from http://www.ahrq.gov/professionals/quality-patient-safety/quality-resources/tools/literacy/index.html

Agency for Healthcare Research and Quality. (2016). *TeamSTEPPS® strategies and tools to enhance performance and patient safety*. Retrieved from http://www.ahrq.gov/professionals/education/curriculum-tools/teamstepps/index.html

American Academy of Physician Assistants. (2006). *Q&A about physician assistants: The most commonly asked questions about PAs*. Retrieved from http://www.gidoctor.net/client_files/file/Physician-Assistants.pdf

American Association of Colleges of Nursing. (2016). *Home page*. Retrieved from http://www.aacn.nche.edu/

American Association of Colleges of Osteopathic Medicine. (2016). *Home page*. Retrieved from https://www.aacom.org/

American Association of Colleges of Pharmacy. (2016). *Home page*. Retrieved from http://www.aacp.org/Pages/Default.aspx

American Dental Education Association. (2016). *Home page*. Retrieved from http://www.adea.org/

American Pharmacists Association. (2014). *Pharmacists' patient care processes*. Retrieved from http://www.pharmacist.com/sites/default/files/files/PatientCareProcess.pdf

American Recovery and Reinvestment Act (ARRA) of 2009, Pub. L. No. 111-5, 123 Stat. 115, 516 (2009).

American Society of Health-System Pharmacists. (2010). *2015 ASHP health-system pharmacy initiative*. Retrieved from http://www.ashp.org/doclibrary/policy/2015/2015goals.aspx

American Society of Health-System Pharmacists. (2016). *Transitions of care resource center*. Retrieved from http://www.ashp.org/menu/PracticePolicy/ResourceCenters/Transitions-of-Care

American Society of Health-System Pharmacists, & the American Pharmacists Association. (n.d.). *ASHP-APhA medication management in care transitions best practices*. Retrieved from http://media.pharmacist.com/practice/ASHP_APhA_MedicationManagementinCareTransitionsBestPracticesReport2_2013.pdf

Anderson, G. (2005). *U.S. still spends more on health care than any other country* [Press release]. Retrieved from http://www.jhsph.edu/news/news-releases/2005/anderson-health-spending.html

Association of American Medical Colleges. (2016). *Home page*. Retrieved from https://www.aamc.org/

Association of Schools of Public Health. (2016). *Home page*. Retrieved from http://www.aspph.org/

Avoid Readmission through Collaboration. (2013a). How ARC measures improvement. Retrieved from http://www.avoidreadmissions.com/arc-action-network.html

Avoid Readmission through Collaboration. (2013b). *Initiatives*. Retrieved from http://www.avoidreadmissions.com/improving-transitions-of-care/initiatives.html

Balaban, R. B., Weissman, J. S., Samuel, P. A., & Woolhandler, S. (2008). Redefining and redesigning hospital discharge to enhance patient care: A randomized controlled study. *Journal of General Internal Medicine*, *23*(8), 1228–1233. doi:10.1007/s11606-008-0618-9 PMID:18452048

Brandt, B. F. (2015). Interprofessional education and collaborative practice: Welcome to the 'new' forty-year old field. *The Advisor*. Retrieved from https://nexusipe-resource-exchange.s3.amazonaws.com/IPECP%20-%20Welcome%20to%20the%20New%2040-Year-Old%20Field%20-%20Brandt;%20The%20Advisor.pdf

Brian, J. W., Chetty, V. K., Anthony, D., Greenwald, J. L., Sanchez, G. M., Johnson, A. E., & Culpepper, L. et al. (2009). A reengineered hospital discharge program to decrease rehospitalization. *Annals of Internal Medicine*, *150*(3), 178–187. doi:10.7326/0003-4819-150-3-200902030-00007 PMID:19189907

Buring, S. M., Bhushan, A., Broeseker, A., Conway, S., Duncan-Hewitt, W., Hansen, L., & Westberg, S. (2009). Interprofessional education: Definitions, student competencies, and guidelines for implementation. *American Journal of Pharmaceutical Education*, *73*(4), 59. http://www.ncbi.nlm.nih.gov/pmc/articles/PMC2720355/ doi:10.5688/aj730459 PMID:19657492

Calvert, S. B., Kramer, J. M., Anstrom, K. J., Kaltenbach, L. A., Stafford, J. A., & Allen, N. M. (2012). Patient-focused intervention to improve long-term adherence to evidence-based medications. *American Heart Journal*, *163*(4), 657–665. doi:10.1016/j.ahj.2012.01.019 PMID:22520532

Canadian Interprofessional Health Collaborative. (2016). *CIHC overview*. Retrieved from http://www.cihc.ca/about/overview

Centers for Disease Control and Prevention. (2013). *Collaborative practice agreements and pharmacists' patient care services: A resource for pharmacists*. Retrieved from http://www.cdc.gov/dhdsp/pubs/docs/Translational_Tools_Pharmacists.pdf

Centers for Medicare & Medicaid Services. (2016a). *Community-based care transitions program*. Retrieved from https://innovation.cms.gov/initiatives/CCTP/index.html SG – change from 2016 to this.

Centers for Medicare & Medicaid Services. (2016b). *Readmissions reduction program (HRRP)*. Retrieved from https://www.cms.gov/Medicare/Medicare-Fee-for-Service-Payment/AcuteInpatientPPS/Readmissions-Reduction-Program.html

Centre for the Advancement of Interprofessional Education. (2002). *Defining IPE*. Retrieved from http://caipe.org.uk/resources/defining-ipe/

Centre for the Advancement of Interprofessional Education. (2016). *Welcome to CAIPE*. Retrieved from http://caipe.org.uk/

Coleman, E. A., & Boult, C. E. (2003). Improving the quality of transitional care for persons with complex care needs. *Journal of the American Geriatrics Society*, *51*(4), 556–557. doi:10.1046/j.1532-5415.2003.51186.x PMID:12657079

Davidson, R. A., & Waddell, R. (2005). A historical overview of interdisciplinary family health: A community-based interprofessional health professions course. *Academic Medicine*, *80*(4), 334–338. doi:10.1097/00001888-200504000-00005 PMID:15793015

European Interprofessional Education Network. (n. d.). *Our history*. Retrieved from http://www.eipen.eu/geschiedenis_9.html

Foster, A. J., Murff, H. J., Peterson, J. F., Gandhi, T. K., & Bates, D. W. (2003). The incidence and severity of adverse events affecting patients after discharge from the hospital. *Annals of Internal Medicine*, *138*(3), 161–167. doi:10.7326/0003-4819-138-3-200302040-00007 PMID:12558354

General Pharmaceutical Council. (2016). *What does a pharmacist do?* Retrieved from https://www.pharmacyregulation.org/raising-concerns/raising-concerns-about-pharmacy-professional/what-expect-your-pharmacy/what-does-0

Health Resources and Services Administration. (2016). *Health literacy*. Retrieved from http://www.hrsa.gov/publichealth/healthliteracy/

Institute for Healthcare Improvement. (2016). *IHI triple aim initiative*. Retrieved from http://www.ihi.org/engage/initiatives/TripleAim/Pages/default.aspx

Institute of Medicine. (1972). *Educating for the health team*. Retrieved from https://nexusipe-resource-exchange.s3.amazonaws.com/Educating_for_the_Health_Team_IOM_1972.pdf

Institute of Medicine. (2001). Crossing the quality chasm: A new health system for the 21st century. Retrieved from http://iom.nationalacademies.org/~/media/Files/Report%20Files/2001/Crossing-the-Quality-Chasm/Quality%20Chasm%202001%20%20report%20brief.pdf

Interprofessional Education Collaborative. (2016). *Resources*. Retrieved from https://ipecollaborative.org/Resources.html

Jacomino, M., Bamdas, J. M., Keller, K., Hamlin, E., Hawkins, M., Gordon, S., & Ouslander, J. G. (2015). An innovative interprofessional education program for university medical, nursing, and social work students learning in teams during sessions and visits with geriatric mentors. *Journal of Interprofessional Education & Practice*, *1*(3-4), 100–103. doi:10.1016/j.xjep.2015.10.003

Jencks, S. F., Williams, M. V., & Coleman, E. A. (2009). Rehospitalizations among patients in the Medicare fee-for-service program. *The New England Journal of Medicine*, *360*(14), 1418–1428. doi:10.1056/NEJMsa0803563 PMID:19339721

Kilcup, M., Schultz, D., Carlson, J., & Wilson, B. (2003). Postdischarge pharmacist medication reconciliation: Impact on readmission rates and financial savings. *Journal of the Journal of the American Pharmacists Association*, *53*(1), 78–84. doi:10.1331/JAPhA.2013.11250 PMID:23636160

Kohn, L. T., Corrigan, J. M., & Donaldson, M. S. (Eds.). (2000). *Institute of medicine: To err is human: Building a safer health system*. Washington, DC: National Academies Press.

McDaniel, A., & Robertson, K. (1995). Interdisciplinary professional education: A collaborative clinical teaching project. *American Journal of Pharmaceutical Education*, *59*(2), 131–136.

National Center for Education Statistics. (n. d.). *What is NAAL?* Retrieved from https://nces.ed.gov/naal/

National Center for Interprofessional Practice and Education. (2015). *About the national center*. Retrieved from https://nexusipe.org/informing/about-national-center

National Coordinating Council for Medication Error and Prevention. (2016). *About medication errors*. Retrieved from http://www.nccmerp.org/about-medication-errors

Naylor, M. D., & Keating, S. K. (2008). Transitional care: Movement from one care setting to another. *The American Journal of Nursing*, *108*(S9), 58–63. doi:10.1097/01.NAJ.0000336420.34946.3a PMID:18797231

Parker, R. (2000). Health literacy: A challenge for American patients and their healthcare providers. *Health Promotion International*, *15*(4), 277–283. doi:10.1093/heapro/15.4.277

Patient Protection and Affordable Care Act, 42 U.S.C. § 18001 (2010).

Payne, R. A., & Avery, A. J. (2011). Polypharmacy: One of the greatest prescribing challenges in general practice. *The British Journal of General Practice*, *61*(583), 83–84. doi:10.3399/bjgp11X556146 PMID:21276330

Pinquart, M., & Sorensen, S. (2003). Differences between caregivers and noncaregivers in psychological health and physical health: A meta-analysis. *Psychology and Aging*, *18*(2), 250–267. doi:10.1037/0882-7974.18.2.250 PMID:12825775

Project RED. (2014). *Project RED (re-engineered discharge)*. Retrieved from http://www.bu.edu/fammed/projectred/

Rozich, J. D., & Resar, R. K. (2001). Medication safety: One organization's approach to the challenge. *Journal of Clinical Outcomes Management*, *8*(10), 27–34.

Schulz, R., Newsom, J., Mittelmark, M., Burton, L., Hirsch, C., & Jackson, S. (1997). Health effects of caregiving: The caregiver health effects study: An ancillary study of the cardiovascular health study. *Annals of Behavioral Medicine*, *19*(2), 110–116. doi:10.1007/BF02883327 PMID:9603685

Script Your Future. (2014). *Script your future program*. Retrieved from http://www.scriptyourfuture.org/wp-content/uploads/2014/11/lessons_learned.pdf

Script Your Future. (2016). *Tools*. Retrieved from http://www.scriptyourfuture.org/tools/

Sebaaly, J., Parsons, L. B., Pilch, N. A., Bullington, W., Hayes, G. L., & Easterling, H. (2015). Clinical and financial impact of pharmacist involvement in discharge medication reconciliation at an academic medical center: A prospective pilot study. *Hospital Pharmacy*, *50*(6), 505–513. doi:10.1310/hpj5006-505 PMID:26405342

Silo Mentality. (2016). In *Business Dictionary.com*. Retrieved from http://www.businessdictionary.com/definition/silo-mentality.html#ixzz3yZpAGcrA

Society of Hospital Medicine. (2015). *Project BOOST® mentored implementation program*. Retrieved from http://www.hospitalmedicine.org/BOOST/

Stanton, M. P., & Lammon, C. A. (2008). The "wins" of change: Evaluating the impact of predicted changes on case management practice. *Professional Case Management*, *13*(3), 161–168. doi:10.1097/01.PCAMA.0000319970.61358.9a PMID:18562911

Starr, B., & Sacks, R. (2010). *Improving outcomes for patients with chronic disease: The medication adherence project (MAP)*. Retrieved from http://www.nyc.gov/html/doh/downloads/pdf/cardio/cardio-map-tools-manual.pdf

Tam, V. C., Knowles, S. R., Cornish, P. L., Fine, N., Marchesano, R., & Etchells, E. E. (2005). Frequency, type and clinical importance of medication history errors at admission to hospital: A systematic review. *Canadian Medical Association Journal*, *173*(5), 510–515. doi:10.1503/cmaj.045311 PMID:16129874

The Joint Commission. (2016). *National patient safety goals effective January 1, 2016*. Retrieved from http://www.jointcommission.org/assets/1/6/2016_NPSG_AHC.pdf

The Joint Commission. Joint Commission Center for Transforming Healthcare, & Joint Commission Resources. (n. d.). *Transitions of care: The need for a more effective approach to continuing patient care*. Retrieved from http://www.jointcommission.org/assets/1/18/Hot_Topics_Transitions_of_Care.pdf

The University of Texas at Austin. (n. d.). *Physician role*. Retrieved from http://www.healthipe.org/healthcare-roles/physician

Think Florida. (n. d.). *Home page*. Retrieved from http://think-florida.org

University of Hawai'i at Hilo. (2012). *College of pharmacy awarded $14.3 million to develop system to save healthcare costs* [News release]. Retrieved from http://hilo.hawaii.edu/news/press/release/1196

University of Washington. (2016). *Center for health sciences interprofessional education, research, and practice*. Retrieved from http://collaborate.uw.edu/about/about-us.html

World Health Organization. (2010). *Framework for interprofessional education and collaborative practice*. Retrieved from http://apps.who.int/iris/bitstream/10665/70185/1/WHO_HRH_HPN_10.3_eng.pdf?ua=1

World Health Organization. (2016). *Patients for patient safety*. Retrieved from http://www.who.int/patientsafety/patients_for_patient/en/

Zillich, A. J., Snyder, M. E., Frail, C. K., Lewis, J. L., Deshotels, D., Dunham, P., & Sutherland, J. M. et al. (2014). A randomized, controlled pragmatic trial of telephonic medication therapy management to reduce hospitalization in home health patients. *Health Services Research*, *49*(5), 1537–1554. doi:10.1111/1475-6773.12176 PMID:24712335

KEY TERMS AND DEFINITIONS

Health Literacy: The degree to which individuals have the capacity to obtain, process, and understand basic health information needed to make appropriate health decisions (Health Resources and Services Administration, 2016).

Interprofessional Education: (IPE): Occurs when two or more professions learn with, from, and about each other to improve collaboration and the quality of care (CAIPE, 2002).

Medication Errors: "Any preventable event that may cause or lead to inappropriate medication use or patient harm while the medication is in the control of the healthcare professional, patient, or consumer. Such events may be related to professional practice, healthcare products, procedures, and systems including prescribing; order communication; product labeling, packaging, and nomenclature; compounding; dispensing; distribution; administration; education; monitoring; and use" (The National Coordinating Council for Medication Error and Prevention, 2016).

Polypharmacy: Concurrent prescribing of at least four or five drugs (Payne, & Avery, 2011).

Readmission: Admission to a subsection (d) hospital within 30 days of a discharge from the same or another subsection (d) hospital (CMS, 2016b).

Transitions of Care: Refers to the movement of patients between healthcare practitioners, settings, and home as their condition and care needs change (The Joint Commission, 2016).

Triple Aim: A framework developed by the Institute for Healthcare Improvement that describes an approach to optimizing health system performance (IHI, 2016).

This work was previously published in Healthcare Community Synergism between Patients, Practitioners, and Researchers edited by Valerie C. Bryan and Jennifer Lynne Bird, pages 65-87, copyright year 2017 by Medical Information Science Reference (an imprint of IGI Global).

Chapter 17
Meeting Patients Where They Are:
Using Multimedia and Interactive Voice Technology to Humanize Communication and Engage Patients

Geri Lynn Baumblatt
Emmi Solutions, LLC, USA

ABSTRACT

In this chapter the author describes the challenges of engaging and communicating with patients and how technology can improve communication, elicit honest patient disclosure, and create more productive conversation and help patients engage and partner in their care. The author will also discuss how research with multimedia programs reveals it can help reduce anxiety, improve knowledge, help low health literacy audiences, and contribute to improved outcomes. This chapter will also examine how multimedia decision aid programs can help patients understand their options and complex risk information, while helping them consider their values and preferences so they can truly engage in shared decision making.

INTRODUCTION

Each of us becomes a patient when we interact with the healthcare system. We all want to avoid pain and suffering, feel better, and have a good quality of life. Beyond that, we also want to avoid adverse events, infections, procedures, and unnecessary costly treatments that drive up the cost of care for everyone. And people definitely do not want to accrue medical bills that put them or their family in serious financial jeopardy (Himmelstein, Warren, Thorne, & Woolhandler, 2005).

Yet, despite the high stakes and their own wellbeing, “patients are the most underutilized resource” in healthcare (Safran, 2004). Why is this?

DOI: 10.4018/978-1-5225-1928-7.ch017

Unfortunately, even in the best circumstances, patient-provider relationships are beset with challenges. Over the course of a year, clinicians only have the opportunity to spend mere minutes interacting with patients and family caregivers. The challenges are compounded by the patient-clinician power dynamic, health literacy and literacy challenges, as well as, social, economic, emotional and physical stress, not to mention any pain, fatigue, or challenges caused by an illness.

Many people end up at the mercy of poor health, feeling anything but competent and in control. Illness and disease often robs us of our autonomy and diminishes our volition. The process of seeking treatment or getting diagnosed can also be unnerving. For example, if you have chest pain, are you over-reacting or under-reacting if you go to the emergency department? We often lack the knowledge to evaluate the situation and act. In the face of a diagnosis or procedure we want to feel in control and capable of dealing with our circumstances. Instead, even physicians report feeling carried along by a system that makes it harder instead of easier to act or question events.

As kidney cancer patient and Society of Participatory Medicine board member Peggy Zuckerman explains, "Patients would be more likely to communicate with their doctors, whether electronically or otherwise, if there was real encouragement in communication. Right now, much of it is one-way, physician-to-patient, with the physician setting the rules and the agenda. In most other personal encounters, there is a bit of time to create a tone of collaboration. In a medical setting, the time constraints, the culture of paternalism, and the complexity of information to be dispersed and/or shared makes communication more difficult" (personal communication, April 30, 2015).

Yet, each day patients need to take medications, make challenging lifestyle and behavior changes, remember how to do their physical therapy exercises, and show up for important but intimidating procedures, like colonoscopies.

This chapter will explore how poor communication, knowledge gaps and incomplete understanding (the realm of health literacy) and communication affects the ability, interest and motivation of patients to engage in self-care, even at the most basic level.

Then it will look at how technology such as web-based multimedia programs and interactive voice response (IVR) calls, can empower patients to participate and partner in their care and become owners of their health and wellbeing. These tools create an easy, low effort, and less stressful way for patients and families to understand their health conditions and procedures, ask honest and even embarrassing questions, and create the competency and understanding they need to participate in shared decision making. It will also describe research showing these programs can reduce anxiety and improve knowledge as well as clinical outcomes.

BACKGROUND

The term "patient" stems from Old French *pacient or "patience"* meaning: "quality of being willing to bear adversities, calm endurance of misfortune, suffering, etc." To be "patient" is to "endure without complaint" (Harper, 2001). This is a historical definition, but it connotes deference, powerlessness, and passivity as well as a need to be firm and unyielding, as if to say: do as caregivers say, but do not give in to pain or despair. Only fairly recently do patients no longer see themselves as passive recipients of care or those who are acted upon, but as motivated partners, or even as advocates who must intervene in their care.

As many have noted, the term "patient engagement" implies patients must be activated to engage. Yet, in this fundamentally mutual enterprise, we often fail to provide patients with the most essential tools to participate: a real understanding of their condition, how it will affect their life over time, their treatment options, and the time, ability, and a safe and unintimidating setting to ask meaningful questions about their care.

Leaving Patients to Connect the Dots

Too often, we presume patients know and understand their condition at least at a very basic level. We assume people were previously educated — that there was a moment of level setting, candor, knowledge transfer, and teach-back to confirm understanding. However, in most cases, that either never took place, or the patient, still reeling from the news of a diabetes or cancer diagnosis, simply could not absorb it. Other times, a silent condition like hypertension may not register as important or even real. And the information is often provided at a level many people cannot fully understand, or in a way that leaves it to patients to "connect the dots."

For example, when a patient is diagnosed with type 2 diabetes, simply understanding the concept of blood sugar is new. And when we talk about "sugar", how many people understand this is not limited to refined sugar, desserts, and sugary drinks? Do we truly help them understand how what they eat and their ability to manage diabetes will affect their body over time? It is fairly easy for patients to understand what it means when we say that over time diabetes will affect their eyes and vision. And it can even be fairly straightforward to explain how diabetes affects the nerves in their feet to help them understand why they may not feel a cut or injury that can become infected. But while some people understand an infection can lead to the loss of a foot, or may know of family members this happened to, other times this potential outcome is inferred and not made explicit. This is not to suggest we should frighten people into action, but to ensure they understand what is at stake so their actions are moored in that knowledge.

To go a step further, if a patient is told that over time, diabetes will affect their kidneys and can lead to kidney disease, what does that mean to them? Kidney disease sounds bad, but for most people it is largely an abstraction — organs that sound important but do not confer the same type of immediately understandable benefit like eyesight. How many people understand that "kidney problems" may eventually lead to dialysis, surgery to create a fistula in their arm so they can receive dialysis, or to a potential kidney transplant? And how often is there a clear conversation about how their condition and treatment will affect their longevity?

In the United States, nephrologists often find that a large number of people with diabetes and hypertension never show up when they are referred to a nephrologist. Patients often have no understanding why they are being referred or how important it is. It seems unfair to assume they simply do not care. Instead, patients often reach a point where they need to make decisions about their renal care, and when they hear how their condition has progressed, they often feel blind-sided by a conversation about dialysis.

It is extremely challenging to be candid with people about this kind of information. And these messages need to be repeated multiple times and in various ways to ensure people take it in and know what it means for their day-to-day life. When these dots are not connected to create a unified picture, people *appear* un-engaged. In reality, they are not acting because they do not recognize how their condition, medication, or procedure will affect (or is already affecting) them.

The Challenge of Low Health Literacy

Numerous studies bear out the health literacy gaps that create failures in what should be a smooth connection between knowledge, activation, and action. The study of Fang, Panguluri, Machtinger and Schillinger (2009) measured the health literacy of 183 patients who were taking warfarin (most of them for many years) to prevent a stroke. "When questioned about the drug, however, only 9.3% of the study participants understood that the purpose of their taking warfarin was to prevent stroke. Perhaps even more shocking was the fact that more than 40% of patients surveyed did not know what a stroke was" (Fang et al., 2009). Of course, without basic health education, most people do not know what a stroke is or the diversity of problems it can cause.

When people do not get the knowledge and information about their health in a way they can understand — and what it means in the near and long term — how can we expect them to be activated to engage?

Health literacy research shows that avoiding medical jargon and communicating with patients in plain language is essential. Yet, even when information is understandable, working memory (the ability to remember, process and comprehend information) fails. Pain and illness adds additional burdens to focus, attention, and comprehension. It is no wonder research shows by time patients walk out the door they have already forgotten anywhere from 40% to 80% of what they were told; and much of what is remembered is often incorrect (Kessels, 2003).

Power Dynamics at Play

Patients both rely on and are intimidated by clinicians. Many clinicians make meaningful efforts to mitigate this power dynamic; but patients are often embarrassed to ask questions or voice concerns (Katz, Jacobson, Veldar, & Kripalani, 2007). People often nod their heads as though in agreement, afraid or unable to articulate their concerns. Other times, people silently choose not to take a medication because it previously gave a relative or friend a side effect, like leg pain. As a VP of Clinical Care Management for a U.S. health system explained, "You're asking for personal information from people… But I knew people were leaving medications at the pharmacy and not picking them up. And I knew people wouldn't tell you things like that" (Gerr, Saulsberry, Clark, & Kerns, 2014, p. 25).

Whether consciously or unconsciously, patients often do not respond honestly or withhold information because they want to be viewed positively and create a good impression. This "impression management" (also called "self presentation") means that as patients, we are not reliable (Leary & Kowalski, 1990). Unfortunately, clinicians get a less accurate picture of what patients are and are not willing and able to do. This causes communication gaps, especially around stigmatized topics like eating disorders, tobacco and drug use, as well as more common topics like contraception, acne, and exercise habits (Leary, Tchividijian, & Kraxberger, 1994).

Impression management also plays a role in whether people will make lifestyle changes. For example, people who see themselves as overweight, flabby, or not fit are often embarrassed to be seen working out, putting on a swimsuit, or lifting weights that look light to others at a gym. Termed "physique anxiety," this can be paralyzing but not something people readily admit. A study of overweight women's reactions to exercise programs found the "most powerful influences seemed to be the social circumstances of the exercise setting, especially concerns about visibility, embarrassment, and judgment by others" (Bain, Wilson, & Chaikind, 1989).

Technology can help mediate face-to-face power dynamics. It can address and normalize unspoken patient concerns. It can also facilitate better relationships, create new lines of patient-clinician communication, improve understanding, and empower patents to engage.

SOLUTIONS AND RECOMMENDATIONS

Technology was once thought of as cold and impersonal. Today we know technology and the online world can be deeply engaging. Something as simple as a text message or emoticon can generate experiences of connection and care. A survey of people age 19 to 29 indicated they are so attached to these devices they sleep with their smartphone or tablet in their bed (Schocker, 2013). These devices connect us to the larger world, allowing us to interact with friends, family, and colleagues. They connect us to others with similar interests, health conditions, political views, and help us find everything from romance to employment.

When technological tools and information are designed in partnership with both patients and clinicians, they can become powerful ways to engage patients, and to share understandable, reliable information. This formative research helps ensure this information resonates with their current pain, problems, and even embarrassing concerns.

For decades, patients have been sent home with brochures, booklets, printouts, and discharged with binders full of instructions. These tomes make good doorstops, but reading them feels like a task. They can be an intimidating format even for educated and highly motivated patients. And for those with literacy and reading challenges, they are inaccessible.

People often sit down to read print materials or screens of static online text with a sigh, mustering the energy to begin. Reading takes effort, and stressful clinical information multiplies that burden. So when stressed, scared, ill, and weary patients go home with information critical for them to understand, narrated multimedia or video provides a more approachable format that reduces cognitive load and requires less mental effort. These formats can demonstrate procedural steps and can animate information in an unintimidating and diagrammatic way that anyone can understand. In fact, simplified medical information is preferred regardless of education level (Davis, Crouch, Wills, Miller, & Abdehou, 1990).

Prescribed, Web-Based Multimedia Programs

Multimedia combines voiceover, illustrations, animation, text, and interactions. Consistent with Mayer and Moreno's findings (2003) in the development of cognitive theory of multimedia learning, this type of orchestrated content creates a low-effort experience and enables patients to quickly view a lot of information in an easy-to-understand format.

Multimedia programs can connect with patients in language they understand, at a time when they are ready to learn, and on the devices they already own. This consumer-friendly technology helps patients engage in more productive conversations with their healthcare team and to take action around healthcare events or conditions.

Multimedia can help patients understand newly diagnosed health conditions, how and why to use a device like a nebulizer or CPAP device, or educate people about new skills and behaviors like injecting insulin or breastfeeding. It can help people understand their treatment options and consider their goals, values and preferences. Programs developed in these formats can also help people understand an upcoming test or procedure while augmenting and helping to document more thorough and authentic informed consent.

Multimedia programs can also be part of a technology platform so that clinicians can prescribe the programs to patients. Other times, multimedia programs can be placed on a patient portal. However, when a clinician or a member of the care team, hospital, or health plan recommends and prescribes programs, and each patient receives a personalized and unique access code, this confers a level of importance. This creates a sense of intention and feeling cared for and both patients know they are getting exactly the information their physician wants them to see. The recommendation of the clinicians helps patients recognize the information is essential, helpful, worth their time. Clinicians also know the information the patient views is up to date and relevant; as opposed to the variable information people may come across when doing an online search.

An individualized prescription (often delivered via email as web link) for information that is relevant to that individual can be delivered to a patient before, after, or between clinical encounters.

For example, if a patient is being scheduled for a surgical procedure, a multimedia or video program can be ordered, the patient is notified, they can view the program on any web-enabled device, and the experience can also be tracked. A program can be prescribed when a patient is scheduled for their procedure. It can also be prescribed or automated through an electronic medical record (EMR).

Patients can opt to receive their personalized access code however it is most convenient for them: by email, phone, text message, or a print out. Patients can view programs on any web-enabled device (tablet, desktop computer, laptop, or smartphone) when it is convenient for them. This type of choice autonomy gives people freedom to absorb information in the comfort of their home, where the stress and distraction of the clinical environment and patient-physician power dynamic do not interfere. People are truly "at home" as a person instead of as a "diabetic" or a patient. People can pause, go back, and re-play sections or watch the program as many times as they like. They are in control and can review the information as needed.

This type of web-based information also makes it easy to share it with other family members who often cannot be present to hear the clinician's explanation or instructions. It can also help families co-ordinate care; if an adult child lives half way across the country, without much effort, they can log on, watch, and understand their parent's procedure, recovery, why it is being done, and what the risks and alternatives are, and better plan a visit to help with the recovery.

These types of programs can also be tracked. This way patients can be reminded to start or finish watching a program if they forget. And questions patients type in captured for them in their patient portal or in personalized print summary. On some platforms, any questions the patient has can be typed in, tracked/captured for the clinician, who can then review the patient's questions and better prepare for their next conversation. This type of tracking can also help document best practices, such as providing education for topics like breastfeeding or counseling for smoking cessation.

A personal access code also creates a secure way for patients and clinicians to communicate with each other — a problem so often hindered by privacy concerns, and, in the United States, by compliance with the federal Health Insurance Portability and Accountability Act (HIPAA) of 1996 that protects the confidentiality and security of healthcare information.

Engaging Patients in Meaningful Informed Consent

Helping patients truly understand their procedures and the associated risks and alternatives is the true spirit of informed consent. Multimedia programs can provide more robust informed consent. It can give patients more realistic expectations and give them the knowledge they need to make truly informed decisions, and helps confirm whether a procedure will treat their symptoms and condition.

This helps address the culture of defensive medicine. In the United States, malpractice insurers like Beazley recognize the benefits this more robust patient education and engagement, and provide a reduced premium for hospitals that use this type of engagement technology.

Narrated Animation: Improved Understanding

Most patients have only a very basic understanding of physiology. Without much existing knowledge to build on, clinicians often struggle to help patients understand unfamiliar anatomy, health conditions, and procedures. Without strong visuals, these explanations frequently leave patients lost and confused.

However, when animation is coupled with narration patients can watch and understand key physiology (like how blood moves through the heart), or it can help them grasp more complex information (like ejection fraction). These challenging concepts are often essential to patients understanding their conditions or making decisions about procedures.

Other times, patients need to learn a new skill (like putting on compression stockings, or how to use a device (like a nebulizer). Multimedia demonstrations can provide a significant improvement over a series of static images that can leave out key information and make the reader or viewer do more interpretative work to understand the progression.

Research done by Meppelink, van Weert, Haven and Smit (2015) found that when animation is combined with narration, people with limited health literacy have better recall of the information. Interestingly, narrated information also creates better attitudes to the information. When narration was used to inform people about colon cancer screening, it resulted in better attitudes towards the message itself, which positively influenced screening attitudes. These positive attitudes resulted in stronger intentions to get screened. This is supported by previous research showing multimedia learning leads to increased motivation because of the autonomy, self pacing, and review opportunities (Schunk, Pintrich, & Meece, 2008). Better motivation and attitudes have also been associated with multimedia education. Abdoolatiff and Narod (2009) found students who completed a computer-based science lab performed significantly better on a test measuring understanding of the lab and reported increased motivation and enthusiasm for the material.

In the study done by Meppelink et al. (2015), researchers concluded that voice narration paired with animations "is the best way to communicate complex health information to people with low health literacy." This is essential for reaching the most vulnerable and underserved patients.

The Ease of Listening to a Conversation

Reading demands a high level of effort and concentration. Pain, discomfort, worry about a diagnosis, or the shock of being diagnosed with a serious condition puts people in a state of flight or flight and creates "attentional narrowing," where the brain can only focus on the most frightening statements (Kessels, 2003). These diagnoses can have a profound effect on a patient's emotional state. One study of over 1000 women found 23% of women diagnosed with breast cancer experienced post-traumatic stress disorder (PTSD), with 16.5% still experiencing PTSD two to three months later (Vin-Raviv et al., 2013). The physical and emotional stress makes it challenging for patients to focus, absorb, and remember information or thoughtfully consider treatment options.

With narration, the viewer can listen instead of read. Words are processed in the verbal channel instead of visually. This helps offload the cognitive load placed on the brain to process and understand information. With narration "the processing demands on the visual channel are thereby reduced, so the learner is better able to select important aspects of animation for further processing" (Mayer & Moreno, 2003).

And when narration is friendly, conversational, and empathic, viewers report they can listen to information they otherwise find too overwhelming to read. The voiceover seems to replace or temper patients' own more anxious internal voice that tends to take over when they read.

Conversational narration creates the experience of a well-informed friend is sitting next to people and walking them through the information. Casual conversation is our most familiar and comfortable mode of language and communication. As linguists like John McWhorter (2012, 2013) explain, "pragmatic particles" (also called "discourse particles") such as "well" and "you know" are a common way to indicate empathy. These colloquial moments "help establish a warm shared frame of reference".

According to Clark and Mayer (2011), multiple studies found conversational narration helps learners identify with the content and understand it better than more formal language (pp. 184-185). Casual speech also has a way of reaching out, whereas the technical and clinical language of medicine excludes people and reminds them they are not "in the know," even though the experience of their illness or procedure is often deeply personal.

Understanding Patient Concerns, Reducing Anxiety, and Improving Outcomes

When multimedia content is developed with both patients and clinicians providing input and feedback, the programs can then anticipate common patient questions and concerns. For example, acute back pain can be frightening and seem debilitating, and it is rife with misconceptions. When patients schedule appointments to see their physician for low back pain, at the same time a multimedia program about that topic can be prescribed so they can view it before their appointment. With this pre-appointment education, patients learn back pain usually is *not* serious, imaging is *not* usually needed, and findings like a herniated disc are common and are *not* necessarily the cause of their pain. With these assumptions and worries addressed, the patient is much less likely to arrive in a nervous state, catastrophizing their pain and asking for imaging, which is often unnecessary and counterproductive. Instead, they arrive with their worst fears already allayed.

For a procedure like colonoscopy, there is a lot of procedure-related anxiety because it sounds uncomfortable, unfamiliar, and embarrassing. Patients often cancel or do not show up for scheduled procedures. Patients often worry about something they are too embarrassed to ask about, like an existing hemorrhoid, thinking it may cause serious pain during a colonoscopy. Working with patients when creating this content can help anticipate these types of questions so they can be addressed and normalized. Patients realize that even though the topic felt embarrassing, it must be common enough to address it in a general program.

Of course, the answers to these questions are not always good. In those instances, the conversational narration can level with people, creating a moment of candor. Knowing and feeling like they were told the truth is still less stressful than the anxiety of the unknown.

When topics like hemorrhoids, sex, gas, and bowel movements are addressed, it also makes people feel comfortable to ask other questions.

Content designed with patients have also been shown to reduce patient anxiety and lead to better outcomes. In a study at the University of Chicago Medical Center, the gastroenterology department prescribed a multimedia colonoscopy program to patients when they scheduled them for their procedure. Most of the patients who viewed the program (89%) showed up for their colonoscopy, compared with only 68% of patients who did not watch it (Thomas, Kedia, & Cohen, 2007).

Multimedia programs have also been shown to reduce anxiety and improve outcomes. In a randomized controlled study at Dartmouth-Hitchcock Medical Center, 51 patients were given a standard printed pre-procedural packet. A second group of 52 patients received both the print packet and were also prescribed the multimedia colonoscopy program. Patients' perception of their anxiety level was measured with a state trait anxiety inventory before and after patients reviewed the print packet or the packet plus the multimedia program. Of the patients who viewed the multimedia program, 58% reported reduced anxiety (Parker, Zipurksy, Ma, & Siegel, 2013).

In addition, those who viewed the multimedia colonoscopy program were 11% more knowledgeable. And even though the physicians performing the colonoscopies did not know which patients had watched the multimedia program, analysis found patients who viewed it also required 18% less sedation medication and their procedure times were 14% shorter (Parker et al., 2013). This was further confirmation that those patients were less anxious.

Normalizing the Patient Experience

Helping patients feel comfortable so they will ask the questions weighing on their minds and disclose personal information is key to engagement. Patients often get home and realize they do not understand instructions, what a medication or treatment is meant to do, or when to call about problems or side effects, etc. The onus is then on them to find out, and to admit they do not remember or understand.

Virtual interactions with multimedia and interactive voice response (IVR) phone calls help create a sense of privacy and safety. Research shows people are more likely to honestly self-reveal personal information in a virtual setting (Lucas, Gratch, King, & Morency, 2014). Once another human is no longer present, impression management is diminished. People have a "sense of invulnerability to criticism… and an impression their responses 'disappear' into the computer" (Weisband & Kiesler, 1996, p. 3).

Taking this a step further, multimedia can enable patients to ask questions virtually. The program can even prompt and encourage people to ask questions. This can help patients feel it is safe and acceptable to ask questions, and that it is even something they are invited and expected to do.

For example, it is always difficult to broach the topic of smoking. Clinicians do not like bringing it up, and patients feel ashamed and judged. Even though most people want to quit, it usually takes about seven attempts to quit permanently. And before that final, successful quit attempt, people feel like failures. However, when information about quitting is presented in a virtual environment, when another human is not present, patient viewers are less likely to feel pressured, shamed, or lectured.

Likewise, when it comes to the risks of a procedure, patients and families are often hesitant to ask questions. They may fear it will be interpreted as litigious or as questioning the physician's skill or experience. Multimedia programs can walk patients through risk information at home. Interface design and narration can invite patients to flag risks in virtual setting, which helps them feel safe and normalizes it. The technology can also enable the physician's office to receive any flagged risk in advance so they have time to prepare for the conversation with the patient before their next meeting.

Creating a Safe, Honest Environment

As discussed above, virtual interactions have been shown to make people feel safe and they are more likely to honestly disclose information. Personalized, interactive voice response (IVR) phone calls can also be used to reach out and provide small doses of information to help keep patients and family members on point with daily tasks and to collect information like outstanding patient questions, new symptoms or side effects.

Research shows patients are comfortable engaging with IVR calls across a variety of health conditions. In a study done by Piette et al. (2013), patients completed 83% of attempted IVR assessments. Participation rates for heart failure and cancer were 90%, 81% for the diabetes, and 71% among patients with depression. That same study found that "older patients had higher call completion rates, even among patients > 75 years of age."

For example, a single IVR call can be used to reach patients to find out if they had a diabetes eye exam. If they have, this information can be reported back to their physician for documentation. If they have not, the IVR call can help patients understand why this is important and a "warm-transfer" can be done so the patient can immediately speak with an office to schedule their exam. This takes advantage of the patient's intention to act, but does not leave it to the patient's motivation or memory to make a separate call to schedule it during business hours.

Other times, a series of IVR calls can be used with our without multimedia programs to help patients engage and more successfully transition from hospital to home. For example, when a patient with heart failure is discharged to home, they and members of their family (both local and remote) can be signed up to receive regular IVR calls for a number of weeks or even months. An automated IVR call series can deliver and reinforce necessary instructions, like making sure they schedule and have transportation to their follow-up appointment. IVR calls can also collect data on patients' status to ensure recovery is progressing. Patients can be asked if they have any questions about taking their medications, or if they have any new symptoms or side effects. In this virtual setting, patients feel safe honestly disclosing personal information like their weight, or admitting they are still confused about the changes to their medications.

In the case of heart failure, patients can be asked if they have a scale to weigh themselves, the call can explain why getting a daily weight is important, ask if they weighed themselves, and how much they weigh each day. The hospital can then get a daily report, and an algorithm can be used to identify if any patients have gained weight over the course of a week (as this is usually an early warning sign of trouble). If they have, this can be noted as a red flag. The hospital staff can then use their human resources more intelligently and efficiently to reach out to those patients to engage them.

In a small study of 20 patents with heart failure most participants 95% said receiving IVR calls helped them feel more connected to their health care team and more confident in performing care plan activities. 90% also felt better prepared to start discussions about their health with their doctor (Zan et al., 2015).

Engaging Patients in Shared Decision Making

Often, there is no single best treatment option for something like low-risks prostate cancer, and patients are ideally invited to take part in shared decision making (SDM). SDM is a process where the provider helps the patient understand the decision, its consequences, and then helps them apply their values and preferences in order to make the best decision for that individual. This can be very challenging. And decision aids are tools that can be used during or between clinical encounters to help walk patients through this information in a more understandable and unbiased way.

The benefit of decision aids generally is well documented. In its review of the impact of decision aids, the Cochrane Collaboration reviewed 115 randomized controlled studies. When decision aids were compared to usual care, patients who used decision aids were more knowledgeable and had much more realistic expectations. 74% of people had more realistic expectations, 31% were less passive in decisions, with fewer people left undecided (Stacey et al., 2014).

Unfortunately, clinicians often view patients as unwilling or unable to engage in SDM. For example, a survey of 106 gastroenterologists found that 34% were enthusiastic about SDM and 47% were actually skeptical of it, with only 12% stating they have a "systemic, consistent, and formally documented approach to SDM" (Siegel et al., 2015). In contrast, a survey of 460 patients with a serious digestive disease, namely ulcerative colitis (UC), across a wide age range (19 to 81) found that most patients (87%) wanted to share treatment decision-making with their doctors. In fact, the majority (98%) also wanted more than just a basic understanding of UC (Thompson et al., 2016). A systematic review of patient preferences for shared decisions found that 71% of patients want to be involved in decisions (Chewning et al., 2012).

Patients are often very interested to understand their condition or options. Many people are simply overwhelmed and have no idea where to begin asking questions or discussing their preferences. They lack the orientation and understanding to participate in a clinical conversation. As one mother explained, "When we were told my four year old son had Crohn's, our world flipped upside down. The attending doc… saw the mom-panic in my eyes, sat down, put his feet up on my son's bed and settled in for a nice long chat. However, I didn't have any idea what to ask." (personal communication, Sept 11, 2014). This sense of feeling both panicked and adrift is common. Yet we expect patients to settle in for a conversation when they are neither oriented nor calm. What is often interpreted as unwillingness or inability of patients to participate may be the healthcare system's failure to give people the understanding and support they need to engage.

Anxiety about a condition or treatment options can continue to exist even when patients have been living with a condition for many years. Helping people consider all the treatment options for a condition like ulcerative colitis (UC) is challenging. UC impacts patients' quality of life and increases their risk of colon cancer. Despite having serious problems for many years, people with UC are often afraid to learn about surgical treatment, which usually involves getting a temporary or permanent ostomy (where a bag is placed over an opening on their abdomen to collect feces). People tend to underestimate their emotional resilience and ability to adapt and bounce back from things that seem unimaginable, like an ostomy or learning to self-inject a medication.

This is a known challenge in SDM that social psychologists have termed: "immune neglect," because people think it will take longer and be harder for their so-called psychological immune system to cope and adapt. People often refer to an ostomy bag it as a "poop bag" and cannot imagine living with it, let alone that it could provide a better quality of life. In fact, research shows that not only do people with colostomies report the same moods and similar levels of life satisfaction as those who do not have them, but "overall life satisfaction and quality of life increased with time for patients with permanent, but not temporary, ostomies" (Smith, Lowenstein, Rozin, Sherriff, & Ubel, 2007).

Unfortunately, this leads people to make poor decisions. A UK study found increased UC-related mortality when treating UC with colectomy [ostomy] surgery was only considered as a last resort (Roberts, Williams, Yeates, & Goldacre, 2007). Delaying surgery for UC to the point of last resort also increases post-op complications (Randall et al., 2010). Therefore, it is essential to help UC patients consider treatments they fear and put off. Unfortunately, fear of UC surgery tends to persist even when others who have gotten an ostomy say how it much better their life is now — even that they wished they had done it years earlier. People are often too scared to read about it online or research surgery on their own.

This was borne out by a study done by Thompson et al. (2016) of 460 UC patients, which found that patients' second biggest concern after the risk of developing colon cancer was surgery to remove their colon, resulting in a temporary or permanent ostomy. In fact, 78% of the patients said they would consider surgery only as a last resort. The article discussion concludes that, "De-mystification of colectomy, and in particular of ileostomy-related and colorectal cancer-related concerns, can dramatically change patient perception of colectomy by directly addressing their 'fear of the unknown'." The same study found that most UC patients (85%) indicated they would find it most helpful to view a web-based decision aid prior to meeting with their doctor to discuss their treatment options.

One benefit of multimedia programs that play like a video or movie is that it is effortlessness to allow the program to play on. Even when the program reaches a stressful topic, the program continues to convey information and does not rely on the viewer's volition to keep moving through it. The format reverses the equation, so that instead of making an effort to keep reading, the patient-viewer needs to make an effort to stop or pause the program – essentially creating a "default effect."

As per self-determination theory, because this type of program is usually viewed at home, there is also time and opportunity to support autonomy by acknowledging emotions that accompany new diagnoses or treatment decision, providing rationale in a way that the patient does not feel judged and minimizes pressure (Deci & Flaste, 1996, p. 101). For example, since most UC patients are resistant to hearing about surgery, a multimedia program can validate and normalize their anxiety and aversion to surgery. The program can acknowledge that for most people surgery to remove the colon is a daunting topic and something that is often thought of as a last resort – creating a moment of empathy.

A multimedia program can provide context, in this case as to why surgery can be a good option at some point and why people should talk with their doctor about when it would be a viable option for them. The animations of the different surgical options (ileostomy or "J-pouch"; see example in Figure 1) demonstrate the procedures in a format that demystifies them and is more understandable than still drawings and less frightening than real video footage.

Figure 1. Example from explanation of J-pouch surgery
© 2014 Emmi Solutions, LLC. Treatment Options for Ulcerative Colitis program

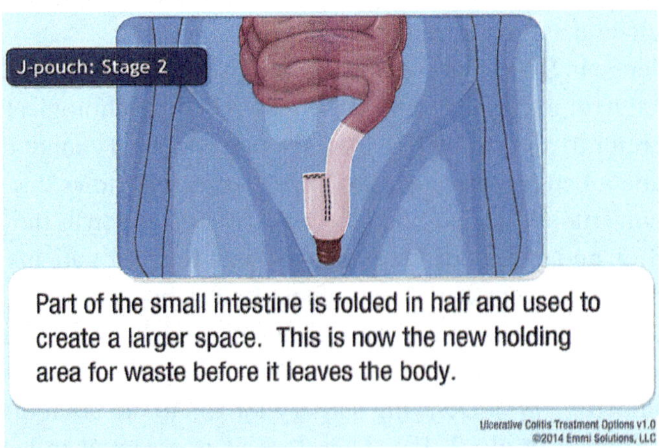

Pressure is minimized and patient autonomy is created when a program provides opportunities to decide whether they want more in-depth information about topics such as the risks of ileostomy or J-pouch surgery, and what life is like afterward. Participants do not feel like information about surgery is being forced on them and are then interested to hear more in-depth information.

While clinicians may often ask patients if they would like more information about a treatment, the interpersonal dynamic may intrude. Patients may feel they would be asking for too much of a clinician's time, or they may feel too overwhelmed to try and absorb it in the office setting. In other cases, they may feel pressured or like they are being a "bad patient" if they decline to hear more information.

Research shows most patients hold back showing emotions like sadness in front of providers. But in a virtual setting people are more likely to display more intense emotions (Lucas et al., 2014). Being able to review an online program at home gives patients the latitude to view it when distractions are minimal, and in a private setting where they are not regulating or suppressing emotions.

In this private setting, multimedia can also take the time to walk patients through thought exercises. For example, this can walk women through various scenarios to help them think about how they would feel wearing a prosthetic under a party dress or bathing suit, how they would feel changing in a gym locker room, how it would impact activities like swimming, and each woman's relationship with her partner.. This is a more emotionally engaging experience that moves beyond the facts of treatment pros, cons, and tradeoffs to help women think about what the reality of day-to-day life would be like. These preferences are uniquely personal and not typically elicited as part of a standard clinical assessment. Research shows that patients who use decision aids that include these types of explicit values clarification exercises are more likely to choose an option congruent with their values (Stacey et al., 2014).

If the patient's doctor is not aware of how she feels about these matters, a treatment might be selected based on criteria that are less important to her. If the doctor assumed a woman wanted to preserve her breast, whereas the patient just wanted to deal with the problem once and for all and avoid the inconvenience of radiation therapy, the doctor might recommend a lumpectomy when a mastectomy might be a better fit. Clinicians cannot predict each patient's unique preferences. Every patient is different and the possible reasons patients and their families may opt for counter-intuitive or unexpected treatment decisions are impossible to predict.

Research shows when clinicians assume they know what patients prefer, they are often wrong. In a study done by Montgomery et al. (2007), physicians thought most women (71%) with breast cancer would rank conserving their breast as a top treatment goal. But when women were surveyed, only seven percent reported it was a top goal for them. And while no physicians in this study (zero percent) believed women would be very concerned about avoiding a prosthetic breast, 33% of patients placed great importance on this. This disconnect between clinician assumptions and reality would send many women down a treatment pathway that does not reflect their goals and would potentially leave them with a greatly diminished quality of life. This mismatch is sometimes called a "preference misdiagnosis."

Interactive capabilities can help patients think through and more document their concerns, goals, and preferences at home where they feel comfortable disclosing what is often very sensitive information (see Figure 2). This creates a better starting point for the conversation with their treatment team.

Decision science continues to investigate virtual interactions to help patients understand not just their preferences, but also the trade-offs of treatment options. Interactive, dynamic slider bars may help people grasp trade-offs to make treatment choices more in line with their values. Instead of asking people what matters to them or having them check or rank it, sliders that adjust based on each other's position as people pull them out or push them back help people understand what is important to them and how this

Figure 2. Example of patient values clarification interaction
© 2012 Emmi Solutions, LLC. Early-stage Invasive Breast Cancer: Considering Your Treatment Options program

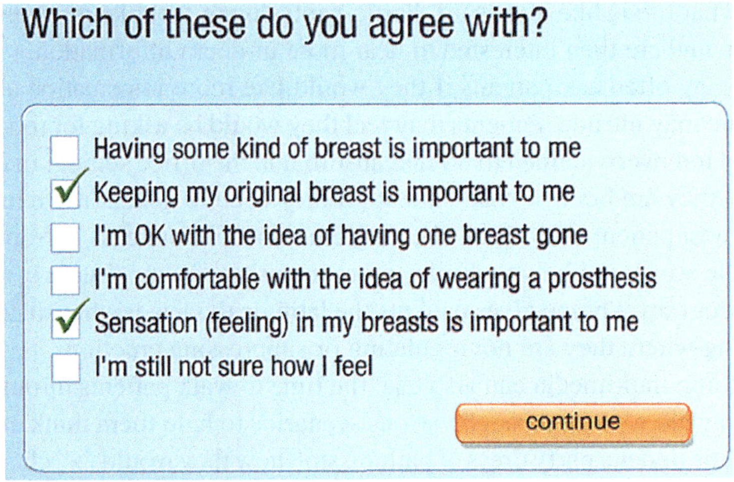

then maps to their treatment options. In work done by Witteman et al. (2012), this kind of interactive exercise reduced the number of patients who experienced discordance between their choices and their stated values from 23% down to 14%.

FUTURE RESEARCH DIRECTIONS

The research and patient feedback on virtual interactions with IVR calls and multimedia program are encouraging. While some outcomes have already been measured, such as patient attendance at procedures and shorter procedure times for colonoscopy, the opportunity to measure numerous other outcomes after patients interact with virtual tools is fertile ground. For example, many patients who view decision aids for chronic hip, knee, and low back pain indicate they are now leaning away from surgery and toward less aggressive treatment like physical therapy. But finding out what treatment patients actually receive is key to understanding to the full impact of these tools and to understanding what kind of training clinicians need so they do not deter or mitigate their impact.

Anecdotally, clinicians often report better experiences when patients use these tools as well. In an era of clinician burnout, it is essential physicians feel they have tools and resources to improve their conversations and help them with the challenges engaging patients in processes that informed consent and shared decision making pose. A growing body of evidence indicates patients who receive this type of multimedia program arrive with a better base understanding of the physiology, their condition, what it means, and what the treatment or procedure entails. Instead of feeling lost, they have better questions rooted in information their provider knows is reliable. There is also opportunity to assess to what degree these tools can improve patient and physician satisfaction, and whether it creates more efficient visits.

Dr. Corey Siegel, Director of the IBD Center at Dartmouth-Hitchcock Medical Center describes his encounters with patients to discuss treatment options for Crohn's disease after they view a multimedia decision aid: "They understand the stakes and are more comfortable being involved in decisions since they have a better grasp of the issues. People are also more comfortable asking me questions" (personal communication, July 19, 2013). It would be valuable to study how and to what degree multimedia tools improve the quality of patient-physician conversations and whether it affects clinicians' perceptions of patients' understanding and their willingness to engage in SDM.

CONCLUSION

Multimedia programs and IVR can help break down patient-clinician communication barriers, reduce patient anxiety, and improve competence, understanding, relational dynamics and autonomy, to create more productive and empowered patients. These tools can create better and more engaging experience for patients, providers, and caregivers. Once patients get information in a way they can understand, review, and share outside of the clinical setting, this gives them the orientation, foundation, privacy, and confidence they need to engage more fully in their care and are empowered to ask the questions that matter to them; and this engagement is an essential for a meaningful and valuable healthcare experience.

REFERENCES

Abdoolatiff, S., & Narod, F. B. (2009). Investigating the effectiveness of computer simulations in the teaching of "atomic structure and bonding". In *Chemistry Education in the ICT Age* (pp. 85-100).

Bain, L. L., Wilson, T., & Chaikind, E. (1989). Participant perceptions of exercise programs for overweight women. *Research Quarterly for Exercise and Sport*, *60*(2), 134–143. doi:10.1080/02701367.1989.10607428 PMID:2489834

Chewning, B., Bylund, C., Shah, B., Arora, N. K., Gueguen, J. A., & Makoul, G. (2012). Patient preferences for shared decisions: A systematic review. *Patient Education and Counseling*, *86*(1), 9–18. doi:10.1016/j.pec.2011.02.004 PMID:21474265

Clark, R., & Mayer, R. (2011). *E-Learning and the Science of Instruction: Proven Guidelines for Consumers and Designers of Multimedia Learning*. New York: Pfeiffer. doi:10.1002/9781118255971

Davis, T. C., Crouch, M. A., Wills, G., Miller, S., & Abdehou, D. M. (1990)... *The Journal of Family Practice*, *31*(5), 533–538. PMID:2230677

Deci, E. L., & Flaste, R. (1996). *Why We Do What We Do: Understanding Self-Motivation*. New York: Penguin Books.

Fang, M. C., Panguluri, P., Machtinger, E. L., & Schillinger, D. (2009). Language, literacy, and characterization of stroke among patients taking warfarin for stroke prevention: Implications for health communication. *Patient Education and Counseling*, *75*(3), 403–410. Retrieved from http://www.ajmc.com/journals/supplement/2014/a465_ma14_transitions/a465_mar14_owen_s81t91/P-3#shash.SfblJhR1.dpuf doi:10.1016/j.pec.2008.12.009 PMID:19171448

Gerr, R., Saulsberry, K., Clark, M., & Kerns, C. (2014). *The Shared Accountability Care Model: Keeping Patients Activated, In-Network, and Brand Loyal*. The Advisory Board Company.

Harper, D. (2001). *Online Etymology Dictionary*. Retrieved from http://www.etymonline.com/index.php?term=patience&allowed_in_frame=0

Health Insurance Portability and Accountability Act. (1996). *CMS.gov*. Retrieved from https://www.cms.gov/Regulations-and-Guidance/HIPAA-Administrative-Simplification/HIPAAGenInfo/downloads/hipaalaw.pdf

Himmelstein, D. U., Warren, E., Thorne, D., & Woolhandler, S. (2005, February). MarketWatch: Illness And Injury As Contributors To Bankruptcy. *Health Affairs*. Retrieved from:http://content.healthaffairs.org/content/early/2005/02/02/hlthaff.w5.63/suppl/DC1

Katz, M. G., Jacobson, T. A., Veldar, E., & Kripalani, S. (2007). Patient Literacy and Question-asking Behavior During the Medical Encounter: A Mixed-metholds Analysis. *Journal of General Internal Medicine*, *22*(6), 782–786. doi:10.1007/s11606-007-0184-6 PMID:17431697

Kessels, R. P. (2003). Patients' Memory for Medical Information. *Journal of the Royal Society of Medicine*, *96*(5), 219–222. doi:10.1258/jrsm.96.5.219 PMID:12724430

Leary, M. R., & Kowalski, R. M. (1990). Impression management: A literature review and two-component model. *Psychological Bulletin*, *107*(1), 34–47. doi:10.1037/0033-2909.107.1.34

Leary, M. R., Tchividijian, L. R., & Kraxberger, B. E. (1994). Self-presentation can be hazardous to your health: Impression management and health risk. *Health Psychology*, *13*(6), 461–470. doi:10.1037/0278-6133.13.6.461 PMID:7889900

Lucas, G. M., Gratch, J., King, A., & Morency, L. (2014). It's only a computer: Virtual humans increase willingness to disclose. *Computers in Human Behavior*, *37*, 94–100. doi:10.1016/j.chb.2014.04.043

Mayer, R., & Moreno, R. (2003). Nine Ways to Reduce Cognitive Load in Multimedia Learning. *Educational Psychologist*, *38*(1), 43–52. doi:10.1207/S15326985EP3801_6

McWhorter, J. (2012). Gosh, Golly, Gee. *New Republic*. Retrieved from htttp://www.newrepublic.com/article/politics/magazine/103945/romney-language-mcwhorter

McWhorter, J. (2013, February). Txting is killing language. JK!!! *TED2013*. Retrieved from http://www.ted.com/talks/john_mcwhorter_txtng_is_killing_language_jk#t-126831

Meppelink, C., van Weert, J., Haven, C. J., & Smit, E. G. (2015). The Effectiveness of Health Animations in Audiences with Different Health Literacy Levels: An Experimental Study. *Journal of Medical Internet Research*, *17*(1), e11. doi:10.2196/jmir.3979 PMID:25586711

Montgomery, A. A., Emmett, C. L., Fahey, T., Jones, C., Ricketts, I., Patel, R. R., & Murphy, D. J. et al. (2007). Two decision aids for mode of delivery among women with previous caesarean section: Randomised controlled trial. *BMJ (Clinical Research Ed.)*, *334*(7607), 1305. doi:10.1136/bmj.39217.671019.55 PMID:17540908

Parker, S., Zipurksy, J., Ma, H., & Siegel, C. (2013, October). Randomized controlled trial demonstrates a web-based multimedia program used prior to first-time colonoscopy decreased patient anxiety, sedation requirement and procedure time while increasing knowledge. Dartmouth-Hitchcock Medical Center, Geisel School of Medicine at Dartmouth. *Poster presented at the Meeting of the American College of Gastroenterology*, San Diego, CA.

Piette, J., Rosland, A., Marinec, N., Striplin, D., Bernstein, S., & Silveira, M. (2013). Engagement With Automated Patient Monitoring and Self-Management Support Calls. *Medical Care*, *51*(3), 216–223. doi:10.1097/MLR.0b013e318277ebf8 PMID:23222527

Randall, J., Singh, B., Warren, B., Travis, S., Mortensen, N., & George, B. (2010). Delayed surgery for acute severe colitis is associated with increased risk of postoperative complications. *British Journal of Surgery*, *97*(3), 404–409. doi:10.1002/bjs.6874 PMID:20101648

Roberts, S., Williams, J., Yeates, D., & Goldacre, M. (2007). Mortality in patients with and without colectomy admitted to hospital for ulcerative colitis and Crohn's disease: Record linkage studies. *British Medical Journal*, *17*(7628), 1033–3. doi:10.1136/bmj.39345.714039.55 PMID:17977817

Safran, C. (2004). *United States House Ways and Means Health Subcommittee testimony*. Washington, D.C.

Schocker, L. (2013). Young People Are Sleeping With Their Phones. Their Parents Are Sleeping With People. Retrieved from http://www.huffingtonpost.com/2013/09/16/sleep-phone-tablet-bed_n_3924161.html

Schunk, D. H., Pintrich, P. R., & Meece, J. L. (2008). *Motivation in education: Theory, research, and applications*. Upper Saddle River, New Jersey: Pearson/Merrill Prentice Hall.

Siegel, C., Lofland, J., Naim, A., Gollins, J., Walls, D., Rudder, L., & Reynolds, C. (2015). Gastroenterologists' Views of Shared Decision Making for Patients with Inflammatory Bowel Disease. *Digestive Diseases and Sciences*, *60*(9), 2636–2645. doi:10.1007/s10620-015-3675-z PMID:25939543

Smith, D. M., Lowenstein, G., Rozin, P., Sherriff, R. L., & Ubel, P. A. (2007). Sensitivity to disgust, stigma, and adjustment to life with a colostomy. *Journal of Research in Personality*, *41*(4), 787–803. doi:10.1016/j.jrp.2006.09.006 PMID:17940585

Stacey, D., Légaré, F., Col, N. F., Bennett, C. L., Barry, M. J., Eden, K. B., & Wu, J. H. C. et al. (2014). Decision aids for people facing health treatment or screening decisions. *Cochrane Database of Systematic Reviews*, *January*. doi:10.1002/14651858.CD001431.pub4 PMID:24470076

Thomas T., Kedia, P. & Cohen, R. D. (2007). Impact of an Internet-based educational program on colonoscopy attendance and quality (abstract). *American Journal of Gastroenterology* Supplement S454.

Thompson, K. D., Connor, S. J., Walls, D., Gollins, J., Stewart, S. K., Bewtra, M., … & Siegel, C. A. (2016). Patients with ulcerative colitis are more concerned about complications of their disease than side effects of medications. *Inflamm. Bowel Dis.*, 22(4), 940-947.

Vin-Raviv, N., Hillyer, G. C., Hershman, D. L., Galea, S., Leoce, N., Bovbjerg, D. H., & Neugut, A. I. et al. (2013). Racial Disparities in Posttraumatic Stress After Diagnosis of Localized Breast Cancer: The BQUAL Study. *Journal of the National Cancer Institute*, *107*(7). doi:10.1093/jnci/djt024 PMID:23434900

Weisband, S., & Kiesler, S. (1996, April). Self disclosure on computer forms: Meta-analysis and implications. Proceedings of the SIGCHI conference on human factors in computing systems (pp. 3-10). ACM.

Witteman, H. O., Scherer, L. D., Angott, A. M., Ubel, P. A., Dickson, M., Holtzman, L. G.,... Zikmund-Fisher, B. J. (2012). Hold My Hand: Explicitly Showing Tradeoffs and Fit Between Values and Options Helps People Make Choices Concordant With Their Stated Values. Proceedings of 34th. Chicago: Annual Meeting of The Society for Medical Decision Making. Retrieved from https://smdm.confex.com/smdm/2012az/webprogram/Paper7417.html

Zan, S., Agboola, S., Moore, S. A., Parks, K. A., Kvedar, J. C., & Jethwani, K. (2015). Patient Engagement With a Mobile Web-Based Telemonitoring System for Heart Failure Self Management: A Pilot Study. *Journal of Medical Internet Research*, *3*(2), e33. doi:10.2196/mhealth.3789 PMID:25842282

KEY TERMS AND DEFINITIONS

Attentional Narrowing: The brain tends to focus on the most frightening statements. This focus draws all or most of an individual's attention, and it becomes difficult for him or her to listen to and absorb any other information.

Cognitive Load: The amount of mental effort and resources the brain's limited short-term memory needs to process and understand information.

Default Effect: A phenomenon where people leave an existing choice, setting, or state (such as a media program continuing to play) in place because changing it requires an active decision and effort (such as clicking "pause").

Immune Neglect: Also called "immune bias." People tend to underestimate their own ability to cope and adapt to challenging or negative events. This bias leads to poor decision-making.

Impression Management (Self Presentation): Whether consciously or unconsciously, patients may not respond honestly or withhold information because they want to be viewed positively and create a good impression on the clinician or healthcare worker.

Information Therapy: When clinicians or healthcare teams prescribe patient-friendly, trusted information to people that is relevant to their condition, medical decision, or procedure at that point in time.

Interactive Voice Response (IVR) Phone Calls: Scheduled, automated phone calls that use speech recognition and keypad responses to understand their responses and dynamically interact with them. Information can also be collected with this type of system.

Preference Misdiagnosis: When a clinician assumes they know what a patient would prefer regarding their treatment, does not ask the patient about their preferences, and the clinician's assumption is often wrong. Also referred to as a "silent misdiagnosis."

Progressive Disclosure: A design technique to prevent users from getting overwhelmed by information, where the information is sequenced across multiple screens and becomes more detailed as the user moves through it.

Shared Decision Making: A process where the provider helps the patient understand the decision, its consequences, and then helps them apply their values and preferences in order to make a decision.

This work was previously published in Transformative Healthcare Practice through Patient Engagement edited by Guendalina Graffigna, pages 139-162, copyright year 2017 by Medical Information Science Reference (an imprint of IGI Global).

Chapter 18
Active and Healthy Aging:
Satisfaction with Health Services by Elderly Patients in Turkey

Emine Özmete
Ankara University, Turkey

ABSTRACT

This study aims to investigate the difficulties experienced by elderly persons in accessing healthcare services and their satisfaction with issues as regards the healthcare system. In this study, qualitative research was carried out to assess the difficulties regarding the healthcare delivery system and satisfaction with the healthcare services. This qualitative research was performed through in-depth interviews with 6 men and 4 women aged 65+ years, in Ankara, the capital city of Turkey. It was discovered that elderly persons required the support of others to access a doctor, a health institution or hospital and the care and support of others for the regular intake of their drugs with increasing age. They were satisfied with the current family physician program. The most significant challenges experienced by elderly persons regarding the healthcare delivery system included crowded hospitals, difficulty walking, the unavailability of wheel chairs, and inadequate assistance from support staff.

INTRODUCTION[1]

Since the very beginning, human beings have strived hard to find ways to live healthy and even eternally. Developments in the second half of the past century and the effects of advancements in the fields of health and technology onto the quality of life for human beings prove that humanity's goal of "longevity" has been achieved. In 30-35 years, one out of every four Turkish citizens will be older than 65 years (TurkStat, 2014). In developed countries, the current rate of people older than 65 is one out of seven, and the same group will comprise a quarter of the total population in only 15 years. This has spurred on the conversation surrounding the "aging" process for the elderly population. By 2050, the number of "older elderly persons" will be six times more than that of "young elderly persons" above the age of 65. It is anticipated that the oldest population of elderly persons (aged 80 years and above) will increase

DOI: 10.4018/978-1-5225-1928-7.ch018

by 160% globally by 2040, more than all other populations of elderly persons. Today, the average age is above 40 years in certain European countries, Canada, and Japan. In Monaco, average age exceeds 50 years, the highest in the world. Today, the average age around the world is 29.4 years, and 30.7 years in Turkey (TurkStat, 2014; WHO, 2015).

In addition, life expectancy at birth is increasing by the day. This, in turn, contributes to the global growth rate of the elderly population. Life expectancy at birth for women is the longest in Japan. Average life expectancy at birth for Japanese women is 86 years. Life expectancy at birth in Turkey is an average of 78 years. This span is 75.3 years for men and 80.7 years for women (TurkStat, 2015). Rapid aging is associated with dramatic changes in family structure, employment patterns, and migration movements. On the other hand, increase in the elderly population is generally considered to be associated with an increase in healthcare expenditures as well. In 2050, healthcare expenditures as a share of GDP will be doubled due to the increase in the elderly population. Health expenditures in Turkey were 6.1% of GDP in the previous years (2008), yet this percentage increased to an annual rate of 7.1% between 2000 and 2010 (OECD, 2015).

Increase in life expectancy around the world and in Turkey has also increased the need for meeting the social, cultural and economic needs of the elderly population as well as the reorganization of health and care services. Active and healthy aging practices have been initiated at the sectorial level in many countries around world. Endeavors such as the reorganization and standardization of services, mutual workforce exchanges among countries, and benchmarking systems have been accelerated within the scope of this process, which consider long life to be a risk. In order for a given country to improve its fight against aging, it is imperative that the same country review the applications in other countries with experience and techniques in place and develop a model compatible with its own economic and social conditions. As of 2100, life expectancy at birth will be 100 years throughout the world. In addition to the growth of the elderly population, the empowerment of women, the fight against poverty and protecting the planet from factors such as global warming are also conversations that are coming to the fore. Both individuals and governments will have to deal with the reorganization of the healthcare delivery system and social security expenditures. Therefore, there will be a need for balance between the resources allocated by the public and private sectors. The gap between the actual life course and life expectancy will require developmental tasks to be redefined in social terms. As for healthcare, there is a growing need for increasing the number of healthy years in a lifespan and revising the organization healthcare services (Lis, Reichert, Cosack, Billings and Brown, 2008; WHO, 2015). Herein, we are faced with the concepts of healthy and active aging as part of a comprehensive universal approach. This study aims to draw attention to the importance of the concept of healthy aging as elderly populations are growing around the world and in Turkey and to explain the execution of health services geared toward the elderly, healthcare satisfaction and commonly faced problems.

BACKGROUND

There is a direct correlation between the development levels of countries and health. In developed countries, society's health status is considered to be a natural consequence of socio-economic development. Development in the field of health is the most significant indicator of investment in human capital. The 21 targets listed in the World Health Organization's declaration titled "Health for All by the year 2000" for a level of health that would permit all individuals in society to lead a socially and economically pro-

Box 1.

Target: Healthy Aging. By the year 2020, people over 65 should be able to enjoy their full health potential and play an active social role. • There should be an increase of at least 20% in life expectancy and in disability-free life expectancy at age 65 years. • There should be an increase of at least 50% in the proportion of people 80 years of age who live in a home environment, are able to meet their own needs, and maintain self-esteem and a place in society.

ductive life have been important determiners for health policies in Europe since the 1980s. One of these targets was set to focus on healthy and active aging and is explained as such (WHO, 2011):

The aim of healthcare services is to keep individuals alive while maximizing their physical, mental, and psycho-social capacity, making them feel happier by protecting them against potential health problems, and thereby improving their life quality. Healthcare services rank as a high priority in the national social policies of many countries with an aim of emphasizing the importance of human health in order to raise healthy societies. For this purpose, improving health and life quality, and eliminating inequality in the healthcare system have been set as objectives. The objective of ensuring easy access to healthcare services and improving life quality, especially for elderly persons, in a multidimensional fashion has become a major topic of discussion (WHO, 1999).

Aging is not a new notion in the globalized world. However, each day this concept is further complicated by new problems, and there is a need for new service models. All countries have had to face the issue of growing economic and social demands that occur during the aging process. Due to the world's changing conditions, the developing healthcare system, and cultural and social changes, aging and related issues have come to dominate the agenda of services (European Union, 2014). On the other hand, in consequence of the development of technology and healthcare services, the average life expectancy has increased. Old age is often unmanageable for elderly persons due to the change in needs and consumption habits, difficulties in meeting economic and social needs, and the prevalence of medical conditions such as dementia and Alzheimer's disease (Kinsella and He, 2009).

Achieving the goal of health for all means "increasing the number of healthy individuals in society, an increase in healthy individuals' capacity to absorb information, and development in their cognitive and physical skills". Preparing for old age, effectively benefiting from healthcare services starting from infancy and continuing through every stage of life, and adopting a healthy lifestyle are the most important criteria for being a healthy elderly person. The increase in elderly populations and rapid demographic change both around the world and in Turkey is increasing the need for active and healthy aging with each new day (Lis, Reichert, Cosack, Billings and Brown, 2008).

As recommended by the World Health Organization based on the objectives listed above, the concept of "active aging" means "the process of optimizing opportunities for health, participation and security in order to enhance quality of life as people age." "Health" is the key concept in this definition. Active aging allows people to realize "their potential for physical, social, and mental wellbeing throughout the life course" and ensures their participation in society in accordance with their needs, requests, and capacities/skills, "while providing them with adequate protection, security and care when they need." (Paul, Ribeiro and Teixeira, 2012). The World Report on Ageing and Health published in 2015 by the World Health Organization defines the concept of healthy aging as the process of maintaining and optimizing functional abilities (capacity) that ensure wellbeing in old age (WHO, 2015). Healthy aging is a matter that must be examined with a holistic approach based on lifespan and functional status.

In addition, the key aspects of the active aging model, which includes healthy aging, can be listed as follows:

1. That the individual be in control of their daily life based on their own preferences and rules, that they be able to make their own decisions, and that they have the autonomy to be able to handle this process.
2. Independence is the capacity to be functional in daily life, and to live independently in society without requiring help from others or with a little help from others.
3. Quality of life is the status of life perceived by the individual in the place they live, in the value system, and in the cultural structure in connection to individual expectations, goals and standards. Quality of life, which is a comprehensive concept, includes aspects such as the individual's physical health, psychological state, level of independence, social relationships and beliefs.
4. Life expectancy is the years during which the individual can live in a healthy manner without disabilities or diseases (Paul, Ribeiro ve Teixeira, 2012; WHO 2015).

Thus, it is understood that active aging includes both objective and subjective conditions from the individual's life, does not simply focus on old age, and is described with various indicators based on different stages of life (Figure 1).

Active aging includes the concept of healthy aging and may also be commonly used to have a similar meaning to successful aging. Successful aging is a more comprehensive approach that includes the concepts of active aging and healthy aging. Successful aging implies a lack of disease, maintaining functional capacity and active participation in life. Individuals who show no loss or barely any loss of function compared to their own age group, and who don't lose their connection to life are defined as "successful" elderly individuals. Individual factors such as sports or exercising, adequate and balanced nutrition, maintaining successful social relationships, traveling and active living are important in realizing successful aging. On the other hand, improving health services, quick and easy access to these

Figure 1. Active aging and life cycle approach

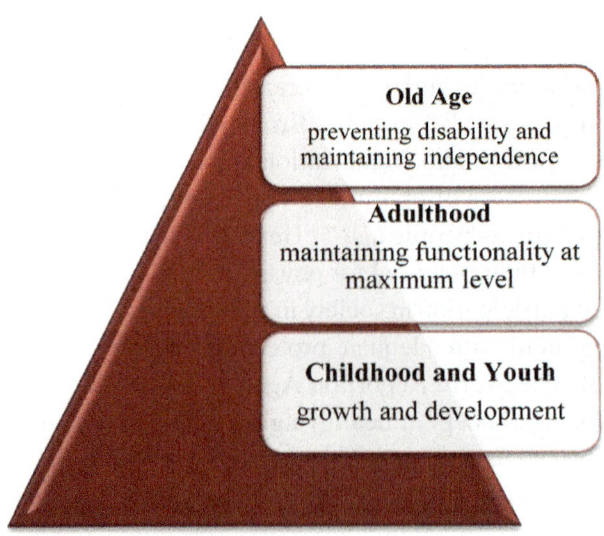

services by the elderly, affirmative action toward older persons in providing health services, determining the problems faced in accessing health services and reorganization of the services comprise the environmental factors at the macro level for active and healthy aging. Successful aging has certain standards. These standards include:

1. Having no diseases and having no addictions associated with a disease.
2. Being able to use cognitive and physical functions.
3. Actively participating in life (Rowe and Kahn, 1998).

Elderly people have become and will continue to be the focus of health policies and social policies in every country due to the growing elderly population. An essential issue that concerns every individual in society is the opportunity to access reliable and quality health services. Today, countries that have adopted the social welfare approach are considered to be liable for provision of active, efficient, and adequate healthcare services as a basic human right to the entire society or for taking the necessary measures (National Institute on Aging, 2011). Services aiming to preserve and improve health, prevent pathogenesis, diagnose and treat patients as early as possible, prevent disabilities, provide disabled persons with medically and socially therapeutic services, and ensure people to live a quality, happy, and long life are collectively considered healthcare services. Healthcare services can also be defined as the total efforts of various types of healthcare professionals for the diagnosis and treatment of diseases and preserving people's current health status within a range of health institutions and organizations. The main goal of healthcare services is to provide society with said services at the required level of quality, timing, and lowest possible cost (UNFPA, 2012).

In many countries, the healthcare delivery model in practice today has not kept pace with the changing epidemiology and health needs of the population. The focus often remains on building new hospitals, buying expensive new equipment and upgrading acute service delivery structures. The management of care processes remains, to a large extent, focused around episodic care needs. However, population aging requires a different approach, involving a shift from acute, episodic and hospital centric care to the management of chronic conditions, building age-friendly hospitals, the delivery of continuity of care across different care settings and providers, and a strong role for primary care professionals such as general practitioners (Colombo, 2015).

In conjunction with the growing elderly population, the need for health and care services increases due to the high prevalence of diseases occurring during old age. Nevertheless, the scope of the services to be planned for old age should be revised in line with the characteristics of old age. Important steps that can be taken to achieve that end include providing the elderly, which as a group has been considered the most disadvantaged group in terms of health, with facilitated access to healthcare services and equal opportunities, generalizing practices focused around wellbeing, ensuring that hospitals maintain accessible physical conditions, accompanying elderly individuals inside the hospital, providing care after being discharged from the hospital, and planning home care.

The quality of healthcare services within the larger system, the problems experienced by the elderly in accessing the services, and their satisfaction with the services along with social, emotional, and environmental factors contribute to the level of life quality experienced during the aging period. In the healthcare delivery system, a main challenge will be the management of complex combinations of chronic conditions. In many OECD countries, more than half of individuals aged over 65 years have more than one chronic condition, and many individuals aged 75 and older have three or more. Health and social care systems are still grappling with how to manage the diversity and uniqueness of this complex combination of diseases and care needs in an effective way, in relation to how to organize care teams, how to identify the right metrics for measurement, or how to equip health professionals with the skills they need to address changing population structures and epidemiological profiles (OECD, 2015; Colombo, 2015).

The anticipated requests posed by the elderly population regarding healthcare services will increase unless the prevalence of chronic diseases in elderly persons is decreased by strategies that promote and improve health. It is evident that the requirement for the workforce to provide the elderly with services will be on the rise as the healthcare demands of older people increase. Today, as with many other countries, there are only a limited number of healthcare professionals in Turkey with specialization to serve the elderly. It is important to employ healthcare professionals and support personnel with the knowledge and skills required to meet the demand for healthy aging. On the other hand, age-friendly hospital studies have just started. This study has been conducted to understand the implications of this situation for the elderly in the healthcare delivery system, to prove the difficulties experienced by elderly persons in accessing healthcare services and their satisfaction with issues as regards the healthcare delivery system.

MAIN FOCUS OF THE CHAPTER

The decline of health in old age is usually the result of chronic diseases. Most of these are diseases that are preventable or deferrable by adopting healthy habits. For this reason, physical activity and good nutrition become more important for health and wellness in later years. Other health problems can be effectively managed especially if diagnosed early. As individuals age, even if their capacity declines, with a supportive environment, they can go where they need to go when needed and do what they want to do. Countries have certain areas to work on to achieve active and healthy aging and improve health policies. The first of these is the increase in the elderly population and the diversity of health services required during old age by younger elderly persons and older elderly persons. For this reason, with the functional status of older individuals in mind, the areas that the policies should primarily be focusing on include elderly care, meeting the increasing demands regarding health services, the retirement system and social services (WHO, 2015).

Both the World Health Organization and the United Nations define the chronic diseases increasing in parallel with the aging of the world's population as the 21st century's most important health issue. 40% of the European population older than 15 years suffers from a chronic disease. This percentage increases with the age categories and Europeans who reach the age of retirement are at high risk for developing at least one chronic disease. According to the World Health Organization, one out of three Europeans who have reached the age of retirement suffers from at least two chronic diseases. The distribution of diseases has undergone changes due to the increasing level of development and expected lifespan in Turkey, in parallel with the world. When the distribution of death causes according to disease groups at the national level in Turkey are compared to those in developed and developing countries, it is observed that non-communicable chronic diseases comprise 78.7% of all deaths. This rate increases up to 86% in the European Union and developed countries. In Turkey, ischemic heart disease (21.7%) and cerebrovascular diseases (15.0%) are the leading diseases that lead to death (Healthy Aging and Chronic Disease Report, 2012).

According the active ageing index in practice in European Union countries, the average active ageing index score obtained from 28 European Union countries was 33.9. Among the European Union countries, the country with the highest active ageing index score was Sweden (44.9) followed by Denmark (40.3) and the Netherlands (40.0). The countries with the lowest active ageing index scores were Greece (27.6), Poland (28.1) and Hungary (28.3). While Denmark and Finland share the lead for independent living, one of the domains of the active ageing index, Sweden was the leader in the capacity for active ageing and employment domains, and Ireland was first in terms of participation in society. On the other hand, Slovenia, Poland, Latvia and Romania were last in terms of employment, participation in society, independent living and capacity for active ageing, respectively.

When the difference in men and women is European Union countries is considered in terms of the active ageing index, it is observed that while the active aging index score is higher in men in most countries, the active ageing index score in Finland, Estonia and Latvia is higher in women than in men. When the active ageing index data from 2010 and the data from 2014 were compared in terms of the domains of employment, participation in society, independent living and capacity for active ageing, it was determined that there was general improvement in active aging in European Union countries, and that the scores obtained in 2014 increased in all domains (EU, 2015).

According to the 2015 report of the global aging index, in which the general living conditions and levels of wellbeing are evaluated, Turkey placed 75th among 96 countries. Switzerland, Norway and Sweden were the top three countries. The USA placed 9th in the index in terms of the wellbeing of the elderly, while Afghanistan placed last. When the subcategories of elderly wellbeing are considered, Turkey ranked 35th in terms of matters related to income security such as retirement income and per capita income, 40th in terms of matters related to having an active environment such as social ties, physical safety and citizenship, and 52nd in terms of health status explained with variables such as life expectancy, health and psychological wellbeing at age 60. According to the global aging index, elderly persons in Turkey are most behind in the domain of capacity level, explained by employment status, having a profession and level of education. Turkey ranks 93rd in this category. This is why it is important to offer individuals the opportunities and technologies for lifelong learning and support individual productivity (Scobie et al., 2015).

The "Profile of Retired Persons in Turkey" (2012) conducted with 3400 retirees by the Turkish Association of Retired Persons investigated individuals' competence of independent living, physical and psychological health status, and whether or not they were benefiting from healthcare. The mean age of the participants was 60.8 years. In the study, while 59.2% of the retired individuals reported their physical activity as good or at a normal level for a retired person, close to a quarter (24.3%) of the retired individuals reported their physical activity as poor, and 7.4% reported their physical activity as very poor. Retired individuals reported that they do not struggle with hair care (77.5%), bathing (72.1%), and going to or getting out of bed (71.5%), but mostly struggle and receive help with climbing stairs (23.1%) and going to the doctor (15.4%). Retired individuals reported that they do not struggle with preparing meals (65.0%) or washing dishes (66.7%), but mostly receive help with home care and cleaning (10.2%) and small repairs around the house (10.8%). While nearly half of the retired individuals (48.6%) reported their physical health as good, 42.1% reported their physical health as poor. The most commonly occurring diseases included rheumatic diseases (56.8%), cardiovascular diseases (45.0%), visual disorders (35.5%), bone-related diseases (30.0%), nervous system disorders (23.4%) and digestive system diseases (21.8%). The majority of retired individuals included in the study (90.6%) were using walking aids. 87.4% were using hearing aids. Considering the fact that participant mean age was 60.8 years, these rates could be regarded as negative in terms of healthy aging.

The Life Satisfaction Survey is conducted by the Turkish Statistical Institute (TurkStat) each year in every province of Turkey, and a significant part of this survey is the section covering satisfaction with the healthcare and social security services. For the purposes of the present study, the satisfaction with healthcare and social security services was assessed by the author as based on the data collected with the Life Satisfaction Surveys conducted in 2012, 2013, and 2014. The level of satisfaction felt by individuals 65 years of age and above regarding healthcare services has been explained within the context of a range of topics.

First, the general satisfaction with healthcare services has been explained according to the age groups, using the data collected in the years 2012, 2013, and 2014:

The percentage of individuals aged 65 years and older who were "very satisfied" and "satisfied" with healthcare services, was 86.76% for the year 2012. The percentage of those "not satisfied" and "not satisfied at all" was very low (4.48%). In 2013, the percentage of individuals aged 65 years and older who were "very satisfied" and "satisfied" with the healthcare services was 84.94% for the year 2013 and 84.72% for the year 2014.

Regarding the satisfaction with the physical examinations at healthcare institutions by the year; it was observed that 77.63% of individuals aged 65 years and older were satisfied with said service in 2012. The percentage increased to 78.39% in 2013 and decreased to 71.04% in 2014. The percentage of individuals aged 65 years and older who were not satisfied with the physical examinations at healthcare institutions was 20.06% in 2012, 20.08% in 2013, and 27.21% in 2014.

The satisfaction felt by aging individuals regarding the behavior of physicians toward patients was investigated based on the data collected with the Turkey Life Satisfaction Survey carried out by TurkStat. To determine the level of satisfaction, the answers given to the question "Is there a problem with the behavior of physicians toward patients?" were assessed. The percentage of individuals aged 65 years and older who stated that there was a problem with the behavior of physicians toward patients was 17.08% in 2012, 9.77% in 2013, and 10.61% in 2014. The percentage of individuals aged 65 years and older who stated that there was no problem with the behavior of physicians toward patients and that they were satisfied with the behavior of physicians was 80.71% in 2012 and increased to 88.69% in 2013 and 87.27% in 2014.

Satisfaction regarding the behavior of nurses/caregivers toward patients was assessed with the following question: "Is there a problem with the behavior of nurses/caregivers toward patients?" 14.42% of individuals aged 65 years and older said there was a problem with the behavior of nurses/caregivers toward patients in 2012. The percentage decreased to 7.96% in 2013 and increased to 10.82% in 2014. In other words, the satisfaction felt by individuals aged 65 years and older regarding the behavior of nurses/caregivers toward patients was 82.61% in 2012, 89.55% in 2013 and 86.76% in 2014. It was observed that satisfaction with the behavior of both the physicians and the nurses/caregivers slightly decreased in 2014.

Satisfaction regarding the number of physicians and healthcare professionals was assessed with the following question: "Do you think that the number of physicians and healthcare professionals is sufficient?" More than half (53.55%) of the individuals aged 65 years and older thought that the number of physicians and healthcare professionals was sufficient in 2012. This percentage decreased to 45.38% in 2013 and 42.1% in 2014.

In order to assess satisfaction regarding physical examination and analysis prices at healthcare institutions, the TurkStat Life Satisfaction Survey asked participants the following question: "Is there a problem with physical examination and analysis prices at healthcare institutions?" The ratio of individuals aged 65 years and older who suggested that there was a problem with physical examination and analysis prices at healthcare institutions was 31.0% in 2012. This percentage of dissatisfaction increased to 36.44% in 2013 and 37.3% in 2014. Thus, as with the other age groups, an annual decrease was observed in the level of satisfaction felt by those aged 65 years and older regarding physical examination and analysis prices at healthcare institutions (satisfaction rates: 54.88% in 2012, 44.85% in 2013, 45.66% in 2014).

The treatment and drug expenses of individuals aged 65 years and older have mostly been reimbursed by the Social Security Institution (84.77% in 2012, 81.82% in 2013 and 84.19% in 2014).

The TurkStat Life Satisfaction Survey assessed the level of satisfaction regarding the quality of healthcare services with the following question: "Is there a problem with the quality of healthcare services?" According to the 2012 data, 81.03% of individuals aged 65 years and older thought there was no problem with the quality of healthcare services.

Furthermore, it was observed that elderly individuals were satisfied with making appointments for physical examinations and analyses and did not think there were any problems regarding this matter. The percentage of those who were satisfied increased with each year, starting from 82.61% in 2012 to 84.59% in 2013 and 84.06% in 2014.

The ratio of elderly individuals who suggested that there was a problem with drug prices was 31.99% in 2012, 33.66% in 2013, and 40.85% in 2014.

The TurkStat Life Satisfaction Survey investigated the level of satisfaction with the cleanliness of healthcare institutions by asking, "Is there a problem with the cleanliness of the healthcare institutions?" It was observed that the opinions of individuals aged 65 years and older regarding the cleanliness of healthcare institutions gradually grew more positive. While 10.76% of the elderly individuals thought there was a problem with the cleanliness of healthcare institutions in 2012, the percentage decreased to 8.4% in 2013 and increased to 8.91% in 2014. In other words, while the percentage of those who did not think there was a problem with the cleanliness of healthcare institutions was 85.96% in 2012, 88.96% in 2013, and 88.21% in 2014.

According to the results of the TurkStat Life Satisfaction Survey in 2013, the percentage of satisfaction felt by all age groups regarding healthcare services in Turkey was 74.7%. The percentage of those who thought services were moderately satisfactory was 10.6%, and 14.7% were not satisfied with healthcare services (these results were calculated by the author using data from the TurkStat Life Satisfaction Survey, 2012; 2013; 2014).

Though studies that aim to determine the health conditions of the elderly in Turkey are common, there are very few studies aiming to determine the challenges faced by the elderly in accessing health services. The Life Satisfaction Survey, the results of which were mentioned above, aims to measure the general life satisfaction of all age groups. The survey also aims to present satisfaction or dissatisfaction with health services through the quantitative research method. These results and quantitative data do not fully explain the challenges experienced by elderly patients receiving healthcare. For this reason, this study aims to determine the challenges older persons face and the matters with which they are satisfied using the qualitative research method.

METHOD

The qualitative research method was employed for this study, which aims to investigate the difficulties experienced by elderly people in accessing healthcare services and their satisfaction with the healthcare delivery system.

Qualitative research separates social reality from physical reality. It has been suggested that physical reality is independent from personal interpretations, yet the social reality is formed by personal interpretations. Therefore, it is generally accepted that social reality is involved with both objectivity and subjectivity, that it differs depending on each individual's mode of perception, and that the data only becomes meaningful once interpreted. An observation/interview is required to investigate satisfaction as a reflection of the interaction between the individual and their environment or to investigate how problems occur, and said observation/interview can only be interpreted using the qualitative method (Balnaves and Caputi, 2001). This study has used the qualitative research method to determine the challenges the elderly face as a disadvantaged and vulnerable group in society and in accessing services and the matters with which they are satisfied. In this way, considering the challenge in determining topics specific to older persons and the scarcity of studies on satisfaction/dissatisfaction with health services which include all age groups, this study has attempted to determine challenges or matters of satisfaction specific to the elderly using the qualitative research method.

This study on healthy aging examines how elderly individuals view healthcare services. For this purpose, the study focuses on two basic questions:

1. Are elderly individuals satisfied with healthcare services? If so, what specifically are they satisfied with?
2. What difficulties do elderly individuals experience in accessing healthcare services?

In addition to these two basic questions, two other questions were included, one regarding individual health status and another regarding personal habits, in order to understand the process of healthy aging:

3. Do you have any chronic diseases that require you to take regular medication?
4. How do you spend the day? Do you play sports or exercise?

The interview technique was utilized in the qualitative research process. Interviewing is the most frequently used method in qualitative research and can be defined as a social interaction, which includes asking the participant previously prepared questions and systematically recording the answers. Semi-structured interview forms were used for this study. The semi-structured interview form was composed of open-ended questions and the questions were listed in accordance with the interview guide (Martin and Bridgmon, 2012).

The deep interview technique was used as the method of qualitative data collection. A total of 10 elderly individuals (6 men, 4 women) aged 65 years and older were interviewed in order to collect information. The interviews were realized in a time period of 40 to 50 minutes.

The interviews conducted with the semi-structured interview forms including the aforementioned open-ended questions aimed to collect information that could be used to interpret issues such as health problems, exercise and activity levels, thoughts on their lives and healthy aging, satisfaction/dissatisfaction with healthcare services, and difficulties in accessing healthcare services.

The intended population of the study was women and men aged 65 years and older residing in the city of Ankara (capital city of Turkey). Participants were recruited to the study on a volunteer basis. The elderly individuals were interviewed at the institutions where they were receiving healthcare services, or at their homes. In accordance with the purpose of the study, in order for objective assessments to be made regarding health services, the older persons who participated in the study were selected from a pool of elderly patients who routinely benefited from health services and who were periodically admitted to the hospital for check-ups. The elderly individuals were briefed on the research before the interview; their consents were obtained, and they were ensured that they would be able quit the interview anytime they wanted to and that the information they might provide during the interview would be used solely for research purposes based on principles of confidentiality. The information collected through the interviews has been disclosed in accordance with the purpose of the study.

Participants

Due to ethical considerations, code names were used instead of the true names of the participants. General information regarding the participants is provided in Table 1. In this study, 6 men and 4 women aged 65 years and older were interviewed. The participants were aged 66-84 years. While all the men were at least primary school graduates, 2 women were literate and 2 women were illiterate. The men were predominantly retired workers or civil servants. The women were housewives. Only one individual worked as a tradesman. All the participants had social security. The women were not employed, thus they benefited from their spouse's social security packages (Table 1).

It was observed that not having the opportunity to attend school, especially as a woman, leads to challenges in old age as with all stages of life:

I grew up in a village. I could not attend school because I had to work in the fields. That is how it was back then. I am not literate. I have difficulty going places. I even have a hard time signing my name. (Z.G., 80, female)

Table 1. General information regarding the participants

Participants	Gender	Age	Education	Occupation
M.M.	Men	75	Secondary school	Retired white collar
C.G.	Men	84	Primary school	Retired blue collar
M.A.	Men	75	Secondary school	Retired white collar
Ş.Ş.	Men	70	Secondary school	Retired white collar
M.A1.	Men	73	University	Retired teacher
C.Ş.	Men	70	Primary school	Tradesman
Z.G.	Women	80	Illiterate	Housewife
Y.H.	Women	70	Literate	Housewife
F.Ş.	Women	72	Illiterate	Housewife
N.G.	Women	66	Literate	Housewife

23.9% of the elderly population in Turkey (2013) is illiterate, while 41.2% are primary school graduates, and 4.7% are college or university graduates. The education status of the elderly population varies significantly by sex (TurkStat, 2014a). The education status of the elderly individuals interviewed within the scope of this study is similar to that of the elderly population in Turkey.

Healthy Aging: Satisfaction vs. Difficulties Regarding Access to Healthcare Services

This section covers whether or not the elderly individuals have chronic diseases that require taking regular medication, how healthy they feel, how they spend the day, whether or not they play sports or exercise, their satisfaction/dissatisfaction with healthcare services, and the difficulties they experience.

Chronic Diseases

Conditions such as cognitive impairment, immobility, instability, urinary/fecal incontinence, and insomnia as well as cardiovascular diseases, respiratory problems, pressure sores, genitourinary conditions, diabetes mellitus, thyroid, delirium, dizziness, and stroke, the diagnoses and treatments of which have gained importance, are prevalent in old age. Therefore, old age is a period marked with an increase in the prevalence of chronic diseases and dependence, that has particular healthcare requirements, that necessitates the planning of long-term post-treatment care. In old age, due to worsened health conditions, functional abilities are limited and dependence on others in engaging with daily life activities is increased. In this study, all the enrolled elderly individuals suffered from the aforementioned chronic diseases:

I was born in 1940. I suffer from cardiac insufficiency. I need to take frequent rests due to my condition. I need to take my medication regularly, and sometimes I forget to take them on time. (M.M., male)

I suffer from cardiac insufficiency. I can no longer go out by myself. I have trouble walking. I am unable keep up with medication or doctor-related errands. My children take care of them. They replace my medication when I run out. It is better if someone reminds me to take my medication or gives them to me. (C.G., 84, male)

I am 75 years old now. I have kidney failure. I have to go to the hospital frequently. (M.A., male)

I suffer from cardiac insufficiency. I feel I don't have enough strength to do anything. It is very hard to be old. (Ş.Ş., 70, male)

I have heart disease and diabetes. My son and daughter-in-law have taken care of me since my spouse's death. I actually have three kids. I regularly use insulin injections and cardiac drugs. I wish my wife was still alive. I forget about my diseases when I spend time with my grandchildren. It makes me happy. I feel healthy. (M.A1., 73, male).

I have a slipped disc and diabetes. I haven't been able to move much in the last week since my herniated disc worsened. I avoid going to the doctor alone. Because I have had difficulty walking, I go to the hospital more often nowadays. I am looking for a hospital that can treat both my herniated disc and diabetes. I want to be better, and I try to take my drugs regularly. (N.G., 66, female)

I have hypertension. I have too much blood. My blood values are high. I also have a coagulation disorder and osteoporosis. I take care of things myself. I feel strong enough to. I am not dependent on others. I am going through a good time of life. I feel healthy for now. Even if I do not always do a good job, I always take care of things myself. (Z.G., 80, female)

I don't feel healthy at all. I have been smoking since I was a kid. I have many conditions induced by smoking. I need to see a doctor at least once a month. I experience shortness of breath. I have cardiovascular occlusion and diabetes. (C.Ş., 70, male)

I feel exhausted, and I cannot see. I can't say I'm that healthy. One of my eyes doesn't see, and I have hearing problems. I also have hypertension. I have to take my medication regularly. My children buy my drugs. I have five children. Every month I stay with a different child. I pay a monthly fee to whoever is hosting me that month. They provide for my hospital and drug expenses. They take me to the doctor. (F.Ş., 72, female)

I have osteoporosis. I suffer from gastrointestinal problems. I have no other diseases, no hypertension and no diabetes. I don't take my osteoporosis medication. I drink a lot of milk and eat a lot of yogurt. I don't go to the doctor for myself. I am taking care of my 85-year-old spouse. He has Alzheimer's and frequently falls. I give him his drugs regularly and on time. I give him fruits and vegetables. I get his drugs from the family doctor. I cannot leave him home alone. I cannot take him to the doctor alone. My children are far away. (Y.H., 70, female)

As is seen, the majority of the participants had cardiovascular diseases along with renal failure and gastrointestinal conditions. The individuals aged 66-84 years reported at least one health condition that required regular drug use. It is understood that they generally needed care and expected support from others for the regular intake of their drugs and going to a doctor. Especially as age increases, women and those who are older require more attention. Secondary aging effects such as smoking were also evident. It is striking that the 70-year-old woman participant took care of her 85-year-old spouse, without taking care of herself or going to the doctor

In the context of aging and gender, women assume approximately 70% of tasks related to caring for elderly individuals around the world. Among elderly couples, women usually take care of their spouses since women usually live longer and are younger than their spouses. Caring for the elderly is generally the responsibility of the elder daughter in the event that there is no spouse or if the man cannot take care of his spouse. It has been observed that in families that have both adult daughters and adult sons, the adult daughters assume two times the responsibility that the adult sons assume in caring for elderly parents (Özmete, 2015).

How They Spend the Day and Whether They Play Sports or Exercise

72-year-old F.Ş. reports that she raised 5 children, was a full-time mother, did not realize how fast the years passed went by because of how busy she was, felt alone after losing her spouse, but finds things to do by herself each day.

I wake up at 11 o'clock. I have my breakfast after I do my prayers. After spending some time for personal care and basic needs, I begin to knit decorative baby shoes (F.Ş. presented a gift of decorative baby shoes to the researcher during the interview as well). I talk with my daughter-in-law and grandchildren a lot. I sing ditties. I don't do sports and I am not accustomed to do so. Now I have diseases. I am at the end of my life. As I await death, I try to live my life to the fullest. I am always moving around in the house, and I would like people around me. I don't like to be alone. Sometimes I am terribly moved by the passing of my spouse. He comes to me in my dreams and tells me it's not time yet, and that I should wait a little longer.

An 80-year-old woman (Z.G.) said that she currently lives alone, but that if she needed care, she would like to live with her children and be cared for by them.

I live alone at home. I live by myself but I don't feel lonely. My children live near me, and I visit them whenever I want. I go out and walk around. I watch TV. I try to help my children with their errands and take care of my grandchildren. I cannot sit around and do nothing since I used to be very busy. I don't do sports, but I have daily occupations.

66-year-old female participant N.G. reported that she got along well with her children, that she had grandchildren who were employed or who were students, that she took care of them, and that she did her best to help them out. She explained how she spends the day as follows:

I wake up to do my prayers in the morning. I prepare breakfast. I have breakfast with my spouse. Then I don't understand how the time goes by. I start preparing lunch. Generally, my children visit since they live so close. Occasionally, I try to walk but I'm unable to do it regularly; old age, you know. I have always wanted to learn how to swim, and if I knew how to, I would swim more frequently. I also always wanted a house with a garden. I wish I had a garden to occupy myself with and get my hands dirty.

73-year-old male retired teacher M.A1, who stays with his son and daughter-in-law, reported that he would be very happy if his wife was still alive, yet he is happy to live with his son and daughter-in-law. He wants them to always be the ones who take care of him. He asks for help first from his son, and sometimes from his daughter-in-law and grandchild. M.A1. summarized a normal day as follows:

I don't regularly play sports or exercise. When I wake up in the morning, I read the newspaper until my daughter-in-law has prepared breakfast. Then I have breakfast with my daughter-in-law and grandchildren. After breakfast, I take the grandchildren to school. After that I go to the park, where my friends are. We chat together. At noon, when the call to prayer goes off, we go to the mosque all together. After that I go back home. I watch TV with my daughter-in-law. In the evening, I go to the school to pick up my grandchildren. By the time we get back home, my son is usually already back. We have dinner. After watching TV and chatting with my son a little, I go to sleep.

Reporting that in the last three years since he lost his spouse, he has felt like he doesn't belong to this world, that he doesn't quite enjoy anything, and that he has had many diseases due to smoking, 70-year-old male participant C.Ş. summarized his routine day as follows:

I wake up early in the morning; I don't sleep after the morning prayers. I read the Quran. After breakfast, I go to my market. I own a small market. I spend most of my day at the mosque and the market. Occasionally I go out for visits. Sometimes I meet up my friends. I like to spend time with my grandchildren and children.

70-year-old Y.H., who takes care of her 85-year-old spouse with Alzheimer's reported that she was responsible for all the work at home, that she could not hire a caregiver, and that it is hard to find a reliable person and caregivers are economically costly.

I spend the entire day caring for my spouse. I wake up early in the morning. We have breakfast at the same time every day. I give him his medication, clean the house, cook, and wash the clothes and dishes. My neighbors visit me. I chat with them. I go out to buy bread and do some shopping, and quickly return back. The day is over before I know it, and I usually feel tired.

It was observed that the individuals in this study with reported medical conditions such as cardiac insufficiency and renal failure did not play sports or exercise due to their health problems, and they did not have such habits in the past either.

The interviewed individuals did not have habits of regularly playing sports or exercising. It is understood that they did not have such habits in the past either. The statements of the participants once again underscore the importance of adopting sports and exercise habits and raising awareness regarding the importance of adopting these habits at an early age. It is understood that doing one's prayers is a part of daily life for elderly individuals. Especially for the men, going to the mosque is a common practice for mobility, seeing friends, and praying. Furthermore, the men get out more frequently for the purposes of seeing friends, going to the mosque, going to the park, or walking the grandchildren to school. The women spend more time at home. In fact, women spend most of their time at home or in the neighborhood their entire lives, and this is not associated with aging. Therefore, it is understood that women are more akin to accept and adapt to an inactive life. For men, the loss of the role as a worker accelerates the acceptance of the phrase "I am old now!"

Satisfaction with Healthcare Services and Difficulties Experienced

In this part of the study the participants were asked about their satisfaction with healthcare services and the difficulties they experienced, separately. However, their replies included both the satisfactory components and the difficulties they faced. Therefore, the views that include both aspects are provided below.

70-year-old Y.H., who had osteoporosis and gastrointestinal conditions, and took care of her 85-year-old spouse with Alzheimer's disease, reported her views regarding the healthcare system as follows:

My spouse is a retired worker. We used to only be able to go to the Social Security Institution (SSI) hospitals. If we wanted to go to a state hospital, we had to be referred from a SSI hospital. Now we are able to go to any hospital in any city just by showing our identity cards. We can choose our hospital and doctor. Furthermore, the elderly does not have to wait in lines anymore. We can go directly to see a doctor for physical examination. It is hard to find a specialist doctor with experience in every hospital. You need to see different doctors just to be diagnosed with a single disease. I don't have the strength to do that on my own. I don't know where to go or how to make an appointment. It is very hard to bring my spouse to see a doctor. His movements are slow, he falls down, and I'm unable to walk him around inside the hospital. I need help from others. When he needs to be hospitalized, it is hard to find him a bed. Even if there is a bed, you need to be in communication with the doctors. These are our challenges. I am very happy with our family doctor. I can get our medication quickly, and the pharmacist is also helpful. They guide us in how to treat our diseases.

A 75-year-old retired male civil servant (M.M.) with cardiovascular disease explained:

Doctors are considerate when they have time. They are polite. Sometimes there are many patients. I cannot find a seat when I go to the hospital. I am old. I cannot stand up. I cannot find a wheelchair when I need to go somewhere else in the hospital for an analysis. There is nowhere to hold onto. Fortunately, I have relatives, but who would help me out if I didn't? I ask those working at the hospital. They say they will help but I only end up waiting. They say another patient took the wheelchair, and I will have to wait. Everything ends up taking longer than it should.

84-year-old C.G., who has cardiovascular disease, explained his views regarding the services provided at the healthcare institutions as follows:

My daughter deals with the process of getting me admitted to the hospital. Anyways, I'm unable to come by myself. I have difficulty walking. I cannot stabilize my balance. I use a wheelchair to get everywhere. The stretchers here are so high that I have difficulty climbing onto them. My daughter is unable to help on her own. The personnel are busy. My hands are weak, so I'm unable to much wait on them. I always need someone to accompany me during analyses. Otherwise everything takes longer. I cannot do anything without the help of my daughter.

Required to go to the hospital frequently due to renal failure, 75-year-old M.A. reported his satisfaction with healthcare services and the problems he faces as follows:

I have no complaints about this hospital. The doctors and nurses do their best and show concern. The staff is good. But I went to the polyclinic of another hospital. I could not get a physical examination because I didn't schedule an appointment with the hospital. I am an old person; I don't know where to call. My eyes cannot see the numbers or buttons on a phone. I cannot do it by myself. Sometimes I wait at the polyclinic for hours. It would be helpful to have the assistance of someone accompanying me who could help me with my procedures, tell me what is required. That would help older people like me. I come here alone. Sometimes I confuse the polyclinics. I do not know where to go. I try to find places by asking people as I go.

A 70-year-old retired male civil servant (Ş.Ş.) with cardiovascular disease reported his satisfaction with the healthcare services as follows:

Polyclinics are very crowded. The doctors try to show interest and respect. But they get tired too. Sometimes personnel speak harshly. We are old people. We are their elders. We wouldn't be here if we didn't have a problem. I want them to show respect and understanding. My ears don't hear. Sometimes they provide information regarding my disease, but they talk too fast and I cannot understand them. Sometimes they hardly say anything. They just hand me some papers and give me minimal information. Most personnel are not helpful. They say something like "I don't work in this department," and they go away. Also the toilets are very low here; there is nothing to hold onto. My knees are in pain. I have trouble bending over.

Thanks to the improvements in the healthcare services, individuals are able to go to any hospital in any city, and individuals aged 65 years and older are allowed to receive physical examinations without waiting in lines within the scope of affirmative action. The fact that elderly individuals have limited mobility in hospitals, difficulties regarding physical accessibility, and the need elderly individuals have for a patient consultant or an accompanying person requires the reorganization of healthcare services for elderly persons. As can be understood from the reports provided by the participants, elderly individuals experience problems related to making doctor's appointments, lack of information/inability to find where to go in the hospital, lack of physical strength to go to the relevant units, problems associated with physical accessibility including with toilets, and lack of attention by the support personnel due to patient crowd/intensity.

FUTURE RESEARCH DIRECTIONS

With the increase in the elderly population around the world and in Turkey, determining the social, cultural, economic and healthcare related needs of the elderly population has become important. In addition, easy access to protective and preventive therapeutic health services is important in terms of active and healthy aging. In the studies conducted to this day, generally quantitative research has been performed regarding the satisfaction of all age groups with health services. Whereas, the challenges elderly population faces in accessing health services and the matters with which they are satisfied should be evaluated with the characteristics of this group in mind. This study has used the qualitative research method to determine the challenges the elderly face in accessing health services and the matters with which they are satisfied. Qualitative research is an effective method in presenting social realities specific to this group that cannot be presented with quantitative data. On the other hand, qualitative research reveals data supporting the formation of question structures for future quantitative research plans. In order to determine the challenges older persons face in terms of health services and the matters with which they are satisfied, quantitative research must be conducted on a larger scale, and the subject must be presented with quantitative evidence.

CONCLUSION

The aim of healthcare services is to keep the individual alive while maximizing their physical, mental, and psycho-social capacity, making them feel happier by protecting them against potential health problems, and thereby improving their quality of life. Healthcare services rank as a high priority in the national social policies of many countries with an aim of emphasizing the importance of human health in order to raise healthy societies. For this purpose, improving health and life quality, and eliminating inequality in the healthcare system have been set as objectives. The objective of ensuring easy access to healthcare services and improving life quality, especially for elderly persons, in a multidimensional fashion has become a major topic of discussion.

As recommended by the World Health Organization based on the objectives listed above, the concept of "active aging" means "the process of optimizing opportunities for health, participation and security in order to enhance quality of life as people age." Active aging allows people to realize their potential for physical, social, and mental wellbeing throughout the life course and ensures their participation in society in accordance with their needs, requests, and capacities/skills, while providing them with adequate protection, security and care when they need.

The factors that affect healthy aging include individual determinants such as the individual's educational status, employment status, economic status, genetic factors, attitudes and behaviors regarding healthy aging, and where they live as well as the social environment in which they live, interpersonal relationships, social structure, and the provision of healthcare services.

Today (2014), the percentage of individuals aged 65 years and older in the general population has increased to 8%. There are 9,063,677 citizens aged 60 years and older and 6,192,962 citizens aged 65 years and older. There are 1,315,845 citizens aged 80 years and older, who we call "the older elders." The average life expectancy at birth increased from 66 years in the year 2000 to 75 years in 2014. Pursuant to a study conducted by the World Health Organization as regards the basic health indicators in the European Region, it was predicted that average life expectancy at birth would increase to 77.2 in 2020, with 74.5 years for men and 80.0 for women (WHO, 2014). As can be understood from the above data, Turkey has rapidly entered into a process of becoming an aging society. This underscores the importance of arrangements and interventions with an aim to increase the number of healthy years in a lifespan.

Healthy and active aging is an approach that should be given attention throughout one's life as a whole and at every stage of life. It is harder to become a healthy and active elderly individual and develop individual attitudes and behaviors towards that end once the individual has gotten old. Therefore, from a perspective of lifelong learning, individuals should be encouraged to gain the habit of participating in sports activities and exercising beginning in the childhood period, making it a part of their life, and adopting it as a life style. Societies aim to have a healthy generation that is active and productive, distanced from smoking and other substances, gets adequate and balanced nutrition, participates in society and gets involved in volunteer work with an attitude of social sensitivity and social responsibility.

The needs of the elderly take on increased importance due to the increase in the average life expectancy at birth. Readiness for assuming a productive and valuable role at an advanced age is a phenomenon that should be explained on both the individual and societal levels. The youth should be supported in their preparations for their old age period. Preparation for a socially productive and healthy old age requires taking steps lifelong learning and providing equal opportunities for the elderly to participate in social and economic activities.

One of the most basic factors to attain healthy and active aging is to raise the level of health literacy in Turkey based on an awareness of healthy and active aging. Health literacy is an individual's capacity to obtain, interpret, and understand basic health information and services so as to protect and improve one's health and find cures for impaired health. 4,924 individuals from 12 regions participated in the Turkish Health Literacy Survey (2014) and it was discovered that 64.6% of the participants had inadequate or problematic health literacy. The general health literacy index of Turkey was determined to be 30.4 (Durusu-Tanriover et al., 2014). Considering that the mean age of the participants of the survey was 41.4 years, it is evident that in 20 years there will be an elderly population with inadequate capacity to obtain, interpret, and understand basic health information and services so as to protect and improve their health, and find cures for their impaired health. Therefore, education and awareness activities should be urgently initiated in order to raise society's awareness of healthy and active aging. Data and evidence regarding healthy and active aging should be produced in Turkey similar to the active aging surveys conducted in European countries which reveal changes over the years. Both in order to implement the Turkish Healthy Aging Action Plan and Implementation Program and also in accordance with the present study, it is understood that there is a need to determine the active and healthy aging index in Turkey. The evidence that will be obtained in this way is also important for the revision of the healthcare services to be provided to the elderly.

Along with the individual factors, structural factors such as the service plan and composition of the services are also determinative for healthy and active aging. 6 men and 4 women aging 65 years and above were interviewed within the scope of the present study on healthy aging and the experienced problems. Accordingly:

- The educational levels of the female participants were lower than those of the male participants. The male participants were at least primary school graduates and have been employed. Only two female participants were literate, while two women were illiterate. The female participants were never employed and were included in the social security system via their spouses.
- The elderly individuals had chronic diseases such as cardiovascular diseases, cardiac insufficiency, diabetes, renal failure, respiratory tract diseases, and vision and hearing problems that were prevalent in old age. They needed to see a doctor or be admitted to a health institution frequently (at least once a month).
- They needed someone's assistance in order to get to a doctor or a health institution.
- As age advances, they needed someone's attention and support to be able to take their medication regularly. Delays in replacing the finished drugs and forgetting the time of drug intake prevents regular intake.
- Matters regarding healthcare services considered to be satisfactory:
    - They thought that doctors were attentive and respectful.
    - They thought that access to physical examinations in any city and in any hospital was a significant improvement.
    - They were pleased that those aged 65 years and older had the opportunity to have physical examinations without having to wait in line.
    - They were happy with the family physician program.
- Difficulties experienced regarding healthcare services:
    - The hospitals were crowded, they couldn't find a seat, they couldn't walk, they couldn't find wheelchairs, and support personnel did not provide sufficient assistance.
    - They needed someone to accompany them during analyses and to access the units of the hospital. They were not able to resolve the procedures by themselves.
    - They had difficulty finding specialist doctors with experience, making different appointments with different doctors, and showing up for analyses and appointments with different doctors on different days.

- They experienced difficulty finding a spare bed in the inpatient units when necessary. They needed to talk to the department heads or clinical chiefs to resolve this, but it was difficult for them.
- The toilets were not suitable for elderly individuals and the stretchers were too high.
- Especially the elderly individuals with vision and hearing disabilities complained that the personnel did not act in an understanding manner.

As is seen, the expectations of elderly individuals with regard to the healthcare services underscore the need for units that would take care of elderly individuals using a holistic approach with attention, support, respect, and understanding. Therefore, polyclinics that specialize in the medical branch known as Geriatrics to evaluate the elderly using a holistic approach must be popularized in hospitals. In addition to geriatric specialists, these polyclinics should employ a team of specialists from other branches of medicine, including Ophthalmology, Otorhinolaryngology, Neurology, Psychiatry, Cardiovascular Diseases, Physical Medicine and Rehabilitation, and Infectious Diseases etc. Upon geriatric assessment by the geriatric specialists, the elderly individual should be referred to another specialist, as necessary, in the same polyclinic without the need for being referred to other units. Furthermore, there is a significant need for someone to accompany elderly individuals in the hospital. It is evident that elderly individuals experience difficulty completing admission, appointment, analysis, and physical examination processes. Therefore, hospital attendants should be employed. The challenges faced by elderly individuals most frequently were the insufficient number of healthcare professionals and the prices of drugs etc. due to increased healthcare expenditures during a time of economic loss. The burden of chronic diseases on total healthcare expenditures is gradually increasing as the elderly population grows. Therefore, implementing the "Care Assurance/Insurance System" as used in developed countries, which have already faced the needs of elderly populations, in order to readily finance the healthcare expenditures of elderly individuals, will decrease the burden of future healthcare expenditures for both the individual the state. For example, the compulsory care insurance system (the Social Long-term Care Insurance [LTCI]) was implemented in Germany in 1995 based on the infrastructure prepared by the intergenerational agreement in 1956.

Unless the chronic diseases of the elderly are not mitigated by strategies aimed at improving and developing health, elderly individuals' demands of the healthcare systems will only increase. It is obvious that the need for labor force to serve elderly individuals will increase with the increased demand for medical care by elderly individuals. Today the number of healthcare professionals specialized in old age is limited as with many other countries. It is important to employ healthcare professionals and support personnel equipped with the knowledge and skills necessary to meet elderly individuals' needs for healthy aging. Together with the growing the elderly population, health policies and social policies will focus on elderly individuals in all countries today and in the future.

REFERENCES

Balnaves, M., & Caputi, P. (2001). *Introduction to quantitative research methods an investigative approach* (p. 272). USA: Sage Publication.

Colombo, F. (2015). Health systems are still not prepared for an ageing population. In P. Love (Ed.), *Ageing: debate the issues*. OECD.

Durusu-Tanriover, M., Yildirim, H. H., Demiray-Ready, F. N., Çakır, B., & Akalin, H. E. (2014). *Turkey health literacy research*. Ankara: Health –Union Pub.

European Union. (2014). The 2015 ageing report: underlying assumptions and projection methodologies. *European Economy*, 8.

European Union. (2015). *European summit on ınnovation for active and healthy aging* (Final Report).

Healthy Aging and Chronic Disease Report. (2012). *Healthy aging and chronic disease report*. Ankara: Association of Evidence Based Medicine Pub. Retrieved from http://www.kanitadayalitip.org/yayinlar/sa%C4%9Fl%C4%B1kl%C4%B1%20ya%C5%9Flanma%20toplant%C4%B1%20raporu.pdf

Kinsella, K., & He, W. (2009). An aging world: 2008. U.S. Census Bureau, International Population Reports, Washington, DC: Government Printing Office.

Lis, K., Reichert, M., Cosack, A., Billings, J., & Brown, P. (Eds.). (2008). *Evidence-based guidelines on health promotion for older people*. Vienna: Austrian Red Cross.

Martin, W. E., & Bridgmon, K. D. (2012). *Quantitative and statistical research methods: from hypothesis to results*. UK: Jossey- Bass.

National Institute on Aging. (2011). *Global health and aging*.

OECD. (2015), *Ageing: debate the ıssues*. Paris: OECD Publishing. Doi:10.1787/9789264242654-en

Özmete, E. (2015). The reflection of gender inequality in aging: Psycho-social, economic and cultural evidences for caregiver and care receiver. *Journal of Gender and Women Studies: KIMLIK*, *1*(Spring).

Paul, C., Ribeiro, O., & Teixeira, L. (2012). Active ageing: an empirical approach to the who model. *Current Gerontology and Geriatrics Research.* doi:10.1155/2012/382972

Population Institute. (2016). Demographic Vulnerability: Where Population Growth Poses the Greatest Challenges. Retrieved from https://www.populationinstitute.org/external/Final-DVI-report.pdf

Rowe, J. W., & Kahn, R. L. (1998). *Successful aging: The Mac Arthur Foundation Study*. New York: Dell Publishing.

Scobie, J., Amos, S., Beales, S., Dobbing, C., Gillam, S., & Knox-Vydmanov, C. et al. (2015). *Global age watch index*. London, UK: HelpAge International.

Turkey Retired Profile Research. (2012). *Turkey retired profile research*. Ankara: Association of Turkey Retirees General Center Education and Cultur Pub.

TurkStat. (2014). *Population registration system data based on address*. TurkStat. Retrieved 5 from www.tüik.gov.tr

TurkStat. (2014a). Elderly people with statistics 2014. *TurkStat Bulletin* (March 18, 2015). Retrieved from www.tuik.gov.tr/PreHaberBultenleri

TurkStat. (2015). Life Expectancy Tables 2013-2014. *TurkStat Bulletin* (October 7, 2015). Retrieved from http://www.tuik.gov.tr/PreHaberBultenleri.do?id=18618

UNFPA. (2012). *Ageing in the 21st century: a celebration and a challenge*. New York: United Nations Populations Fund.

WHO. (1999). *Health21: The health for all policy framework for the WHO European region*. European Health for All Series. Retrieved from http://www.euro.who.int/__data/assets/pdf_file/0010/98398/wa540ga199heeng.pdf

WHO. (2011, July). *The new European policy for health – Health 2020: Vision, values, main directions and approaches*. World Health Organization. EUR/RC61/9, EUR/RC61/Conf. *Doc.* (Vol. 2, p. 18).

WHO. (2014). *Core health indicators in the WHO European Region 2014, special focus, health 2020 targets indicators*. World Health Organization.

WHO. (2015). *World report on ageing and health. Luxemburg*. World Health Organization.

ADDITIONAL READING

Agren, G., & Berensson, K. (2006). *Healthy aging: a challenge for Europe*. Stockholm: The Swedish National Institute of Public Health.

Aiken, L. R. (1995). *Aging*. Londra: Sage Publication.

Arizona Department of Health Services. (2013). *2014-2018 Arizona healthy aging plan: a framework to support healthy living and functional health for older Arizonan residents*. Arizona, USA: Arizona Department of Health Services Bureau of Tobacco & Chronic Disease.

European Commission. (2012). *Active ageing and solidarity between generations 2012 edition a statistical portrait of the European Union 2012*. Eurostat.

Grey, A., & Rae, M. (2007). *Ending aging: the rejuvenation breakthroughs that could reverse human aging in our life time*. New York: St. Martin's Griffin.

Hansson, R. O., & Carpenter, B. N. (1994). *Relationships in old age*. New York: The Guilford Pres.

ILC. (2015). *Active aging: a policy framework in response to the longevity revolution*. Rio de Janeiro: International Longevity Centre Brazil.

Lawton, M. P. (1990). Aging and performance of home tasks. *Human Factors*, *32*(5), 527–536. PMID:2074107

Myers, T. S. (1989). *How to keep control of your life after 50*. Lexington, Massachusetts: Lexington Books.

OECD. (2014). *OECD family database*. OECD - Social Policy Division - Directorate of Employment, Labor and Social Affairs. Retrieved from http://www.oecd.org/social/family/database

Tufts Health Plan Foundation. (2015). *Highlights from Massachusetts healthy aging data report: community profiles 2015*. USA: Massachusetts Healthy Aging Collaborative and Tufts Health Plan Foundation.

Zaidi, A. (2015, July). Active aging indicators. *Paper presented at United Nation Economic Commission OEWG,* Brussels.

Zastrow, C. (2008). *Introduction to social work and social welfare: Empowering people.* Canada: Thomson Brooks/Cole.

KEY TERMS AND DEFINITIONS

Active Aging: The process of maximizing conditions such as participation in society, social integration, safe life environment, and being healthy for individuals starting at an early age.

Aging: Aging occurs as the result of accumulating disorders in the body's structure and functions. Aging is an unpreventable chronological, social and biological process.

Health Literacy: The level of capacity required to understand, obtain and process health information and services in order for individuals to make effective and appropriate decisions regarding health.

Health Policies: Policies that will primarily focus on providing solutions for the changing health problems and needs of vulnerable groups and that will ensure the reorganization of health services accordingly.

Health Services for the Elderly: A type of health service that is considerate of the healthcare needs of the elderly, takes affirmative action, and includes age-friendly hospital practices with the increasing elderly population in mind.

Healthy Aging: Ensuring equal opportunity in access to protective-preventive and therapeutic health services during all life stages so that individuals adopt an active lifestyle and age in a healthy manner.

Societal Aging: An increasing rate of elderly population aged 65 and older in a society.

ENDNOTE

1 This study supported by Ministry of Health, General Directorate of Improvement of Health.

This work was previously published in the Handbook of Research on Healthcare Administration and Management edited by Nilmini Wickramasinghe, pages 384-406, copyright year 2017 by Medical Information Science Reference (an imprint of IGI Global).

Chapter 19
The Value of Measuring Patient Engagement in Healthcare:
New Frontiers for Healthcare Quality

Guendalina Graffigna
Università Cattolica del Sacro Cuore, Milan, Italy

Serena Barello
Università Cattolica del Sacro Cuore, Milan, Italy

ABSTRACT

The concept of patient engagement offers a unique opportunity to inform our understanding of patients' ability to be active in managing their care. However, unless promoting the active role of patients is today identified as a priority to promote care quality, a wide debate still exists on how to translate this principle into practice and how to assess initiatives aimed at increasing the level of patient participation in their care. Measuring patient engagement along the care course might ensure that the medical care truly serves patients' needs, priorities, and preferences. Unless the measurement of patient engagement is today a big issue for policy makers and healthcare practitioners, only few scientifically validated assessment tools currently exist to identify patients' level of involvement in their healthcare. In this chapter authors review the main validated tools currently available in the scientific community devoted to assess the patients' ability and availability to be actively engaged in their care, with a particular focus on the recently developed Patient Health Engagement Scale, specifically designed to assess the emotional and psychological adaptation of patients along their care process and their level of engagement in the healthcare management.

INTRODUCTION

Western healthcare systems are today facing some of the greatest challenges of their history. Population growth, breakthroughs in the treatment and management of chronic disease conditions and changes concerning the levels of patients' health needs and expectations have led to a system that is increasingly under pressure and financially unsustainable (Beaglehole et al., 2008; Blinded et al., 2013; Wiederhold

DOI: 10.4018/978-1-5225-1928-7.ch019

et al., 2013). In considering how best to develop an effective system that delivers quality care and value for health consumers – and one that is able to meet future care demand – the role that patients play has become ever more important: giving them back a starring role is today a priority for health policies both at an ethical and pragmatic levels.

Indeed, increasing evidence has demonstrated that patients' engagement in their health and healthcare is a key solution for leading innovative actions in the complex and mutable context of healthcare delivery and organization (Graffigna et al., 2015a). The term patient engagement encompasses a number of related concepts, including patient-centered care and shared decision-making, all of which build on the idea of involving patients as full partners in their care and health-related decisions. Patient engagement, indeed, aims at giving (back) a leading role to patients and taking them on board for a more efficient and effective process of care delivery. Under this broad umbrella term, there is evidences that patient engagement is linked with fewer adverse events, better patient self-management, fewer diagnostic tests, decreased use of healthcare services and shorter lengths of stay in hospitals. Particularly, researches have showed that those patients who are more active and engaged in their care more frequently reports better clinical outcomes (Hibbard & Greene, 2013), higher quality of life (Barello & Graffigna, 2014a), higher satisfaction with their care relationships (Becker & Roblin, 2008; Alegría et al., 2009), healthier behaviors (Hibbard et al., 2007), more effective self-management skills (Skolasky et al., 2008) and treatment adherence (Green & Hibbard, 2012). Furthermore, empirical researches have demonstrated how patient engagement may contribute to a reduction of healthcare costs and to better economically sustainable organizational processes (Coulter & Ellins, 2007; Berwick et al., 2008; Hibbard et al., 2013).

In this chapter, moving from a review of current literature about the healthcare requirements to face the ongoing societal and economic challenges, we shall introduce the concept of "person-centered care", such as a new approach to healthcare organization able to acknowledge the complex psycho-social needs and identities representation of care recipients. We shall also discuss how this broader vision – which encompass that one merely focused on "patients" such as healthcare clients – is crucial in the context of integrated care.

Adopting a multifaceted definition of patient's engagement is in this light very important, to acknowledging not only the cognitive and behavioral components of this patients' attitude to healthcare, but also to become aware of the role that the patients' emotional adjustment to their diagnosis and to the new medical regimen may play in fostering or hindering patients' ability to accomplish self-management. Another crucial aspect to move steps forward towards the effective reform of healthcare is adopting procedures to assess the needs of engagement of the patients: currently, only a few dedicated assessment tools exist to help clinicians in diagnosing the level of engagement of their patients, and thus their needs and expectations in order to manage their care in a more satisfactory and effective way. The chapter reviews the principal ones and then deepens the feature of a new tool dedicated to measure the patients' ability to psychologically adjust to their disease and to engage in its management: the Patient Health Engagement Scale (PHE-s; Graffigna et al., 2015a). The chapter concludes with some concrete advices to assess patients' engagement in the clinical setting and use this "diagnosis" to improve the care process.

BACKGROUND: CULTURAL AND ORGANIZATIONAL IMPLICATIONS OF PATIENT ENGAGEMENT

To adequately address the challenges related to chronic care processes, questioning current care models is today required. Present healthcare processes are more often designed to respond to the acute needs of individuals, rather than to anticipate and shape patterns of care for long-term chronic conditions (Berwick et al., 2008). The long-term treatment of chronic conditions requires a revision of classical models of care in order to guarantee sustainable care services. To address this requirement, and consequently to successfully manage patients and their own care, a better synergy between healthcare organizations and territorial services is necessary. Acute conditions are primarily treated within the traditional hospital or clinical settings for short period of time. On the contrary, chronic conditions need long-term approach to care: this should result in a more synergic connection between services (inside and outside the hospital settings) by taking advantage of all the resources (psychological, social and pragmatic) that are present in the territory the patients belong to. Integrated care and home-based care models are currently considered as a potential solution to improve quality and sustainability of healthcare services, particularly when the management of chronic conditions is concerned (Kodner & Spreeuwenberg, 2002). However, to achieve the goal of an integrated system of care, the role of the patients and the lenses through which healthcare actors look at them, need to be questioned and revised. Indeed, in this context, patients have to become main actors in the care environment by acquiring the needed motivation, knowledge and skills to face the medical course in partnership with a proactive care team. Furthermore, an integrated model of chronic care implies the systematic consideration of all the potential resources or hindrances to care management that are present in the territory. Moving towards an effective integrated care model requires the previous assessment of all the organizational, social and human factors that are implied in the complex system of care, both inside and outside the classical institutional boundaries of the hospital. Thus, not only it is important to achieve a fluid synergy among all the healthcare services dislocated on the territory in order to improve their effective communication and collaboration; but it becomes also crucial to sustain the fruitful interdisciplinary collaboration among all the different healthcare professionals involved along the patients' care journey management. Furthermore, extremely important is acknowledging the role that unformal network of caregivers may play along the care process. Peers may offer important support to patients both at the pragmatic and at the affective level and they should be considered healthcare partners in the spectrum of an integrated model of care. Thus, their presence, their action and their role should be questioned in order to contribute to healthcare systems innovation, in the direction of a really systematic and fruitful dialogue between healthcare organizations and the territory they belong to.

In the practice, linking healthcare services (as well as hospital and primary care organizations) means considering whose missions are overlapping across the spectrum of care delivery. This requires a coordinative behavior among health service suppliers and actively engaged patients to work as a system for gaining health goals. In this scenario promoting patients' engagement appears crucial: if empowered and made aware of the importance of their active role along their care journey, patients may become a fundamental ingredient to favoring the achievement of an effective and efficient integrated model of care.

TOWARDS A "PERSON-CENTERED" APPROACH TO HEALTH AND CARE

As stated above, the idea of engagement expresses the goal of a maximum acknowledge of the patients' role in the care process. However, in the practice, this is still far to be realized. Curious to be noticed, the words we use to advocate for engagement are still anchored to a "*passivizing*" approach of medical care. We still speak of "*patients*", and we argue that "*they have to be engaged*" in the care process. These linguistic expressions are a sort of paradox (and very often our language and the terms we choose to indicate concept and practices tell us a lot of our implicit conventions and assumptions!).

The word patient originally meant 'one who suffers'. This English noun comes from the Latin word patients, the present participle of the deponent verb, *patior*, meaning 'I am suffering,' and akin to the Greek verb *πάσχειν* (= *paskhein*, to suffer) and its cognate noun *πάθος* (= *pathos,* to feel). As a matter of fact, today the most recurrent conceptualizations and use of the patient engagement concept implicitly evoke an asymmetric relationship between an "*expert*" (i.e. the healthcare professionals) and a "*lay*" person who have to be changed in some extent, namely made more responsive, more adherent to prescriptions, more activated in the care management, etc. Conceptualizations, thus, that appear a reparatory answer to the still "passivizing" approach of medical care, within a healthcare system that has not yet succeeded in the concretization of a real patient-centered approach to medicine. A part from the rhetoric claims that we share with the literature, in the practice the patient is still often considered "*a disease carrier*", and the focus is still on the illness treatment, rather than on the person in its whole.

Given the scenario of integrated care highlighted above, to circumscribe the representation of recipients of care to the mere identity of patients appears reductive. The concept of patients, well advocated by the patient centered movement in medicine, refers to the prominent consideration of all the manifestations of the disease that the individual is carrying and to its psychosocial correlates (i.e., the "illness", Leventhal et al., 1997). However, in an integrated model of care, where the individuals who need and receive care are not only registered in an institutional context of care but they are back in their social context and integrated in their community, this representation needs to be revised. Indeed, along their chronic management of care, such "patients" need to find a new balance between their healthcare requirements and their previous roles, commitments and life routines. In other words, in order to become effective and sustainable, integrated model of care have to acknowledge that the recipients of the healthcare services are often *also* workers, partners, family members, community members, sons, daughters, and so on. Recipients of care are thus *persons*, not only patients. They are individuals who play several social roles, and the patient role is only one of them. Thus, referring to healthcare clients in the terms of "persons" better acknowledges the psycho-social complexity of their health needs and expectations: this acknowledgement is a fundamental precursor of the translation of patient's engagement from a mere claim to a real guidance of practice. Persons that are more complex than "patients". Persons incarnate different social roles, different desires, different aspirations in their public and private life. Roles that have to be acknowledged and sustained even after the occurrence of a diagnosis, even after that an individual is labelled "patient", in a very passivizing medical language. Thus, passing a sense of control on one own disease and cure process – not only at the behavioral level, but foremost at the cognitive and emotional levels – appears to be crucial for guaranteeing a true engagement of people towards their health and care.

Given an integrated care scenario, thus, a new paradigm shift in medicine has to be advocate: that one towards a "person-centered care". Speaking about "person centered care", in sum, means adopting a more holistic, critical and ethical approach to medical care and to the recipient of such interventions: it means to become aware of the complex and fluid identity projects that patients are carrying and to understand how a changed health status may impact on such life projects. The claim for a broader and more positive conceptualization of patient engagement would lead to a more genuine consideration of "patients" as "persons", who are carrier of histories, desires, needs, preferences and projects for their present and the future life: projects that – at least at the emotive levels – shouldn't made impossible by the disease, but – at the maximum – reconfigured and reoriented, in the *eudaimonic* development of a new self-representation.

In the practice, realizing a "person-centered" vision of care requires to adopt a holistic approach towards individuals: this vision deeply challenge the past dominant bio-medical paradigm, by refocusing healthcare organizations from a doctor-centered practice – where the health practitioner is considered the knowledge holder –, to a model of care where listening to the "persons' voice" and making them main actors of their medical course is fundamental to align health services provisions and care expectations. The shift towards person-centered sensibility in healthcare should re-oriented medicine's objectives: in this perspective, taking care of persons means not only dealing with disease treatment and technical procedures but also implies a full consideration of the whole person's life projects and illness experience – that is the emotional and relational patient's needs concerning his/her own care. In other words, a person-centered care approach advocates for a more comprehensive understanding of care recipients, not only as carriers of organic dis-functionalities, but as whole persons involved in a sociocultural context and featured by unique life histories, experiences, and expectations of health and care.

PROMOTING PATIENTS ENGAGEMENT: THE KEY TO ACHIEVE A PERSON CENTERED MODEL OF CARE

Currently, several definitions of patient engagement exist, addressing different aspects of such experience (Barello et al, 2014a).

Some scholars focused on the analysis of the organizational and cultural elements that may hinder or sustain patients' engagement, mainly addressing the role of doctor-patient relationship in the process. For instance, Dearing and colleagues (2005) states that developing engagement means to foster a client-therapist working alliance that may help the client gaining a more realistic understanding of the nature, process, and expected outcomes of treatment. Other scholars pointed at the shared decision making strategies as a crucial asset to enhance patients' engagement in their care. Davis and colleagues (2007), for instance, agree that patient's engagement is the result of patients becoming informed partners in their care, including a recasting of the care relationship where clinician enact the role of adviser, and patients - or designated surrogates for incapacitated patients - serving as the locus of decision making. Other scholars adopted a more holistic analysis of the organizational and contextual factors in play in the patients' engagement process. Mahmud (2004), for instance, sees engagement as an organizational process that leads to a revision of the healthcare priorities in the direction of empowering people to provide input in decisions that affect their lives encourages support for those decisions, which in turn improves the public's trust and confidence in the healthcare system. Finally, Mc Bride and colleagues (2007) also point at the importance of informal care and define engagement as the element that will allow, at different levels, the wider community to have a say in the future direction of their health.

These definitions of patients' engagement have the value of systematizing some of the relational and organizational dynamics that happen in the management of chronic care and that may result in important levers for patients' engagement. However, on the other side, these definitions tend to oversimplify the experience of engagement itself, by representing it as an "on-off" status, that may be present or absent, instead of acknowledging the dynamic and complex psycho-social roots of such patients' experience.

In this light, other authors, neglected the analysis of organizational and contextual factors that contribute to the development of engagement to primarily focus on the inter-individual components of patients' engagement experience. These authors, thus, advocated that understanding how the illness experience influences the way patients feel and function in their daily lives is essential for developing appropriate care pathways. Authors interested in the inter-individual dimensions of patient engagement tended to problematize the dynamic development of such experience, by pointing at engagement as a complex psycho-social process which develops in time according to specific stages or experiential positions.

According to these scholars, promoting patient active participation in healthcare presupposes to have a holistic vision of the individual. Effective disease management implies to consider that multiple experiential dimensions interact when a patient faces his/her illness course. These dimensions could be synthetized as follows:

- **Behavioral Dimension:** Connected to all the activities the patient acts out to face the disease, basing on its emotional and cognitive reaction.
- **Cognitive/Knowledge Dimension:** Connected to the need to know, understand and make sense of the disease, its treatments, its possible developments, its monitoring;
- **Emotional Dimension:** Connected to the need to psychologically and emotionally manage (and adjust to) the onset of the disease and new life condition linked to it.

However, scholars often tended to address only one of this psycho-social components of engagement in their definition, by neglecting the others.

For instance, Légaré and colleagues (2013) mainly focused on the cognitive dimensions of engagement. They detected in patients' level of knowledge and literacy about their health status and their medical prescriptions, the most important resources for patients' engagement. The ability of searching for health information, of decoding such information and of using them, thus, is considered by this authors the essence of engagement.

Gruman and colleagues (2010) and Hibbard and colleagues (2009), further than patients' health literacy, focused on their behavioral abilities to enact effective self-care behaviors. The ability to manage health and healthcare, throughout conscious and "consumeristic behaviors" is considered by these authors such an indicator of patients' ability to self-determinate their health status, and thus, of them being well engaged in their care. Particularly Hibbard and colleagues (2009) developed the concept of "activation" to underline the importance of addressing patients' ability to enact engagement conducts and to participate in their care management. Hibbard also stated that patient activation is a function of the patients' confidence in their own knowledge and ability to participate in the care process.

PROMOTING PATIENTS' ENGAGEMENT: THE ROLE OF THE EMOTIONAL ELABORATION OF THE DISEASE

The emotive and psychodynamic component of engagement has been less addressed so far, although scholars agree on the role of patients' emotions in hindering or sustaining patients' engagement (Street et al., 2005; Hibbard & Mahoney, 2010; Meglic et al., 2010; Barello et al., 2014a). Graffigna and colleagues

(2014a) try to address this component of engagement by stating that engagement is a "*process-like and multi-dimensional experience, resulting from the conjoint cognitive, emotional and conative enactment of individuals towards their health management. In this process patients go through four subsequent phases (blackout, arousal, adhesion and eudaimonic project). The unachieved synergy among the different subjective dimensions (think, feel, act) at each stage of the process may inhibit patients' ability to engage in their care*". Theses authors exemplified the role of emotions as a fundamental component of patients' engagement in some specific pathological areas such as diabetes (Graffigna et al., 2014b) and cardiovascular diseases (Barello et al., 2015a). Patients' experience of their illness(es) and the emotional elaboration of the health condition is recognized to affect the patients' strategies for dealing with their health care experience. Promoting patient active participation healthcare means fostering the patient's advancement in the process of emotional elaboration and adjustment of his/her own illness condition (i.e. patient engagement). Only supporting this aspect, the patient will be able to enhance his/her disease management skills (i.e. patient activation).

The interaction among these three dimensions impact the patients' attitudes toward the disease condition and the ways of disease management. The failure of this interaction might explain patients' resistance and barriers in effectively managing their disease condition. Each dimension, indeed, allows to discover specific unmet needs that patients might experience in several domains of their daily life. Addressing those needs might enhance the level of patient engagement in the disease care and positively impact on clinical outcomes.

For instance, in the diabetic patient lack of health literacy and behavioral skills for managing treatments associated to the emotional burden related to the diagnosis might affect the capacity of individuals of effectively coping with the diabetes care process.

MEASURING PATIENT ENGAGEMENT: A FUNDAMENTAL FOR PROMOTING HEALTHCARE QUALITY

The fast pace of change in the healthcare system requires patients to be more and more aware of their care options and be active agents in evaluating options about where and when to seek care. Patients are no longer passive recipients of care; instead, they are empowered consumers of medical products and services and are recognized to be real partners in the process by which those products/services are developed. Patients increasingly act as advocates for new treatments, and many be fully engaged in making decisions about their care. In this context, patients strongly require clinicians to be helped in meeting their health goals (Stewart, 2001).

However, unless promoting the active role of patients is today identified as a priority to promote care quality, a wide debate still exists on how to translate this principle into practice and how to assess initiatives whose goal is to increase the level of patient participation in their care (Coulter & Dunn 2002).

If we want patient engagement to mean real partnership between patients and health providers on mutually-agreed health plans, healthcare systems need to find effective ways to measure the quality and the effect of this collaborative process. These interventions should work towards medical outcomes and care procedures that the patient understands and has had an opportunity to help determine. Measuring patient engagement along the care course might ensure that the medical care truly serves the patient's needs, priorities, and preferences.

Measuring patient engagement in healthcare is a crucial step for improving patient's care experience and outcomes. In this contexts patient-reported experience measures (PREMs), might support this process. This kind of measures is important because we should not assume that every individual in a specific socio-demographic group is the same when engaging with taking decision about heath and treatments, acquiring new health information, participating in health-promoting behaviors, following treatment prescriptions, or even interacting with the health professional during a clinical consultation. To assume that all patients will respond to these situations in the same way is counterproductive. That's why it is important to measure the level of patient engagement to understand these differences. Particularly, measuring patient engagement might have different aims and is a fundamental condition for:

- Population segmentation and risk stratification to target interventions;
- Designing customized care pathways according to the unique patient's needs;
- Evaluating the quality and quantity of intervention to support the active role of patients in their care process;
- Measuring the performance of health care systems and evaluating the effectiveness of care interventions.

From a strategical point of view, it is fundamental to establish not only why administering assessment for patient engagement, by also to reason about when and which patients have to be included. Indeed, the timing of patient engagement measurement might vary depending on the patients' disease and illness history, the setting of care, the socio-cultural context the patient belongs to and the patients' ability to self-report.

Moreover, clinicians should consider that assessing the level of patient engagement could follow two main logics (Figure 1):

- On the one hand, a "*linear logic*" might suggest to administrate measures for patient engagement in crucial turning points of the care process (i.e. diagnosis, treatment decision making, hospital discharge, clinical follow-ups...);
- On the other hand, a "*processual logic*" might encourage clinicians to administrate patient engagement measures when critical events occur in the disease course. These events could be both clinical-related (i.e. new symptoms, disease relapse, unexpected new diagnosis…) and patients' context-related (i.e. caregivers' disease or death, changes in the patients' psychological status, changes in the patients' social context…). These events might deeply impact on the ability of patients to be active participants of their care and on their availability in engaging in treatment/care decisions.

THE CURRENT MEASUREMENT TOOLS FOR ASSESSING PATIENT ACTIVE ENGAGEMENT IN THEIR CARE

Unless the measurement of patient engagement is today a big issue for policy makers and healthcare practitioners and the need for defining criteria to assess interventions devoted to meaningfully include individuals in their care constitutes a priority for healthcare, only few scientifically validated assessment tools currently exist to help identify patients' level of involvement in their healthcare.

Figure 1. Linear vs. processual logics in patient engagement measurement

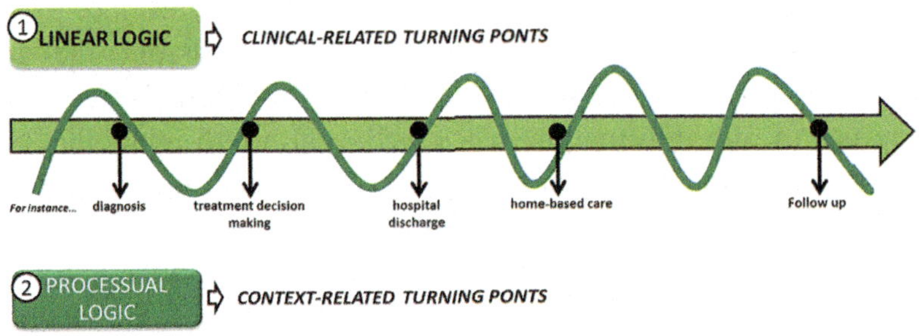

More in depths, the scientific literature provides practitioners of very few instruments specifically developed to assess these crucial aspects in the patients' care experience. The following paragraphs are aimed at offering readers a brief overview of the main assessment tools - currently available in the scientific community – devoted to assess the patients' ability and availability to be actively engaged in their care, with their main characteristics and psychometric properties. These instruments can be grouped into two main categories: some instruments collapse in the group of measures aimed at assessing the patients' ability to self-manage the health condition; another category is, on the other hand, constituted by instruments dedicated to assess the patients' engagement experience along their care management journey. Let's see them in more details.

MEASURING THE PATIENTS' ABILITY TO SELF-MANAGE THEIR HEALTH AND HEALTHCARE

The Patient Activation Measure (PAM)

Developed by Hibbard and colleagues (2005; 2012) and recently validated in Italy (Graffigna et al., 2015b), the 13-item Patient Activation Measure is an interval-level, unidimensional Guttman-like measure that contains items measuring self-assessed knowledge about chronic conditions, beliefs about illness and medical care, and self-efficacy for self-care. The PAM focused on physical conditions, and it was designed to measure activation as a broad construct. PAM can be a valuable instrument when the aim of assessment is to evaluate the current patients' behavioral skills in managing the disease and the care prescriptions.

The Altarum Consumer Engagement (ACE) Survey

ACE (Duke et al., 2015) is a 15-question survey measures consumer behavior in managing their own health and making health care decisions. This instrument consists of four valid subscales (commitment, informed choice, navigation, ownership) each indicative of a unique aspect of engagement. According to these premises, ACE is an insightful tool when clinicians need to evaluate the ability of patients in facing current health decision making processes basing on their knowledge and skills for care management

The Partners in Health (PIH) Scale

Developed by Battersby and colleagues (2003), the PIH is a generic assessment scale for patients managing their chronic medical conditions, that is relevant to the primary health care setting. The scale consists of 11 items aimed at measuring the patients' features regarding the following dimensions: (1) Knowledge of the condition and various treatment options; (2) Ability to negotiate a plan of care; (3) Engagement in activities that protect and promote health; (4) Monitoring and management of the symptoms and signs of the clinical condition(s). Both patients and health professionals judged the scale as acceptable and easy to use, and the health professionals endorsed its clinical utility

The Patient Enablement Instrument (PEI)

The Patient Enablement Instrument (PEI) – developed by Howie and colleagues (1998) is designed to capture the patients' ability to understand the nature of their problems and cope with their illness. The PEI was developed to be used in primary care and is to be completed by the patient after consultation. This tool addresses six questions regarding a patient's recent visit, and, assess the following areas: how much they felt able to (1) cope with life, (2) understand their illness, (3) cope with their illness, (4) keep healthy, (5) felt confident about their health, and (6) able to help themselves. The scale was found to be reliable (Cronbach's $\alpha = 0.897$). Scores were categorized to indicate low (0–4), medium (score 5–9), and high enablement (10–12)

The Self-Management Ability Scale (SMAS)

Developed by Cramm and colleagues (2012) and based on the self-management of well-being (SMW) theory (Steverink et al., 2005), the 30-item Self-Management Ability Scale (SMAS) measures self-management abilities (SMA). The 30-item SMAS consists of six five-item subscales. Each sub-scale assesses one of the six core abilities to form the composite construct of self-management: (1) to take initiatives (be instrumental or self-motivating in realizing aspects of well-being); (2) to invest in resources for long-term benefits; (3) to maintain variety in resources (achieve and maintain various resources for each dimension of well-being); (4) to ensure resource multi-functionality (gain and maintain resources or activities that serve multiple dimensions of well-being simultaneously and in a mutually reinforcing way); (5) to self-efficaciously manage resources (gain and maintain a belief in personal competence to achieve well-being); and (6) to maintain a positive frame of mind. Each of these abilities directly relates to the dimensions of well-being specified in the SPF theory: physical well-being (comfort and stimulation) and social well-being (affection, behavioral confirmation, and status)

MEASURING PATIENTS' ENGAGEMENT PSYCHOLOGICAL EXPERIENCE: THE PATIENT HEALTH ENGAGEMENT SCALE (PHE-s)

These different assessment tools described above are widely used to measure patients' health literacy and level of behavioral competence in self-management. They are thus mainly oriented towards the cognitive and behavioral components of patients' self-management. However, as stated above, growing acknowledgement is played to the emotional and psychodynamic components of the patients' illness experience that appears to be the first movers of patients' confidence and ability to acquire information about their health status and to master self-management behaviors. The emotional component of engagement, conceived as the patients' process of elaboration and adjustment to the disease, has also been demonstrated to be a crucial mediator of patients' activation and adherence (Graffigna et al., 2015c; Graffigna et al., in press).

The patient's illness experience is recognized to be mutable and unstable across time. This aspect impacts on the patient's both availability and ability to actively engage in his/her process of care management. Although healthcare professionals and scholars agree in recognizing the importance of the emotional elaboration of the patients' illness journey in the chronic care management process (Barello et al., 2015), so far validated tools to assess this aspect have been neglected.

To our knowledge an original contribution in this direction is given by the recently developed Patient Health Engagement scale (PHE-s). The PHE-s developed by Graffigna and colleagues (2015a) is a measure of patient engagement psychological experience that is grounded in rigorous conceptualization and appropriate psychometric methods. The scale consists of 5 ordinal items and was developed based on the authors' conceptual model of patient engagement (PHE model), which features four evolutionary stages along a continuum of engagement (Figure 2).

The PHE model, offers clinicians a general picture of the patients' global attitudes toward their health conditions and treatment management. Particularly, it describes an evolutionary process of patient engagement featuring four subsequent phases (i.e. *blackout*; *arousal*; *adhesion*; *eudaimonic project*). According to this model, patient engagement appears to be a function of the patients' emotional elaboration toward their health and care management.

According to this model, patient engagement is a dynamic and evolutionary psychological process that involves the recovery of life projectuality - even with the disease. This process also features peculiar ways of interaction and decisional negotiation between the patient and the healthcare that depends strongly on the phase of the process through which the patients is passing. This evolutionary view of the patient engagement process suggests that a fully engaged patient results from a series of psychological

Figure 2. The process of patient engagement as described in the PHE model (Graffigna et al., 2014a)

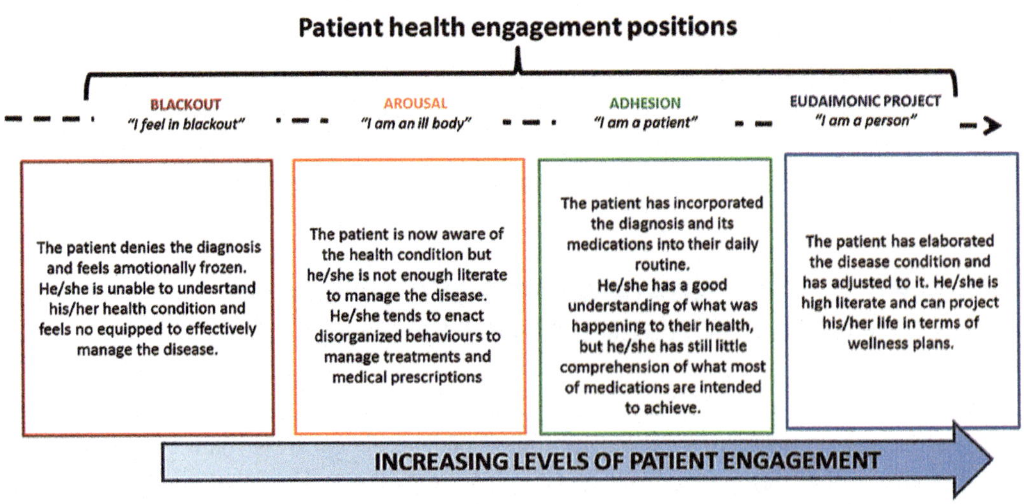

reframing of his/her health condition and that the success of the patient in advancing along the process depends on how he/she succeeded in the previous phases. The last position of the engagement process (i.e., eudaimonic project) culminates in a patient that has gained a positive approach to health management and has recaptured an active role in society by re-establishing plans for wellness. Such patient has succeeded in incorporating disease management into his/her life. In particular, the four positions of engagement featured by the PHE model may be summarized as it follows.

Blackout

This position is typical of patients at the beginning of their care journey, usually at the moment of the diagnosis or in the occurrence of a relapse or worsening of their clinical condition. The urgency and perceived drama of these moments creates in patients a state of emotional, behavioral, and cognitive blockage ("*blackout*"). Patients describe themselves as psychologically frozen, shocked by the disease, unable to face and manage it. Patients thus perceive the disease and its management out of their control. They feel like "in suspension," as they are looking forward to obtain a ruling from someone. In this phase patients tend to be passive and to delegate their cure to their reference healthcare professional. Patients are disengaged in this moment, but the emotional elaboration of their condition start from this, thus this initial experience is crucial to then evolve in the journey of engagement.

In this initial position patients describe their diagnosis as distressing and unacceptable. They perceive strongly negative emotions and tend whether to refuse the disease (by denying the symptoms and their recurrence) or to depressively experience it, as the end of their positive trajectory of life. Patients in this stage cannot easily elaborate the received information about the disease (cognitive blindness) and as a consequence they also feel blocked in acting (behavioral freezing) and managing their disease. Patients in this phase tend to be completely absorbed in their illness experience and often experience difficulty attending to the needs of their private and social life due to a focus on the management of their disease and its treatment. In this phase, the patients' quality of life strongly depends on the effectiveness in controlling/reducing the side effects connected to treatments and clinical stability.

Arousal

In the position of *"arousal"*, patients have acquired and initial understanding of their health condition and of the medical requirements to manage them. They have also elaborate a first adjustment to their disease, although if they are still far from having accepted it. At the emotional level patients still appear distressed and very preoccupied for their health condition: as a result they are hyper-attentive to every signal in their bodies (emotional alert) that they tend to overestimate and to refer to their diagnosis, even when this is not appropriate. Patients in this position perceive symptoms as an "alarm" that worries the patient and may cause overwhelming emotional reactions. Patients are equipped with more information about their health condition compared to the previous phase, although their health literacy is still superficial and fragmented (superficial knowledge). Moreover, they feel behaviorally unable to manage their disease and treatment prescriptions effectively (behavioral disorganization).

Adhesion

In this position patients have moved some progress along their emotional elaboration of the disease. This position of engagement is often experienced by patients in a more advanced stage of their medical journey and it appears function of the broader spectrum of health knowledge (cognitive adhesion) which the patients have acquired from their reference healthcare professional or autonomously searching for health information. Patients in this position have accepted their disease and their new identity of "patient". They also have developed the basic behavioral skills (formal adherence) to effectively comply with medical prescriptions. They also feel sufficiently confident in their own emotional strength to cope with their disease. Although already manifesting a satisfactory level of activation, patients in this position are not really autonomous in managing the rules necessary to be healthy (i.e., healthy life style and correct medication regimen). The ability of these patients to cope with their disease and its management is challenged when some change happens in their daily routine (i.e., when going to holiday, when travelling for work…). Since patients in this position have not fully elaborated and integrated their disease condition yet, they find also difficult to completely accept the rationale behind the medical requests of changing their lifestyle or of their new medication regimen. Accordingly, patients revealed the need to continuously hang on their reference healthcare professionals' authority, which they conceive as a «life-line», waiting for the time when they will be able and self-confident to self-manage.

According to the specificities of this status, the patient's quality of life depends mainly on the fulfillment of the patient's healthcare needs and on the responsiveness of the healthcare provider. The patient's wellness is closely associated with the experience of a healthcare system that is truly attuned to the care expectations of the patient.

Eudaimonic Project

Finally, in the "*eudaimonic project*" position, patients have fully accepted their health condition and the successfully integrated their new identity of "patients" in a more complex and broader self-representation. They have elaborated the idea that the disease occurrence has impacted greatly on their life routines but that it is still possible (and legitimate) to maintain some sort of positive self-realization in their private life (elaboration). Patients in this experiential position became able to recognize internal resources that are useful for acquiring a positive approach to life and to health, despite the diagnosis, and that become the base for a full engagement in their self-management. Patients gradually become co-constructors of their health and capable of enacting a meaningful health management, which allows them to improve their quality of life. Patients are able to effectively search for appropriate information about their disease conditions and medications. This allows them to give full sense to their health experience (sense making) and effectively enact healthy behaviors, in due time, even when contexts change (situated practices). Patients have also developed a new perspective about their disease, which can now be thoughtful and integrated in a wider life project. They also become able to make some reasonable but still satisfactory plan for their near feature, in the light of the new health condition and maybe despite shorter expectations of life. According to this experiential position, patients are the managers of their own care, and they can mobilize healthcare services proactively when there is a need. Moreover, they can advocate for the health of their community (e.g., raising concerns to policymakers, helping others navigate the health care system, and advancing healthcare quality and equity). The patient in this phase becomes an experienced testimonial of good self-care practice who is able to become a caregiver of others similar to him/her. Given the patients' reconquered possibility to consider themselves as whole persons despite their disease condition, their quality of life depends strongly on their renewed ability to make realistic life decisions that are consistent with the influence of their disease on their life. This position of the model is considered as the full realization of patients' engagement, also at the level of the emotional elaboration and acceptation of the disease. This is the position to which patients should tend along their emotional journey of disease management and adjustment to their illness.

APPLICATION OF THE PHE-S IN CLINICAL SETTINGS

The Patient Health Engagement Scale (PHE-s), based on this model, allows to briefly and easily assess the level of emotional elaboration of a patient concerning his/her health condition by simply asking five straight forward questions. This set of questions — and the alternative of answers that the model offers — may orient clinicians, managers, and other professionals in dealing with interventions aimed to sustain patients' self-care abilities in assessing primary psychological needs and care expectations. Basically, the PHE-s questions the patients' stage of psychological elaboration about the changed health condition and of their engagement needs (way of "feeling" when reflecting on health status). This instrument is today the only one specifically dedicated to assess the degree of emotional elaboration and adjustment reached by the patient concerning his/her own health condition when engaging in health management. The specificity of this scale lays in the fact that it allows not only to assess the current patient's attitude towards his/her health condition, but also to forecast the patient's risk for disengagement in health management and thus to design preventive targeted intervention to optimize care pathways.

The PHE-s is a patient self-administrable questionnaire developed with the aim of diagnosing the level of patient engagement in their healthcare process that is function of his/her degree of emotional elaboration of the new health condition. This tool allows clinicians to move from a style of interaction that is clinician-directed and focuses on patients' adherence to treatments, to one that supports patients' motivation and autonomy in the care process, matches patients' level of engagement, and ultimately increases engagement. The information from the PHE-s might help guide the discussion and the action plan for care. Figure 3 shows the instruction form to be presented to the patient before asking him/her to fill out the questionnaire. Figure 4 shows the complete PHE-s.

The clinician who is in charge when administering the scale to the patient has to introduce and explain to the subject the aim of the questionnaire by specifying that to be effective in answering the proposed questions, the patient should refer to how he/she is currently living/experiencing his/her health status; The response options featuring this instrument (i.e. ordinal scale) allow patients to easily mirror with the current emotional states related to their disease condition. The ordinal structure of the response options also allows subjects to position themselves along an experiential continuum. Finally, the 7 response options for each item allow patients to position themselves in "intermediate" points (also for avoiding the social desirability mechanism). These 7 positions can be easily converted into a "patient engagement" scoring by following the instructions offered by the conversion table (Figure 5).

Finally, the clinician has to support the patient during the administration of the instrument in order to clarify possible doubts when filling out the questionnaire. The PHS-s has been constructed moving from 5 items with points (rang) of an ordinal categorical nature, instead of a quantitative-metric logic as usually adopted in psychometrics scales. The final scoring, thus, have to keep into account the ordinal origin of items answers. In order to calculate the PHE score, the most correct choice at the methodological level

Figure 3. Instruction form for introducing the PHE-s to the patient (Graffigna et al., 2015a)

Following, you will find 5 statements that describe how a person might feel when thinking about his/her disease. Each sentence can be completed by indicating one of the 4 states or the intermediate points between two states. Please, indicate the state that better describes you by indicating the corresponding position.

Following an example to help you in answering the questions

Example 1
When I think about my health status...

I feel sad		I feel anxious		I feel resigned		I feel relaxed
●	○	○	○	○	○	○

if you were sad when thinking about you disease, you would indicate the first position

Example 2
When I think about my health status...

I feel sad		I feel anxious		I feel resigned		I feel relaxed
○	●	○	○	○	○	○

if you were in an intermediate position between sadness and anxiety when thinking about you disease, you would indicate the second position

Figure 4. The PHE-s (Graffigna et al., 2015a)

Thinking about my health status…

1	I feel in blackout		I am in alarm		I am aware		I feel positive
	o	o	o	o	o	o	o
2	I feel dazed		I am in trouble		I am conscious		I feel serene
	o	o	o	o	o	o	o
3	When I think about my illness I feel overwhelmed by emotions		I feel anxious every time a new symptom arises		I got used to my illness condition		Despite my illness I perceive coherence and continuity in my life
	o	o	o	o	o	o	o
4	I feel very discouraged due to my illness		I feel anxious when I try to manage my illness		I feel I adjusted to my illness		I am generally optimist about my future and my health condition
	o	o	o	o	o	o	o
5	I feel totally oppressed by my illness		I am upset when a new symptom arises		I feel I have accepted my illness		I can give sense to my life despite my illness condition
	o	o	o	o	o	o	o

Figure 5. Conversion table for calculating the PHE-s score

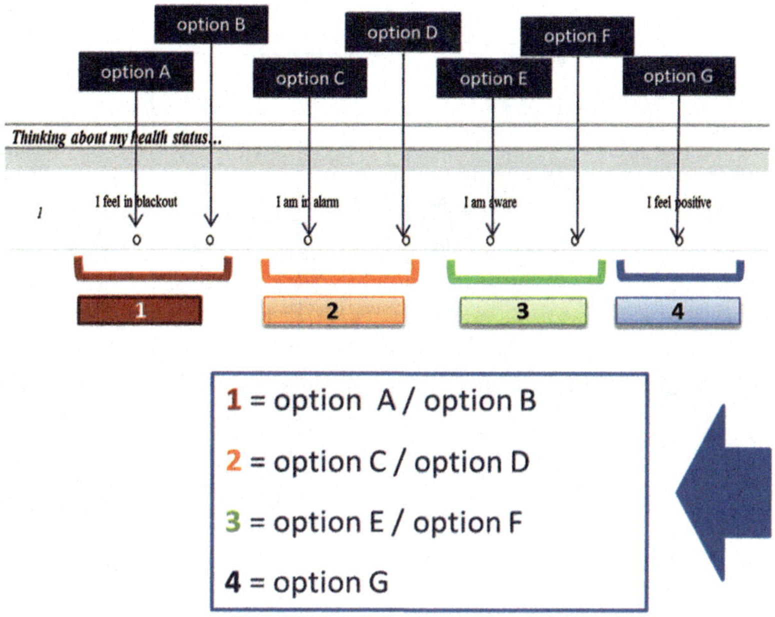

would be considering the metrical factor resulting from the not-linear analysis of principal components (CATPCA). This statistical technique requires an advanced knowledge of data-mining procedures and the use of dedicated software. This would not be possible in the applied clinical settings and during the daily clinical practices. Thus, during scale validation procedures, a simpler approach was used, in order to make the PHE-s usable from the larger group of patients and healthcare professionals interested in assessing the emotional adjustment of patients along their engagement process. The two best adequate indexes to synthetize ordinal data are the median and the mode. In the PHE-s validation study (Graffigna et al., 2015a) the linear correlation between the metric factor of CAPTCA and, respectively, mode and median have been calculated. Both correlations resulted high (i.e. correlation with mode=.91; correlation with median= -96). For ordinal data, the median score is considered a more robust and reliable index and, differently from the mode, it is always univocally defined. Thus the median has been adopted as the index to calculate the PHE-s score. To obtain the PHE-s level, the median of the row PHE-s scores should be calculated. And with a simple conversion it is possible to transform the row PHE-s scores in the corresponding patient's engagement position (Figure 6).

THE PHE SCALE AS A GUIDELINE FOR CLINICAL ACTIONS

When clinicians have to face a diagnostic process, they might proceed according to different logics. On the one hand, they can follow a "top-down" approach where the diagnosis determines an intervention (i.e. clinical, pharmacological...). In this case the diagnosis is based on predetermined criteria which are part of the clinician's expertise. Diagnosing patient engagement following this logic means to administrate the questionnaires and collect data and information in order to plan an intervention aimed at "correcting" dysfunctional behaviors or knowledge which might hinder the active role of patients in the care process.

Figure 6. Procedure to calculate the PHE-s level

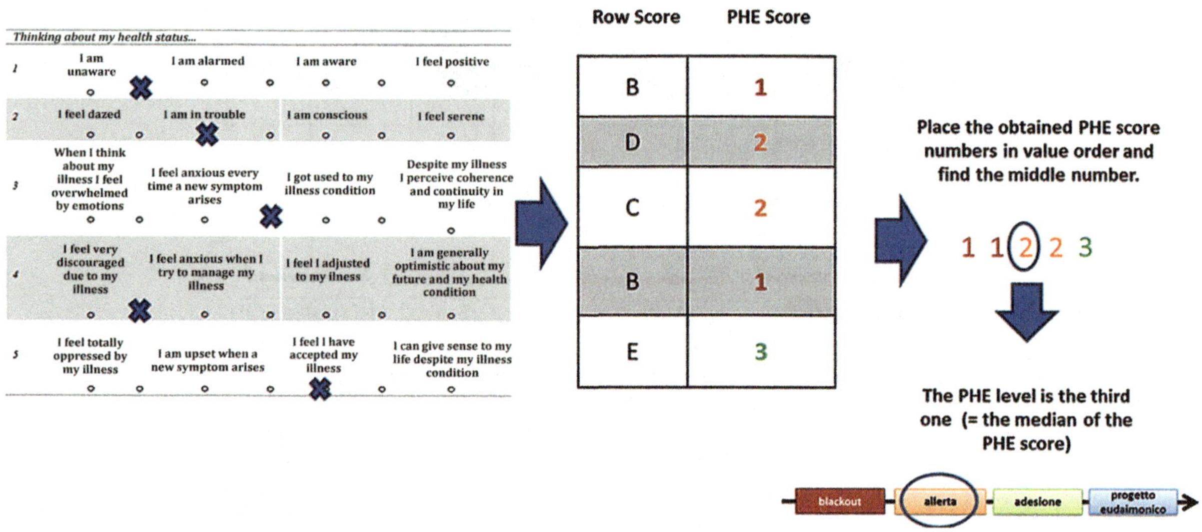

On the other hand, another logic might guide the clinician's action when assessing the patient engagement level. In this case, the clinician and the patients are considered both expert actors of the care process. Diagnosis and intervention are guided by a circular logic which results in the definition of a therapeutic and relational contract between the patient and the provider. The diagnosis represents - in this case - a starting point for guiding the clinical encounter and establishing a shared plan for care. It is conceivable as a moment of patient's self-awareness (and empowerment) concerning his/her capacity and availability to actively engage in the care process. The diagnostic phase is a first occasion to promote the patients' change. In this sense, we can say that the assessment has a therapeutic value *per sé* (Provenzi et al., 2016). However, it is important to consider the diagnostic moment as the first step for planning a shared plan for intervention basing on the information collected by administering the questionnaires.

In particular, when defining a shared plan of intervention basing on the level of patient engagement assessed in the diagnostic moment, means questioning different strategical aspects:

- First of all, clinicians have to think about the style of interaction more suitable for each level of engagement. This means reflecting upon the best way of relationship with each patient in order to better fine tune with his/her illness experience and role expectation in the care process.
- Second, effective patient engagement requires to carefully plan the quality and the quantity of information and knowledge the patients is able to receive and use along the care experience. Having in mind the level of patient engagement and activation might orient clinicians in selecting the most effective information to be provided to improve the patients' active management of the care prescriptions.
- Finally, planning a co-constructed intervention for patient engagement, also implies to define the best timing for intervening and the frequency of interaction with the patients to effectively support them.

The PHE-s allows to evaluate patients in a holistic way by collecting multiple information regarding all the experiential dimensions involved in the patient engagement experience. However, by combining this with the other instruments today available, practitioners might obtain a comprehensive overview about the patient's level of skills, knowledge and emotional acceptance of his/her health condition. In particular, the adoption of the PHE-s (alone or in combination with the other tools) may guarantee to have not only a superficial measure of what patients do or know when dealing with the disease management, but also a deeper understanding of the emotional dynamics underlining the adjustment of patients to the disease condition and the acceptance of his/her new patient identity. Catching this last aspect – that is the patient illness experience – should be considered as a reading key for health practitioners to fine tune with their patients when taking decisions about healthcare (Barello & Graffigna, 2015b).

For instance, when patients receive a PHE-s score of "*Blackout*", the clinicians should be aware that, in order to improve their level of engagement, patients need to overcome the emotional confusion connected to the disrupting critical event. In this scope, a trusted relationship with the healthcare provider is crucial for overcoming the blackout phase. The healthcare professional is asked to scaffold patients in this phase and offer solidarity by making an empathic response and educating them about their health. This informative action is expected from the referential healthcare professional who becomes, since the moment of the diagnosis, the privileged spokesperson for the patient along the care process. If patients fail to build a solid relation with the healthcare provider, their emotional behavioral responses may become dysfunctional, often leading to patients' dropout.

In other cases, when patients receive a PHE-s score of "*Arousal*", they manifest to have acquired a basic understanding of their diagnosis and of their health status, but they are still overwhelmed by negative emotions linked to the diagnosis. Patients in this phase, in order to move forward in their engagement journey, need to be supported in emotionally and pragmatically copying with the change related to the health condition. With patients in this PHE-s positions, healthcare professionals have to legitimate patients in asking for help and be open to answer all the questions and doubts they may have. Furthermore, healthcare professional should provide a "how to do" list with practical situations and ways to face them in the daily management of health for planning an reminding screenings.

When patients receive a PHE-s score of "*Adhesion*" they have reached a good adjustment to their disease, although they are not able to approach it in a positive light and thus they do not have enough personal resources to completely mange medical prescriptions. At this stage, healthcare professionals are claimed to train problem-solving skills and sustain patients' motivation towards self-management. They also should promote a therapeutic alliance aimed to sustain patients' initiatives and motivation to be autonomous. Empowering sessions are also welcome with patients tailored healthy behavior tracking.

The PHE-s score of "*Eudaimonic Project*" indicates patients who fully accomplished their engagement journey: they have successfully elaborated their new healthcare conditions and adjusted to it. They learned the information and the skills necessary to cope with the disease and the medical prescriptions. They also matured a positive approach to health and life, recognizing how the "patient role" is only referring to a new identity of the individual, additional to previous role and commitment. These patients need to be sustained in this positive approach to healthcare, they need support for succeed in this renewed balance between healthcare needs and quality of life needs. Healthcare professionals are claimed to health coaching, goal setting and support these patients in planning and achieving positive health plans. Healthcare systems should promote at distance relationship and remote communication with a referential healthcare professional. Patients and caregivers' participation to make their voice reflected in healthcare organizations governance should also be accomplished at this stage.

CONCLUSION

From what we defined a "person-centered" approach to integrated care, assessing the level of patient engagement is an essential component of a successful strategy for improving patients' experience. Eliciting feedback from patients regarding their attitudes towards their health status affords an opportunity to highlight and address aspects of care that need improvement and to monitor performance with regard to meeting patient expectations in the delivery of care. Furthermore, being able to assess the level of emotional elaboration of the disease and the patient psychological adjustment to its management is crucial to sustain not only effective clinical interventions but also to allow patients to maintain positive and satisfactory life trajectories and their successful engagement in care management.

At present few dedicated tools exist to assess the level of patients' engagement. Although the emotional and psychodynamic component of the engagement experience is recognized by health scholars to play an important role in sustaining or hindering patients' ability to managing their disease, so far only one dedicate tool exists to diagnose the emotional mindset of patients along their engagement journey. In this chapter we have described and discussed the specificities of the Patients Health Engagement Scale (PHE-s), developed in order to assess patients' engagement also in its emotional component. Since previous empirical study have showed how the level of patients' elaboration of the disease is an antecedent and mediator of patients' activation towards self-management, becoming able to assess it may help in forecasting patients' ability in improving their skills to cope with the disease and the medical prescriptions in daily life. This may lead to the planning of better personalized and, thus, more effective healthcare interventions. However, the PHE-s may be useful also when used to measure the effectiveness of clinical interventions. Particularly, measuring the level of patient engagement after an educational session, after a medical consultation, or even after service delivery reorganization may be an important asset to account for the made changes and achieved goals.

Furthermore, if combined with other validated tools, the PHE-s may contribute to the deeper and more complete assessment of patients' healthcare needs and priorities, together with their quality expectations towards the healthcare systems.

Moving steps forwards in the practice of measuring healthcare effectiveness in engaging patients should be envisaged as a crucial goal to concretely reform services and to make them better effective and sustainable at the economic level.

REFERENCES

Alegría, M., Sribney, W., Perez, D., Laderman, M., & Keefe, K. (2009). The role of patient activation on patient–provider communication and quality of care for US and foreign born Latino patients. *Journal of General Internal Medicine*, *24*(3), 534–541. doi:10.1007/s11606-009-1074-x PMID:19842003

Barello, S., & Graffigna, G. (2014b). Engaging patients to recover life projectuality: An Italian cross-disease framework. *Quality of Life Research: An International Journal of Quality of Life Aspects of Treatment, Care and Rehabilitation*, *24*(5), 1087–1096. doi:10.1007/s11136-014-0846-x PMID:25373927

Barello, S. & Graffigna, G. (2015b). Patient engagement in healthcare: pathways for effective medical decision making. *Neuropsychogical Trends,* 2015, 53.

Barello, S., Graffigna, G., Savarese, M., & Bosio, A. C. (2014a). Engaging patients in health management: Towards a preliminary theoretical conceptualization. *Psicologia della Salute*, *3*(3), 11–33. doi:10.3280/PDS2014-003002

Barello, S., Graffigna, G., Vegni, E., Savarese, M., Lombardi, F., & Bosio, A. C. (2015a). 'Engage me in taking care of my heart': A grounded theory study on patient–cardiologist relationship in the hospital management of heart failure. *BMJ Open*, *5*(3), e005582. doi:10.1136/bmjopen-2014-005582 PMID:25776041

Battersby, M. W., Ask, A., Reece, M. M., Markwick, M. J., & Collins, J. P. (2003). The Partners in Health scale: The development and psychometric properties of a generic assessment scale for chronic condition self-management. *Australian Journal of Primary Health*, *9*(3), 41–52. doi:10.1071/PY03022

Becker, E. R., & Roblin, D. W. (2008). Translating primary care practice climate into patient activation: The role of patient trust in physician. *Medical Care*, *46*(8), 795–805. doi:10.1097/MLR.0b013e31817919c0 PMID:18665059

Berwick, D. M., Nolan, T. W., & Whittington, J. (2008). The triple aim: Care, health, and cost. *Health Affairs*, *27*(3), 759–769. doi:10.1377/hlthaff.27.3.759 PMID:18474969

Coulter, A., & Dunn, N. (2002). After Bristol: putting patients at the centre. Commentary: Patient centered care: timely, but is it practical? *British Medical Journal*, *324*(7338), 648–651. doi:10.1136/bmj.324.7338.648 PMID:11895824

Coulter, A., & Ellins, J. (2007). Effectiveness of strategies for informing, educating, and involving patients. *BMJ: British Medical Journal*, *335*(7609), 24–27. doi:10.1136/bmj.39246.581169.80 PMID:17615222

Davis, R. E., Jacklin, R., Sevdalis, N., & Vincent, C. A. (2007). Patient involvement in patient safety: What factors influence patient participation and engagement. *Health Expectations*, *10*(3), 259–267. doi:10.1111/j.1369-7625.2007.00450.x PMID:17678514

Dearing, R. L., Barrick, C., Dermen, K. H., & Walitzer, K. S. (2005). Indicators of client engagement: Influences on alcohol treatment satisfaction and outcomes. *Psychology of Addictive Behaviors*, *19*(1), 71–78. doi:10.1037/0893-164X.19.1.71 PMID:15783280

Duke, C. C., Lynch, W. D., Smith, B., & Winstanley, J. (2015). Validity of a New Patient Engagement Measure: The Altarum Consumer Engagement (ACE) Measure™. *The Patient-Patient-Centered Outcomes Research*, *8*(6), 559–568. doi:10.1007/s40271-015-0131-2 PMID:26097010

Graffigna, G., Barello, S., Bonanomi, A., & Lozza, E. (2015a). Measuring patient engagement: Development and psychometric properties of the Patient Health Engagement (PHE) scale. *Frontiers in Psychology*, 2015, 6. PMID:25870566

Graffigna, G., Barello, S., Bonanomi, A., Lozza, E., & Hibbard, J. (2015b). Measuring patient activation in Italy: Translation, adaptation and validation of the Italian version of the patient activation measure 13 (PAM13-I). *BMC Medical Informatics and Decision Making*, *15*(1), 1. doi:10.1186/s12911-015-0232-9 PMID:26699852

Graffigna, G., Barello, S., Bonanomi, A., Menichetti, J. (in press). The Motivating Function of Healthcare Professional in eHealth and mHealth Interventions for Type 2 Diabetes Patients and the Mediating Role of Patient Engagement, *Journal of Diabetes Research*.

Graffigna, G., Barello, S., Libreri, C., & Bosio, C. A. (2014b). How to engage type-2 diabetic patients in their own health management: Implications for clinical practice. *BMC Public Health*, *14*(1), 648. doi:10.1186/1471-2458-14-648 PMID:24966036

Graffigna, G., Barello, S., Riva, G., & Bosio, A. C. (2014a). Patient Engagement: The Key to Redesign the Exchange Between the Demand and Supply for Healthcare in the Era of Active Ageing. *Active Ageing and Healthy Living: A Human Centered Approach in Research and Innovation as Source of Quality of Life, 203*, 85

Graffigna, G., Barello, S., & Triberti, S. (2015c). *Patient Engagement: A Consumer-Centered Model to Innovate Healthcare*. Berlin: DeGruyter Open. doi:10.1515/9783110452440

Greene, J., & Hibbard, J. H. (2012). Why does patient activation matter? An examination of the relationships between patient activation and health-related outcomes. *Journal of General Internal Medicine*, *27*(5), 520–526. doi:10.1007/s11606-011-1931-2 PMID:22127797

Gruman, J., Rovner, M. H., French, M. E., Jeffress, D., Sofaer, S., Shaller, D., & Prager, D. J. (2010). From patient education to patient engagement: Implications for the field of patient education. *Patient Education and Counseling*, *78*(3), 350–356. doi:10.1016/j.pec.2010.02.002 PMID:20202780

Hibbard, J. H. (2009). Using systematic measurement to target consumer activation strategies. *Medical Care Research and Review*, *66*(1 Suppl.), 9S–27S. doi:10.1177/1077558708326969 PMID:19052169

Hibbard, J. H., & Greene, J. (2013). What the evidence shows about patient activation: Better health outcomes and care experiences; fewer data on costs. *Health Affairs*, *32*(2), 207–214. doi:10.1377/hlthaff.2012.1061 PMID:23381511

Hibbard, J. H., Greene, J., & Overton, V. (2013). Patients with lower activation associated with higher costs; delivery systems should know their patients' scores. *Health Affairs*, *32*(2), 216–222. doi:10.1377/hlthaff.2012.1064 PMID:23381513

Hibbard, J. H., & Mahoney, E. (2010). Toward a theory of patient and consumer activation. *Patient Education and Counseling*, *78*(3), 377–381. doi:10.1016/j.pec.2009.12.015 PMID:20188505

Hibbard, J. H., Mahoney, E. R., Stock, R., & Tusler, M. (2007). Do Increases in Patient Activation Result in Improved Self-Management Behaviors? *Health Services Research*, *42*(4), 1443–1463. doi:10.1111/j.1475-6773.2006.00669.x PMID:17610432

Howie, J. G., Heaney, D. J., Maxwell, M., & Walker, J. J. (1998). A comparison of a Patient Enablement Instrument (PEI) against two established satisfaction scales as an outcome measure of primary care consultations. *Family Practice*, *15*(2), 165–171. doi:10.1093/fampra/15.2.165 PMID:9613486

Kodner, D. L., & Spreeuwenberg, C. (2002). Integrated care: Meaning, logic, applications, and implications–a discussion paper. *International Journal of Integrated Care*, 2002, 2. PMID:16896389

Légaré, F., & Witteman, H. O. (2013). Shared decision making: Examining key elements and barriers to adoption into routine clinical practice. *Health Affairs*, *32*(2), 276–284. doi:10.1377/hlthaff.2012.1078 PMID:23381520

Leventhal, H., Benyamini, Y., Brownlee, S., Diefenbach, M., Leventhal, E. A., Patrick-Miller, L., & Robitaille, C. (1997). Illness representations: theoretical foundations. In *Perceptions of health and illness* (Vol. 2, pp. 19-46).

Mahmud, S. (2004). Citizen participation in the health sector in rural Bangladesh: Perceptions and reality. *IDS Bulletin*, *35*(2), 11–18. doi:10.1111/j.1759-5436.2004.tb00116.x

McBride, T., & Korczak, V. (2007). Community consultation and engagement in healthcare reform. *Australian Health Review*, *31*(5), 13–15. doi:10.1071/AH070S13 PMID:17402899

Meglic, M., Furlan, M., Kuzmanic, M., Kozel, D., Baraga, D., Kuhar, I., & Brodnik, A. et al. (2010). Feasibility of an ehealth service to support collaborative depression care: Results of a pilot study. *Journal of Medical Internet Research*, *12*(5), e63. doi:10.2196/jmir.1510 PMID:21172765

Provenzi, L., Menichetti, J., Coin, R., & Aschieri, F. (2016). (in press). Psychological assessment as an intervention with couples: Single case application of collaborative techniques in clinical practice. *Professional Psychology*.

Rask, K. J., Ziemer, D. C., Kohler, S. A., Hawley, J. N., Arinde, F. J., & Barnes, C. S. (2009). Patient activation is associated with healthy behaviors and ease in managing diabetes in an indigent population. *The Diabetes Educator*, *35*(4), 622–630. doi:10.1177/0145721709335004 PMID:19419972

Skolasky, R. L., Mackenzie, E. J., Wegener, S. T., & Riley, L. H. III. (2008). Patient activation and adherence to physical therapy in persons undergoing spine surgery. *Spine*, *33*(21), E784–E791. doi:10.1097/BRS.0b013e31818027f1 PMID:18827683

Steverink, N., Lindenberg, S., & Slaets, J. P. J. (2005). How to understand and improve older people's self-management of wellbeing. *European Journal of Ageing*, *2*(4), 235–244. doi:10.1007/s10433-005-0012-y

Stewart, M. (2001). Towards a global definition of patient centered care: The patient should be the judge of patient centred care. *British Medical Journal*, *322*(7284), 444. doi:10.1136/bmj.322.7284.444 PMID:11222407

Street, R. L. Jr, Gordon, H. S., Ward, M. M., Krupat, E., & Kravitz, R. L. (2005). Patient participation in medical consultations: Why some patients are more involved than others. *Medical Care*, *43*(10), 960–969. doi:10.1097/01.mlr.0000178172.40344.70 PMID:16166865

KEY TERMS AND DEFINITIONS

Illness Experience: Disease refers to a specific clinical entity characterized by a disturbance in the structure or function of any part, organ, or system of the body. Illness is a broader concept that refers to any condition that a person views as sickness (Eisenberg, 1977). Leventhal and colleagues identified five dimensions of the illness experience: 1) identity of the illness – connecting the symptoms with the illness and having an understanding of the illness; 2) timeline – duration and progression of the illness; 3) causes – perceived reason for the illness; 4) consequences – what will be the physical, psychosocial and economic impact of the illness; 5) controllability – can the disease be controlled or cured?

Measuring Patient Experience: Ensuring that care is person-centered is one of six essential aims for achieving high-quality health care. The use of assessment measures to query patients about their experiences of health and healthcare management is the best and often only way to examine whether the experiences deemed essential for high-quality, person-centered care actually take place.

Patient Activation Measure: Developed by Hibbard and colleagues, the 13-item Patient Activation Measure is an interval-level, unidimensional Guttman-like measure that contains items measuring self-assessed knowledge about chronic conditions, beliefs about illness and medical care, and self-efficacy for self-care. The PAM focused on physical conditions, and it was designed to measure activation as a broad construct.

Patient Activation: Patient activation can be defined as the degree of patient baheviour as an active agent in the management of his/her own health including developmental stages: 1) believing the patient role is important, 2) having the confidence and knowledge necessary to take action, 3) actually taking action to maintain and improve one's health, and 4) staying the course even under stress.

Patient Engagement: Process-like and multidimensional experience, resulting from the conjoint cognitive (think), emotional (feel) and conative (act) enactment of individuals towards their health management. Patient engagement can be characterized by how much information flows between patient and provider, how active a role the patient has in care decisions, and how involved the patient or patient organization becomes in health organization decisions and in policy making.

Patient Health Engagement Scale: developed by Graffigna and colleagues, this is a measure of patient engagement that is grounded in rigorous conceptualization and appropriate psychometric methods. The scale consists of 5 ordinal items and was developed based on the authors' conceptual model of patient engagement (PHE model), which features four positions along a continuum of engagement (i.e., blackout; arousal; adhesion; eudaimonic project).

Patient Participation: Patient participation means to involve patients in the decision making process regarding health issues and also it is a strategy aimed at encouraging patients to participate in improving patient safety.

This work was previously published in Promoting Patient Engagement and Participation for Effective Healthcare Reform edited by Guendalina Graffigna, pages 192-214, copyright year 2016 by Medical Information Science Reference (an imprint of IGI Global).

Chapter 20
The Patient-Centered Medicine as the Theoretical Framework for Patient Engagement

Borghi Lidia
University of Milan, Italy

Galli Federica
University of Milan, Italy

Vegni Elena Anna Maria
University of Milan, Italy

ABSTRACT

The present contribution will describe the origin, development and main characteristics of the patient-centered medicine; the literature on patient-centeredness, in particular in the field of chronic disorders, will be discussed and the importance of this approach underlined; arguments about the importance of patient-centered medicine as theoretical frame founding and supporting the concept of patient engagement will be highlighted, considering that only within this medical epistemology the patient's engagement can find a full and complete expression.

INTRODUCTION

Engagement is a relatively new concept, as far as the healthcare system is concerned. Its application is very interesting and useful in a variety of different health contexts, not only in regard to patient care, such as the management of chronic diseases, but also as a possible concept at an organizational level. The issue of "patient engagement" is often linked to other concepts as those of patient activation, patient participation, patient's adherence, and patient empowerment. The term is frequently used to convey different meanings and a unique definition is missing. The aim of this chapter is to introduce a theoretical discussion of the concept connecting it, in a pure conceptual view, to the framework of patient-centered medicine (PCM). In our view, a fruitful and actual patient engagement may be better realized within

DOI: 10.4018/978-1-5225-1928-7.ch020

the theoretical framework of the PCM. It is difficult to conceive the engagement of a patient without considering the existence of at least two actors playing in a healthcare context, in a communicative and relational exchange. The importance of engaging patient and the ways to reach this involvement could not be seen out of the doctor-patient relationship. To support this view, we will describe the origin of PCM, its conceptual evolution, and the related practice in order to better involve patients in the management of their illness conditions. Patients are increasingly facing with multiple chronic disorders (comorbidity) and more and more aware of their rights; moreover an increased lay health literacy favor a more conscious public of people not passive but actively requiring to the health care system. This (r) evolution in the domain of care concerned all the western healthcare organizations all over the recent years, generating new issues both at the level of doctor-patient relationship and at organizational level (public health systems). We will discuss PCM and patient engagement in this modified environment. But, because the relations between doctor and patient is a core issue in the theoretical framework of PCM, the patient engagement may be reached in a relational view only assuming the PCM as a conceptual setting of the medical practice.

BACKGROUND

Patient centered medicine is above all a revolution in medicine, a method that changes the way of practicing medicine, the way in which physicians communicate and relate with their patients during medical consultations and the role that these two actors play within the visit. It originated and spread from North America and northern Europe during the 1970s.

This way of relating to a patient has its roots on the theoretical thinking of two British psychoanalysts Michael Balint and his wife Edin, who coined the term "patient-centered medicine" in 1969. Balint (1969) wrote "there is another way of medical thinking which we call 'patient-centered medicine'. Here, in addition to trying to discover a localizable illness or illnesses, the doctor also has to examine the whole person in order to form what we call an 'overall diagnosis'. This should include everything the doctor knows and understands about his patient; the patient, in fact, has to be understood as a unique human-being. The illness which can be described in terms of a 'traditional diagnosis' is either an incident like a broken leg, or a part like accident proneness which makes better sense if understood in terms of the whole" (Balint, 1969).

Balint, as a psychoanalyst, described a form of psycho-therapeutic intervention that general practitioners could use for people who had disorders that were partially or wholly psychosomatic; but the revolution in her thoughts and words went beyond: a new way of understanding the complaints reported by the patients, not in terms of pathology, but in terms of the unique individuality of the patient was described (Balint, 1957). In this sense, the new concept contrasted with the "doctor-centered care", by allowing patients more control of the medical visit, and from "disease-centered care", by focusing not only on the disease but also on the patient who suffers (Bensing, 2000).

The development of this method should be viewed in light of a revolution in the model of medicine, an epistemological change shifting the science of medicine from a biological reductionist approach - the biomedical model - to a bio-psychosocial point of view. This shift was theorized by the American psychiatrist George L. Engel, who in 1977 posited a new epistemological paradigm expanding the biomedical model. The bio-psychosocial perspective (Engel, 1977, 1981) constitutes the theoretical frame of patient-centered medicine, presenting it as a broadening of the scope of medicine from organic disease, focused on diagnosis and treatment, to also encompass the patient's experience of disease. In the bio-psychosocial model (Engel, 1977, 1981), disorders are conceptualized as existing at a number of interacting, hierarchical levels (from biological to psychological and social levels). According to this point of view, every patient has a story that demonstrates the interactions among the biologic, psychological, and social components of his or her life.

Engel (1977) wrote that the bio-psychosocial model would "take into account the patient, the social context in which he lives, and the complementary system devised by society to deal with the disruptive effects of illness".

These changes in the medical epistemology have significant impacts on the clinical method with a shifting from disease-centered to patient-centered perspective.

The disease-centered method has been, so far, the dominant model in medical practice; as previously stated, it is based on the biomedical paradigm in which patients' reports of their medical conditions are read as the expression of disease processes and the clinical method focuses on identifying standard disease entities and numeric entities, and on this basis proposes an evidence based therapeutic treatment. This clinical method has several strengths according to McWhinney (1989, 1993): it is simple, clear, verifiable and allows not only formulation of diagnostic hypotheses but, as the disease is the effect of a cause that is biologically identifiable and given the constancy of the cause-effect relations, also allows clinicians to identify a prognosis. Nevertheless, in the past few years, it has been criticized for oversimplifying the problems of illness, assuming that disease is fully accounted for by deviations from the norm of measurable biological variables and not taking into account the patient's perspective.

Development of the concept of patient-centeredness is closely linked to these perceived limitations in the disease-centered method of practicing medicine. As we have discussed above, patient-centered medicine gives clinicians a more complex goal to achieve during the process of caring for the patient.

The complexity is the result of various factors. First, it considers the patient as a unique person with his/her own experience of the disease and with an active role in the care process; it integrates the traditional understanding of disease with each patient's point of view on his condition, moving from TO CURE the disease centered medicine TO CARE. As Kleinman (1989) stated, beyond the dimension of the "disease", intended as the doctor's understanding of the biomedical disorders, there is the "illness", that refers to the patient's subjective experience of feeling sick. Patient-centered medicine deals with the non-biological aspects of the disease: even personal, psychological and social aspects are recognized as current and important, so that the tasks of the consultation are focusing not only on disease but also on the "patient agenda", his/her personal illness experience, which may be broken down into four main factors (his/her feelings, his/her ideas about the illness, the impact of his/her problems on his life, his/her expectations about what should be done and his desires) (Moja & Vegni, 2000).

Secondly, the patient-centered method suggests that communication and relational skills and techniques are a core professional competence to be used by clinicians; for example, interviewing skills and communication techniques are proposed in order to achieve the comprehension of the patient's agenda, e.g. attentive listening, open questions, paraphrasing and asking for understanding.

Thirdly, it also takes into account the perspective of the physician with the own emotional experience.

These concepts outline that the main differences between the two clinical methods are played out in the context of the doctor-patient relationship, where the content and style of the relationship is defined as "an abstraction embodying the activities of two interacting systems (persons)" (Szasz & Hollender, 1956). The relationship between doctor and patient is no longer a means to make a diagnosis, but it becomes the aim of the medicine itself. The relationship is recognized as part of a process where the patient is the protagonist, the only true expert of his own health.

So it can be said that a clinical consultation that is patient-centered elicits and explores patients' expectations, feelings, and illness beliefs, and tries to activate the patient to take some control in the medical visit (Platt et al., 2001).

The patient-centered perspective promotes changes not only in the field of the clinical practice, but also, in the fields of education and research. In particular, new modes of teaching and learning, e.g., the use of role-playing and videotaping, are proposed as tools necessary for real understanding of the importance of doctor-patient communications and relationships. In the field of research, and in particular in the outcome of research, the evaluation of the results of health interventions in clinical practice, patient-centered medicine has been the basis of various studies quantifying the state of health, not only through clinical outcomes but also through measurements of outcomes reported by the patient - the so-called patient-reported outcomes. Ample literature has found associations between the patient-centered model of communication and patient satisfaction (Kinmonth, Woodcock, Griffin, Spiegal, & Campbell, 1998; Kinnersley, Stott, Peters, & Harvey, 1999; Rosenberg, Lussier, & Beaudoin, 1997; Williams, Weinman, & Dale, 1998; McMillan et al., 2013; Rathert, Wyrwich, & Boren, 2012), treatment adherence (Rosenberg et al., 1997; Safran et al., 1998; Street, Makoul, Arora, & Epstein, 2009), medical outcomes (Arora, 2003; Kaplan, Greenfield, & Ware, 1989; Maisiak, Austin, West, & Heck, 1996; Rao, Weinberger, & Kroenke, 2000; Rosenberg et al., 1997; Robinson, Callister, Berry, & Dearing, 2008; Ekman et al., 2012) and decreased rates of malpractice claims (Levinson, Roter, Mullooly, Dull, & Frankel, 1997). Furthermore, clinician failure to elicit and discuss patient expectations predicts dissatisfaction with the visit and the persistence of symptoms (Jackson, Kroenke, & Chamberlin, 1999; Kravitz, Callahan, Azari, Antonius, & Lewis, 1997).

A synthetic overview of this long and ongoing process may be that PCM grounds on the biopsychosocial context, and lies on the exploration of the so-called patient's agenda (the interplay of ideas and interpretations, expectations and desires, feelings and personal context the patient brings with him/her during the medical encounter) by the mean of specific communication techniques (Moja & Vegni, 2001). The achievement of such professional skills between doctor and patient is the outcome of structured educational/academic interventions. Academic curriculum or post-graduate education should be planned taking into consideration such a goal (Street & de Haes, 2013). Unfortunately, the Italian context is not representative of a widespread and common training on communication skills for health professionals (with some rare exception), while in English speaking countries this issue is widely addressed (e.g., Fortin, Dwamena, Frankel, & Smith, 2012; Stewart et al., 2003). Within this scenario, the contribution to the spread of patient-centered medicine has been led by the new challenges the healthcare system has to face and the new outcomes the medicine has to deal with.

CHRONICITY AND MULTIMORBIDITY: NEW CHALLENGES FOR MEDICINE

Besides cultural and epistemological changes, there are other important factors and contemporary forces that have bolstered the shift towards the origin of the patient-centered method within the wider biopsychosocial paradigm transformation. The growing demands for quality and safety in health care have refocused attention on patient outcomes. Moreover, the shift stems from the attempt to cut health care costs and is expressed in particular in the field of general practice. For example, in the United States, serious concerns about the excessive price of medical care have resulted in consideration of whether shifting care from the subspecialist to the primary care physician could reduce costs (Bardes, 2012). Last but not least, and probably most interesting as far as this contribution is concerned, the increase in prevalence and incidence of chronic disease, as well as the increase of the aging population, played a crucial role in the need for a new medical model.

Chronic conditions are defined as illnesses that last longer than three months and are not self-limiting. Common examples of chronic conditions are diabetes, asthma, congestive heart failure, stroke, low back pain and arthritis. Most of these diseases have major physical, psychological, social and financial consequences and impact the lives of individuals and their families in many ways. From the societal perspective, chronic diseases are a major source of health care utilization (Vlieland, 2002). At a younger age, chronic conditions are increasing also as consequence of the development of specialized pediatric intensive care unit care (PICU). On one hand, PICU contributed to the improved survival rates for critically ill children, but on the other historical data suggest that pediatric critical care may have exchanged mortality for morbidity over the last several decades, with a prevalence of new morbidity that is 4.8%, twice the mortality rate (Pollack et al., 2014). In the most cases, the transition from childhood/adolescent care to adult care is guaranteed.

In all developed countries, chronic conditions are spreading as consequence of the increase of the aging population (Beaglehole et al., 2008; Wiederhold, Riva, & Graffigna, 2013). On adults, data from US report that nearly half of the adult population is affected from chronic conditions with one-fourth of all adults have multiple (2 or more) chronic conditions (Ward, 2013). In the US population, studies projecting the prevalence of chronic conditions in upcoming years estimate an increase of diabetes by more than 80 percent, of Parkinson's disease by 30 percent and Alzheimer is projected to increase by 40 percent. The National Cancer Institute projects that by 2020 there will 30 percent cancer survivors more than in 2010 (Dall et al., 2013).

A chronic medical condition is often comorbid with other medical and/or psychopathological disorder(s): it has been demonstrated that over 50% of depressed patients show multiple chronic medical conditions as well (Wells, Rogers, Burnam, Greenfield, & Ware Jr, 1991), with additional consequences for health care services and primary care providers for costs, treatment planning and outcome. Multi-morbidity has been defined as the "most common chronic condition", and its prevalence progressively increases with age, affecting more than 60% of people aged 65 or older (Barnett et al., 2013).

These conditions result in numerous adverse health outcomes, increased health care needs, and subsequently higher medical costs. These patients are more likely to be admitted to hospital, have poorer quality of life, and receive multiple drugs with consequent difficulties in adherence (Marengoni et al., 2011). In the past, strategies have focused on preventing and ameliorating a single disease at a time; however, the large percentage of people with two or more conditions, or multiple chronic conditions, has added a level of complexity to developing intervention strategies. Moreover, the presence of physical and mental multi-morbidity also significantly impacts the costs of health care, with estimates of increasing costs by at least 45% for each person with a chronic physical disease and a co-morbid mental health problem (Naylor et al., 2012).

Patients with multi-morbidity have the most complex health needs, but due to the traditional disease-oriented approach in healthcare, they risk facing highly fragmented care that may lead to partial, ineffective, and potentially inadequate interventions.

As illustrated above, health care systems around the world have been worldwide modeled around the epistemology of the disease model. This presumes a series of assumptions such as: organ or system-based pathology cause disease, symptoms are "caused" by the underlying disease, the treatment is focused on removing the underlying cause of pathology and it is identical for everyone. The patient is simply the holder of the disease, which is the same for everyone. The doctor is the only holder of the medical knowledge to be transmitted to the patient, in a hierarchical way. This approach to disease fails to detect differences in patients' needs, does not take into account patient expectations, beliefs, impact on function, quality of life and his/her relational and inner world. The traditional disease-oriented approach does not take into account the overall health status of patients with multi-morbidity, since it is focused on a single disease and neglecting fundamental aspects of health, like frailty and functional ability as well as cognitive and affective state.

It is immediately clear how chronic diseases are extremely complex and how they can be better understood within a bio-psychosocial perspective, and therefore, that the most suitable clinical method to approach chronic disease is the patient-centered method. In this complex context new approaches to improve care are needed, with the aim to diminish suffering of patients, improving their quality of life and satisfaction of the clinicians, and the concept of engagement seems to be particularly promising in this model.

DRAWING THE ROADMAP TOWARDS PATIENT ENGAGEMENT, PATIENT-CENTRED MEDICINE AND CHRONIC DISEASE

We know that the patient-centred approach is built on several premises such as the fact that patients often do not seek healthcare only because a symptom, that usually bring more than one concern to their clinicians, that empathic communication allows patients to experience the clinician's compassionate presence (Fortin et al., 2012). Setting up the clinical interview in a way attuned with the emotional and personal status of the patient is the *sine qua non* of the patient-centred approach, the fast track in the direction of patient engagement. This is exceedingly true in the case of chronic disorders (Eaton, Roberts, & Turner, 2015), when the patient is usually older and forced to cope with multiple disabling conditions.

The increase of chronic disease and multi-morbidity poses new questions and challenges to the traditional health system and doctor-patient relationship. Complexity of care in patients with multimorbidity requires the involvement of a large number of healthcare providers and resources. Rethinking the doctor-patient relationship based on the traditional disease-centered model by shifting to a patient-centered model may be the common ground for promoting new methods for care management. The Picker Institute (Gerteis, Edgman-Levitan, Daley, & Delbanco, 1993) in partnership with patients and families, conducted a multiyear research project and identified eight characteristics of care as the most important indicators of quality and safety, from the patients' perspective: respect for the patient's values, preferences, and expressed needs; coordinated and integrated care; clear, high-quality information and education for the patient and family; physical comfort, including pain management; emotional support and alleviation of fear and anxiety; involvement of family members and friends, as appropriate; continuity, including through care-site transitions; and access to care. Care that achieves these goals is deemed to be patient-centered (Mead & Bower, 2000).

We consider the patient-centredness as "the" method to be used in each doctor-patient encounter, the essential tool in the hands of the health professionals towards a fruitful PE, mostly in the case of chronic disorders. De Haes (2006) brilliantly evidenced some different meanings and conceptual background of the PCM, outlining the importance of tailoring care according to patient's peculiarities. Communication in the medical encounter has several functions: building relationships, information gathering, information provision, making decisions, responding to emotions, managing uncertainty and last, but not least, enabling patient self-management (Moja & Vegni, 2000; Street & De Haes, 2013). We wonder if it might be useful to tailor PCM interventions bearing in mind some characteristics of the patients' adjustment to the illness course towards a better PE.

As we pointed out, there is no shared consensus on the definition of patient engagement, but the general consensus is that it is related to the importance of taking an active role in one's health, having knowledge, skills, and confidence to manage health/chronic conditions and performing health-promoting behaviors. The term "engagement" is also used in very different contexts as marketing and consumer behavior literature to describe the attitude of a consumer toward a brand, product, service, or even media event (Gambetti & Graffigna, 2010).The adoption of the term engagement in the healthcare field is recent and indicates a renewed partnership between patient and healthcare professional involved in the health and care management (Hibbard, Stockard, Mahoney, & Tusler, 2004; Coulter, 2012).

The difficulties in the definition of PE are related to the existence of several constructs having indefinite boundaries or handled interchangeably because not having (often) a clear-cut definition: shared decision making, patient participation, involvement, empowerment or activation, self-management, compliance or adherence are examples of constructs linked to PE, but not exhaustive of the meaning we confer to PE. We agree with Graffigna, Barello and Triberti (2015b) that PE is an umbrella concept encompassing all the previous definitions, without replacing them (Barello & Graffigna, 2015).

The role of patient engagement in chronic disease care is increasingly being cited as critical for improving health outcomes and reducing costs. A recent review of the literature on chronic diseases and patient engagement (Simmons, Wolever, Bechard, & Snyderman, 2014) supported the link between improved outcomes and patient engagement, demonstrating that relatively short interventions can increase and promote positive health outcomes. Moreover, specific behavioral targets and their tracking appear essential to assess the role of patient engagement over time to achieve positive health outcomes. In contrast, poor patient engagement is a risk factor for worse chronic disease outcomes. In this framework, early identification of individuals who are low in patient engagement coupled with tailored behavioral interventions to enhance participation may provide a reasonable and low cost target for personalized health care innovation (Simmons et al., 2014). In other words, the adjustment of a patient to changed health conditions is a long and complex psychological process where the personality, the age, the familial, social and cultural context of life of *that* patient play a critical role.

Graffigna et al. (2015b) described patient engagement as the final outcome of a long process encompassing emotional, cognitive, and behavioral reframing of the patient's health condition (PHE model), where the success of each phase depends on the success of the previous one. In the last phase of the model the patients successfully reframed the pathological condition, incorporating it into their life projects, where they are no longer overwhelmed by their health conditions. By our perspective, it is difficult to think that the engagement of the patient can be realised without passing through an empathic dyadic exchange realised in healthcare contexts, without a sound patient-doctor alliance, and overlooking the building of a trustworthy relationship. The patient-centred medicine may be seen as characterised by two main streams (Liberati et al., 2015): the first one is *dyadic* and pertains to the more traditional stream belonging to the approach having as main objective the exploration both of patient's objective disease and symptoms and their subjective illness experience (patient's agenda). The second one is *organizational* and is addressed to identify organizational and system-level facilitators of and barriers to PCC. Both could be an interesting and valuable frames within which to conceptualize the patient engagement. But, to address our main aim in this contribution, the conceptual grounding of patient engagement in the context of a patient-centredness medicine, we focus on the dyadic, relational view of PCM exploring its fundamental role to reach a fruitful and real engagement of the patient.

The Patient Health Engagement (PHM) model (Graffigna et al., 2015b) suggests that the patients steadily get over changes in their health condition through the so-called "patient journey". It means that the patient adjusts to a changed health condition through a process articulated in four steps characterised by specific emotional, behavioural and cognitive factors. The first one is the "Black out": the patient in this stage appears overwhelmed by the illness experience, blocked and with a passive attitude toward the healthcare system (e.g., it might be preferred a paternalistic approach by the physician). In the second step, the patient is in "Arousal": it means to be "hyper-attentive" to every signal in their body, but also to be better informed about their health condition, even though in a superficial manner and in a way that does not allow the self-management of their disease and treatment. The third step is the "Adhesion": the patient acquires a broader spectrum of behavioural skills to cope with their illness, starting to perceive the importance of their role. The final step is the "Eudaimonic project": the patients fully accept their condition, are no more overwhelmed by illness and are prone to become "partner" with the healthcare system in managing the changed health condition.

Health professionals should always bear in mind the existence of a process of psychological modification and adaptation to changed health conditions, and PE might be better realised if grounded on the different steps of this process on the basis of PCM framework, considering 1) The other (the patient) as a necessary subject of information regarding the personal and changing perspective about being ill; 2) The necessary relational and communication skills tailored on the basis of the patient journey; and 3) Taking into account the relevance of the physician's inner experience of being with a patient who will never recover. A possible challenge in the connection between the patient engagement journey and the patient centred medicine may be that of conceptualizing a specific way of interacting with the patient (goal to reach, communication skills to use, personal reaction of the doctor) during each stage of the journey as it has been done as far as the concept of process of patient education with his/her motivational levels and readiness to act (Prochaska & Di Clemente, 1982; Grüninger, 1995). In each critical point of the patient engagement during a chronic illness the principles of PCM could represent a guide for the physician's work with patients. Communication skills are the principal way in the direction of decoding and labelling the psychological state of *that* patient in *that* clinical situation. Communication skills may be taught, learnt and practised, and most of all may aid the identification of the stage the patient is experiencing and his/her agenda to tailor every exchange we have with the specific characteristics of *that* patient, always in the direction of PE. If the patient is allocated in the "black-out" stage any attempt towards active engagement may result ineffectual. In that stage, the patient seems to be overwhelmed by emotions: it is not the time for acting, planning, giving statistics. It is the time to dedicate a lot of effort to empathic reflection, stating partnership, legitimating and respectful support. We have to wait the awkward transition to the "Arousal" stage to broaden the repertoire of communicative skills and techniques: tactful questioning skills (we recommend in this stage open questions), facilitation and active listening, eliciting patients view of the problem, surveying the field may be very useful in this stage to accompany the patient to shift from passive to active role in the coping with illness. With the transition to "Adhesion" the patients are gradually more aware of the primary role to undertake in coping with illness: it may be especially helpful negotiating priorities, focusing and more directive comments. Once it has been reached the final stage of the "Eudaimonic project" probing, challenging, checking back and summarizing have to be used to strengthen the active role of the patients and their complete and informed engagement. The connection between PCM and PE seems to be a promising practical way to discover, giving achievable goals in the doctor-patient relations and interesting challenges for clinical and experimental research.

SOLUTIONS, RECOMMENDATIONS AND FUTURE DIRECTIONS

Facing the new challenges that are arising in health care, such as the spread of chronic disease, aging population, the need of reducing health care costs, and looking at the possible answers as the health resource optimization and the spread of good health practice, the concept of patient engagement may be a keystone.

Achieving effective patient engagement could reduce health care costs in the sense that patients would decrease the demand for check-ups or general practitioner consultations, or the phenomenon of doctor shopping because of being better able to manage their own disease and treatment and to implement good health practices.

In this context, the promotion of patient activation and satisfaction, treatment adherence, and medical outcomes are critical issues, in particular when dealing with chronically ill patients, and are concepts intimately related to patient engagement, that we consider an umbrella concept encompassing several meanings and objectives that may be reached through the aid of PCM.

Nevertheless, in the opinion of the authors, all of these concepts remain "orphan" without the conceptual framework of patient-centered medicine, that means *in primis* tailored care accordingly to the exploration of the patient's agenda by specific communication techniques. Only within a patient-centered method of care a fruitful engagement can be fully realized. Patient-centered medicine entails a shifting by the classical outcomes (e.g. adherence, patient satisfaction) to new ones, such as promoting an active role of the patients in their healthcare or evaluating patient engagement, to allow a real full share-decision making and to facilitate health literacy. Helping patients to be more active in medical consultations change centuries of physician-dominated dialogues to dialogues that engage patients as active participants. This change has become possible thanks to the epistemological, clinical and methodological revolution brought in by patient-centered medicine. In regards to the health system, the adoption of a patient-centered care entails a review of the educational system in healthcare to achieve a patient-centered working method. Patient-centered methods of care could be taught in the context of structured training programs.

Lines of research for the future should go in the direction of measuring patient engagement after the fulfillment of patient-centered interventions. It opens to several lines of research considering all the different constructs PE is made, the steps the patients experience in the adjustment process to chronic illness and the different instruments the PCM makes available to health professionals. To the best of our knowledge, no study has been conducted that correlates measurements of patient engagement, such as the Patient Activation Measure (PAM) (Hibbard et al., 2004) or the Patient Health Engagement (PHE) (that is the first instrument specifically aimed to measure engagement) (Graffigna, Barello, Bonanomi, & Lozza, 2015a), with classic measures of patient-centeredness, like the Roter Interaction Analysis System (RIAS) (Roter, 1991; Roter & Larson, 2002) or the Patient Centred Score Sheet (PCSS) (Henbest

& Stewart, 1989). If patient engagement will found to be directly associated with measures of patient-centeredness, it could be supported the authors' hypothesis of considering PE as a new goal for PCM.

Another important field for future research, in a framework shifting from and individual to a familiar and societal context, is to consider what means to engage a third party in the care process and how this may be inserted in a patient-centered visit. In particular conditions, as the frail elderly, diseases that severely limit individual capacity and autonomy (e.g., dementia), and pediatric conditions, the role of the third party becomes more and more crucial: in these particular conditions engaging the caregivers in the patients' journey is a new challenge and try to achieve this goal within a patient-centered clinical consultation seems to be not enough: consultations should become also caregiver-centered and familiar-centered in a wider, social perspective.

CONCLUSION

If PE represents a new goal for the medicine, the PCM may be considered an epistemological framework towards this objective. The public healthcare system may benefit in terms of reduction of costs: engaged patients in a patient-centered perspective are more satisfied, more compliant, less prone to instigate legal action in case of medical error, more engaged in their social context, and so on. New lines of research entails the measurement of PE and PCM, and the promotion of good health practices in the framework of patient-centered consultations, assessing the impact on outcomes, both in clinical, patient-reported and social terms.

REFERENCES

Arora, N. K. (2003). Interacting with cancer patients: The significance of physicians' communication behavior. *Social Science & Medicine*, *57*(5), 791–806. doi:10.1016/S0277-9536(02)00449-5 PMID:12850107

Balint, E. (1969). The possibilities of patient-centred medicine. *The British Journal of General Practice*, *17*(82), 269–276. PMID:5770926

Balint, M. (1957). *The doctor, his patient and the illness*. London: Tavistock Publications.

Bardes, C. L. (2012). Defining "patient-centered medicine". *The New England Journal of Medicine*, *366*(9), 782–783. doi:10.1056/NEJMp1200070 PMID:22375968

Barello, S., & Graffigna, G. (2015). Patient engagement in healthcare: Pathways for effective medical decision making. *Neuropsychological Trends*, *17*(1), 53–65. doi:10.7358/neur-2015-017-bare

Barnett, K., Mercer, S. W., Norbury, M., Watt, G., Wyke, S., & Guthrie, B. (2012). Epidemiology of multimorbidity and implications for health care, research, and medical education: A cross-sectional study. *Lancet*, *380*(9836), 37–43. doi:10.1016/S0140-6736(12)60240-2 PMID:22579043

Beaglehole, R., Epping-Jordan, J., Patel, V., Chopra, M., Ebrahim, S., Kidd, M., & Haines, A. (2008). Improving the prevention and management of chronic disease in low-income and middle-income countries: A priority for primary health care. *Lancet*, *372*(9642), 940–949. doi:10.1016/S0140-6736(08)61404-X PMID:18790317

Bensing, J. (2000). Bridging the gap.: The separate worlds of evidence-based medicine and patient-centered medicine. *Patient Education and Counseling*, *39*(1), 17–25. doi:10.1016/S0738-3991(99)00087-7 PMID:11013544

Coulter, A. (2012). Patient engagement—what works? *The Journal of Ambulatory Care Management*, *35*(2), 80–89. doi:10.1097/JAC.0b013e318249e0fd PMID:22415281

Dall, T. M., Gallo, P. D., Chakrabarti, R., West, T., Semilla, A. P., & Storm, M. V. (2013). An aging population and growing disease burden will require a large and specialized health care workforce by 2025. *Health Affairs*, *32*(11), 2013–2020. doi:10.1377/hlthaff.2013.0714 PMID:24191094

De Haes, H. (2006). Dilemmas in patient centerdness and shared decision making: A case for vulnerability. *Patient Education and Counseling*, *62*(3), 291–298. doi:10.1016/j.pec.2006.06.012 PMID:16859860

Eaton, S., Roberts, S., & Turner, B. (2015). Delivering person centred care in long term conditions. *British Medical Journal*, *350*(feb10 14), 181. doi:10.1136/bmj.h181 PMID:25670186

Ekman, I., Wolf, A., Olsson, L. E., Taft, C., Dudas, K., Schaufelberger, M., & Swedberg, K. (2012). Effects of person-centred care in patients with chronic heart failure: The PCC-HF study. *European Heart Journal*, *33*(9), 1112–1119. doi:10.1093/eurheartj/ehr306 PMID:21926072

Engel, G. L. (1977). The need for a new medical model: A challenge for biomedicine. *Science*, *196*(4286), 129–136. doi:10.1126/science.847460 PMID:847460

Engel, G. L. (1981). The clinical application of the biopsychosocial model. *The Journal of Medicine and Philosophy*, *6*(2), 101–124. doi:10.1093/jmp/6.2.101 PMID:7264472

Fortin, A. H., Dwamena, F. C., Frankel, R. M., & Smith, R. C. (2012). *Smith's Patient Centered Interviewing: An Evidence-Based Method: An Evidence-Based Method*. McGraw Hill Professional.

Gambetti, R. C., & Graffigna, G. (2010). The concept of engagement: A systematic analysis of the ongoing marketing debate. *International Journal of Market Research*, *52*(6), 7. doi:10.2501/S147078531020166

Gerteis, M., Edgman-Levitan, S., Daley, J., & Delbanco, T. (1993). *Through the patient's eyes: Understanding and Promoting Patient-Centered Care Paperback*. San Francisco: Jossey-Bass.

Graffigna, G., Barello, S., Bonanomi, A., & Lozza, E. (2015a). Measuring patient engagement: Development and psychometric properties of the patient health engagement (PHE) scale. *Frontiers in Psychology*, 2015, 6. PMID:25870566

Graffigna, G., Barello, S., & Triberti, S. (2015b). *Patient engagement: a consumer-centered model to innovate healthcare*. Warsaw, Poland: DeGruyter Open. doi:10.1515/9783110452440

Grüninger, U. J. (1995). Patient education: An example of one-to-one communication. *Journal of Human Hypertension*, *9*(1), 15–25. PMID:7730996

Henbest, R. J., & Stewart, M. A. (1989). Patient-centredness in the consultation. 1: A method for measurement. *Family Practice*, *6*(4), 249–253. doi:10.1093/fampra/6.4.249 PMID:2632300

Hibbard, J. H., Stockard, J., Mahoney, E. R., & Tusler, M. (2004). Development of the Patient Activation Measure (PAM): Conceptualizing and measuring activation in patients and consumers. *Health Services Research*, *39*(4p14 Part 1), 1005–1026. doi:10.1111/j.1475-6773.2004.00269.x PMID:15230939

Jackson, J. L., Kroenke, K., & Chamberlin, J. (1999). Effects of physician awareness of symptom-related expectations and mental disorders: A controlled trial. *Archives of Family Medicine*, *8*(2), 135–142. doi:10.1001/archfami.8.2.135 PMID:10101984

Kaplan, S. H., Greenfield, S., & Ware, J. E. Jr. (1989). Assessing the effects of physician-patient interactions on the outcomes of chronic disease. *Medical Care*, *27*(3 Suppl.), S110–S127. doi:10.1097/00005650-198903001-00010 PMID:2646486

Kinmonth, A. L., Woodcock, A., Griffin, S., Spiegal, N., & Campbell, M. J. (1998). Randomised controlled trial of patient centred care of diabetes in general practice: Impact on current wellbeing and future disease risk. *British Medical Journal*, *317*(7167), 1202–1208. doi:10.1136/bmj.317.7167.1202 PMID:9794859

Kinnersley, P., Stott, N., Peters, T. J., & Harvey, I. (1999). The patient-centredness of consultations and outcome in primary care. *The British Journal of General Practice*, *49*(446), 711–716. PMID:10756612

Kleinman, A. (1989). *The illness narratives: suffering, healing, and the human condition*. New York: Basic Books.

Kravitz, R. L., Callahan, E. J., Azari, R., Antonius, D., & Lewis, C. E. (1997). Assessing patients' expectations in ambulatory medical practice. *Journal of General Internal Medicine*, *12*(1), 67–72. doi:10.1007/s11606-006-0010-6 PMID:9034949

Levinson, W., Roter, D. L., Mullooly, J. P., Dull, V. T., & Frankel, R. M. (1997). Physician-patient communication: The relationship with malpractice claims among primary care physicians and surgeons. *Journal of the American Medical Association*, *277*(7), 553–559. doi:10.1001/jama.1997.03540310051034 PMID:9032162

Liberati, E. G., Gorli, M., Moja, L., Galuppo, L., Ripamonti, S., & Scaratti, G. (2015). Exploring the practice of patient centered care: The role of ethnography and reflexivity. *Social Science & Medicine*, *133*, 45–52. doi:10.1016/j.socscimed.2015.03.050 PMID:25841094

Maisiak, R., Austin, J., West, S., & Heck, L. (1996). The effect of person-centered counseling on the psychological status of persons with systemic lupus erythematosus or rheumatoid arthritis. A randomized, controlled trial. *Arthritis and Rheumatism*, *9*(1), 60–66. doi:10.1002/art.1790090111 PMID:8945114

Marengoni, A., Angleman, S., Melis, R., Mangialasche, F., Karp, A., Garmen, A., & Fratiglioni, L. et al. (2011). Aging with multimorbidity: A systematic review of the literature. *Ageing Research Reviews*, *10*(4), 430–439. doi:10.1016/j.arr.2011.03.003 PMID:21402176

McMillan, S. S., Kendall, E., Sav, A., King, M. A., Whitty, J. A., Kelly, F., & Wheeler, A. J. (2013). Patient-centered approaches to health care: A systematic review of randomized controlled trials. *Medical Care Research and Review*, *70*(6), 567–596. doi:10.1177/1077558713496318 PMID:23894060

McWhinney, I. (1989). The need for a transformed clinical method. In M. Stewart & D. Roter (Eds.), *Communicating with medical patients*. London: Sage.

McWhinney, I. (1993). Why we need a new clinical method. *Scandinavian Journal of Primary Health Care, 11*(1), 3–7. doi:10.3109/02813439308994894 PMID:8484077

Mead, N., & Bower, P. (2000). Patient-centredness: A conceptual framework and review of the empirical literature. *Social Science & Medicine, 51*(7), 1087–1110. doi:10.1016/S0277-9536(00)00098-8 PMID:11005395

Moja, E. A., & Vegni, E. (2000). *La visita medica centrata sul paziente*. Milano: Cortina Editore.

Naylor, C., Parsonage, M., McDaid, D., Knapp, M., Fossey, M., & Galea, A. (2012). *Long-term conditions and mental health: the cost of co-morbidities*. London: The King's Fund and Centre for Mental Health.

Platt, F. W., Gaspar, D. L., Coulehan, J. L., Fox, L., Adler, A. J., & Weston, W. W. et al.. (2001). "Tell me about yourself": The patient-centered interview. *Annals of Internal Medicine, 134*(11), 1079–1085. doi:10.7326/0003-4819-134-11-200106050-00020 PMID:11388827

Pollack, M. M., Holubkov, R., Funai, T., Clark, A., Berger, J. T., Meert, K., & Jenkins, T. L. et al. (2014). Pediatric Intensive Care Outcomes: Development of New Morbidities During Pediatric Critical Care. *Pediatric Critical Care Medicine, 15*(9), 821–827. doi:10.1097/PCC.0000000000000250 PMID:25226501

Prochaska, J. O., & Di Clemente, C. C. (1982). Transtheoretical therapy: Toward a more integrative model of change. *Psychotherapy (Chicago, Ill.), 19*(3), 276–288. doi:10.1037/h0088437

Rao, J. K., Weinberger, M., & Kroenke, K. (2000). Visit-specific expectations and patient-centered outcomes: A literature review. *Archives of Family Medicine, 9*(10), 1148–1155. doi:10.1001/archfami.9.10.1148 PMID:11115222

Rathert, C., Wyrwich, M. D., & Boren, S. A. (2013). Patient-Centered Care and Outcomes A Systematic Review of the Literature. *Medical Care Research and Review, 70*(4), 351–379. doi:10.1177/1077558712465774 PMID:23169897

Robinson, J. H., Callister, L. C., Berry, J. A., & Dearing, K. A. (2008). Patient-centered care and adherence: Definitions and applications to improve outcomes. *Journal of the American Academy of Nurse Practitioners, 20*(12), 600–607. doi:10.1111/j.1745-7599.2008.00360.x PMID:19120591

Rosenberg, E. E., Lussier, M. T., & Beaudoin, C. (1997). Lessons for clinicians from physician-patient communication literature. *Archives of Family Medicine, 6*(3), 279–283. doi:10.1001/archfami.6.3.279 PMID:9161356

Roter, D., & Larson, S. (2002). The Roter interaction analysis system (RIAS): Utility and flexibility for analysis of medical interactions. *Patient Education and Counseling, 46*(4), 243–251. doi:10.1016/S0738-3991(02)00012-5 PMID:11932123

Roter, D. L. (1991). *Roter Interaction Analysis System: Coding Manual*. Baltimore, USA: Johns Hopkins University.

Safran, D. G., Taira, D. A., Rogers, W. H., Kosinski, M., Ware, J. E., & Tarlov, A. R. (1998). Linking primary care performance to outcomes of care. *The Journal of Family Practice, 47*(3), 213–220. PMID:9752374

Simmons, L. A., Wolever, R. Q., Bechard, E. M., & Snyderman, R. (2014). Patient engagement as a risk factor in personalized health care: A systematic review of the literature on chronic disease. *Genome Medicine*, *6*(2), 16. doi:10.1186/gm533 PMID:24571651

Stewart, M., Brown, J. B., & Weston, W. W., NcWhinney, I. R., McWilliam, C.L., & Freeman, T.R. (2003). Patient-centered medicine-Transforming the clinical method. Bristol, UK: Radcliffe medical Press.

Street, R. L. Jr, & De Haes, H. (2013). Designing a curriculum for communication skills training from a theory and evidence-based perspective. *Patient Education and Counseling*, *93*(1), 27–33. doi:10.1016/j.pec.2013.06.012 PMID:23890580

Street, R. L. Jr, Makoul, G., Arora, N. K., & Epstein, R. M. (2009). How does communication heal? Pathways linking clinician–patient communication to health outcomes. *Patient Education and Counseling*, *74*(3), 295–301. doi:10.1016/j.pec.2008.11.015 PMID:19150199

Szasz, T. S., & Hollender, M. H. (1956). A contribution to the philosophy of medicine: The basic models of the doctor-patient relationship. *A.M.A. Archives of Internal Medicine*, *97*(5), 585–592. doi:10.1001/archinte.1956.00250230079008 PMID:13312700

Vlieland, V. T. P. (2002). Managing chronic disease: Evidence-based medicine or patient centred medicine? *Health Care Analysis*, *10*(3), 289–298. doi:10.1023/A:1022951808151 PMID:12769416

Ward, B. W. (2013). Prevalence of multiple chronic conditions among US adults: Estimates from the National Health Interview Survey, 2010. *Preventing Chronic Disease*, 2013, 10. PMID:23618545

Wells, K. B., Rogers, W., Burnam, A., Greenfield, S., & Ware, J. E. Jr. (1991). How the medical comorbidity of depressed patients differs across health care settings: Results from the Medical Outcomes Study. *The American Journal of Psychiatry*, *148*(12), 1688–1696. doi:10.1176/ajp.148.12.1688 PMID:1957931

Wiederhold, B. K., Riva, G., & Graffigna, G. (2013). Ensuring the best care for our increasing aging population: Health engagement and positive technology can help patients achieve a more active role in future healthcare. *Cyberpsychology, Behavior, and Social Networking*, *16*(6), 411–412. doi:10.1089/cyber.2013.1520 PMID:23751102

Williams, S., Weinman, J., & Dale, J. (1998). Doctor-patient communication and patient satisfaction: A review. *Family Practice*, *15*(5), 480–492. doi:10.1093/fampra/15.5.480 PMID:9848436

KEY TERMS AND DEFINITIONS

Bio-Psychosocial Model: The bio-psychosocial model is a general model stating that biological, psychological and social factors, all play a significant role in human functioning in the context of disease or illness. It posits that, health is best understood in terms of a combination of biological, psychological, and social factors rather than purely in biological terms.

Chronic Disease: The term chronic is usually applied when the course of the disease lasts for more than three months. A chronic condition is a persistent or otherwise long-lasting in its effects or a disease that comes with time.

Disease-Centered Medicine: Disease-centered method is based on the biomedical paradigm in which patients' reports of their medical conditions are read as the expression of disease processes and the clinical method focuses on identifying standard disease entities and on this basis proposes an evidence based therapeutic treatment.

Health Literacy: It is the ability to obtain, read, understand and use healthcare information to make appropriate health decisions and follow instructions for treatment.

Patient Agenda: It is a key concept of the patient-centered medicine. Patient's personal illness experience becomes a critical aspect of the care process in its four principal dimensions (feelings, ideas, the impact of problems on their lives, expectations).

Patient Reported Outcome: It is a measurement of health status directly reported by the patient.

Patient-Centered Medicine: The patient-centered medicine deals with the non-biological aspects of the disease: even the personal, psychological and social aspects are recognized as current and important, so that the tasks for the consultation are focusing not only on disease but also on patients' illness experience.

This work was previously published in Promoting Patient Engagement and Participation for Effective Healthcare Reform edited by Guendalina Graffigna, pages 25-39, copyright year 2016 by Medical Information Science Reference (an imprint of IGI Global).

Chapter 21
LiveWell – Promoting Healthy Living and Wellbeing for Parkinson Patients through Social Network and ICT Training:
Lessons Learnt and Best Practices

Maged N. Kamel Boulos
University of the Highlands and Islands, UK

Emmanuel Ifeachor
Plymouth University, UK

Javier Escudero
Edinburgh University, UK

Peng Zhao
Plymouth University, UK

Camille Carroll
Plymouth University, UK

Pedro Costa
INOVAMAIS – Serviços de Consultadoria em Inovação Tecnológica, S.A., Portugal

Gerhard Doppler
Bit media e-solutions GmbH, Austria

Laura Carrasco Marín
Asociacíon Parkinson Madrid, Spain

Luiza Spiru
Ana Aslan International Foundation, Romania

Kristin Helga Guðmundsdótti
Samvil ehf. Fjarkennsla.com, Iceland

Marija Kosem
Splošna bolnišnica Brežice, Slovenia

ABSTRACT

About 1.2 million people in Europe have Parkinson's disease (PD). PD patients often suffer from social exclusion and depression due to progressive lack of control over the disease. Eventually, most require constant care, leading to huge socioeconomic burdens. To partially tackle this issue, 7 partners in 7 countries participated in LiveWell (EU-funded project, 2012-14) to develop an innovative Web-based

DOI: 10.4018/978-1-5225-1928-7.ch021

education, training and social community platform targeting PD patients, carers and clinicians. This paper describes LiveWell from conception to completion, presents lessons learnt over the course of the project, and highlights some identified main areas of best practice. The Project Consortium might not have had the chance to implement everything learnt in the current outputs, but these lessons and guidelines can be later used to improve LiveWell, and can also be generalised to benefit similar e-health services. The combination of appropriate online education and social communities could help patients and carers cope positively with PD, promoting social inclusion and better outcomes.

1. BACKGROUND: MOTIVATION AND MAIN CHALLENGES THAT LIVEWELL IS ATTEMPTING TO ADDRESS

About 1.2 million people in Europe (127,000 people in the UK or 1 in 500 people) have Parkinson's disease (PD). Its main symptoms include tremors and stiffness, which affect daily activities. PD patients often suffer from social exclusion and depression due to the progressive lack of control over their condition. Eventually, most of them require constant care, leading to huge socioeconomic burdens (Gustavsson et al., 2011; Kowal et al., 2013).

Furthermore, almost half of all EU and UK patients show limited health literacy. This poses an additional challenge when developing online education material for those patients to help them better cope with, and self-manage, their condition (Kamel Boulos, 2013). One common question the Livewell Project Consortium often receives regarding the education and training component of Livewell is 'why are you 'reinventing the wheel' when there are already so many quality (best evidence) online resources out there for PD patients and their carrers?' Our answer is that while there are many existing excellent resources, they are mostly targeting users with high/sophisticated reading levels (high literacy and (digital) health literacy levels)—Figure 1.

Livewell attempts to address this issue, and also adds a component of social networking and peer support to its educational provision to help patients and their carers combat social isolation and depression. Research evidence also shows that Internet use and online social engagement can protect against health literacy decline during ageing (and hence result in better health outcomes), independent of cognitive decline (Kobayashi et al., 2015).

Figure 1. Google search results for 'Parkinson's disease' filtered by reading (comprehension) level as at 12 September 2014 (for more information about this particular Google search filter, please see http://googlesystem.blogspot.co.uk/2010/12/google-shows-reading-levels-for-search.html)

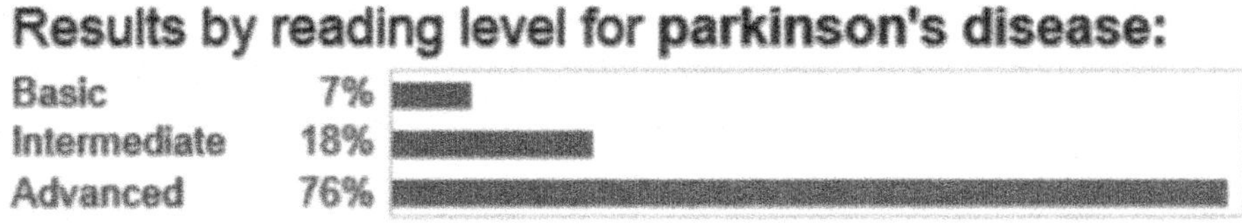

Furthermore, people with Parkinson's disease face a number of usability and ergonomics challenges in relation to using ICT interfaces, caused by their tremors and muscle stiffness, and requiring special design considerations when developing online services for them (Begnum, 2010). This paper presents a review of the authors' approach to developing the EU-funded Livewell platform and service for Parkinson's disease patients and their carers.

2. PROJECT OVERVIEW (2012-2014): OBJECTIVES AND METHODS

Livewell (Promoting Healthy Living and Wellbeing for Parkinson Patients through Social Network and ICT Training; http://www.livewell-community.eu/ and https://www.facebook.com/Livewellcommunity) is a 24-month, seven-partner (Table 1), EU-funded project under the Lifelong Learning Programme—LLP (October 2012 – October 2014). The main aim is to develop an innovative Web-based Training and Social Networking System that targets the following audiences:

- **Parkinson's Disease Patients:** to help them better self-manage their condition and to promote their well-being and inclusion;
- **Caregivers:** to provide access to information, training and greater online community support; and
- **Healthcare Professionals:** to enable them to monitor patient's participation in activities to improve rehabilitation; to access patient-completed clinical symptom checklists; and to securely communicate with patients online (via private asynchronous messaging).

The Web-based platform has two main components:

- **Training with e-Learning Contents:** Offering information packages featuring interactive training contents, games / exercises and quizzes.
- **Social Community:** Serving as a learning, discussion and patient diary/logging (clinical symptom checklists, etc.) platform by facilitating interactions between PD patients, carers and clinicians, within the confines of privacy. It enables the exchange of ideas within a well-tuned online community, as well as peer-to-peer support.

2.1. Methods

To design and develop the platform, the Livewell team started by conducting a comprehensive *needs analysis and desk research exercise*.

Table 1. Partners in the Livewell Project Consortium

1. INOVA+ (Portugal), *co-ordinator*
2. Plymouth University (UK)
3. Parkinson Association of Madrid (Spain)
4. Bitmedia e-Solutions GmbH (Austria)
5. Ana Aslan International Foundation (Romania)
6. Samvilehf. Fjarkennsla.com (Iceland)
7. BrežiceGeneral Hospital (Slovenia)
In addition, Parkinson's Disease Associations in all seven countries were involved in some way in the project (e.g., Parkinson's UK (PUK) and Cure Parkinson's Trust helped with recruitment of participants in UK).

2.1.1. Desk Research

Initial desk research was carried to understand the limitations observed among older users, especially those with motor or cognitive impairments, when using electronic devices.

Changes in perceptual, cognitive, psychomotor and physical skills must be borne in mind when designing devices and interfaces for older people (Caprani et al., 2012). For example, declines in perceptual abilities often result in older adults having vision and hearing problems (Hourcade and Berkel, 2008). In this sense, declines in visual perception have prompted recommendations for adjusting the way information is displayed in user interfaces designed for older adults. Some of these include increasing the size, brightness and contrast of visual elements, and avoiding colour coding using short-wavelength colours (Hourcade and Berkel, 2008).

As adults get older, their cognitive abilities decline, including processing speed and their working and episodic memory (Hourcade and Berkel, 2008). Keeping the use of text, colour and icons simple can significantly reduce confusion and increase ease of use. The impairment of older persons' attention skills can also lead to further complications in the use of the computers and tablets, if distracting information is presented on the screen (Caprani et al., 2012). Overall, these factors tended to be disregarded by developers in the past. Furthermore, little work had been carried out to evaluate the users' cognitive abilities and little is known about the impact of cognitive factors on Web design and how exactly this can affect a user's understanding of content (Crabb et al., 2012). However, these factors may play a crucial factor in the cognitive accessibility of the information (Kamel Boulos, 2005; Crabb et al., 2012).

Physical problems can also occur as a result of ageing and age-related diseases (Caprani et al., 2012). Such problems, combined with cognitive and perceptual challenges, affect the performance of older adults in fine motor tasks, including pointing, grasping, and reaching. There is a decline in the speed, accuracy and consistency of their movements, especially for complex tasks. A number of studies have shown that older adults have difficulty using computer pointing devices (Hourcade and Berkel, 2008). This can result in difficulties grasping a mouse and adequately positioning it on an element (Guillaume and Nadine, 2010; Phiriyapokanon, 2011). Even in healthy ageing, there is an overall decrease in the speed of movement, and older users may find it difficult to make precise selections of small interface targets (Caprani et al., 2012).

Touch screens are claimed to provide more intuitive ways of interaction (Phiriyapokanon, 2011), as they can incorporate large virtual buttons. In general, items can be large on the screen, making them easier to see and to select accurately (Caprani et al., 2012; Phiriyapokanon, 2011). At the same time, the use of virtual buttons on the screen means that older users do not require as much strength to select a target and do not have to divide their attention between keypad and screen (Caprani et al., 2012).

Nonetheless, interacting with touch screens is challenging for tremor patients due to a lower input accuracy caused by their tremor symptoms. It has been suggested that continuous movements are able to lower these symptoms, but still they may need more attempts to select a target than a healthy subject (Mertens et al., 2012). Additionally, people with motion impairments may find it difficult to keep their finger over the target to select it accurately (Mertens et al., 2012).

Therefore, considering the specific requirements of older people and patients with Parkinson's disease, a number of strategies have been suggested in the past to facilitate the use of computers and tablets:

- The simplest strategy involves making targets larger. A similar approach involves making the active area of targets larger than their visual area (Hourcade and Berkel, 2008).
- Tapping small icons may be challenging for older people or patients with tremor. An alternative to "tapping" may be "touching". It may come into contact with the touch screen outside the target and may also be lifted outside the target, but at some point in between it has to touch the target. Although "touching" provides a different way to interact with the device, the use of targets 50% larger than standard-sized ones may enable 65–84 year olds to achieve similar accuracy rates to those achieved by the other age groups when tapping on standard-sized targets. Thus, the simple strategy of making targets larger may be sufficiently effective to enable an older user to interact with the device (Hourcade and Berkel, 2008).
- It is also important to reduce scrolling whenever possible and allow for slower response times (Caprani et al., 2012).
- Older adults had more difficulties in keeping a mental representation of the menus and options in the applications. Thus, the structure of the menus and their presentation must be very clear (Zhou et al., 2012).
- When designing for finger input in touch screens, it is important to note that a font size big enough to be read may be too small for fingertip tapping. On the other hand, a too-large font may result in scrolling and poorer overview of functions per screen (Zhou et al., 2012).
- Older people might gain better understanding from word-based than graphic-based interfaces. They may gain benefits from sans-serif fonts, short line lengths and left justified text. Following a moving text (marquee style) might increase cognitive effort and should be avoided (Phiriyapokanon, 2011).
- Finally, it is essential to pay attention to the readability ('reading with understanding') of the text used in such interfaces to ensure that the content is not only visually or physically accessible, but also cognitively accessible. In this sense, the content needs to be checked against the expected literacy levels of both patients with potential cognitive impairment and their lay carers (Kamel Boulos, 2005; Crabb et al., 2012).

Our desk research results are available in full at http://www.livewell-community.eu/system/files/LiveWell-desk%20research-final%20version.pdf (http://www.webcitation.org/6TGrxdMw4).

2.1.2. Identification of Requirements

In parallel, we carried out a study to identify the needs of end-users by surveying a representative sample of prospective users: patients (n=27), caregivers (n=21) and healthcare professionals (n=43) from the different partners' countries, in addition to the above mentioned desk research (review of relevant literature and related projects). Findings of the needs analysis exercise can be downloaded in full at http://www.livewell-community.eu/system/files/LiveWell-needs-analysis-final%20version.pdf (http://www.webcitation.org/6TGs2jgvo). They helped shape Livewell's specifications.

The Project Consortium has identified some areas of good practice in relation to *needs analysis and desk research exercise* (Table 2).

Table 2. Areas of good practice in relation to Livewell's needs analysis and desk research exercise

- Always involve users/all stakeholders (or a representative sample of them) from an early stage, to prevent 'designers' blindness' and improve user acceptance later on.
- A survey of relevant literature and related projects can serve as a good (albeit partial) proxy to understanding real users' needs and requirements.
- PD patients and carers' needs and requirements (in terms of educational PD content and interface usability/content presentation) are unique. It is imperative to understand and address them in any online service targeting these audiences.

2.1.3. Development of Training and Educational Contents in Seven Languages

Livewell's educational material was designed to meet the identified needs. We adapted materials from known good sources (e.g., PUK patient information resources in PDF format, with PUK's kind permission).

Improvements over original PUK material include:

- We improved the readability of the latter (to match lower patient and carer reading levels);
- Added meaningful photos involving a real PD patient actor and their family (Figure 2); and
- Added interactivity and knowledge testing quizzes at various points throughout the material.

Figure 2. Livewell features meaningful photos (involving a real PD patient actor and their family), interactivity and knowledge testing quizzes

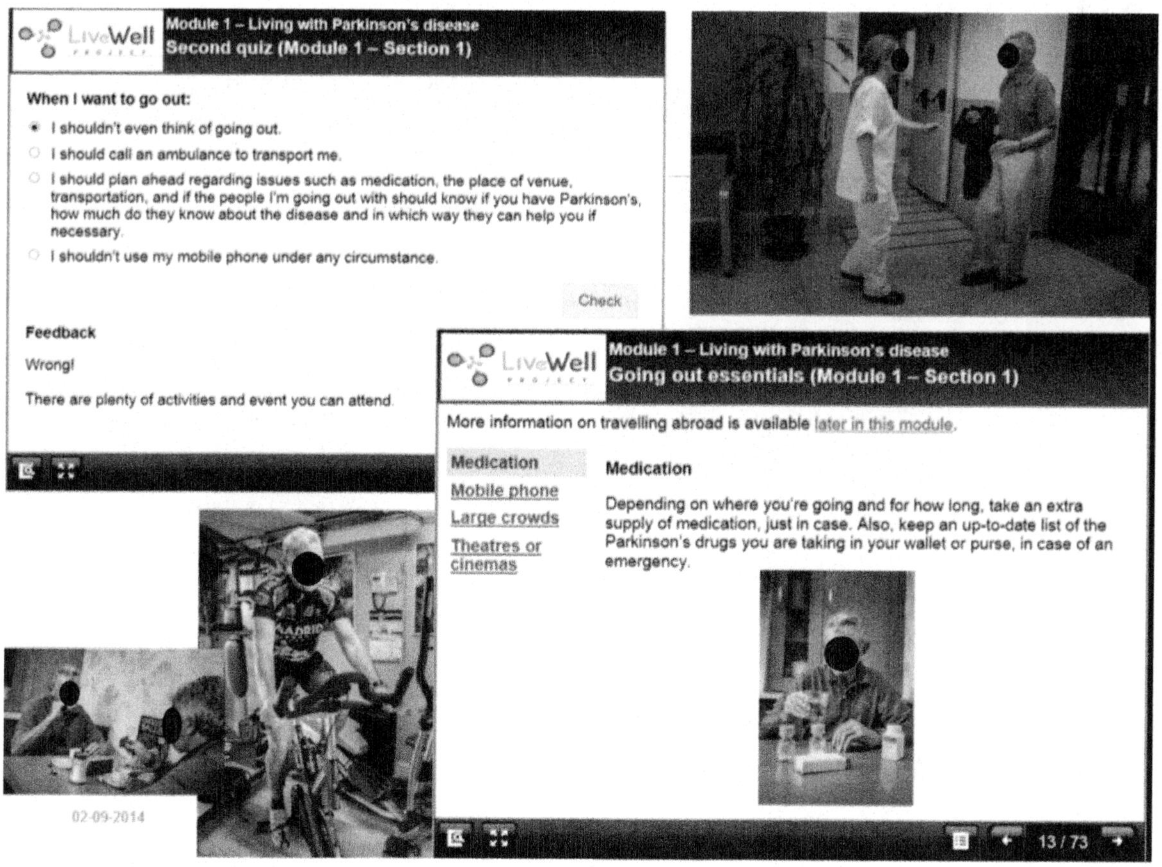

The material was then translated to six additional EU languages (German, Icelandic, Portuguese [International], Romanian, Slovenian and Spanish) besides English, and care was taken during the translation to ensure that the different language versions are also readable (with understanding) by the majority of users operating in those languages (Figure 3).

The Project Consortium has identified some areas of good practice in relation to *training and educational contents development* (Table 3).

2.1.4. Platform Development (Software/ICT Component)

The project consortium decided early in favour of using open source technology for both the online platform and educational content authoring. The decisions were taken to use Drupal (https://www.drupal.org/) as open source content management system, and add to it the necessary functionality for activity tracking and Parkinson's Association (administrators) management. As with the education and training content, the rest of the platform interface (in Drupal) has also been translated to six additional EU languages besides English.

Figure 3. Livewell's e-learning contents in seven EU languages. Users can switch between languages by using the country flags buttons (top right corner on Livewell's Web site) before starting a module

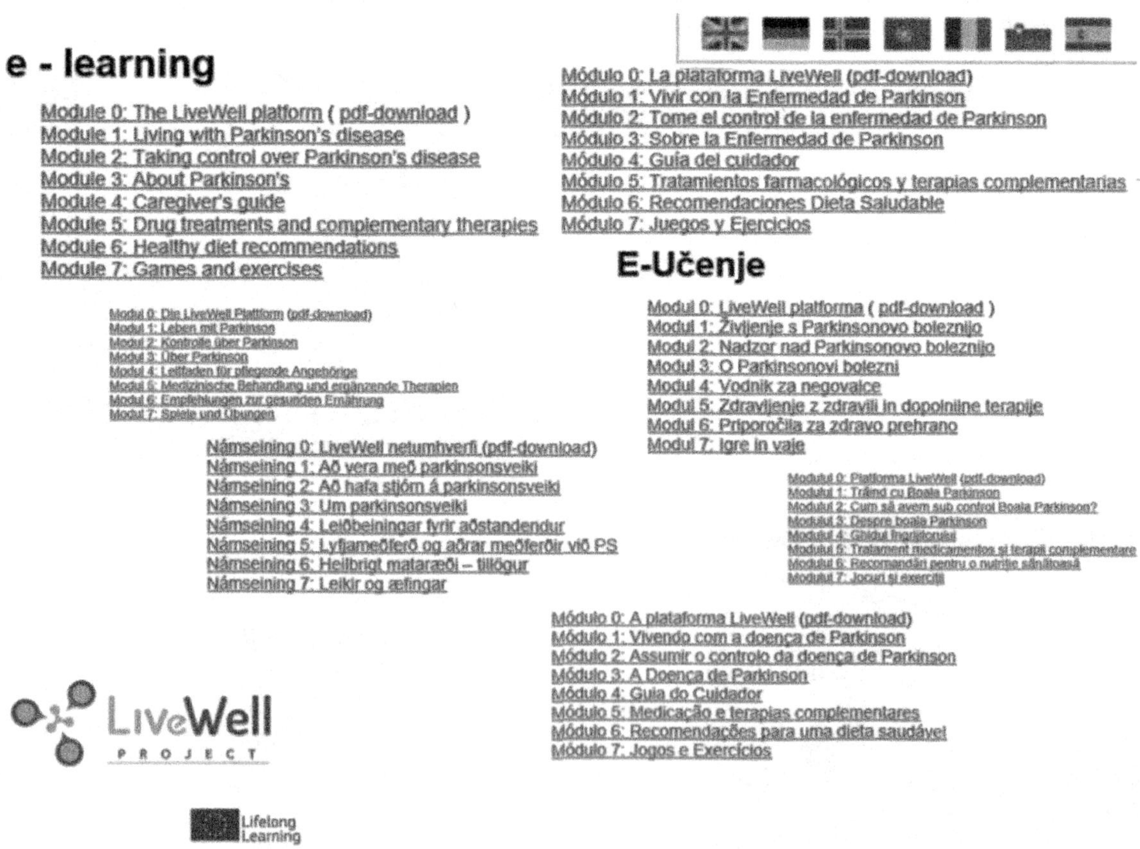

Table 3. Areas of good practice in relation to Livewell's training and educational contents development

• The use of meaningful visuals and photos can help patients and carers relate better and more closely with the content presented to them. However, the production of such photos can prove costly and time-consuming, and also requires the full written consent of all involved actors to use their photos online. This photography exercise was carried out by Parkinson Association of Madrid (Spain). • Knowledge testing quizzes must provide feedback/explanation after marking user's answer. • Online health education material based on the latest, best medical evidence is still pretty useless if it fails to address the essential (digital) health literacy needs and reading (with understanding) levels of the target audiences. Make sure your content is readable and cognitively accessible by your target audiences (hence the need to fully understand those audiences and their profiles before starting to write content for them)! Avoid medical jargon and complex sentences. Use readability formulae as a guide (Kamel Boulos, 2005), and test your material with a sample of your readers (readers' panel). • Have tiered, tagged packages tailored according to user level: Clearly label and tag (in metadata) content for target audiences, and produce different sets for different audience levels. In our case, we have only produced one set for newly diagnosed PD patients and new carers. More experienced patients who have had the disease for longer periods would need different/additional education and training material, specially tailored for them.

For content authoring, the project consortium opted for Xerte (http://www.nottingham.ac.uk/xerte/index.aspx), an open-source, advanced HTML5 (http://www.w3.org/TR/html5/) technology developed at the University of Nottingham, which allows online authoring and publishing, and provides features for content export and re-import (see additional information about our choice of a content authoring tool at http://www.slideshare.net/sl.medic/liv-wellporto-magedwp325oct12).

Both Drupal and Xerte systems were installed on the same physical server. An alternative offline distribution version (of only the education and training content) was also produced on USB key (Figure 4).

However, the use of open source technology also had some disadvantages (stability and reliability issues). One example is a "mixed content warning" displayed as soon as the Web site is opened via 'https://' due to 'http://' references to scripts and CSS (cascading style sheets) files used across the platform. Another example is to do with Xerte modules that (sporadically) stop working without any known reason, but most probably after making some edits or using "special" non-Latin characters. These problems might get fixed in future releases of the packages in question, as developers from the open source community around the world attempt to address them and improve the software.

Figure 4. Offline distribution using USB key. The key includes educational content and all Xerte software necessary to run it to maintain interactivity without Internet connection

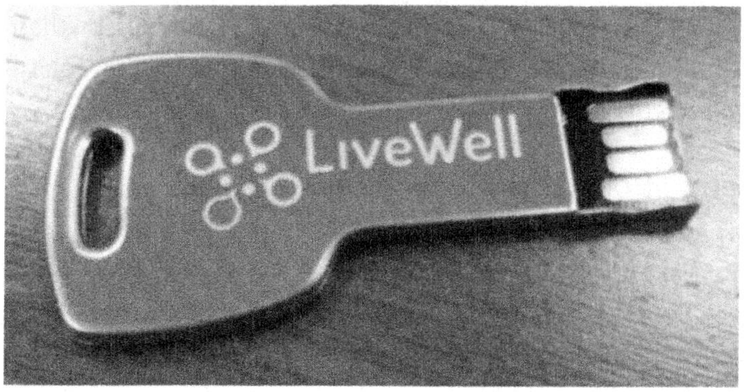

Livewell's user data confidentiality, privacy and security are ensured as follows:

- Little information about users is stored by the system. We never store any unnecessary personal information such as real full name, social security number and date of birth, etc., to eliminate the risk of such information falling into the hands of other users or intruders. Self-registration (for the clinical diary/checklists [Figure 5] and messaging components of Livewell) only asks for a username (nickname), e-mail address and an initial password. As soon as the user clicks on a link sent to the supplied e-mail address, the user account gets activated, allowing the person to write and receive in-platform messages to/from other users.
- The secure 'HTTPS' protocol should be ideally used for the user's diary and messaging functionalities.
- A user's e-mail address is never shown to other users of the platform.
- The feature of "activity logging" contains more patient sensitive data, such as diary entries, answers to clinical checklists (Figure 5) or learning activities. Therefore, we introduced a user management process for Parkinson's Associations (as administrators of groups of patients) with the following provisions:
    - One user is assigned a special role to be manager of a Parkinson's Association;
    - This user gets an additional "Admin" menu with the following two features:
        - Ability to invite other users (already known to him/her outside the system via the corresponding Parkinson's Association) either as patients or as health professionals to own Association on Livewell (these invited users receive an invitation mail, which has to be confirmed by clicking a link in it); and
        - Assign patients (from own Association) to health professionals (again of own Association).
    - Individual health professionals are able to see the details and activities of only those patients assigned to them.

By this "grouping" of users under Parkinson's Associations, putting the management process into the hands of Association administrators, we have managed to effectively silo and protect users from different Associations as far as user activity features are concerned. However, the internal messaging can still be used to communicate with any other user of the system if the username (nickname on the system) of the target user (message recipient) is known to the sender (e.g., given to them by their Association's Admin).

The Project Consortium has identified some areas of good practice in relation to *platform development (software/ICT component)* (Table 4).

2.1.5. Livewell Testing / Formative Evaluation Methods

- **Pre-Pilot Testing (2013):** This exercise was mainly conducted for usability testing purposes (involved only eight potential end-users who tried an early version of the first two educational modules). Their feedback informed, and was incorporated into, the development of the final version of Livewell.

Figure 5. A patient-completed clinical symptoms checklist in Livewell

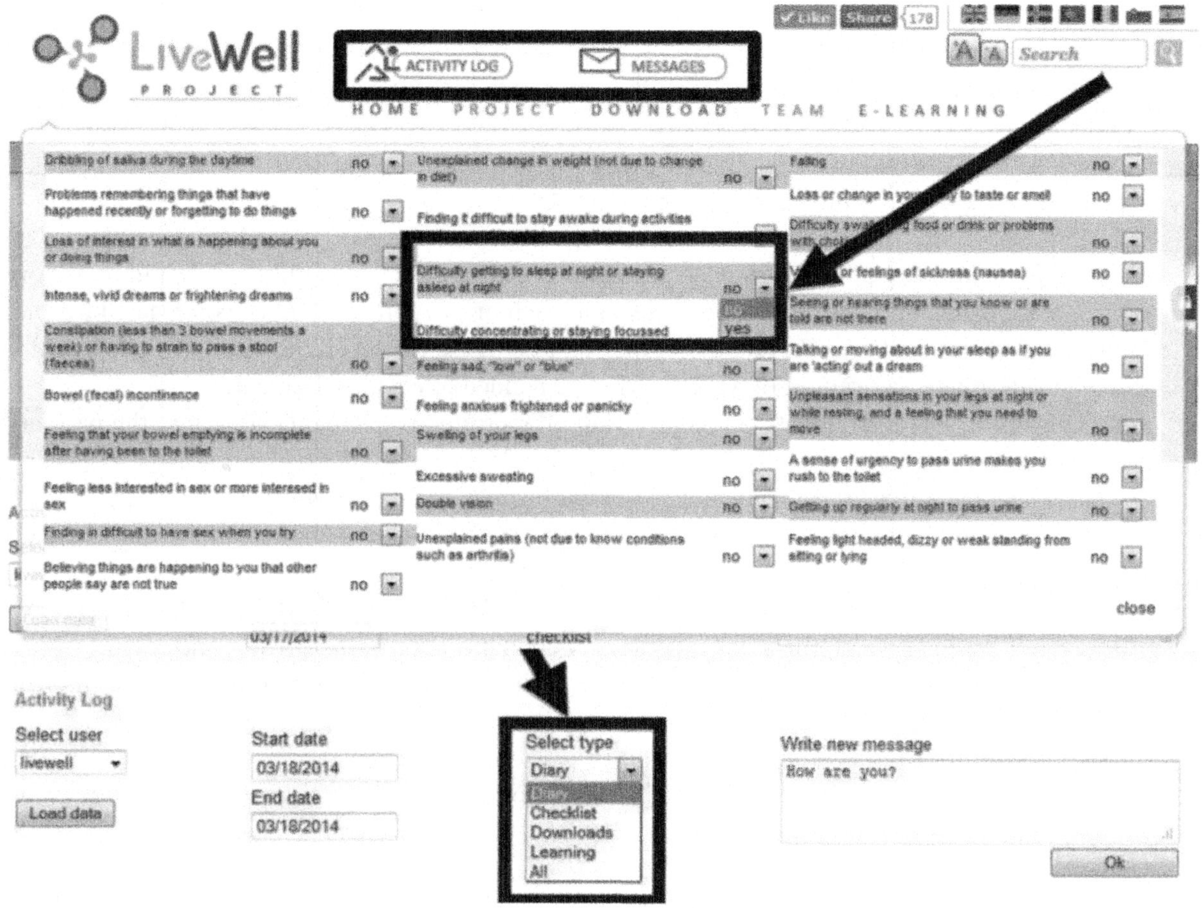

Table 4. Areas of good practice in relation to Livewell's platform development (software/ICT component)

• Offer a 'system manual' for new users: An introductory module (Module 0: http://www.livewell-community.eu/system/files/module_0_The_LiveWell_platform_EN.pdf [http://www.webcitation.org/6TGs7vipE - also available in other supported languages]) that can also be printed (being supplied in PDF) proved very useful for new users to learn about how the education content and rest of the platform work and how various actions, e.g., answering quizzes, can be taken by the user.
• HTML5 enables a single deployment to be accessed by different device form factors (e.g., a smartphone, a tablet, a laptop or a desktop computer) without the need to reformat content for each device. It is also non-proprietary (unlike Adobe Flash) and is a W3C (World Wide Web Consortium) standard.
• Open source ensures systems are future-proof and not dependent on any costly proprietary options or updates, but might require higher technical skills to install and debug.
• Thanks to the use of Xerte, it is easier to export our e-learning content or parts of it as standards-compliant, reusable learning objects (RLOs) or sharable content objects (SCOs) to serve in other learning programmes, projects and contexts.
• Always ensure vulnerable users' (patients and carers) privacy and security are well preserved in online e-health platforms.
• Develop a comprehensive social media strategy (with plans in place for community fostering, regular updates and comments moderation) to 'tell the world' about your developments and reach out to, and engage, more prospective users (see Livewell's page on Facebook: https://www.facebook.com/Livewellcommunity).
• Ensure sustainability beyond project duration (end of funding in October 2014 in our case). Entrust ownership to relevant bodies, e.g., PD Charities, capable of maintaining and regularly updating the content. To address this issue, the Livewell team released all its PD educational content under the Creative Commons (BY,NC,SA) open license (https://creativecommons.org/licenses/by-nc-sa/3.0/). We have also compiled a 'how-to' manual (in PDF) to explain step-by-step (with screenshots) the process of content updating within Xerte to interested PD Charities and Associations wishing to undertake this task in the future. Furthermore, we are offering a 'module dump' of the latest version of all of our modules (all seven languages) in Xerte for third parties willing to deploy the content on their own Xerte server installation.

- **Pilot Testing, Summer 2014:** At seven centres across Europe, involving about 100 PD patients (stages I to IV of the disease), 60 caregivers and 10 healthcare professionals. The objective of the pilot testing was to find out 'how useful potential end users find the platform and the training contents' or in other words, 'whether the platform and the training contents are meeting the needs of end users'.

The steps involved in the pilot testing are:

- Ethical approvals were obtained by each partner prior to the start of the pilot testing phase, following the established regulations and procedures in each of the partners' seven countries. Informed Consent and Confidentiality Agreement forms, as well as the LiveWell brochure and other helpful documentation (e.g., a printout of Module 0) were handed to each participant;
- Initial (1st) Livewell demonstration meeting with all recruited participants at each of the partners' institutions;
- End users are then given the chance to use the platform at home (1-2 weeks);
- Online questionnaire to provide feedback following the above steps – the link to the questionnaire (in user's language) was sent to all users by email (for questionnaire details, see the English version at https://docs.google.com/forms/d/1ebNDbS8ulkD40BKeXBZIMfgBdQCOpeuyobi2SYRPIDE/viewform?usp=send_form or http://www.webcitation.org/6TGsEkRl0); and
- Follow-up (2nd) meeting in the form of a focus group with only select participants at each of the partners' institutions.

The Project Consortium has identified some areas of good practice in relation to *service development and testing* (Table 5).

3. RESULTS AND RECOMMENDATIONS FOR FUTURE DEVELOPMENTS

The report covering the full evaluation results of the project (including participants' statistics) has been marked as private/confidential (to be shared only internally among project partners and with the European Commission), so we are not able to share the full details in a public article. Instead, below, we provide some important highlights extracted from that report. Interested readers might still be able to receive a full copy of the results by submitting a request to the Project Coordinator (contact details can be found at http://www.livewell-community.eu/menu-home/contact-us).

Table 5. Areas of good practice in relation to Livewell's service development and testing

• Developing e-health ICT interventions without full target users' involvement from an early stage should be avoided! Iterative development/testing (*cf.* our pre-pilot testing phase in 2013) helps ensure user involvement (and that users' needs are properly addressed) and reduce development costs. In Livewell, we only had the chance to conduct one iteration with a single pre-pilot testing (development/testing cycle), but two or three iterations where resources permit would have been better. • Our online pilot testing questionnaire was created using Google Docs/Forms. Google Docs/Forms is a handy and free tool for creating questionnaires, but data might reside on, or transit through, servers outside the EEA (European Economic Area). In Livewell, we did not use internal questionnaire checks and validation measures, e.g., to ensure users are not providing inconsistent or out of range answers (e.g., someone entering their age as 300), or taking the questionnaire more than once (by same user). This is better avoided in the future where possible (where resources permit the development of a better questionnaire with proper checks and validation measures).

3.1. Positive Feedback: What Many of the Pilot Participants as Well as Our 'External Project Evaluator' (an Independent EU Firm) Liked

- **Content:** Available in seven EU languages, the modules are clearly structured and include comprehensive information about their respective topics. Each module starts with an overview about what the user can expect to learn in the module. It also gives information to whom this module is addressed (caregiver and/or patient). Each module ends with a summary of achieved learning outcomes.
- **Presentation:** The design of the slides is clear. The slides are not overloaded (some patients disagree--see later). A good mixture of information, further links, pictures and quizzes ensures that people do not get easily tired, even when the number of slides per module is quite high.

3.2. What Some Participants Did Not Like, and Suggestions for Improvement and Future Work

These were mostly usability issues, many of which are due to current Xerte package limitations, e.g., lack of a user-controllable font size changing button in the modules' navigation panel. There were also some educational-content-related issues, including an issue about content usefulness for users with already an advanced degree of knowledge about PD. There was also a routine workflow integration issue raised by some clinicians (UK). Some details of these issues, as well as recommendations for improvement are provided below.

Getting a user name and password (for the messaging, communication and activity logging parts of Livewell that require users to log in) was not easy and did not always work. One patient described the situation, saying: "*It took a long time to find out what was going to happen (in contrast setting up an account from almost any online shopping site is much quicker)*". This is an area of Livewell that should be improved.

The communication tools were judged as not so much relevant for some of the patients and caregivers that are not daily users of the Internet or computers. Interaction with health professionals can be interesting but need to be better explained inside the platform. Some patients and carers expressed concern that there is no way for them (no directory) to identify the correct usernames of other registered members in order to be able to send them messages. (This was partly 'by design' to protect users from receiving unsolicited messages from other unknown users [see above].)

Nurses from UK had a routine practice integration issue in that they have no time to spare in their already very busy schedule to use the proposed online system to regularly read and respond to messages and monitor patients' activity logs. But they could see great value in patients bringing with them to the consultation printouts of their completed Livewell checklists and diary (Figure 5). Methods for better routine workflow integration should be further investigated and the system refined accordingly (if there are resources and funds to do so in the future).

Some slide links were broken. A few slides were missing or would not appear (Xerte issue). There were some typos here and there, and some text portions/questions are written in a rather poor English (for the English language version of the modules). These issues should be easy to rectify.

The main Web site (Drupal-based platform) has two buttons for increasing and decreasing font size, but these do not apply to the Xerte modules (in the modules, font can only be changed either via key board [Ctrl+/-] or touch [pinch to zoom]). This inconsistency was felt to be a bit odd and confusing.

For some patients, the font size and/or spaces between lines were too small. They were reading the text with difficulty, perhaps also because, in their view, there was too much text per page. Patients suggested that text should only occupy 2/3 of each whole page. Font size changing button(s) would also give users more easy control in such situations, provided that scroll-bars can be automatically offered when the text is made too large by the users and can no longer fit into the available slide space, to give users a visual cue about any 'hidden' text in such situations and how to access it (via scroll bars). A 'read aloud' function of slide text (text to speech) might be helpful for some readers (the current HTML5 implementation can integrate well with existing screen readers, but a dedicated built-in function/button would come in very handy).

Some patients with more serious tremor could not click the mouse in a precise manner to navigate through each module. The software might "collapse" after multiple imprecise mouse clicks. Patients suggested that they would better use keyboard buttons, if offered, and/or a different presentation that minimises the need for clicking. Current presentation was found by some participant groups to be more appropriate (usability wise) for caregivers who do not have tremors.

A good number of patients and carers were already familiar with Livewell's module contents and the provided disease information. They were expecting to discover new information and/or learn about new PD findings and new treatments, but could not find any. Our content needs to be explicitly labelled as primarily designed for *newly* diagnosed patients and *new* carers, and a separate set developed for those with more advanced information needs.

Other important perceived deficiencies and suggestions include:

- The modules are currently lacking a decent free text search facility that searches across all modules at one time to dig up all the relevant info in one go, e.g., to instantly find slides about 'back pain'.
- A module slide bookmarking function would be a desirable feature to quickly return/jump to favourited slides within modules at a later time.
- As far as content is concerned, the 'external project evaluator' pointed out that 'Module 6: healthy diet recommendations' could benefit from the inclusion of additional links to some appropriate recipes, to inspire readers, so that they do not get the feeling that they are very limited in their nutrition options.
- Also, the Plymouth team (Kamel Boulos) proposed the use of trackable Kinect exergames, specially tailored for PD patients within some of the modules (Kamel Boulos, 2012). (Kinect now also works on PCs, so these proposed exercise games need not be exclusive to the Xbox 360 and Xbox One game consoles.)

4. LIMITATIONS

This paper summarised our experience in implementing Livewell as a free online service for Parkinson's disease patients and their carers. In realising the different components of the Livewell platform, the project team drew extensively on the established best research evidence in the field of health informatics/ digital health, as well as their own past experience in delivering related large health ICT projects, such as the eCAALYX EU-funded project (http://ecaalyx.org/ – Plymouth University's parts were led by the corresponding author on this article), among others.

Extensive user testing (including testing for scalability and under various conditions and evaluating for statistically-significant efficacy and clinical/health outcomes, by conducting a trial involving a large number of end users over a longer period) was not possible, given the project's relatively short duration (24 months) and limited budget (a grand total of only 291K Euros shared by seven Partner Organisations over the whole project duration). Furthermore, the EU LLP (Lifelong Learning Programme) under which the Livewell project was funded has a specific mission and requirements, where focus is not on conventional informatics/ICT research as such (http://ec.europa.eu/education/tools/llp_en.htm). All these factors combined limited the sort of research evidence that could be generated from the Livewell project (in addition to the public sharing restrictions that are in place for some of the project results, as is common in many EU-funded projects and their deliverables).

Subject to securing additional funding in the near future, a further cycle (or more than one) of development and user evaluation is warranted and could indeed provide valuable results, with more robust and generalisable research evidence for other health ICT solution developers to benefit from. Nevertheless, we believe that many of the rather general/generic principles and guidelines for best practices presented in the current article could still be of value to students and developers studying and working in the area of health ICT.

5. SUMMARY DISCUSSION AND CONCLUSION

This paper reported some of the lessons learnt by the Livewell Consortium over the duration of the project (2012-2014), and highlighted the main identified areas of best practice. We might not have had the chance to implement in full, in the project's current online outputs, all the above mentioned best practices and everything learnt or suggested by the participants in our pilot evaluation, but these lessons and best practice guidelines remain very helpful. They can be later used to inform and improve a future version of the Livewell service (if new funds can be secured for this purpose), and can also be in part adapted and generalised to benefit other similar e-health/online patient education services.

We believe that the combination of appropriate online education/training and social communities could help patients and caregivers cope positively with PD, promoting social inclusion and better disease management. Our findings echo those of the Ages 2.0 EU-funded project (http://www.ages2.eu/), which similarly reported that training older people in social media carries the potential of improving wellbeing and combatting isolation (http://www.webcitation.org/6WnQhGK6v). Ultimately, we want to further develop the Livewell Online Social Community following the ParkinsonNet (Netherland; http://www.parkinsonnet.info/) approach (Bloem, 2014), optimise the service to better suit the existing busy workflows of healthcare professionals, address all the identified usability issues (including implementing a search function across all modules), and integrate some trackable Kinect exergames specially tailored for PD patients within the education and training modules.

5.1. Competing Interests

The authors declare that they have no competing interests.

5.2. Authors' Contributions

MNKB conceived and led the writing of this manuscript with inputs from EI, JER, PZ, CC, PC, GD, LC, LS, KH and MK.

ACKNOWLEDGMENT

This project has been funded with the support from the European Commission. This publication reflects the views only of the author, and the Commission cannot be held responsible for any use which may be made of the information contained herein. Project Number: 527943-LLP-1- 2012-1-PT-GRUNDTVIG-GMP.

REFERENCES

Beaudet, L., & Ducharme, F. (2013). Living with moderate-stage Parkinson disease: Intervention needs and preferences of elderly couples. *The Journal of Neuroscience Nursing*, *45*(2), 88–95. doi:10.1097/JNN.0b013e3182828ff4 PMID:23422694

Begnum, M.E.N. (2010). Challenges for Norwegain PC-users with Parkinson's disease - a survey. LNCS: Computers Helping People with Special Needs, 6179: 292-299 (Springer). doi:10.1007/978-3-642-14097-6_47

Bloem, B.R. (2014). Revolutionising management of chronic disease: the ParkinsonNet approach. BMJ, 348:g1838. doi:10.1136/bmj.g1838

Caprani, N., O'Connor, N. E., & Gurrin, C. (2012). Touch Screens for the Older User. In A. Cheein (Ed.), *Fernando A.* Assistive Technologies. InTech; doi:10.5772/38302

Crabb, M., Hanson, V. L., & Cobley, A. (2012). Cognitive Usability: Using Human Factors to Influence Future Online Usability Requirements. Presented at the DE2012 conference. http://www.slideshare.net/mikecrabb/cognitive-usability-using-human-factors-to-influence-future-online-usability-requirements

Guillaume, L., & Nadine, V. (2010). Influence of age and interaction complexity on touch screen. In: *Proceedings of the 2010 12th IEEE International Conference on e-Health Networking Applications and Services (Healthcom)*, pp. 246 –253. doi:10.1109/HEALTH.2010.5556560

Gustavsson, A., Svensson, M., Jacobi, F., Allgulander, C., Alonso, J., Beghi, E., & Olesen, J. etal. (2011). Cost of disorders of the brain in Europe 2010. *European Neuropsychopharmacology*, *21*(10), 718–779. doi:10.1016/j.euroneuro.2011.08.008 PMID:21924589

Hourcade, J. P., & Berkel, T. R. (2008). Simple pen interaction performance of young and older adults using handheld computers. *Interacting with Computers*, *20*(1), 166–183. doi:10.1016/j.intcom.2007.10.002

Kamel Boulos, M. N. (2005). British Internet-Derived Patient Information on Diabetes Mellitus: Is It Readable? *Diabetes Technology & Therapeutics*, *7*(3), 528–535. doi:10.1089/dia.2005.7.528 PMID:15929685

Kamel Boulos, M. N. (2012). Xbox 360 Kinect Exergames for Health. *Games for Health Journal*, *1*(5), 326–330. doi:10.1089/g4h.2012.0041 PMID:26191998

Kamel Boulos, M. N. (2013). Social media and mobile health (Chapter 13, under Part B: Taking action to create and strengthen health literacy-friendly settings). In: Ilona Kickbusch, Jürgen Pelikan, Franklin Apfel and Agis Tsouros (Editors). THE SOLID FACTS - Health Literacy. Copenhagen, Denmark: World Health Organization Regional Office for Europe, pp. 63-67. http://www.euro.who.int/__data/assets/pdf_file/0008/190655/e96854.pdf

Kobayashi, L. C., Wardle, J., & von Wagner, C. (2015). Internet use, social engagement and health literacy decline during ageing in a longitudinal cohort of older English adults. *Journal of Epidemiology and Community Health*, *69*(3), 278–283. doi:10.1136/jech-2014-204733 PMID:25428933

Kowal, S. L., Dall, T. M., Chakrabarti, R., Storm, M. V., & Jain, A. (2013). The current and projected economic burden of Parkinson's disease in the United States. *Movement Disorders*, *28*(3), 311–318. doi:10.1002/mds.25292 PMID:23436720

Mertens, A., Hurtmanns, J., Wacharamanotham, C., Kronenbürger, M., Borchers, J., & Schlick, C. M. (2012). Swabbing: Touchscreen-based input technique for people with hand tremor. *Work J. Prev. Assess. Rehabil.*, *41*, 2405–2411. doi:10.3233/WOR-2012-0474-2405 PMID:22317077

Phiriyapokanon, T. (2011). Is a big button interface enough for elderly users? Towards user interface guidelines for elderly users. LAP Lambert Academic Publishing. Based on thesis by same author at http://www.diva-portal.org/smash/get/diva2:416488/FULLTEXT01.pdf

Zhou, J., Rau, P.-L. P., & Salvendy, G. (2012). Use and Design of Handheld Computers for Older Adults: A Review and Appraisal. *International Journal of Human-Computer Interaction*, *28*(12), 799–826. do i:10.1080/10447318.2012.668129

This work was previously published in the International Journal of Healthcare Information Systems and Informatics (IJHISI), 10(3); edited by Joseph Tan, pages 24-41, copyright year 2015 by IGI Publishing (an imprint of IGI Global).

Section 4
Patient Education

Chapter 22
Knowledge in Action: Fostering Health Education through Technology

Theresa J. Barrett
New Jersey Academy of Family Physicians, USA

ABSTRACT

This chapter will explore the possibilities and the challenges presented by technology in the area of patient education. Beginning with an overview of the use of the medical record in patient care, the chapter will move on to discuss the evolution of electronic health records (EHR) and the emergence of health information technology in the education of patients. Emerging technologies, the primary care physician's role in creating tailored education plans for their patients, as well as the importance of self-directness in learning both for the physician and the patient will also be discussed. The chapter will conclude with an overview of information and health literacy and how these impact shared-decision making and patient activation (the ability to be engaged in one's own health care). The overall goal of the chapter is to present how physicians and patients can use technology in order to facilitate better patient care and improve patient outcomes.

INTRODUCTION

The rapid growth of technology has had a profound impact on the doctor-patient relationship. Gone are the days when a patient walked passively into a physician's office and waited to be told what was wrong and how their care was going to be managed. Today, patients visit their doctor armed with scores of print-outs from web searches about their disease, or the disease they think they have. They have researched medications or treatment options. They have downloaded an app that monitors their blood pressure or blood sugar and they bring progress reports to their office visits or have them sent through a secure email system. Physicians search through reams of data to determine what information can be best used to educate the patient, and then wonder if the patient will be willing to work as a member of the health care team in the management of their disease. Information used to educate patients is no more than a

DOI: 10.4018/978-1-5225-1928-7.ch022

mouse click or an app away. Channeling the right information into an education plan tailored to each patient's individual need is one more challenge for today's busy primary care physician. Overcoming this challenge is one of the best hopes for improved patient and community health.

FROM INK TO BYTES: THE EMERGENCE OF THE ELECTRONIC HEALTH RECORD

Patient case records have existed since ancient times. One of the earliest known records comes from the Edwin Smith Surgical Papyrus (Wilkins, 1964).[1] When the papyrus manuscript (circa 3000-2500 B.C.) was finally translated in 1930 by James H. Breasted, it was found to be part of a surgical treatise and contained 48 patient case histories systematically arranged by injury and divided into sections: title, examination, diagnosis, and treatment (Wilkins, 1964).

In fifth century Greece, patient case records evolved significantly under the guidance of Hippocrates and his followers (Reiser, 1991a). Case records had two main purposes in the Hippocratic literature: demonstration of the natural cause of the illness and the description of the illness' clinical course through close observation of the patient's symptoms (Reiser, 1991a). Hippocratic cases were recorded chronologically and followed a set format. The record began with the preceding cause of the illness and the presenting symptoms of the patient. Next recorded were the actions taken by the patient and the resulting symptoms that prompted the patient to seek care. This was followed by notes on the progress of the illness. Such progress notes were only included in the patient record when there was an important change in symptoms. Case reports concluded with disclosure of the results of the case, which was often death (Reiser, 1991a). The chronologic order of the case gave the Greek physician insight as to when therapeutic action should be taken and focused attention on the symptoms that would most predict the outcome, as a tenet of Greek medicine was not to initiate therapy which would have no effect on the course of the illness (Reiser, 1991a).

In the seventeenth century, sickness was thought to be caused by a single mechanism recognized since the time of Hippocrates, namely the disruption of the equilibrium of the four main building blocks of the body (blood, phlegm, black bile, yellow bile) (Reiser, 1991a). Thomas Sydenham, a seventeenth century physician, recognized that there was a pattern to the symptoms his patients presented with and he began to hypothesize that illnesses could be categorized by their characteristic symptoms (Reiser, 1991a). With this premise, Sydenham began to develop a universal classification of diseasethat has become the basis for the diagnostic process in modern medicine (Reiser, 1991a).

In the nineteenth century physicians in the major teaching hospitals began to maintain permanent medical records as a method of teaching patient cases to medical students (Gillum, 2013; Siegler, 2010). At that time, standards and quality measures had yet to be developed. Cases were prepared retrospectively as an aid to individual memories with the technique of documentation reflective of the individual writing the case (Craig, 1990). Patient case records were free-form with varying levels of quality (Siegler, 2010). Records were bound in leather volumes and kept serially, with different records kept by the surgical, medical, and outpatient services (Gillum, 2013). Data on patients was hard to retrieve, widely scattered, and often incomplete (Gillum, 2013).

The inconsistent quality and sub-standard completion of records prompted medical boards to restructure the medical record in the late 1800s (Siegler, 2010). These changes reflected the need to manage and preserve patient information. As a result of the restructuring, all interventions experienced by the patient while in the hospital were kept in a single history, with a standard method of collecting and ordering the clinical data (Reiser, 1991b). [2] Forms, graphs, and tables dominated the patient record with little room left for narrative descriptions (Siegler, 2010). This fixed structure was met with some controversy as physicians felt constrained by only being able to write procedure notes and observations, but eventually physicians found a way around these constrictions and began to document their opinions and findings through what eventually became today's progress notes (Siegler, 2010).

In the early 1900s, Henry S. Plummer, a physician at the Mayo Clinic, was dissatisfied with the way patient records were kept and turned to models from business and industry as a means to address the problem of scattered and disorganized data (Camp et al., 2008). Plummer research resulted in the "dossier model," which remains the foundation for medical records at the Mayo Clinic today (Camp et al., 2008). In Plummer's model, each patient who entered the Clinic received a serial number that they maintained throughout all subsequent visits (Camp et al., 2008). All information about the patient was kept in an envelope with the patient's personal number, with any new information added to the original chart, which was stored in a central location (Camp et al., 2008).

From the 1920s through the 1970s and into the 1980s, medical records remained paper-based, and even with improvements in record-keeping, data storage and retrieval was a growing challenge. The introduction of the computer in the 1960s gave some hope that this technology would result in better diagnoses, record-keeping, and management of health services (Reiser, 1991b). However, as time passed, people came to realize that developing the proper computer programs was a challenge.Software and hardware were expensive, and the resistance of administrative and clinical staff to change meant that the potential of this technology was not going to be recognized quickly (Reiser, 1991b).

Despite these issues, the search for a better way to document and manage patient information continued. In the late 1960s, Larry Weed, MD introduced the Problem Oriented Medical Record (POMR) (Weed, 1968). Weed proposed that the medical record should contain a complete list of each patient's problems. This list would become an active "table of contents" for the patient's chart that could be updated at any time by any member of the healthcare team (Weed, 1968). The POMR provided for the inclusion of a patient history, patient data, medical information, and feedback loops. This structure created an organizational framework for the development of a computerized record-keeping system (Fitzmaurice, Adams, & Eisenberg, 2002). The POMR consists of four core components: a defined database of information, a problem list, an action plan for each problem, and progress note on each problem (Kernisan, 2013). Today, the POMR is the international standard for the organization of the entire medical record for both in-patient and out-patient services (Hummel & Evans, 2012).

As technology continued to evolve, hospital departments began to experiment with computerized admissions procedures and computerized master patient indexes (VanFleet, 2010). Healthcare institutions began to develop clinical workstations, which encompassed not just the clinical elements of care, but also the administrative, financial, research (i.e., outcomes and clinical trials), and scholarly (i.e. digital libraries, drug information databases) elements of patient care (Shortliffe, 1999). At the core of the clinical workstation was the patient's medical record in electronic form (Shortliffe, 1999). Unfortunately, the promise offered by the electronic medical record was locked within stand-alone systems that did not communicate with each other, rather like a state highway system that did not cross or connect with any other states' highway system (VanFleet, 2010). Rising medical costs, inconsistent quality of care, and issues of patient safety mandated that these individual systems be connected to improve the effectiveness and efficiency of health care (Chaudhry et al., 2006; Institute of Medicine, 2001; VanFleet, 2010).

The U.S. Department of Health and Human Services Agency for Healthcare Quality and Research (AHRQ) supported the development and evaluation of electronic patient records through the 1970s and 80s (Fitzmaurice et al., 2002). One AHRQ study examined the use of the Summary Time-Oriented Record (STOR) to provide information to physicians (Whiting-O'Keefe, Simborg, Epstein, & Warger, 1985). Research showed that the use of this system allowed physicians to better predict the future symptoms of their patients and what the patients' laboratory results would be (Whiting-O'Keefe et al., 1985). A study of a computerized record summary system conducted at Northwestern University provided evidence that suggested that patients who had computerized records experienced better care and outcomes (Rogers, Harring, Wortman, Waston, & Goetz, 1982).

This need to connect electronic record systems and use the data within them to improve the quality of care provided to patients led to the emergence of health information technology (Health IT) and spurred continuous improvement in the area of electronic health records (EHR). EHRs are seen as the next step to enhance patient care by improving the accuracy and clarity of medical records thus reducing medical errors; reducing the duplication of tests and delays in treatment; and making information available to physicians and patients so they can both make well informed decisions (CMS.gov, 2012). It is believed that when Health IT is fully integrated into the delivery of healthcare substantial improvements in quality and safety as compared to paper records will result (Office of the National Coordinator for Health Information Technology, 2013).

Innovative thinking and new technologies have advanced medicine and the medical record. However, with that advancement the voice and the personality of the patient began to fade. Once Laennec invented the stethoscope in 1816 (a technological leap of the time), the nature of case histories was altered yet again (Reiser, 1991a). The essence of the patient was replaced with detailed descriptions of anatomic changes (Reiser, 1991a) and the relationship between physician and patient changed.

TECHNOLOGY AND THE PATIENT

From the patient's perspective, technology is a means to learn more about their health issues and sharpen the questions that they ask when they talk with their doctor (Fox & Jones, 2009). For physicians, technology means being able to provide personal, patient-centered care while also providing population-based care in the context of the patient-centered medical home (Bailey, 2011). When physicians have access to complete and accurate information provided through health information technology, patients receive better care (HealthIT.gov, 2014). Electronic health records provide that information, improving the physician's ability to diagnose diseases and reduce or even prevent medical errors while improving patient outcomes (HealthIT.gov, 2014).

Impact on Physician-Patient Relationship

When using an EHR, the physician must either simultaneously or alternately interact with both the patient and the computer (Street et al., 2014). This constant switching of attention from patient to screen and back influences the quality of the physician/patient communication and the patient's involvement in the encounter (Street et al., 2014). Richard Gilliam, MD (2013) from the Departments of Medicine and Community and Family Medicine at Howard University, in Washington, DC said:

... physicians must not allow technology to devalue the doctor-patient relationship and a continuity of care in which the patient as person maintains a place in the memory of a clinician, not merely a computer. The electronic health record/electronic medical record must enable this relationship, not interfere with it... (p. 856)

For EHRs to enable the patient-physician relationship, physicians must learn skills that will allow them to seamlessly interact with both the patient and the computer. The physician needs to learn how to provide room for the patient's voice to be heard so that he or she can understand the patient's subjective view of their illness (Andreassen & Nilsen, 2013). EHRs are designed to improve health, defined by the World Health Organization (2006) as "...a state of complete physical, mental and social well-being and not merely the absence of disease or infirmity..." (p. 1). The terms "physical, mental and social well-being" only have meaning when the patient and the physician are communicating with each other and the patient is engaged in their care (Andreassen & Nilsen, 2013).

According to an Institute of Medicine (IoM) report on patient engagement, patients should not only be the healthcare systems unwavering focus, they should be its fully engaged agents of change (Olsen, Saunders, & McGinnis, 2011). The IoM report further stated that the quality of health care should not be judged on scientifically-based clinical decisions alone, but on whether the patient's personal preferences and circumstances were taken into account (Olsen et al., 2011). Listening to the patient should be the beginning of every patient encounter (Olsen et al., 2011). Listening, not just hearing, is critical for patients and physicians to achieve patient-centered care (Rifkin & Lazris, 2014).

Technology, Self-Directedness, and Education

One of the responsibilities of primary care physicians is to educate their patients, their patients' families, and their communities in matters of health (AAFP, 2011). Providing patients with current and complete information enhances the doctor/patient relationship and empowers patients to participate in their care (AAFP, 2011). A study by the Pew Internet and American Life Project (Fox & Jones, 2009) found that while 61% of American adults look online for health information, 86% of survey respondents stated they would ask a health professional, such as a doctor, when they need information or assistance in dealing with health or medical issues.

Despite the changes precipitated by the growth of Internet as a source of medical information, physicians remain a vital part of the health-search and decision making process (Fox & Jones, 2009). It is vital that physicians stay current not only on clinical topics, but also know how to best educate their patients about those topics. Physicians must be able to determine their patients' levels of health literacy and identify barriers to learning (AAFP, 2011). Being able to provide education to patients requires physicians to evaluate materials that already exist or to develop new materials that meet their patients' needs. In turn, patients must learn how to articulate their needs, and feel comfortable doing so. To this end, both physician and patient must be self-directed learners.

Self-Directed Learning

Malcom Knowles, an American educator, defined self-directed learning (SDL) as the process whereby "individuals take the initiative, with or without the help of others, in diagnosing their learning needs, formulating learning goals, identifying human and material resources for learning, choosing and implementing appropriate learning strategies, and evaluating learning outcomes" (Knowles, 1975, p. 18). Other researchers in adult education have presented alternate definitions of SDL. Brockett and Hiemstra (1991) defined SDL as a combination of two processes: an external process focused on education merged with the internal characteristics of the learners. SDL was also presented an external and internal process by Brookfield (1986). For Guglielmino (1977), SDL was part of a learning continuum, with the ability to be self-directed present in some degree in each person. Candy (1995) describes SDL as a concept that embodies personal autonomy and empowerment which is usually not associated with other forms of learning.

SDL has two separate but related dimensions; the external education process and the internal characteristics of the learners (Brockett & Hiemstra, 1991). In the first dimension, the external education process, the learner takes responsibility for planning, implementing, and evaluating their learning. The second dimension focuses on the preference or desire of the learners to take responsibility for their learning.

Brookfield (1986), like Brockett and Hiemstra (1991), also saw SDL as involving both external and internal processes. Externally, SDL requires setting goals, finding resources, implementing strategies, and evaluating the outcomes. Internally, SDL requires a change in consciousness. The learner understands knowledge contextually and sees the moral code governing behavior as a cultural construct. With this altered perspective, learners examine ways in which they can change their personal and social worlds.

Candy (1991) viewed SDL as a goal and a process. Candy, like Knowles (1980), saw SDL as a continuum where the teacher was in control at one end and learner was in control at the other end, with the control shifting between teacher and learner based upon the situation. Guglielmino (1977) too saw SDL as part of a learning continuum, where the ability to be self-directed was present to some degree in each person regardless of where they were on that continuum. From the perspective of a goal, Candy (1991) saw SDL as a way for the learner to exhibit personal autonomy, where Guglielmino (1977) felt that the personality characteristics of the learners ultimately determined whether SDL would take place in a given situation.

Garrison (1997), Grow (1991), and Spear (1988) presented other definitions of SDL.

Garrison defined SDL as a learning approach that motivates the learners to assume responsibility and control of the cognitive and contextual processes of learning, thereby constructing meaningful learning outcomes. The definition of SDL put forth by Grow is based upon the amount of choice that learners have in a given instructional situation. Spear described SDL as a process that gives learners control over the means and goals for learning. Spear felt that while the reasons for learning do not need to be under the control of the learners, once the decision is made to learn, the authority of what and how to learn lies with the learners.

Characteristics of Self-Directed Learners

SDL has been identified as a characteristic of being an adult (Brockett & Hiemstra, 1991; Brookfield, 1986; Guglielmino, 1977; Knowles, 1975). Four reasons have been identified for why adults choose to learn:

1. To adapt to or transmit culture,
2. To understand or develop expertise or special knowledge,
3. To vitalize organizations and societies, and
4. To achieve personal fulfillment (Owen, 2002).

The characteristics that identify self-directed learners have been the subject of much analysis, with the most frequently cited characteristic being the willingness and ability to accept responsibility to learn on one's own (Brockett & Hiemstra, 1991; Brookfield, 1986; Candy, 1991; Garrison, 1997; Grow, 1991; Guglielmino, 1977; Hiemstra, 1994; Knowles, 1975). Another important characteristic of the self-directed learner is the ability to reflect on what one has learned (Brookfield, 1986; Confessore & Kops, 1998; Fenwick & Tennant, 2004; Schon, 1983). Self-directed learners do not uncritically accept and internalize information, rather they assess, reflect, and evaluate what they learned (Confessore & Kops, 1998). Schon (Schon, 1983) stated that when presented with a problem, adults reflect in action to solve that problem. It is through reflection that adult learners construct a personal meaning which results in action (Fenwick & Tennant, 2004).

Self-directed learners exhibit the characteristics of persistence, independence, and initiative (Guglielmino, 1977). They are curious and see problems as challenges, not obstacles (Guglielmino, 1977). Self-directed learners are self-confident, organized, have basic study skills, and enjoy learning (Guglielmino, 1977).

Candy (1991) criticized the conventional profiles of self-directed learners. He felt the profiles failed to portray the intellectual, emotional, and moral aspects of autonomous learning. Rather than start with the profile of what an autonomous adult learner might look like, Candy suggested that researchers should start with the profile of an autonomous person and then determine what that person would be like as a self-directed learner. Candy developed 14 characteristics of autonomous learners based upon this approach. According to Candy (1991) autonomous learners:

1. Take the initiative, with or without help, to assess their learning needs.
2. Select appropriate sources for assistance and can temporarily surrender independence for the sake of practicality in learning.
3. Develop, through inquiry and reflection, the criteria to evaluate the learning being undertaken.
4. Question the justification for rules, procedures, and assumptions that might otherwise be taken for granted.
5. Refuse to agree or comply with what others (teacher) demand when it seems unacceptable.
6. Make reasoned choices among various learning options based on personally significant purposes and ideas.
7. Review the process of learning continuously and makes strategic adjustments when necessary.
8. Conceive goals, plans, and policies independent from pressure from others to do so.
9. Develop understanding of phenomena to such an extent as to be able to explain them under circumstances other than how the phenomena were first conceived.
10. Form opinions and beliefs independently, yet are willing to give up or alter those beliefs when contrary evidence is presented.
11. Pursue a learning goal with determination and excitement without being influenced by external factors.
12. Determine what is of personal value distinct from what may be expedient or convenient.
13. Accept alternative points of view as valid and are willing to deal with objections or criticisms to personal goals without becoming threatened or angry.
14. Demonstrate a realistic appraisal of personal limitations and shortcomings, tempered by positive awareness of strengths, abilities, and motivations as learners (pp. 133-134).

Importance of Self-Directedness in Learning

Toffler (1971) cited psychologist Herbert Gerjuoy's assertion that "tomorrow's illiterate will not be the man who can't read; he will be the man who has not learned how to learn" (p. 375). The benefits of knowing how to learn, in other words in being a self-directed learner, are clearly documented in the literature. Self-directed learners develop skills that allow them to be critical thinkers, to cope with change, and to be more self-confident (Abdullah, 2001; Garrison, 1997; Tough, 1971).

Self-directedness allows learners to develop the abilities to transfer knowledge and study skills from one situation to another (Hiemstra, 1994) and to apply the basic concepts learned to real world problems (Dynan, Cate, & Rhee, 2008). Self-directed learners are pro-active, learn better than passive learners, have better retention, and have developed the skills to be lifelong learners (Dynan et al., 2008; Knowles, 1975). Being self-directed allows learners to stay current in a world where information and knowledge are constantly changing (Hiemstra, 1994).

Self-Directness in Adults

Cyril Houle, a long-time Professor of Adult Education at the University of Chicago, has been credited with playing a central role in advancing the knowledge around self-directed learning both through his own writings and his influence over two of his students: researchers Allen Tough and Malcolm Knowles (Brockett & Donaghy, 2005). With the publication of his seminal work, *The Inquiring Mind,* Houle (1961) changed the way people thought about adult learning (as cited in Hiemstra, 2003). Houle's research revealed that adults who participated in continuing education fell into three groups: goal-oriented learners who used learning as a means to an end, activity-oriented learners who used learning as a form of fellowship or to meet new people, and learning-oriented learners who learned for the enjoyment of learning (as cited in Brockett & Hiemstra, 1991).

Ten years later, Tough (1971) undertook reseach on why adults learn by examining their participation in learning projects. He determined that the learners decided

1. Whether or not to take on a learning project,
2. What they needed to learn,
3. Why they needed to learn it,
4. What resources they needed, and
5. Whether to continue or stop learning.

Brockett and Hiemstra (1991) stated that some of the major reasons for undertaking a learning project were preparation for a job, the need to solve a specific problem, gain knowledge or skill, or satisfy curiosity.

As Tough was developing his theories of adult learning projects, Knowles began to promote his theory of andragogy (as cited in Hiemstra, 2003). Knowles (1980) defined *andragogy* as "the art and science of helping adults learn" (p. 43), as opposed to pedagogy, "the art and science of teaching children" (p. 43). He eventually came to view andragogy and pedagogy as two ends of a spectrum, where pedagogy represented a dependent learner and andragogy an independent learner, regardless of the learners' ages.

Knowles developed assumptions regarding the characteristics of adult learners (Merriam, Caffarella, & Baumgartner, 2007). These assumptions, the core of andragogy, are different from the assumptions undergirding pedagogy. Knowles asserted that as individuals mature they,

1. Move from being dependent to being self-directed;
2. Gather vast experiences that influence their learning, and attach more meaning to learning from experience than from learning passively;
3. Become ready to learn when they realize the need to deal with real-life problems; and
4. Want to be able to apply their learning immediately (Knowles, 1980). Later Knowles (2005) added two more assumptions:
5. Adults need to know why they need to learn before they undertake the task of learning, and
6. Internal motivators for learning are more potent than external ones.

Self-Directedness in Physicians

Physician self-directedness has been recognized as an essential skill if physicians are to maintain competence and improve quality (Jennett, Jones, Mast, Egan, & Hotvedt, 1994). SDL is not only a hallmark of best practice in professional education; it is one of the most effective methods for improving physician performance (Kaufman & Mann, 2010; Mamary & Charles, 2003).

Moore (2008) synthesized the processes that physicians progress through when they engage in learning into five learning stages. These stages are

1. Recognizing the learning opportunity,
2. Searching for resources,
3. Engaging in learning to have an opportunity to improve,
4. Testing what was learned, and
5. Incorporating that learning into practice.

Self-Directed Patients

With the emergence of the patient-centered medical home and patient-centered care, the prescriptive days of a physician telling a passive patient what to do are rapidly fading into history. Both health care systems and the healthcare professionals who work within them, have come to realize that they really can't tell a patient to "do" anything (Funnell, 2000). The motivation to change, to take medication, or to do something different must come from within each individual patient (Funnell, 2000). The patient must not only be at the center of their health care, they must be actively involved in learning about and managing their health issues. Patients must develop the ability to be self-directed.

Self-directed learners take responsibility for their own learning. Whether a physician or a patient, when self-directed learners determine if they need to learn theywill seek out the resources that they need in order to accomplish their goal. There are few other life issues that demand such attentiveness as understanding and making decisions about one's health (Valente, 2011).

Self-directed individuals are increasingly turning to the Internet as a source of information about their health or the health of a family member. This fact is supported by The Pew Research Center's Internet & American Life Project, which has shown that more patients and their caregivers are accessing online resources, search engines, and social networks to get answers to their health questions and then acting on the information they find (Pew Research Center, 2015). For example, in one of the Project's surveys participants were asked if the online information they found concerning a health question indicated the need to consult a medical professional (Fox & Duggan, 2013). Forty-six percent of the respondents indicated that this was the case, while 38% determined that what they found was something they could manage at home. Of the 46% of respondents who consulted a medical professional, 41% stated that the medical professional confirmed what they had determined based on their own research.

Valente (2011) found that issues relating to heredity, age, and an awareness of the relationship between health and mortality motivated older adults to take greater control of their health through SDL. Another motivating factor for older adults to engage in SDL was the recognition of a correlation between independence and health (Valente, 2011). Other studies have shown that adults engage in SDL to learn about their diagnosis, identify resources related to their own condition or that of a person/child they are caring for, discover possible treatment alternatives, manage or learn more about medications, and as preparation for discussions with their physician (Fox & Duggan, 2013; Fox, Duggan, & Purcell, 2013; King, 2014; Rager, 2003).

A health event is typically the trigger which begins the self-directed learning cycle for the adult patient or caregiver (Valente, 2011). The cycle may start with the individual first accessing information on the Internet or by seeking out a health professional (Fox & Duggan, 2013; Valente, 2011). What follows is a process of learning and collaboration between the patient/caregiver and the health professional as information is acquired, treatment options discussed and assessed, and adjustments made to care (Valente, 2011).

Self-Directedness and Information Literacy

The ability to be a self-directed learner requires a degree of information literacy. In an era where the world is literally at our fingertips, being information literate is an essential skill for navigating the world. Information literate people do not drown in the flood of data surrounding them, but know how to find, evaluate, and use information – whether the information comes from the Internet, a book, a film, or any other possible resource –to make a decision or solve a problem (ACLR, 1989).

Information literate people know what resources to use when they want specific information (Norman & Skinner, 2006). These are the people who have learned how to learn (ACLR, 1989). Information literate people develop search strategies, execute them, and then filter the results to gain the knowledge they need (Norman & Skinner, 2006). If one considers the World Wide Web as a vast library of information with over 8 billion resources, knowing how to develop and execute a search for information and then knowing how that information is organized becomes a critical skill (Norman & Skinner, 2006). Information literate people are prepared to be lifelong learners because they know where to find the information they need for any task or any decision (ACLR, 1989).

Becoming an information literate patient means developing the skills to find health information and analyze the source of the information (Henwood, Wyatt, Hart, & Smith, 2003). The next step is being able to communicate the results of the information search to a healthcare professional (Henwood et al., 2003). Self-directedness and information literacy are necessary steps toward health literacy.

FROM INFORMATION LITERACY TO HEALTH INFORMATION LITERACY

Health literacy has been defined as "the degree to which individuals have the capacity to obtain, process, and understand basic health information and services needed to make appropriate health decisions" (Ratzan & Parker, 2000, p. vi). Being health literate allows patients to navigate their way through the healthcare system (including filling out complex forms and locating providers and services); understand mathematical concepts such as probability and risk; share personal information, such as health history, with their healthcare provider; and engage in self-care and chronic-disease management (US Department of Health and Human Services, n.d.). Being health literate is an important aspect to maintaining good health.

A study of health literacy in adults found that the majority of U. S. adults (53%) have intermediate health literacy skills and approximately 36% have basic or below basic skills (Kutner, Greenberg, Jin, & Paulsen, 2006). Only 12% of U.S. adults have proficient health literacy skills (Kutner et al., 2006). Research has shown that low health literacy skills are associated with higher mortality, increased hospitalizations, poorer self-management of chronic diseases, less effective communication between doctor and patient, and overall poorer outcomes (Bostock & Steptoe, 2012; Busch, Martin, DeWalt, & Sandler, 2015; DeWalt, Berkman, Sheridan, Lohr, & Pignone, 2004; Mitchell, Sadikova, Jack, & Paasche-Orlow, 2012).

As patients are asked to assume more responsibility for their own health care, health literacy problems have grown (Ratzan & Parker, 2000). Even people with advanced literary skills can be overwhelmed when faced with health literacy tasks, such as being familiar with a medical term, understanding how their body works, needing to interpret numbers or risks to make a health related decision, or facing a serious illness or condition that requires complicated self-care (US Department of Health and Human Services, 2008).

Over one-third of people have trouble reading and understanding basic medical information (Kutner et al., 2006). When engaging patients, it is important for the physician to ensure that the patient has a sufficient level of knowledge and understanding so that they can make informed decisions regarding their health care (AAFP, 2011). Effective use of technology can aid physicians in helping their patients to become more health literate.

Technology can improve health literacy (Scher, 2012). It allows information to be delivered to a patient in a way they can understand. Patients can receive customized information in their native language, with complete illustrations regarding disease management, patient education, instructions for medications or caregiving, and appointment information all as a result of advancements in technology (Scher, 2012).

Computer programs and mobile apps also help improve health literacy. Patient can go online to learn how to count calories or check the fat content of their food. The Plain Language Medical Dictionary (www.lib.umich.edu/plain-language-dictionary) allows a patient to select a complicated medical term and obtain its definition in clear, concise, non-technical English (Malpani, 2012). Another free app, WebMD (http://www.webmd.com) contains a first-aid guide, a symptom checker for common diseases, and an extensive database of drug information with warnings about possible adverse drug interactions (Malpani, 2012).

TECHNOLOGY'S IMPACT ON THE MEDICAL ENCOUNTER

EHRs and consumer e-health tools are changing the way patients and physicians interact with each other (Ricciardi, Mostashari, Murphy, Daniel, & Siminerio, 2013). Patients are using technology to speed up the discovery of information and sharpen the questions they might ask their physician during an office visit (Fox & Jones, 2009). In one survey on the use of technology, 66% of patients looked online for information on a specific medical program or disease, while 55% looked for information on a certain medical procedure or treatment (Fox & Jones, 2009). Secure email platforms give patients a faster way to ask questions of their physician or another member of the health care team (Ernst, 2013). Patients today use technology to manage their health, access their medical records, and perform a variety of health-related tasks.

Physicians routinely search for clinical information online, use Web-based medical records, and communicate with colleagues and patients through secure Web-based platforms (Silverman, 2012). Technology has provided physicians with a foundation for smart, personalized health management systems that allow for discreet physiological monitoring, early event detection, point-of-care diagnosis, and minimally invasive therapies (Lymberis, 2005). The ability to interact with patients online, both prior to and after the office visits, has the potential to improve and deepen medical care (Silverman, 2012).

Computers in the Exam Room

The use of EHRs introduces a third party into the physician-patient relationship, the computer. The use of computer technology and EHRs hold promise for the delivery of better patient care; however the computer is just one more tool in the toolbox that physicians use to care for their patients. Like any tool, it must be used effectively to accomplish the goal for which it was intended.

The heart and art of medicine rests on a foundation of strong doctor-patient communication (Ha, Anat, & Longnecker, 2010). The introduction of the computer to capture patient data during the medical encounter has been found to impact effective communication by disrupting the postural, verbal, and visual interaction between the patient and the physician (Frankel et al., 2005). While computers can improve the accuracy and quality of the information gathered during the medical encounter, clinicians and patients must figure out how to maintain a personal connection when the computer becomes part of the physician-patient relationship (Frankel et al., 2005).

The way physicians use computers in the exam room can have a negative effect on patient-centered care by decreasing the quality of the dialogue between the physician and the patient (Margalit, Roter, Dunevant, Larson, & Reis, 2003). Training physicians on how to effectively use EHRs would overcome the distance created by the computer (Margalit et al., 2003). It has been shown that once physicians have been trained on the use of computers in the exam room, patient satisfaction scores increased as communication improved (Nagy & Kanter, 2007). In many studies the use of EHRs has been shown to have a positive impact on patient outcomes (O'Connor et al., 2011; Reed et al., 2012).

Examples of successful use of EHR technology exist. In a study of patients with diabetes, EHR use was associated with improvements in control among patients whose diabetes was not well controlled and in less testing among those patients who were already meeting recommended guideline targets (Reed et al., 2012). In another study, the use of clinical support tools embedded in the EHR resulted in glucose control and some aspects of blood pressure control in patients with diabetes (O'Connor et al., 2011). It is thought that a collaborative approach to using the EHR could enhance shared-decision making and empower patients to participate in their own care (Margalit et al., 2003).

Beyond the EHR, there are also computer programs which can assist physicians in providing better information to patients and improve their health literacy in the process. For example, drawMD (www.drawMD.com) is an IPad app containing a library of anatomical images and drawing templates. Physicians use the app to provide better explanations of conditions or procedures to their patients in a simple, interactive way, eliminating medical jargon and bridging language and understanding barriers (Malpani, 2012). AliveCor's (http://www.alivecor.com) Heart Monitor app turns a smartphone into a one-lead ECG through electrodes contained on the back of the phone's case to monitor a patient for an irregular heartbeat, while the SpiroSmart app (available for download in both the iPhone and android app store), developed at the University of Washington, uses the phone's built-in microphone and lip reverberations to assess lung function (Lippman, 2013).

Smart phones and tablets are changing the way physicians and patients collaborate in the treatment and management of disease. An annual market research study (Manhattan Research, 2014) focused on how physicians in the U.S. use digital media, mobile devices, the Internet and other technologies to provide patient care found that 47% of physicians have used a smart phone to show images or videos to their patients and more than one-third recommend a health app to a patient. In addition, one in five physicians surveyed stated they monitor patients remotely (Manhattan Research, 2014).

Physician use of mobile technology in the exam room has had a positive influence over patients. One study (Comstock, 2013) found that patients whose physicians use mobile apps during the patient encounter were more likely to use apps themselves. This same study revealed that 33% of study participants stated that either they or their physicians accessed a mobile device at the point of care. The right app, and the associated behavior change, provide for a more personalized physician-patient connection that can extend beyond the exam room (Hoaglin, 2014).

Beyond the Exam Room

Mobile technology has allowed physicians to continue to care for their patients even outside of the office. In one program, patients with congestive heart failure used telehealth (the use of electronic information and telecommunications technologies) to engage inhome monitoring of blood pressure, weight, pulse oximetry and heart rate (Kulshreshtha, Kvedar, Goyal, Halpern, & Watson, 2010). Data was uploaded daily and decision support software alerted physicians to patients who needed attention. As a result of this program, hospital admissions dropped by 44% compared with usual care. Another program called Care Coordination/Home Telehealth (Veterans Health Administration) integrated health informatics with home telemonitoring and disease management. The result was a 25% reduction in the number of days patients spent in bed and a 19% reduction in the number of hospital admissions compared to usual care (Darkins et al., 2009).

Many physicians prescribe apps for their patients to help them with managing their health and promote health behavior change (Hoaglin, 2014; Lippman, 2013). Today there are health apps that allow smartphones to act like a medical device, helping patients manage their diabetes or monitor their heart rate (Hoaglin, 2014; Malpani, 2012). It is projected that in 2015, 500 million smartphone users worldwide will be using a health-related app, and by 2017 that number is expected to grow to 26 billion (MIT Technology Review, 2014).

Patients in turn are sharing the data they collect through mobile apps with their doctors. In one study (Manhattan Research, 2013) 70% of physicians reported at least one patient who was providing self-monitoring data, and 75% agreed that self-monitoring led to better patient outcomes. Evidence is growing which supports the use of e-health technology to improve heath and increase patient engagement (Ricciardi et al., 2013).

E-health is helping children cope with chronic illness through educational games which help them learn about their disease and manage it more effectively. A video game designed to empower young cancer patients to fight their disease and stick with their prescribed treatment resulted in 41% higher levels of chemotherapy and a 16% higher use of antibiotics among the game's users (Pogorelc, 2013). These same patients also demonstrated better quality of life, improved knowledge about cancer, and higher belief in their ability to beat the disease (Pogorelc, 2013). Children playing a video game designed to help them better manage their diabetes showed a 77% decrease in diabetes-related emergency and critical care visits than did children in the control group (Kato, 2010).

Disease management apps can have a major impact on patient-physicians communication. Rather than trying to answer the question about how they have been feeling during the 15-minute office visit, the patient can now record and show their physician the patterns and features of their everyday life, such as physical activity, diet, quantity and quality of sleep, mood, etc. (Hostetter, 2011). Medical apps extend healthcare outside of the exam room and into people's lives by encouraging people to actively manage their care and partner with their physicians (Hostetter, 2011).

ENGAGING PATIENTS IN THEIR OWN CARE

The first step in engaging patients in their own care is to educate them about their disease based on their needs (Funnell, 2000). Patients want to know how the disease is going to affect them personally. Funnell (2000) stated that the four most important lessons for a physicians to teach are:

1. Helping the patient understand that they do have a problem and it needs to be taken seriously,
2. The patient is in control of managing their illness,
3. The patient has many options for treating their condition and only he or she can decide if the benefits of a certain treatment outweigh the cost, and
4. The patient can change their behavior by setting goals, taking the first steps forward, and figuring out what they are learning about themselves along the way.

Once patients are educated and feel they have more control over their condition, they will be better prepared to take a more active role in their health care. Growing evidence supports the premise that patients who are more involved in their care have better outcomes while incurring lower costs (James, 2013). Shared decision making and patient activation empower patients to be involved.

Shared Decision Making

The concept of shared decision making (SDM) has its roots in a 1982 Presidential Commission Report on ethics in medicine. The report states:

... the Commission sees "informed consent" as an ethical obligation that involves a process of shared decision making based upon the mutual respect and participation of patients and health professionals. Only through improved communication can we establish a firm footing for the trust that patients place in those who provide their health care (President's Commission for the Study of Ethical Problems in Medicine and Biomedical and Behavioral Research, 1982, p. 5).

Sharing decisions between the physician and patient helps ensure that medical care aligns with the patient's values and preferences in situations where there is not one superior course of treatment (Lee & Emanuel, 2013). While the principles of SDM are promoted, the actual practice of SDM lags behind despite the development of numerous patient aids and efforts to support their adoption (Alston et al., 2014).

One reason for this lag in adoption could be the fact that SDM may be a difficult concept for some patients to grasp. Throughout much of history, patients have left health care decisions to the physician whom they trusted (King, 2014). To not do so might insult the physician and leave the patient exposed to criticism from his or her social circle (King, 2014). While sharing knowledge may be perceived to decrease the physician' power, better informed patients could result in a better relationship between doctor and patient and better compliance with treatment plans (Benigeri & Pluye, 2003). The Informed Medical Decisions Foundation states SDM "...honors both the provider's expert knowledge and the patient's right to be fully informed of all care options and the potential harms and benefits" (Informed Medical Decision Making Foundation, 2015, p. para 2).

SDM provides the entire healthcare team, which includes the patient, with many benefits. Among the benefits offered by SDM are greater alignment with patient values, reductions in unnecessary care and costs, reduction in the anxiety associated with the care process, and increased patient knowledge (Lee & Emanuel, 2013). The process of SDM gives patients the support they need to make care decisions that are individualized, while allowing clinicians to feel certain they are prescribing the correct care (Informed Medical Decision Making Foundation, 2015).

The collaborative use of EHR between the physician and patient has the potential to improve shared decision making and involve the patient in their care (Margalit et al., 2003). For example, when patients can input their treatment preferences or concerns into their health record before an appointment their physician can address those issues and in turn provide more individualize care (Ernst, 2013). EHRs used to track patient data allow decision making that is more relevant to the patient (Ernst, 2013). EHRs can identify a patient who is likely to have to make a health decision and facilitate the process of providing information and decision support prior to the patient visit so that the patient is more prepared to talk with their physician (Ernst, 2013).

Patient Activation

Patients must begin to take an active and responsible role in their health care. They must be pro-active in collecting and analyzing information that will help them to make informed decisions about their health care (King, 2014). Patient activation, defined as patients who have the knowledge, skills, and confidence to manage their own heath, is directly related to patient outcomes (Greene & Hibbard, 2011). Studies have shown that older adults who were actively involved in their health care through self-directed learning felt more aware and more sensitive toward their health and the services they received (Valente, 2011). In addition, these adults had more collaborative relationships with their health care professionals which led to treatment plans that worked best for the individual.

Technology can play a large role in patient activation. Using text messaging, interactive websites, and other social media platforms, physicians can provide their patients with instant information and receive feedback from them (Roundtree, Dorsten, & Rief, 2011). They can offer their patients reinforcement and support through the creation of like-minded communities (Roundtree et al., 2011). Patient portals, secure messaging, clinical health summaries, Internet-based resources, self-management tools, decision aids, and mobile applications all provide opportunities to engage both patients and caregivers (HealthIT.gov, 2013).

Active patients are informed patients. However, it may be up to the physician to draw out whether the patient has searched for information in an effort to become more informed. Henwood, Wyatt, Hart, and Smith (2003), researching the factors that facilitate or inhibit an informed patient, found that among the more informed women in the study (those who took steps to learn all they could about their symptoms and possible treatments), there was concern about over-stepping the boundary between physician and patient. The authors found that among the women there was a clear distinction between becoming informed about a condition and feeling able or prepared to disclose what they had learned to their physician (Henwood et al., 2003).

Despite the availability of tools and resources, patient activation levels vary. The Patient Activation Measure (PAM) measures a patient's confidence, belief, and skill for managing their health care (Greene & Hibbard, 2011). Patients at the high end of the PAM scale are engaged and proactive about their health and will follow recommended health behaviors whereas patients at the low end of the scale are usually passive and do not think there is a need for them to play an active role in their care (Greene & Hibbard, 2011). Once physicians understand their patients' level of activation, they can tailor action plans that make sense for the patient (Kamajian, 2014).

EHR data has shown that patients who were more activated had better clinical indicators (Greene & Hibbard, 2011). They were less likely to have been hospitalized or use the emergency department, were less likely to have a high BMI or to smoke, and were more likely to have received preventive care (Greene & Hibbard, 2011). Parchman, Zeber and Palmer (2010) found that participatory (or shared) decision making between the physician and the patient resulted in patient activation, which in turn resulted in improved medication adherence, and control of blood glucose and lipid levels.

It has been shown that greater patient support leads to improved activation (Greene, Hibbard, and, & Overton, 2013). It has also been shown that patients with a higher level of activation report more positive health care experiences than patients with lower levels of activation, even though both were seeing the same physician (Greene et al., 2013). The evidence clearly supports the fact that patients who are engaged in their care have better health care experiences and improved outcomes (Greene & Hibbard, 2011; Greene et al., 2013; Parchman et al., 2010; Valente, 2011).

CONCLUSION

The medical record has evolved through the centuries, always with the patient present in the narrative. Though there was a time when data overshadowed the voice of the patient, the introduction of the electronic health record combined with health care reform and advances in technology has brought the patient back to the center of the medical record. Health IT and the continued growth of the Internet have allowed patients to access their medical records online and physicians and other health care professionals are better able to use EHRs to provide improved patient care (Benigeri & Pluye, 2003).

Consumer e-health tools, such as mobile apps or secure e-mail messaging, along with the expansion of health information technology have created new ways for patients to actively direct and monitor their healthcare (Ricciardi et al., 2013). When patients have the electronic tools to access their health information they are better able to fully participate in their care, coordinate care across multiple providers, self-manage their conditions, and improve communication with their care teams (Ricciardi et al., 2013).

Early research in the field of e-health indicates that both physicians and patients support technology to improve patient care and prefer using computers to share information with one and other (Ricciardi et al., 2013). Through the Internet, patients have access to health education and self-management resources (Kvedar, Coye, & Everett, 2014). They can obtain coaching or personal education materials and participate in online support groups or discussions (Kvedar et al., 2014). Telemedicine, e-health, and asynchronous physician-patient communication create a model of connected care that has the ability to improve access to health care, improve quality, and decrease costs (Darkins et al., 2009).

REFERENCES

AAFP. (2011). *Recommended curriculum guidelines for family medicine residents: Patient education AAFP Reprint No. 284*. Leawood, KS: American Academy of Family Physicians.

Abdullah, M. H. (2001). *Self-Directed Learning. ERIC Digest. (Vol. ED459458)*. Bloomington, IN: ERIC Clearinghouse on Reading English and Communication, Indiana University.

ACLR. (1989). Presidential Committee on information literacy: Final Report. *Association of College and Research Libraries: Publications*. Retrieved from http://www.ala.org/acrl/publications/whitepapers/presidential

ACRL. (2014). What is information literacy. *Association of College and Research Libraries: Introducation to Information Literacy*. Retrieved from http://www.ala.org/acrl/issues/infolit/overview/intro

Alston, C., Berger, Z. D., Brownlee, S., Elwyn, G., Fowler, F. J., Hall, L. K., et al. (2014). *Shared decision-making strategies for best care: Patient decision aids (Discussion Paper)*. Washington, DC: Institute of Medicine.

Andreassen, H. K., & Nilsen, L. L. (2013). User interface and patient involvement. In J. Mantas & A. Hasman (Eds.), Studies in health technology and informatics, Volume 190: informatics, management and technology in healthcare (pp. 21-23). Amsterdam: IOS Press.

Bailey, J. E. (2011). Does health information technology dehumanize health care? *The Virtual Mentor, 13*(3). Retrieved from http://virtualmentor.ama-assn.org/2011/03/msoc1-1103.html PMID:23127322

Benigeri, M., & Pluye, P. (2003). Shortcomings of health information on the Internet. *Health Promotion Journal, 18*(4), 381–386. doi:10.1093/heapro/dag409 PMID:14695369

Bostock, S., & Steptoe, A. (2012). Association between low functional health literacy and mortality in older adults: longitudinal cohort study. *BMJ, 344*, e1602. doi: 10.1136/bmj.e1602

Brockett, R. G., & Donaghy, R. C. (2005). *Beyond The Inquiring Mind: Cyril Houle's connection to self-directed learning*. Paper presented at The Adult Education Research Conference (AERC). Retrieved from http://www.adulterc.org/proceedings/2005/proceedings/brockett.pdf

Brockett, R. G., & Hiemstra, R. (1991). Self-direction in adult learning: Perspectives on theory, research, and practice. Retrieved from http://www-distance.syr.edu/sdlindex.html

Brookfield, S. (1986). *Understanding and faciliating adult learning: A comprehensive anyalsis of principles and effective practices*. San Francisco: Jossey-Bass.

Busch, E. L., Martin, C., DeWalt, D. A., & Sandler, R. S. (2015). Functional health literacy, chemotherapy decisions, and outcomes among a colorectal cancer cohort. *Cancer Control, 22*(1), 95–101. PMID:25504283

Camp, C. L., Smoot, R. L., Kolettis, T. N., Groenewald, C. B., Greenlee, S. M., & Farley, D. R. (2008). Patient records at Mayo Clinic: Lessons learned from the first 100 patients in Dr Henry S. Plummer's Dossier Model. *Mayo Clinic Proceedings*, *83*(12), 1396–1399. doi:10.4065/83.12.1396 PMID:19046561

Candy, P. C. (1991). *Self-direction for lifelong learning: A comprehensive guide to theory and practice*. San Francisco, CA: Jossey-Bass Publishers.

Candy, P. C. (1995). Physician teach thyself: The place of self-directed learning in continuing medical education. *The Journal of Continuing Education in the Health Professions*, *15*(2), 80–90. doi:10.1002/chp.4750150204

Chaudhry, B., Wang, J., Wu, S., Maglione, M., Mojica, W., & Roth, E. et al. (2006). Systematic review: Impact of health information technology on quality, efficiency, and costs of medical care. *Annals of Internal Medicine*, *144*(10), 742–752. doi:10.7326/0003-4819-144-10-200605160-00125 PMID:16702590

CMS.gov. (2012). Electronic Health Records. Retrieved from http://www.cms.gov/Medicare/E-Health/EHealthRecords/index.html

Comstock, J. (2013). Digitas Health: Patients whose doctors use apps use more apps themselves. Retrieved from http://mobihealthnews.com/26642/digitas-patients-whose-doctors-use-apps-use-more-apps-themselves

Confessore, S. J., & Kops, W. J. (1998). Self-directed learning and the learning organization: Examining the connection between the individual and the learning environment. *Human Resource Development Quarterly*, *9*(4), 365–375. doi:10.1002/hrdq.3920090407

Craig, B. L. (1990). Hospital records and record-keeping, C. 1850 - C. 1950, Part II: The development of record-keeping in hospitals. *Archivaria*, *30*(Summer), 21–38. PMID:11616608

Darkins, A., Ryan, P., Kobb, R., Foster, L., Edmonson, E., Wakefield, B., & Lancaster, A. E. (2009). Care coordination/home telehealth: The systematic implementation of health informatics, home telehealth, and disease management to support the care of veteran patients with chronic conditions. *Telemedicine Journal and e-Health*, *14*(10), 1118–1126. doi:10.1089/tmj.2008.0021 PMID:19119835

DeWalt, D. A., Berkman, N. D., Sheridan, S., Lohr, K. N., & Pignone, M. P. (2004). Literacy and Health Outcomes. *Journal of General Internal Medicine*, *19*(12), 1228–1239. doi:10.1111/j.1525-1497.2004.40153.x PMID:15610334

Dynan, L., Cate, T., & Rhee, K. (2008). The impact of learning structure on students' readiness for self-directed learning. *Journal of Education for Business*, *84*(2), 96–100. doi:10.3200/JOEB.84.2.96-100

Ernst, A. (2013). *Shared decision making: Engaging patients to improve health care Health Systems Reform*. Washington, DC: Families USA.

Fenwick, T., & Tennant, M. (2004). Understanding adult learners. In G. Foley (Ed.), *Dimensions of adult learning: Adult education and training in a global era* (pp. 55–73). Berkshire, England: Open University Press.

Fitzmaurice, J. M., Adams, K., & Eisenberg, J. M. (2002). Three decades of research on computer applications in health care: Medical informatics support at the Agency for Healthcare Research and Quality. *Journal of the American Medical Informatics Society*, *9*(2), 144–160. doi:10.1197/jamia.M0867 PMID:11861630

Fox, S., & Duggan, M. (2013). Health Online 2013. *Pew Research Internet Project.* Retrieved from http://www.pewinternet.org/2013/01/15/health-online-2013/

Fox, S., Duggan, M., & Purcell, K. (2013). Family caregivers are wired for health. *Pew Research Internet Project.* Retrieved from http://www.pewinternet.org/2013/06/20/family-caregivers-are-wired-for-health/

Fox, S., & Jones, S. (2009). The social life of health information. *Pew Internet and American Life Project.* Retrieved from http://www.pewinternet.org/files/old-media/Files/Reports/2009/PIP_Health_2009.pdf

Frankel, R., Altschuler, A., George, S., Kinsman, J., Jimison, H., Robertson, N. R., & Hsu, J. (2005). Effects of exam-room computing on clinician-patient communication: A longitudinal qualitative study. *Journal of General Internal Medicine*, *20*(8), 677–682. doi:10.1111/j.1525-1497.2005.0163.x PMID:16050873

Funnell, M. M. (2000). Helping patients take charge of their chronic illnesses. *Family Practice Management*, *7*(3), 47–51. PMID:10947289

Garrison, D. R. (1997). Self-directed learning: Toward a comprehensive model. *Adult Education Quarterly*, *48*(1), 18–33. doi:10.1177/074171369704800103

Gillum, R. F. (2013). From papyrus to the electronic tablet: A brief history of the clinical medical record with lessons for the digital age. *The American Journal of Medicine*, *126*(10), 853–857. doi:10.1016/j.amjmed.2013.03.024 PMID:24054954

Greene, J., & Hibbard, J. H. (2011). Why does patient activation matter? An examination of the relationships between patient activation and health-related outcomes. *Journal of General Internal Medicine*, *27*(5), 520–526. doi:10.1007/s11606-011-1931-2 PMID:22127797

Greene, J., Hibbard, J. H., Sacks, R., & Overton, V. (2013). When seeing the same physician, highly activated patients have better care experiences than less activated patients. *Health Affairs*, *32*(7), 1299–1305. doi:10.1377/hlthaff.2012.1409 PMID:23836747

Grow, G. O. (1991). Teaching learners to be self-directed. *Adult Education Quarterly*, *41*(3), 125–149. doi:10.1177/0001848191041003001

Guglielmino, L. M. (1977). Development of the self-directed learning readiness scale [Ed.D]. University of Georgia, Athens, Georgia. Proquest Dissertations and Theses database. (7806004)

Ha, J. F., Anat, D. S., & Longnecker, N. (2010). Doctor-patient communication: A review. *The Ochsner Journal*, *10*(1), 38–43. PMID:21603354

Health, I. T. gov. (2013). Using e-health tools to engage patients and caregivers. Retrieved from http://www.healthit.gov/sites/default/files/nlc_using_e-healthtools.pdf

Health, I. T. gov. (2014). Improved diagnostics & patient outcomes. *Benefits of EHRs.* Retrieved from http://www.healthit.gov/providers-professionals/improved-diagnostics-patient-outcomes

Healthwise. (2015). What is shared decision making? Retrieved from http://www.informedmedicaldecisions.org/what-is-shared-decision-making/

Henwood, F., Wyatt, S., Hart, A., & Smith, J. (2003). 'Ignorance is bliss sometimes': Constraints on the emergence of the 'informed patient' in the changing landscapes of health information. *Sociology of Health & Illness*, *25*(6), 589–607. doi:10.1111/1467-9566.00360 PMID:12919447

Hiemstra, R. (1994). Self-directed learning. In T. Husen & T. N. Postlethwaite (Eds.), *The international encyclopedia of education* (2nd ed., pp. 1–11). Oxford: Pergamon Press. Retrieved from http://ccnmtl.columbia.edu/projects/pl3p/Self-Directed%20Learning.pdf

Hiemstra, R. (2003). More than three decades of self-directed learning: From whence have we come? *Adult Learning*, *14*(4), 5–8.

Hoaglin, M. (2014). Prescribing an easier pill to swallow with apps. Retrieved from http://www.practicefusion.com/blog/prescribing-easier-pill-swallow-apps/

Hostetter, M. (2011). Health care quality improvement: There's an app for that. *Quality Matters, October/November*. Retrieved from http://www.commonwealthfund.org/publications/newsletters/quality-matters/2011/october-november-2011/in-focus#/3

Houle, C. O. (1961). *The inquiring mind.* Madison, WI: The University of Wisconsin Press.

HRSA.gov. (n.d.). Telehealth. Retrieved from http://www.hrsa.gov/ruralhealth/about/telehealth/

Hummel, J., & Evans, P. (2012). Standardizing the problem list in the ambulatory electronic health record to improve patient care. Department of Health and Human Services.

Informed Medical Decision Making Foundation. (2015). What is shared decision making. Retrieved from http://www.informedmedicaldecisions.org/what-is-shared-decision-making/

Institute of Medicine. (2001). *Crossing the quality chasm: a new health system for the 21st century.* Washington, D.C.: National Academy of Sciences.

James, J. (2013). Patient engagement. People actively involved in their health and health care tend to have better outcomes—and, some evidence suggests, lower costs *Health Policy Brief. Health Affairs.*

Jennett, P., Jones, D., Mast, T., Egan, K., & Hotvedt, M. (1994). The charateristics of self-directed learning. In D. Davis & R. Fox (Eds.), *The physician as learner: Linking research to practice* (pp. 47–65). Chicago: American Medical Association.

Kamajian, S. D. (2014). Patient activation for population health: Shifting from a fee-for-service model toward a proactive, preventive approach with increased engagement. *Osteopathic Family Physician*, *6*(4), 28–31.

Kato, P. M. (2010). Video games in health care: Closing the gap. *Review of General Psychology*, *14*(2), 113–121. doi:10.1037/a0019441

Kaufman, D. M., & Mann, K. V. (2010). Teaching and learning in medical practice: how theory can inform practice. In T. Swanwick (Ed.), *Understanding medical education: Evidence, theory and practice* (pp. 16–36). Hoboken, NJ: Wieley-Blackwell. doi:10.1002/9781444320282.ch2

Kernisan, L. (2013). The problem-oriented medical record. Retrieved from http://thehealthcareblog.com/blog/2013/05/10/the-problem-oriented-medical-record/

King, K. P. (2014). A journey with chronic pain: Self-directed learning as survival. *New Horizons in Adult Education and Human Resource Development*, *26*(2), 5–18. doi:10.1002/nha3.20059

Knowles, M. S. (1975). *Self-directed learning: a guide for learners and teachers*. New York, NY: Association Press.

Knowles, M. S. (1980). *The modern practice of adult education: From pedagogy to andragogy* (Rev. ed.). Englewood Cliffs, NJ: Prentice Hall Regents.

Knowles, M. S., Holton, E. F., & Swanson, R. A. (2005). *The Adult Learner* (6th ed.). Burlington, MA: Elisevier.

Kulshreshtha, A., Kvedar, J. C., Goyal, A., Halpern, E. F., & Watson, A. J. (2010). Use of remote monitoring to improve outcomes in patients with heart failure: A pilot trial. *International Journal of Telemedicine and Applications*, *2010*, 1–7. doi:10.1155/2010/870959 PMID:20508741

Kutner, M., Greenberg, E., Jin, Y., & Paulsen, C. (2006). *The health literacy of America's adults: Results from the 2003 national assessment of adult literacy (NCES 2006–483)*. Washington, DC: National Center for Education Statistics.

Kvedar, J., Coye, M. J., & Everett, W. (2014). Connected health: A review of technologies and strategies to improve patient care with telemedicine and telehealth. *Health Affairs*, *33*(2), 194–199. doi:10.1377/hlthaff.2013.0992

Lee, E. O., & Emanuel, E. J. (2013). Shared decision making to improve care and reduce costs. *The New England Journal of Medicine*, *368*(1), 6–8. doi:10.1056/NEJMp1209500 PMID:23281971

Lippman, H. (2013). How apps are changing family medicine. *Clinician Reviews, 23*(9), 26-31. Retrieved from http://www.clinicianreviews.com/the-publication/past-issues-single-view/how-apps-are-changing-family-medicine/a4b9f63c03dd833345dc1421a2274c53.html

Lymberis, A. (2005). Smart personalized health systems: From gadgets to better health. In C. D. Nugent, P. J. McCullagh, E. T. McAdams, & A. Lymberis (Eds.), Personalized health management systems (Vol. 117, pp. 1-5). Amsterdam: IOS Press. Retrieved from ProQuest ebrary.

Malpani, A. (2012). Using technology to promote health literacy. Retrieved from http://healthworkscollective.com/malpani/61901/using-technology-promote-health-literacy

Mamary, E., & Charles, P. (2003). Promoting self-directed learning for continuing medical education. *Medical Teacher*, *25*(2), 188–190. doi:10.1080/0142159031000092607 PMID:12745529

Manhattan Research. (2013). New Study Reveals That Physicians Embrace Patient Self-Tracking *Taking the Pulse® U.S. 2013*. Retrieved from http://manhattanresearch.com/News-and-Events/Press-Releases/physicians-embrace-patient-self-tracking

Manhattan Research. (2014). Stethoscopes and Smartphones: Physicians Turn to Digital Tools to Boost Patient Outcomes *Taking the Pulse® U.S. 2014*. Retrieved from http://manhattanresearch.com/News-and-Events/Press-Releases/Digital-Tools-to-Boost-Patient-052914

Margalit, R. S., Roter, D., Dunevant, M. A., Larson, S., & Reis, S. (2003). Electronic medical record use and physician–patient communication: An observational study of Israeli primary care encounters. *Patient Education and Counseling*, *61*(1), 134–141. doi:10.1016/j.pec.2005.03.004 PMID:16533682

Merriam, S. B., Caffarella, R. S., & Baumgartner, L. M. (2007). *Learning in Adulthood: A comprehensive guide* (3rd ed.). San Francisco: Jossey-Bass.

MIT Technology Review. (2014). Mobile medical apps: A market on the mov. Retrieved from http://www.technologyreview.com/view/532661/mobile-medical-apps-a-market-on-the-move/

Mitchell, S. E., Sadikova, E., Jack, B. W., & Paasche-Orlow, M. K. (2012). Health literacy and 30-day postdischarge hospital utilization. *Journal of Health Communication: International Perspectives*, *19*(suppl3). doi:10.1080/10810730.2012.715233 PMID:23030580

Moore, D. E. (2008). How physicians learn and how to design learning experiences for them: An approach based on an interpretive review of evidence. In M. Hager, S. Russell, & S. W. Fletcher (Eds.), *Continuing Education in the Health Professions* (pp. 30–62). New York, NY: Josiah Macy, Jr. Foundation.

Nagy, V. T., & Kanter, M. H. (2007). Implementing the electronic medical record in the exam room: The effect on physician-patient communication and patient satisfaction. *The Permanente Journal*, *11*(2), 21–24. PMID:21461089

NCQA. (2015). Patient-centered medical home recognition. Retrieved from www.ncqa.org

Norman, C. D., & Skinner, H. A. (2006). eHealth literacy: Essential skills for consumer health in a networked world. *Journal of Medical Internet Research*, *8*(2), e9. http://www.ncbi.nlm.nih.gov/pmc/articles/PMC1550701/?report=reader doi:10.2196/jmir.8.2.e9 PMID:16867972

O'Connor, P. J., Sperl-Hillen, J. M., Rush, W. A., Johnson, P. E., Amundson, G. H., & Asche, S. E. et al. (2011). Impact of electronic health record clinical decision support on diabetes care: A randomized trial. *Annals of Family Medicine*, *9*(1), 12–21. doi:10.1370/afm.1196 PMID:21242556

Office of the National Coordinator for Health Information Technology. (2013). *Health Information technology patient safety action & surveillance plan*. Washington, DC: Department of Health and Human Services. Retrieved from http://www.healthit.gov/sites/default/files/safety_plan_master.pdf

Olsen, L., Saunders, R. S., & McGinnis, J. M. (Eds.). (2011). *Patients charting the course: citizen engagement in the learning health system*. Washington, DC: The National Academies Press.

One Hundredth and Eleventh Congress. (2009). *American Recovery and Reinvestment Act of 2009*. Retrieved from http://www.gpo.gov/fdsys/pkg/PLAW-111publ5/pdf/PLAW-111publ5.pdf

Owen, T. R. (2002). Self-directed learning in adulthood: a literature review. ERIC - Educational Resources Information Center. (ED461050). Retrieved from http://eric.ed.gov/ERICWebPortal/search/detailmini.jsp?_nfpb=true&_&ERICExtSearch_SearchValue_0=ED461050&ERICExtSearch_SearchType_0=no&accno=ED461050

Parchman, M. L., Zeber, J. E., & Palmer, R. F. (2010). Participatory decision making, patient activation, medication adherence, and intermediate clinical outcomes in type 2 diabetes: A STARNet Study. *Annals of Family Medicine*, *8*(5), 410–417. doi:10.1370/afm.1161 PMID:20843882

Pew Research Center. (2015). Pew Research Internet Project. Retrieved from http://www.pewinternet.org/

Pogorelc, D. (2013). Cigna's healthcare gaming mission: Take a "cancer-fighting" game app global. Retrieved from http://medcitynews.com/2013/08/insurer-cignas-unlikely-mission-taking-a-cancer-fighting-game-app-global/#ixzz2g68Bt5O8

President's Commission for the Study of Ethical Problems in Medicine and Biomedical and Behavioral Research. (1982). *Making health care decisions: The ethical and legal implications of informed consent in the patient-practitioner relationship.* Washington, DC: U.S. Government Printing Office.

Rager, K. (2003). The self-directed learning of women with breast cancer. *Adult Education Quarterly*, *53*(4), 277–293. doi:10.1177/0741713603254030

Ratzan, S. C., & Parker, R. M. (2000). *Introduction, National Library of Medicine Current Bibliographies in Medicine: Health Literacy (Vol. No. CBM 2000-1).* Bethesda, MD: National Institutes of Health, U.S. Department of Health and Human Services.

Reed, M., Huang, J., Graetz, I., Brand, R., Hsu, J., Fireman, B., & Jaffe, M. (2012). Outpatient electronic health records and the clinical care and outcomes of patients with diabetes mellitus. *Annals of Internal Medicine*, *157*(7), 482–489. doi:10.7326/0003-4819-157-7-201210020-00004 PMID:23027319

Reiser, S. J. (1991a). The clinical record in medicine. Part 1: Learning from cases. *Annals of Internal Medicine*, *114*(10), 902–907. doi:10.7326/0003-4819-114-10-902 PMID:2014953

Reiser, S. J. (1991b). The clinical record in medicine. Part 2: Reforming content and purpose. *Annals of Internal Medicine*, *114*(11), 980–985. doi:10.7326/0003-4819-114-11-980 PMID:2024867

Ricciardi, B. L., Mostashari, F., Murphy, J., Daniel, J. G., & Siminerio, E. P. (2013). A national action plan To support consumer engagement via e-health. *Health Affairs*, *32*(2), 2376–2384. doi:10.1377/hlthaff.2012.1216 PMID:23381531

Rifkin, E., & Lazris, A. (2014). *Interpreting health benefits and risks: A practical guide to facilitate doctor-patient communication.* Switzerland: Springer International Publishing.

Rogers, J. L., Harring, O. M., Wortman, P. M., Waston, R. A., & Goetz, J. P. (1982). Medical information systems: Assessing impact in the areas of hypertension, obesity and renal disease. *Medical Care*, *20*(1), 63–74. doi:10.1097/00005650-198201000-00005 PMID:7078276

Roundtree, A. K., Dorsten, A., & Rief, J. J. (2011). Improving patient activation in crisis and chronic care through rhetorical approaches to new media technologies. *Poroi*, *7*(1). doi:10.13008/2151-2957.1081

Scher, D. L. (2012). Can digital health technologies improve health literacy? *The Digital Health Cornor.* Retrieved from http://davidleescher.com/2012/03/27/can-digital-health-technologies-improve-health-literacy/

Schon, D. A. (1983). *The reflective practitioner: How professionals think in action.* U.S.A.: Basic Books.

Shortliffe, E. H. (1999). The evolution of electronic health records. *Academic Medicine*, *74*(4), 414–419. doi:10.1097/00001888-199904000-00038 PMID:10219224

Siegler, E. L. (2010). The evolving medical record. *Annals of Internal Medicine, 153*(10), 671–677. doi:10.7326/0003-4819-153-10-201011160-00012 PMID:21079225

Silverman, B. C. (2012). The "medical encounter 2.0": Practicing medicine in the age of googling, friending and tweeting. *Medical Ethics (Burlington, Mass.), 19*(3), 1–2.

Spear, G. (1988). Beyond the organizing circumstance: A search for methodology for the study of self-directed learning. In H. B. Long et al. (Eds.), *Self-directed learning: application and theory* (pp. 199–221). Athens: Department of Adult Education: University of Georgia.

Street, R. L. Jr, Liu, L., Farber, N. J., Chen, Y., Calvitti, A., & Zuest, D. et al. (2014). Provider interaction with the electronic health record: The effects on patient-centered communication in medical encounters. *Patient Education and Counseling, 96*(3), 315–319. doi:10.1016/j.pec.2014.05.004 PMID:24882086

Toffler, A. (1971). *Future Shock*. New York, NY: Bantam Books.

Tough, A. (1971). *The adult's learning projects: A fresh approach to theory and practice in adult learning* (2nd ed.). Toronto: Ontario Institute for Studies in Educations.

US Department of Health and Human Services. (2008). America's Health Literacy: Why We Need Accessible Health Information An Issue Brief From the U.S. Department of Health and Human Services. Rockville, MD.

US Department of Health and Human Services. (n.d.). What is health literacy? *Quick Guide to Health Literacy*. Retrieved from http://www.health.gov/communication/literacy/quickguide/factsbasic.htm

Valente, J. S. (2011). The role of self-directed learning (SDL) in managing health care: Implications for caregivers. *The Forum, 16*(2). Retrieved from http://ncsu.edu/ffci/publications/2011/v16-n2-2011-winter/valente.php

VanFleet, D. (2010). Heath information management (HIM) history: Past to current day. Retrieved from http://www.rasmussen.edu/degrees/health-sciences/blog/health-information-management-history/

Weed, L. L. (1968). Medical records that guide and teach. *The New England Journal of Medicine, 278*(11), 593–600. doi:10.1056/NEJM196803142781105 PMID:5637758

Whiting-O'Keefe, Q. E., Simborg, D. W., Epstein, W. V., & Warger, A. (1985). A computerized summary medical record system can provide more information than the standard medical record. *Journal of the American Medical Association, 254*(9), 1185–1192. doi:10.1001/jama.1985.03360090075024 PMID:3874972

Wilkins, R. H. (1964). Neurosurgical Classic-XVII: Edwin Smith Surgical Papyrus. *Cyber Museum of Neurosurgery*. Retrieved from http://www.neurosurgery.org/cybermuseum/pre20th/epapyrus.html

World Health Organization. (2006). Constitution of the World Health Organization Basic Documents (54 Supplement 2006 ed.).

KEY TERMS AND DEFINITIONS

Agency for Healthcare Quality and Research (AHRQ): Federal agency whose mission is to produce evidence to make health care safer, higher quality, more accessible, equitable, and affordable, and to work within the U.S. Department of Health and Human Services and with other partners to make sure that the evidence is understood and used.

American Academy of Family Physicians (AAFP): The American Academy of Family Physicians is the national association of family doctors. It is one of the largest national medical organizations, with more than 115,900 members in 50 states, D.C., Puerto Rico, the Virgin Islands, and Guam, as well as internationally. The AAFP was founded in 1947 to promote and maintain high quality standards for family doctors who are providing continuing comprehensive health care to the public.

Centers for Medicare and Medicaid Services (CMS): Federal agency within the U. S. Department of Health and Human Services (DHHS) that administers the Medicare program and partners with state governments to administer Medicaid, the State Children's Health Insurance Program (SCHIP), and health insurance portability standards.

Consumer E-Health: A broad category of electronic tools and services that are primarily consumer oriented but that overlap with health information technology (Ricciardi et al., 2013).

Electronic Health Records (EHR): An electronic version of a patient's medical history maintained by the provider over time, and may include all of the key administrative clinical data relevant to that persons care under a particular provider, including demographics, progress notes, problems, medications, vital signs, past medical history, immunizations, laboratory data and radiology reports The EHR automates access to information and has the potential to streamline the clinician's workflow. The EHR also has the ability to support other care-related activities directly or indirectly through various interfaces, including evidence-based decision support, quality management, and outcomes reporting (CMS.gov, 2012).

Health Information Technology (HIT): Per the HITECH Act, "the term 'health information technology' means hardware, software, integrated technologies or related licenses, intellectual property, upgrades, or packaged solutions sold as services that are designed for or support the use by health care entities or patients for the electronic creation, maintenance, access, or exchange of health information" (111th Congress of the USA, 2009).

Information Literacy: The skills needed to find, retrieve, analyze, and use information (ACRL, 2014).

Patient Activation: Possessing the knowledge, skills, and confidence to be actively engaged in one's own health care (Greene & Hibbard, 2011).

Patient-Centered Medical Home (PCMH): The patient-centered medical home is a way of organizing primary care that emphasizes care coordination and communication to transform primary care into "what patients want it to be." Medical homes can lead to higher quality and lower costs, and can improve patients' and providers' experience of care (NCQA, 2015).

Self-Directed Learning (SDL): The process by which individuals take the initiative, with or without the help of others, in diagnosing their learning needs, formulating learning goals, identifying resources for learning, choosing and implementing appropriate learning strategies, and evaluating learning outcomes (Knowles, 1980).

Shared-Decision Making: Shared decision making (SDM) is a collaborative process that allows patients and their providers to make health care decisions together, taking into account the best scientific evidence available, as well as the patient's values and preferences (Healthwise, 2015).

Telehealth: The use of electronic information and telecommunications technologies to support long-distance clinical health care, patient and professional health-related education, public health and health administration (HRSA.gov, n.d.).

ENDNOTES

1 Named for the Egyptologist, Edwin Smith, who purchased the manuscript in 1862.
2 The medical record was used for billing and administrative purposes as well; however that aspect of the evolution of the medical record is beyond the scope of this chapter.

This work was previously published in the Handbook of Research on Advancing Health Education through Technology edited by Victor C.X. Wang, pages 39-62, copyright year 2016 by Medical Information Science Reference (an imprint of IGI Global).

Chapter 23
Literacy and Decision Making on Health Issues among Married Women in Southwest Nigeria

Adejoke Clara Babalola
Obafemi Awolowo University, Nigeria

ABSTRACT

It has been observed that women lag behind in participating in decision making in Nigeria as the number of women in key positions is nothing to write home about. The study is set to determine the level of women participation in health related decision making and investigate the effect of literacy on women's participation in health related decision making. A random sampling method was used to select three states; and from the three states three Local Government Areas (LGAs) and from the 3 (LGAs) 64 to 68 eligible respondents were selected by purposive sampling technique, making a total number of 600 respondents. Questionnaire was used to elicit information from the respondents.

PRELIMINARIES

It has been observed that women lag behind in participation in decision making in Nigeria as the number of women in political and governmental positions is nothing to write home about. From the Declaration of the Summit of all women politicians held in Abuja on the 28th June 2002, it was observed that the marginalisation of women in Nigeria's patriarchal political system was not a new phenomenon. In fact, it dates back to the Colonial era where women were not even allowed to vote in Northern Nigeria until 1976, and it has continued into the Forth Republic. For instance, out of a total of 11,881 electable positions available during 1999 elections, only 631 women contested. Those that managed to win were a mere 1.62% (181 of the total positions) (Ibrahim and Salihu, 2004). Mejiuni (2012) citing I-IDEA (2000) stated that despite a comparatively large pool of well trained and able women, their absence in major institution of power and decision making processes is particularly striking. UNDP (2006) asserts that:

DOI: 10.4018/978-1-5225-1928-7.ch023

... women have long been under-represented at all levels of governance – as voters, candidates, party leaders, and elected officials, and illiteracy, twice as common among women than men, has impeded women's participation in the political process. Women still hold only 16 per cent of parliamentary seats worldwide. (p.7)

As can be deduced from the quotation above, another factor identified as a hindrance to women's participation in decision making is low level of educational attainment among women. Tsikata and Brown (2001) cited in Kwapong, (2006) stated that the level of education was a major influencing factor in women's level of participation in decision-making. According to UNESCO (2008), total youth literacy rate is 84%, total adult literacy rate is 69% while male is 78% and female 60%. In an online publication, Huebler (2008) while reporting Demographic and Health Survey (DHS) stated that in Nigeria, 55% of the population aged 15 years and older could read and write. According to him, more men (67%) than women (44%) are literate, and the literacy rate is higher in urban (71%) than in rural areas (47%).

The importance of literacy to the health of people especially women cannot be over-emphasised. Given the common recognition of the key roles that women play in fertility planning, infant care/nutrition and health education, female illiteracy can be seen as a major obstacle to health and social development. When a woman is literate, it is expected that it will affect the lives of her entire household. She is able to care for children and husband effectively, prepare for them good and nutritious meals and care for them when they are sick. (LeVine et al., 2000 cited in Wagner 2000).

There have been many studies that demonstrated that there are relationships between women literacy and health by many authors in different countries. Kagitcibasi, Goksen and Gulgoz (2005) examined the effects of the Functional Adult Literacy Programme (FALP) of the Mother-Child Education Foundation in Turkey on the cognitive, personal, familial and social spheres of the lives of women participants. The study revealed that literacy enables women to be self-sufficient in their daily activities. Programme participation contributed to improving women's mobility in the public and provided them opportunities for interactions. The study concluded that functional literacy was a powerful process of transformation, extending from cognitive to non-cognitive gains and from each participant to her immediate environment, and enhancing self-concept and capabilities to function outside the boundary of the community.

Another is the Women's Empowerment Programme organised for women in Nepal through basic literacy, legal literacy, and economic participation activities. It was designed to increase women's literacy, improve the legal environment for females, and encourage women's economic participation in the market. The programmes were based on the notion that women's education and empowerment allow them to become effective agents of change in their households and communities, which in turn enhances the well-being of their families and society at large. Women who had participated in the programmes reported an increase in self-confidence and greater autonomy within their daily lives, and they showed greater involvement in the care of children, reproductive management, and how family income was spent (76% of women surveyed reported using income to alleviate economic hardship in their households). Increases were found in women's involvement in collective community activities and social issues. Participants surveyed, ten years after taking the literacy classes, were found to be still engaged in social actions and income-generating activities, even more than those who had only recently begun attending literacy classes (USAID 1998 as cited in Wagner 2000).

Sandiford et al. (1995) cited in Robinson-Pant (undated) analysed the effects of adult basic education in Nicaragua over a period of ten years, and found a statistically significant drop in infant mortality amongst mothers who had participated in the literacy campaign as compared to those who had not. They also found that the reduced-child mortality rate of adult basic education was greater than for those who had been made literate in primary school.

To confirm this assertion, in Nepal and Bolivia, surveys of around 1000 women (700 adult literacy participants and a control group of 300 non-participants) were conducted over a three-year period. The study revealed that 'improvements in health-related knowledge and behaviour were greater for women who attended literacy and basic education programs'. Positive changes included: seeking medical health for themselves and their sick children, adopting preventive health measures, such as immunisation, and greater knowledge of family planning methods. Another example is in Bolivia, where increased involvement in decision-making in the households among women, who participated in literacy programmes was reported (Burchfield et al., 2002a, 2002b as cited in Robinson-Pant undated).

Also UNESCO (2008) gave the example of People's Action Forum (Zambia) PAF which applies an educational approach known as REFLECT, acronym for "Regenerated Freirian Literacy through Empowering Community Techniques" which provided education to community in rural areas where HIV and AIDS are rife. Through learning basic and essential literacy skills, people come to understand the nature of this pandemic and share the messages of prevention, care and mitigation." Discussing further on programmes UNESCO (2008) gave another example of a programme in Ethiopia, the "Literacy Plus" programme that target rural women and which has led to the increased use of malaria nets. These innovative and successful literacy practices show that when health is at stake, literacy has a major role to play.

An example of literacy education programme is the Adult and Non-Formal Education Association (ANFEAE) (Ethiopia) cited in UNESCO (2008), where a Literacy Plus Programme led to a lot of turnaround in the lives of the people that participated. One of their testimonies is that of Jabu Sithole who could not read or write and it was affecting the health of her children. "I have five children. Each child has a clinic card bearing his or her name. But if one of the children got sick, I did not know which card to take. I had to take the sick child and all five cards and ask the clinic sister to find the right one. The nurses laughed at me. I would delay taking my children to clinic because I was embarrassed and ashamed." But after just three months of attending literacy classes, Jabu could recognise each child's name – her life was beginning to change (UNESCO, 2008). Apart from learning how to read and write Jabu was also able to cope in Kwanibela, an isolated area deep in rural KwaZulu-Natal, South Africa, where there had been little rain, no electricity or phone lines and where only 26 percent of the population is literate, but thanks to The Kwanibela Project, an adult literacy project run by a non-governmental organization called Operation Upgrade, founded in 1996 (UNESCO, 2008).

Kenya launched its national literacy programme in 1978 to meet the needs of 5 million illiterates, increasing by 3 per cent annually. An evaluation conducted some ten years later determined that, in spite of the generally low internal efficiency of the programme, some 70 to 80 per cent of the learners who had received a literacy certificate had indeed achieved at least an average level of performance in reading. The programme had had "a positive effect on the functional knowledge, attitudes and practices of the learners either directly or indirectly. Adults who had completed the programme tended to know more about health, nutrition, agriculture, etc. than the illiterates; they had less traditional attitudes and put new ideas into practice more easily" (Carron et al., 1989 as cited in Bhola and Gómez 2008).

In the same vein, a study of a functional literacy programme in Turkey noted that 'reading even at a very basic level increased the mobility of women in the public domain' which in turn had an impact on accessing health facilities, as one participant described: "Once I went to the hospital. Doctors asked me to go to another ward. I managed to find my way. I managed to read all the signs on the doors and was able to find the ultrasound lab. I did not have to ask anyone. Suddenly I realised I can do things by myself" (Kagitcibasi 2005, as cited in Robinson-Pant undated).

Also Bolivian women who attended literacy and basic education programmes displayed gains in health-related knowledge and behaviour, unlike women who had not participated in such programmes; the former group was more likely, for instance, to seek medical help for themselves and sick children, adopt preventive health measures such as immunization and know more about family planning methods (Burchfield et al., 2002, as cited in UNESCO 2006).

A survey in Nepal found similar effects but was less able to link these to programme participation, because women in the control group of non-participants, like women in the programmes, had been exposed to radio broadcasts and other health interventions. In Mexico, women with no or low literacy had the most difficulty following verbal health explanations by medical personnel. Small scale qualitative studies have provided evidence about how literacy affects cultural beliefs which impact on health. For instance, in interviews with 36 women in two districts of Nigeria, it was discovered that literate women who had circumcised their daughters 'would not do so in future since further reading on the subject had sensitised them to the potential health hazards involved in the practice' (UNESCO, 2006).

The TOSTAN Basic Education Programme in Senegal was developed to improve the educational situation of villagers, particularly women. Its goals are not only to reduce illiteracy, but also to help the population to achieve health and self-development through the use of adapted educational materials. In addition to providing rural people with the opportunity to obtain basic education in their own language, the two-year programme also integrates elements of traditional culture into the curriculum and promotes community ownership and problem-solving to improve living conditions in the villages (TOSTAN 1996 cited in Wagner (2000).

The aim of this paper is to examine the effect of literacy on women's involvement in decision making concerning their children's health and theirs too in Nigeria. This study was therefore undertaken to address the following objectives:

1. To determine the level of women's participation in health related decision making;
2. To investigate the effect of literacy on women's participation in health related decision making.

Research questions:

1. What is the level of women's participation in heath related decision making?
2. What is the effect of literacy on women's participation in health related decision making?

THE SURVEY

The research design for this study is the descriptive survey. A survey design is one in which a group of people or items is studied by collecting and analyzing data from only a few people or items considered to be representative of the entire group (Nworgu, 2006). A survey design is use to gather information from representative sample of the population of interest. Surveys are used to obtain data from individuals about themselves, their households, or about larger social institutions. A descriptive survey is usually interested in collecting data on and describing in a systematic manner, the characteristics, features or facts about a given population. (Nworgu, 2006).Since all women in the south western part of cannot be reached, the study was conducted using samples of women from the population of women in Southwestern part. In carrying out this study, adequate and reliably sampling technique is necessary so as to be able to collect accurate information. Therefore data was collected from women in selected States in South Western part of Nigeria. Their responses to the items on the structured instrument were taken to represent that of all women in Southwestern part of Nigeria. Hence, the adoptions of the descriptive survey design for this study.

A random sampling method of selection was used to select three states namely: Osun, Oyo and Ondo. From each of the selected states, three local government areas were randomly selected making a total of nine Local Government Areas (LGAs) with at least 64 to 68 eligible respondents from each of the selected LGA by purposive sampling technique. 200 eligible women were selected by purposive sampling technique from each of the three states selected making a total number of 600 respondents all together. Eligibility for selection of respondent for this research was based on the fact that they were married or once married and had children. Purposive sampling method was used here because purposive sampling method allows researchers to handpick the cases to be included in the sample on the basis of their judgment of their typicality or possession of the particular characteristics being sort (Cohen, Maniom, & Morrison, 2011). Questionnaire was used to elicit information from the respondents to be able to cover a large number of respondents (Table 1).

DATA ANALYSIS

Data on literacy and decision making on health issues among married women in south-west Nigeria were used for this study. The quantitative data were analyzed using appropriate descriptive and inferential method. Having obtained the data from the eligible respondents, the data were analyzed using STATA

Table 1. Percentage distribution of sample collection procedures

Name of States	Frequency	Percent
Oyo State	200	33.33
Osun State	200	33.33
Ondo State	200	33.33
Local Government Area (LGA)		
Kajola LGA	68	11.33
Oorelope LGA	64	10.67
Ibadan North East LGA	68	11.33
Ife East LGA	68	11.33
Ayedire LGA	68	11.33
Ayedade LGA	64	10.67
Owena LGA	68	11.33
Ondo East	64	10.67
Ondo West	68	11.33
Total	600	100.00

Source: Author's work.

12 software. The analysis involved descriptive analyses in which distribution of the respondents was presented according to their background characteristics. The inferential analysis involved comparison of two variables (dependent and one independent) to establish the relationship that exists between them and to determine the significance of the relationship, and Chi-square tests were used. Research question one was answered using frequencies and percentages. Research question two was answered using frequencies, simple percentages and Chi-square test.

The Table 2 presents percentage distribution of respondents' socio-demographic characteristics. The respondents' were within age 25-34 (34.9%), 35-44 (34.4%) and 45-55 (15.7%) respectively. Overall, two-fifth of the women were into professional/technical/managerial jobs; 38.3% of them were traders;

Table 2. Percentage distribution of respondents' socio-demographic characteristics

	Variables	Frequency	Percentages
Age Group	15-24	54	9.0
	25-34	209	34.9
	35-44	206	34.4
	45-54	94	15.7
	55+ above	36	6.0
	Total	599	100.0
Occupation	Trading	230	38.3
	Artisan	39	6.50
	Health professional	71	11.83
	Farming/unskilled manual	16	2.67
	Professional/Technical/Managerial	242	40.33
	Domestic services/others	2	0.33
	Total	600	100.00
Level of Education	None	132	22.3
	Primary	150	25.3
	Secondary	158	26.7
	Post secondary	152	25.7
Parity (No. of Children)	1-2 children	202	33.7
	3-4 children	304	50.7
	5-6 children	94	15.6
	Total	600	100.0
Religion	Islam	180	30.0
	Christianity	410	68.3
	Others	10	1.7
	Total	600	100.0
Marital Status	Married	554	92.64
	Sep/widow/divorced	44	7.36
	Total	600	100.0

Source: Author's work.

11.8% were health professionals while others; (6.5%) were artisans and 2.7% of the rest were into agricultural/unskilled manual jobs. Fifty percent of the women had an average of four children, 33.7% of them had an average of two children while 15.7% had an average of six children respectively. Analysis by level of education showed that about one-third of these women had no formal education – 22.3%; one-quarter attended primary school - 25.3%; while 26.7% and 25.7% of the rest attended secondary and post-secondary schools respectively. Majority of these women were married (92.64%) with shared religious affiliation with Christians - 68.3% and Muslims - 30.0% respectively.

Research Question One

What is the level of women's participation in health related decision making?

To answer this question, women's responses to the questionnaire were analyzed and presented in table form.

In assessing women's participation in household health, women were asked about who usually make decision on health related issues in their households. The analysis in Table 3 shows that many of the women made joint decision with their husband (41.0%) on health related issues in their households; 32.0% of the women made self-decisions on health related issues within their households while in more than one fourth of the households, only men's (husband) made decision on health related issues within his household in south-western Nigeria.

To answer research question one, women's autonomy on their personal health was accessed. Women were asked whether they made personal decisions on their health and that of their children or their husband made decisions for them. Findings from this study in Table 4, however, revealed that about two – third of women still had their men (husbands) as the sole decision makers on their personal health related issues – 57.5% as against less than half (42.5%) of those who made personal decisions on their health issues. Conversely, about two-third of these women – 59.3% made personal decisions on their child's health in the study area.

Table 3. Percentage distribution of women's' participation on household health

	Variables	Frequency	Percentage
Who Usually Makes Decisions on Health Related Issues in your Households?	Self-decisions	192	32.0
	Husband decisions	162	27.0
	Joint decisions	246	41.0
	Total	600	100.0

Source: Author's work.

Table 4. Percentage distribution of women's autonomy on their personal health

Variables	Frequency (%) Yes	Frequency (%) No	Total
My husband makes decisions on my health issues.	344 (57.5)	254 (42.5)	600
I make my own decisions on my health issues.	438 (73.0)	162 (27.0)	600
I make my own decisions on my children's health.	356 (59.3)	244 (40.7)	600

Source: Author's work.

Still on research question one, the Table 5 assesses women's health seeking behaviour during sickness and pregnancy. The analysis revealed that majority of the women in the study area had a positive health seeking behaviour as almost all of them - 81.0% & 87.6% reported that they went to the hospital when they were sick and pregnant or when their children were sick – 87.6%. However, less than one-fifth of them displayed a negative health seeking behaviour as they reported that they did not visit the hospital when they were sick- 19.0% or pregnant – 15.3%; or taking their children to hospital when they were sick 12.4%. In addition, more than one-fourth of them prefer going to prayer houses during pregnancy – 26.3%.

The Table 6 explicitly examined women's autonomy on their personal health and child's health by assessing the frequency of men's (husbands) decision prevailing over their own decisions on their personal health as well as that of their children. Owing to the fact that the study was conducted in a patriarchal society, the findings showed that husbands' decisions always and sometimes prevailed on their wives decisions with regards to their wives' personal health as reported by 41.7% & 28.0% of the women as against only 30.3% of those who reported that their husbands' decisions never prevailed on their personal health. Only one-third of the women always – 32.2% and sometimes – 30.5% single handedly took personal decisions on their health as against 37.3% of those who have never single handedly taken any personal decision on their personal health.

Research Question Two

What is the effect of literacy on women's participation in health related decision making?

To answer this question, women's responses to the questionnaire were analyzed and presented as shown in table form.

Table 5. Percentage distribution of women health seeking behaviour during sickness and pregnancy

Variables	Frequency (%) Yes	Frequency (%) No	Total
I don't like going to hospital when I am sick.	114 (19.)	486 (81.0)	600
My children are not taking to hospital when they are sick.	74 (12.4)	524 (87.6)	598
I don't like going to hospital during pregnancy.	92 (15.3)	508 (84.7)	600
I prefer going to mission houses when I am pregnant.	158 (26.3)	442 (73.7)	600
My husband does not allow me to go to hospital when I am sick.	90 (15.0)	510 (85.0)	600

Source: Author's work.

Table 6. Percentage distribution of women's autonomy on their child's health

Variables	Always	Sometimes	Never	Total
How often does your husband's decision on your health prevail over your own decision?	248 (41.7)	166(28.0)	180 (30.3)	594
How often do you single handedly take decisions over your own health?	192(32.2)	182(30.5)	22 (37.3)	596
How often do you single handedly take decisions on your child health?	152 (25.5)	238 (39.9)	206 (34.6)	596
How often do you have to wait for your husband's approval before taking decision on your children?	344 (57.5)	114 (19.1)	140 (23.4)	598

Source: Author's work.

In Table 7, women's ability to understand appointment slips, medical forms, medication labels, patients educational materials and hospital clinics signs easily were tested. Ability to perform the task above will afford them the opportunity to take appropriate care of their health. Overall, the Table 7 showed that more than half of women understood appointment slips, medical forms, medication labels, patients educational materials and hospital clinics signs easily while about one fifth (20.0%) of them sometimes understood it easily as against about one-third (30.0%) of women who reported never to understand their appointment slips, medical forms, etc, easily. In addition, more than one-fourth of the women reported difficulty in understanding and filling out medical form.

The Table 8 revealed that less than one-fifth and about one-fourth of women in the study area always and sometimes had difficulty respectively in understanding direction on medication bottles (17.7%), written medical information (18.4%), completing medical forms (22.3%), and getting to their clinic appointment on time (13.7%) as well as learning about their personal medical conditions (19.0). However, more than two-third (more than 60.0%) of these women never experienced or faced any difficulty with reference to understanding direction on medication bottles, written medical information, getting to clinic appointment on time and problems in learning about medical condition etc.

The Table 9 measured women's self confidence in administering medication and following lab instruction correctly. Overall, 61.3% of them were always confident to take their medications correctly; 50.5% of them always confidently filled out medical forms by themselves; 58.3% of them always confidently followed lab instructions correctly; whereas, 32.8% of them always called for someone to read

Table 7. Percentage distribution of respondents' maternal knowledge and literacy

Variables	Always	Sometimes	Never	Total
How often are appointment slips written in a way that is easy to understand?	330 (55.0)	104 (17.3)	166 (27.7)	600
How often are medical forms written in a way that is easy to read?	318 (53.0)	114(19.0)	168 (28.0)	600
How often are medication label written in a way that is easy to understand?	342 (57.0)	108 (18.0)	150 (25.0)	600
How often are patient educational materials written in a way that is easy to understand?	306 (51.0)	118 (19.7)	176 (29.3)	600
How often are hospital clinic signs difficult to understand?	165 (27.7)	164 (27.6)	266 (44.7)	595
How often are appointment slips difficult to understand?	136 (22.7)	156 (26.0)	308 (51.3)	600
How often are medical forms difficult to understand and fill out?	162 (27.1)	144 (24.1)	292 (48.8)	598

Source: Author's work.

Table 8. Percentage distribution of difficulty faced by women in understanding medical information

Variables	Always	Sometimes	Never	Total
How often are directions on medication bottles difficult to understand?	106 (17.7)	120 (20.0)	374 (62.3)	600
How often do you have difficulty in understanding written medical information?	110 (18.4)	138 (23.1)	350 (58.5)	598
How often do you have problems getting to your clinic appointment?	82 (13.7)	132 (22.0)	386 (64.30	600
How often do you have problems completing medical forms because you can't read it?	134 (22.3)	104 (17.3)	362 (60.3)	600
How often do you have problems learning about your medical conditions?	114 (19.0)	96 (16.0)	390 (65.0)	600

Source: Author's work.

Table 9. Percentage distributions of respondents' confidence in following strictly medical or lab instructions

Variables	Always	Sometimes	Never	Total
How often are you unsure on taking your medication correctly?	102 (17.00	130 (21.7)	368 (61.3)	
How confident are you in filling out medical forms by yourself?	302 (50.5)	38 (6.4)	258 (43.1)	598
How confident do you fill you are able to follow instructions correctly?	346 (58.3)	44 (7.4)	204 (34.3)	
How often do you have to call on someone to read out hospital materials?	194 (32.8)	108 (18.2)	290 (49.0)	592

Source: Author's work.

out hospital materials to them as against half of them that never called for someone's help in reading hospital materials to them.

In Tables 10 to 20, the relationship between literacy level and women's participation in literacy related decision making were tested. It was necessary to find out if the level of education at any point has anything to do with women's participation in decision making.

The Table 10 presents the percentage distribution of women's participation by their level of education (literacy). The analysis in aggregate showed a significant relationship between women autonomy and their level of education (χ^2 = 197.078, $p < 0.05$). Thus, the proportion of women who make personal decisions on their health increased consistently with the level of education: no formal education - 21.9%; primary education – 22.3%; secondary education – 24.6% and post-secondary – 31.2%. In the same vein, there is no much significant variation in the proportion of women who made personal decisions on their child's health across level of education except for post-secondary education-27.4%. In all, about two out of five women with no education (40.0%) were prevented from going to hospital by their husband, however, this proportion reduced as women's level of education increased from primary (23.3%) to post-secondary (16.7%).

Analysis of the relationship between women's participation in their households' health and their level of education revealed a significant relationship (χ^2 = 46.5772, $p < 0.05$). The proportion of women who made self-decisions about their households' health issues slightly increased with level of education such that the proportion of women with post-secondary education who made self-decision on their

Table 10. Percentage distribution of women autonomy by level of education

Variables	Level of Education				Total	Chi2 /p-Value
	None	Primary	Secondary	P-Secondary		
My husband makes decisions on my health issues.	64 (18.8)	80 (23.5)	98 (28.8)	98 (28.8)	340	9.799 0.020
I make my own decisions on my health issues.	94 (21.9)	96 (22.3)	106 (24.6)	134 (31.2)	430	26.634 0.000
I make my own decisions on my children's health.	84 (24.0)	84 (24.0)	86 (24.6)	96 (27.4)	350	4.181 0.243
My husband does not allow me to go to hospital when I am sick.	24 (40.0)	14(23.3)	12 (20.0)	10 (16.7)	60	8.112 0.044
Total	278 (21.9)	298 (23.5)	318 (25.1)	374 (29.5)	1268	197.0708 0.000

Source: Author's work.

Table 11. Percentage distribution of women's autonomy on their household health by level of education

	Variables	Level of Education				Total	Chi2 /p-Value
		None	Primary	Secondary	P-Secondary		
Who Usually Makes Decisions on Your Household Health Issues?	Self-decisions	34 (18.1)	36 (19.2)	40 (21.2)	78 (41.5)	188	46.5772 0.000
	Husband decision	38 (23.5)	54(33.3)	52(32.1)	18(11.1)	162	
	Joint decision	60 (24.8)	56 (23.1)	70 (28.9)	56 (23.1)	350	
	Total	132(22.3)	150(25.3)	158 (26.7)	152 (25.7)	592	

Source: Author's work.

households' health issues was 20 percent point greater than the proportion of women in other level of education categories. Also, the study revealed that more than one-fifth of the women with no education (23.5%), primary (33.3) and secondary education (32.1%) have their husbands making decisions on households' health while only about one-tenth of women with post-secondary education (11.1%) have their husbands making sole decisions. In all, there was no significant variation across all level of education in the proportion of women who made joint decisions pertaining to their household health.

From Table 12, the analysis revealed that the rate at which husbands' decisions prevailed over their wives decisions significantly decreased with higher level of education ($\chi^2 = 18.9969$, $p < 0.05$). About one in five women with post-secondary education always had their husbands' decisions prevailing over their health while more than two in five of women with no education (26.8%), primary (30.8%) or secondary (23.3%) always had their husband's decisions prevailing over their health issues. Meanwhile, the proportion of women whose husbands' decisions on their personal health had never prevailed varied and increased steadily with level of education such that 16.7% of women with no education, primary (22.2%), secondary (32.2) and post-secondary (28.9%) had never allowed their husband decisions to prevail over their personal health issues.

From the Table 13, there exists a significant relationship between women's level of education and their ability to single handedly take decisions pertaining to their health ($\chi^2 = 79.3071$, $p < 0.05$). More women with secondary (34.5%) and post-secondary education (37.3), against those with no education (14.6%) and primary (13.6%), are likely to always single handedly take informed decisions on their health. Conversely, the proportion of women who had never single handedly taken personal decision on their health decreased steadily with level of education. The findings revealed an inverse relationship between women autonomy to single handedly taking personal health related decision health and their

Table 12. Percentage distribution of women's' autonomy on their household health by level of education

	Variables	Level of Education				Total	Chi2 /p-Value
		None	Primary	Secondary	P-Secondary		
How Often Does Your Husband Decisions on Your Health Prevail?	Always	64 (26.8)	74 (30.8)	56 (23.3)	46 (19.1)	240	18.9969 0.004
	Sometimes	36 (21.7)	36 (21.7)	42 (25.3)	52 (31.3)	166	
	Never	30 (16.7)	40(22.2)	58 (32.2)	52 (28.9)	180	
	Total	130(22.2)	150(25.6)	156 (26.6)	150 (25.6)	586	

Source: Author's work.

Table 13. Percentage distribution of women's autonomy in taking personal health decision and level of education

	Variables	Level of Education				Total	Chi2 /p-Value
		None	Primary	Secondary	P-Secondary		
How Often Do You Single Handedly Take Decision on your Health?	Always	32 (14.6)	30 (13.6)	82 (37.3)	76 (34.5)	220	79.3071 0.000
	Sometimes	30 (16.7)	66 (36.6)	34 (18.9)	50 (27.8)	180	
	Never	68(36.2)	54(28.7)	40 (21.3)	26 (13.8)	188	
	Total	130(22.1)	150(25.5)	156 (26.5)	152 (25.9)	588	

Source: Author's work.

level of education. The proportion of women with no education who have never single handedly taking personal decision on their health is 10.0% point greater than the proportion of their counterparts with primary education and 20.0% point greater than their counterparts with secondary and post-secondary education respectively.

From the Table 14, the study revealed no significant relationship between women's level of education and their ability to single handedly took decisions pertaining to their child's health ($\chi^2 = 9.2175$, $p > 0.05$). Though not significant, but findings still revealed that more women with primary education (25.6%), secondary (34.5%) and post-secondary education (37.3), compared with those with no education (19.7%), always single handedly taken inform decisions on their child's health.

Findings from this analysis showed that the proportion of women who always waited for husbands approval on any decision was significant and varied slightly with their level of education such that there exists 1.0% increase in the proportion of women with primary and secondary education who waited for their husbands approval and about 15.0% increase in the proportion of those with post-secondary education who waited for their husbands approval on any decision (Table 15). Conversely, the proportion of women who had never waited for husbands' approval on any decision increased consistently with women's level of education such that the proportion of women with no education who had never waited for their husbands increased from 8.8% to 44.1% for women with post-secondary education.

The Table 16 showed the percentage distribution of women health seeking behaviour with level of education. Overall, the findings revealed no significant relationship between women's health seeking behaviour and their level of education ($\chi^2 = 110.9514$, $p > 0.05$). The proportion of women that did not go to hospital (18.5% for primary; 25.9% for secondary) or take their children to hospital (17.1%

Table 14. Percentage distribution of women's autonomy in taking personal health decision on their children and level of education

	Variables	Level of Education				Total	Chi2 /p-Value
		None	Primary	Secondary	P-Secondary		
How Often Do You Single Handedly Take Decisions on Your Child Health?	Always	46 (19.7)	60 (25.6)	62(26.5)	66 (28.2)	234	9.2175 0.162
	Sometimes	38 (25.3)	32 (21.3)	34 (22.7)	46 (30.7)	150	
	Never	48 (23.3)	58 (28.4)	58 (28.4)	40 (19.6)	204	
	Total	132(22.5)	150(25.5)	154 (26.2)	152 (25.9)	588	

Source: Author's work.

Table 15. Percentage distribution of women waiting for approval on any decision taking and level of education

	Variables	Level of Education				Total	Chi2 /p-Value
		None	Primary	Secondary	P-Secondary		
How Often Do You Have to Wait for Your Husband's Approval before Taking Any Decision?	Always	18 (13.2)	20 (14.7)	56(41.2)	42 (30.9)	136	17.7823 0.007
	Sometimes	6(5.3)	8 (7.0)	50 (43.9)	50 (43.9))	114	
	Never	28 (8.2)	52 (15.3)	110 (32.4)	150 (44.1)	340	
	Total	52(8.8)	80(13.6)	216 (36.6)	242 (41.0)	590	

Source: Author's work.

Table 16. Percentage distribution of maternal health seeking behaviour and level of education

	Variables	Level of Education				Total	Chi2 /p-Value
		None	Primary	Secondary	P-Secondary		
Maternal Health Seeking Behaviour	I don't like going to hospital when I am sick.	26 (24.1)	20 (18.5)	28(25.9)	34 (31.5)	108	4.375 0.224
	My children are not taking to hospital when they are sick.	14(20.0)	12 (17.1)	22 (31.4)	22(31.4)	70	3.983 0.263
	When I am pregnant, I do not like going to hospital.	20 (22.2)	16 (17.8)	22 (24.4)	32 (35.6)	90	6.630 0.085
	When I am pregnant, I prefer going to mission house.	38(24.4)	24 (15.4)	38 (24.3)	56 (35.9)	156	17.736 0.000
	Total	98 (23.1)	72 (17.0)	110 (25.9)	144 (34.0)	424	110.9514 0.100

Source: Author's work.

for primary; 31.4% for secondary) among those who were educated did not significantly differ from their counterparts without any formal education (24.1% or 20.0%). Additionally, the proportion of non-educated women that did not go to the hospital when pregnant or proportion of those who preferred going to the prayer houses during pregnancy (22.2% & 24.4%) did not significantly differ from that of their educated counterparts who did not go to the hospital or preferred prayer houses during pregnancy: 17.8% & 15.4% for primary; 24.4% & 24.3% for secondary education.

Individual maternal understanding has been established as a pre-condition for better individual health care. The Table 17 therefore showed a significant relationship between women's level of education and the ease of understanding written appointment slips ($\chi^2 = 96.8542$, $p < 0.05$). More than one-tenth and one-fifth of non-educated women always and sometimes found it easy to understand written appointment slips. Whereas, more than one-fifth of women with primary, secondary and post-secondary education always and sometimes understood easily written appointment slips. Meanwhile, the proportion of women who could not or never easily understood written appointment slips decreased consistently with level of education from 41.5% for no education to 4.9% for post-secondary education.

The Table 18 examined the relationship between women's level of education and ability to easily read written medical forms. The findings showed a significant inverse relationship between women's level of education and their ability to easily read written medical forms ($\chi^2 = 9.2175$, $p > 0.05$). Only

Table 17. Percentage distribution of maternal knowledge and level of education

	Variables	Level of Education				Total	Chi2 /p-Value
		None	Primary	Secondary	P-Secondary		
How Often Are Appointment Slips Written in a Way that Is Easy To Understand?	Always	40 (12.3)	72 (22.1)	90 (27.6)	124 (38.0)	326	96.8542 0.000
	Sometimes	24(23.5)	36 (35.3)	22 (21.6)	20 (19.6)	102	
	Never	68 (41.5)	42 (25.6)	46 (28.1)	8 (4.9)	164	
	Total	132(22.3)	150(25.3)	158 (26.7)	152 (25.7)	592	

Source: Author's work.

Table 18. Percentage distribution of maternal knowledge and level of education

	Variables	Level of Education				Total	Chi2 /p-Value
		None	Primary	Secondary	P-Secondary		
How Often Are Medical Forms Written in a Way that Is Easy To Read?	Always	38 (12.1)	80 (25.5)	96(30.6)	100 (31.8)	314	94.2470 0.000
	Sometimes	22 (19.6)	24 (21.4)	22 (19.6)	44 (39.3)	112	
	Never	72 (43.4)	46 (27.7)	40 (24.1)	8 (4.8)	166	
	Total	132(22.3)	150(25.3)	158(26.7)	152 (25.7)	592	

Source: Author's work.

twelve percent and 19.6% of non-educated women could read written medical form easily, whereas more than one-fourth of women across all level of education always and sometimes read written medical form easily. Meanwhile, the proportion of non-educated (43.4%) women who have never found it easy to read medical form was twice the proportion of their educated counterparts across all levels of education who have never found it easy to read medical forms as well.

Ability to easily read medication label enables women to administer medication correctly either for themselves or for their children. The Table 19 therefore showed that a significant relationship existed between women's level of education and their ability to easily read medication labels ($\chi^2 = 72.1597$, $p < 0.05$). Overall, while only 13.5% and 21.6% of non-educated women always and sometimes read written medication labels easily, more than one-fourth of women with some level of education: 25.3% &39.2% for primary; 27.7% & 25.5% for secondary; 33.5% & 13.7% for post-secondary always and sometimes read medication labels easily respectively. Meanwhile, the proportion of women that have never found

Table 19. Percentage distribution of maternal knowledge and level of education

	Variables	Level of Education				Total	Chi2 /p-Value
		None	Primary	Secondary	P-Secondary		
How Often Are Medication Labels Written in a Way that Is Easy To Read?	Always	46 (13.5)	86 (25.3)	94(27.7)	114 (33.5)	340	72.1597 0.000
	Sometimes	22 (21.6)	40 (39.2)	26 (25.5)	14(13.7)	102	
	Never	64 (42.7)	24 (16.0)	38(25.3)	24 (16.0)	150	
	Total	132(22.3)	150(25.3)	158(26.7)	152 (25.7)	592	

Source: Author's work.

reading written medication labels easily decreased significantly with levels of education from 42.7% for non-educated women to 16.0% for women with post-secondary education.

Ability of the women to understand easily patients' educational material helps them to have more understanding about health related issues and also assist them in taking proper care of their health. The Table 20 therefore showed a significant relationship between women's level of education and their ability to understand patients educational materials easily ($\chi^2 = 98.0871$, $p < 0.05$). The proportion of women with some level of education who always and sometimes understood patients' educational materials was 10.0% point greater among those with primary and secondary education and 20.0% point greater among those with post-secondary education when compared with the proportion of their counterparts with no formal education. Meanwhile, the proportion of non-educated women that did not understand written patients educational materials was about 20.0% point greater than that of their counterparts with primary and secondary education, and more than 30.0% point greater when compared with the proportion of their counterparts with post-secondary education (44.8% versus 8.1%).

The Table 21 presents the relationship between women's level of education and difficulties ever experienced in understanding hospital or clinic signs. Analysis from the table revealed a significant relationship between women's ability to understand hospital or clinic signs easily and their level of education (χ^2= 26.4775, $p < 0.05$). About one third (35.2%) of non-educated women always found it difficult to understand hospital or clinic sign. From the findings, the proportion of those who did not find hospital or clinic signs difficult to understand across all levels of education was 10.0% point greater than that of their counterparts with no formal education.

Difficulties in reading and understanding appointment slips could prevent or hinder women from prompt attendance at hospital or clinics. The Table 22 showed a significant relationship between women's ability to understand appointment slips and level of education ($\chi^2 = 35.4140$, $p < 0.05$). The percentage

Table 20. Percentage distribution of maternal knowledge and level of education

	Variables	Level of Education				Total	Chi2 /p-Value
		None	Primary	Secondary	P-Secondary		
How Often Are Patients' Educational Materials Written in a Way that Is Easy to Understand?	Always	36 (11.9)	72 (23.8)	84(27.8)	110 (36.4)	302	98.0875 0.000
	Sometimes	18 (15.5)	30 (25.9)	40 (34.5)	28 (24.1)	116	
	Never	78 (44.8)	48 (27.6)	34 (19.5)	14 (8.1)	174	
	Total	132(22.3)	150(25.3)	158(26.7)	152 (25.7)	592	

Source: Author's work.

Table 21. Percentage distribution of maternal knowledge and level of education

	Variables	Level of Education				Total	Chi2 /p-Value
		None	Primary	Secondary	P-Secondary		
How Often Are Hospitals or Clinic Signs Difficult to Understand?	Always	56 (35.2)	34 (21.3)	32 (20.1)	37 (23.2)	159	26.4775 0.000
	Sometimes	22 (13.4)	52 (31.7)	48 (29.3)	42 (25.6)	164	
	Never	52 (19.7)	64 (24.2)	78 (29.5)	70 (26.5)	264	
	Total	130(22.2)	150(25.5)	158(26.9)	149 (25.4)	587	

Source: Author's work.

Table 22. Percentage distribution of maternal knowledge and level of education

	Variables	Level of Education				Total	Chi2 /p-Value
		None	Primary	Secondary	P-Secondary		
How Often Are Appointment Slips Difficult to Understand?	Always	50 (37.3)	36 (26.9)	28 (20.9)	20 (14.9)	134	35.4140 0.000
	Sometimes	18 (11.8)	34(22.4)	48 (31.6)	52 (34.2)	152	
	Never	64 (20.9)	80 (26.1)	82 (26.8)	80 (26.1)	306	
	Total	132(22.3)	150(25.3)	158(26.7)	152 (25.7)	592	

Source: Author's work.

of non-educated women who always found it difficult to understand appointment slips (37.3%) was about twice the percentage of educated women, across all levels of education who always found it difficult to understand appointment slips. Conversely, the percentage of women who have never found understanding appointment slips difficult across all level of education was 6.0% point greater than the percentage of their non-educated counterparts who have never found understanding appointment slips difficult.

The Table 23 showed a significant relationship between women's level of education and difficulty encounter in understanding direction on medication bottles ($\chi^2 = 24.6217$, $p < 0.05$). The result revealed that a significant level of difficulty was encountered by non-educated women (39.0%) and showed a decreasing trend in the proportion of primary or secondary educated women who have always or sometimes experienced difficulty in understanding directions on medication bottles (19.5% for primary; 17.1% for secondary). Also, the findings showed an increasing trend in the proportion of women who have never experienced any difficulty starting from non-educated women (19.9%) to those with post-secondary education (29.6%).

From the Table 24, there exists a significant relationship between level of education and difficulty encountered in getting to clinic appointment ($\chi^2 = 109.1324$, $p < 0.05$). The proportion of women who always and sometimes had difficulties in getting to their clinic appointment was higher among non-educated women (42.5% & 35.4%) when compared with their counterparts who had post-secondary education (7.5% & 7.7%). Meanwhile, the proportion of those who had never experienced any difficulty in getting to their clinic appointment was higher among women with post-secondary education (35.6%) and lowest among their non-educated counterparts (11.5%).

Women's ability to complete medical forms correctly assist them in pouring out all their health related issues which will invariably assist medical practitioners to understand their health challenges and

Table 23. Percentage distribution of maternal knowledge and level of education

	Variables	Level of Education				Total	Chi2 /p-Value
		None	Primary	Secondary	P-Secondary		
How Often Are Directions on Medication Bottles Difficult to Understand?	Always	32 (39.0)	16 (19.5)	14 (17.1)	20 (24.4)	82	24.6217 0.000
	Sometimes	26 (22.0)	32 (37.1)	38 (32.2)	22 (18.6)	128	
	Never	74 (19.9)	82 (22.0)	106 (28.5)	110 (29.6)	382	
	Total	132(22.3)	150(25.3)	158(26.7)	152 (25.7)	592	

Source: Author's work.

Table 24. Percentage distribution of maternal knowledge and level of education

	Variables	Level of Education				Total	Chi2 /p-Value
		None	Primary	Secondary	P-Secondary		
How Often Do You Have Problems Getting to Your Clinic Appointment?	Always	42 (42.5)	18 (22.5)	14 (17.5)	6 (7.5)	80	109.1324 0.000
	Sometimes	46 (35.4)	40(30.8)	34 (26.1)	10 (7.7)	130	
	Never	44 (11.5)	92 (24.1)	110 (28.8)	136 (35.6)	382	
	Total	132(22.3)	150(25.3)	158(26.7)	152 (25.7)	592	

Source: Author's work.

Table 25. Percentage distribution of maternal knowledge and level of education

	Variables	Level of Education				Total	Chi2 /p-Value
		None	Primary	Secondary	P-Secondary		
How Often Do You Have Problems Completing Medical Forms?	Always	76 (58.5)	28 (21.5)	18 (13.9)	8 (6.2)	130	137.7401 0.000
	Sometimes	16 (15.7)	32(31.4)	28 (27.4)	2 6 (25.5)	102	
	Never	40 (11.1)	90 (25.0)	112 (31.1)	118 (32.8)	360	
	Total	132(22.3)	150(25.3)	158(26.7)	152 (25.7)	592	

Source: Author's work.

thereby be able to give them proper and adequate treatment. The Table 25 therefore presents a significant relationship between level of education and difficulty in completing medical forms ($\chi^2 = 137.7401$, $p < 0.05$). About two third of non-educated women always have difficulty in completing medical forms. Meanwhile, the proportion of women who always encountered difficulties in completing medical forms decreased as level of education increased: (21.5% for primary; 13.9% for secondary; and 6.2% for post-secondary). Conversely, the proportion of women who had never experienced any difficulty in completing medical forms increased consistently with level of education from no education (11.1%) to post-secondary education (32.8%).

Result from this analysis in the Table 26 found a significant relationship between women's level of education and problems faced in learning about their medical condition ($\chi^2 = 127.1949$, $p < 0.05$). Majority of the non-educated women (60.0%) always found it difficult to understand their medical condition

Table 26. Percentage distribution of respondents' knowledge of personal medical condition and level of education

	Variables	Level of Education				Total	Chi2 /p-Value
		None	Primary	Secondary	P-Secondary		
How Often Do You Have Problems Learning about Your Medical Condition?	Always	66 (60.0)	20 (18.2)	20 (18.2)	4 (3.6)	110	127.1949 0.000
	Sometimes	10 (15.7)	32(33.3)	34 (35.4)	20(20.8)	96	
	Never	56 (14.5)	98 (25.4)	104 (26.9)	128 (33.1)	386	
	Total	132(22.3)	150(25.3)	158(26.7)	152 (25.7)	592	

Source: Author's work.

when compared with their counterparts with primary (18.2%), secondary (18.2%) and post-secondary education (3.6). As shown in the analysis, problems encountered in understanding personal medical condition varied and decreased consistently with level of education.

From the Table 27, forty-four percent of the non-educated women are always unsure whether they are taking their medication correctly or not. The percentage of women that were always unsure whether they were taking their medication correctly decreased with increasing level of education: 28.0% for primary; 20.0% for secondary; and 8.0% for post-secondary. However, as level of education increased, the proportion of women who had never been unsure whether they were taking their medication correctly increased with level of education, ranging from 15.4% for non-educated women to 35.2% for women with post-secondary education.

The Table 28 showed a significant relationship between women's level of education and confidence displayed in filling out medical forms ($\chi^2 = 44.7456$, $p < 0.05$). About one-third of non-educated women have never been confident in filling out medical forms compared to about one-fourth of women with primary and secondary education as against one-fifth of women with post-secondary education. Also, while a little more than one-tenth of women have always been display confidence in filling out medical forms, about one-fourth of their counterparts with primary and secondary education were confident in filling out medical forms as against about one-third of those with post-secondary education.

The Table 29 presents a significant relationship between level of education and women confidence in following medical instructions ($\chi^2 = 58.2462$, $p < 0.05$). The percentage of non-educated women who have never been confident in following medical instruction was 10.0% point greater than the percentage

Table 27. Percentage distribution of respondents' confidence in taking medication correctly and level of education

	Variables	Level of Education				Total	Chi2 /p-Value
		None	Primary	Secondary	P-Secondary		
How Often Are You Unsure You're Taking Your Medication Correctly?	Always	44 (44.0)	28 (28.0)	20 (20.0)	8 (8.0)	100	71.5508 0.000
	Sometimes	32 (25.0)	44(34.4)	36 (28.1)	16 (12.5)	128	
	Never	56 (15.4)	78 (21,4)	102 (28.0)	128 (35.2)	364	
	Total	132(22.3)	150(25.3)	158(26.7)	152 (25.7)	592	

Source: Author's work.

Table 28. Percentage distribution of respondents' confidence in taking medication correctly and level of education

	Variables	Level of Education				Total	Chi2 /p-Value
		None	Primary	Secondary	P-Secondary		
How Confident Are You Filling Out Medical Forms Yourself?	Always	40 (13.4)	70 (23.5)	84(28.2)	104 (34.9)	298	44.7456 0.000
	Sometimes	10 (26.3)	14(36.8)	8 (21.1)	6 (15.8)	38	
	Never	82 (32.3)	64(25.2)	66 (26.0)	42 (16.5)	364	
	Total	132(22.3)	148(25.1)	158(26.7)	152 (25.7)	590	

Source: Author's work.

Table 29. Percentage distribution of respondents' confidence in taking medication correctly and level of education

	Variables	Level of Education				Total	Chi2 /p-Value
		None	Primary	Secondary	P-Secondary		
How Confident Do You Feel You Are Able to Follow the Instructions?	Always	60 (17.7)	72 (21.2)	88(25.9)	120 (35.3)	340	58.2462 0.000
	Sometimes	6 (13.6)	20(45.5)	8 (18.2)	10 (22.7)	44	
	Never	66 (32.7)	56 (27.7)	60 (29.7)	20 (9.9)	202	
	Total	132(22.5)	148(25.3)	156(26.6)	150 (25.6)	586	

Source: Author's work.

of their educated counterparts. Conversely, the proportion of educated women who were confident in taking following medical instructions correctly increased according to the level of education.

The Table 30 presents a significant relationship between women's level of education and frequency of calling for someone's help to read out medical materials ($\chi^2 = 76.1237$, $p < 0.05$). More than one-third of non-educated women have always been calling for someone to help them read out medical materials compare with only 14.0% of their counterparts with post-secondary education. The proportion of those who have never called for someone's help in reading out medical materials consistently varied with increased level of education: 13.1% for no education; 17.2% for primary; 34.5% for secondary; and 35.2% for post-secondary.

SUMMARY AND CONCLUSION

The analysis above showed that many of the women made joint decision with their husbands on health related issues in their households; some of the women made self-decisions on health related issues within their households while in more than one fourth of the households, only men (husbands) made decision on health related issues within their household in south-western Nigeria. Findings from this study also revealed that about two-third of women still had their men (husbands) as the sole decision makers on their personal health related issues as against less than half of those who made personal decisions on their health issues. Boatema (2001) as cited in Kwapong, (2006) observes that women's lives

Table 30. Percentage distribution of respondents' confidence in taking medication correctly and level of education

	Variables	Level of Education				Total	Chi2 /p-Value
		None	Primary	Secondary	P-Secondary		
How Often Has Someone Helped You Read Out Hospital Materials?	Always	68 (36.6)	60 (32.3)	32 (17.2)	26 (14.0)	186	76.1237 0.000
	Sometimes	24 (22.2)	36 (33.3)	26 (24.1)	22 (20.4)	108	
	Never	38 (13.1)	50(17.2)	100 (34.5)	102 (35.2)	290	
	Total	130(22.3)	146(25.0)	158(26.1)	150 (25.7)	584	

Source: Author's work.

are constrained not only by unequal access to land and control of resources but also by their limited ability to participate in decision-making and to exercise autonomy in making decisions that affect them. Also Odufuwa, (2007) study on the roles of women in various decision-making in household private automobile acquisition decision-making in Lagos, Nigeria shows male dominance in decision-making. He further stated that empirical findings reveals that, women's socio-economic profile or background negatively impacts their ability to participate and be involved in household automobile acquisition's decision making. The implication of this is that men may not make decisions that will benefit their wives. On the positive side, majority of the women in the study area had a positive health seeking behaviour as almost all of them - 81.0% & 87.6% reported that they went to the hospital when they were sick and pregnant or when their children were sick – 87.6%, although, more than one-fourth of them preferred going to prayer houses during pregnancy – 26.3%.

Owing to the fact that the study is conducted in a patriarchal society, the findings showed that husbands' decisions always and sometimes prevailed on their wives decisions with regards to their wives' personal health as reported by 41.7% & 28.0% of the women as against only 30.3% of those who reported that their husbands' decisions never prevailed on their personal health. Only one-third of the women always – 32.2% and sometimes – 30.5% single handedly take personal decisions on their health as against 37.3% of those who have never single handedly taken any personal decision on their health. Husbands wield great influence on their wives to the extent that if they were very sick and their husbands forbid them from seeking medical attention, they would comply.

Fortunately, the study found out that the rate at which husbands' decisions prevailed over their wives decisions significantly decreased with higher level of education ($\chi^2 = 18.9969$, $p < 0.05$).

The study therefore found out that there existed a significant relationship between women's level of education and their ability to single-handedly take decisions concerning their health ($\chi^2 = 79.3071$, $p < 0.05$). Analysis of the relationship between women's autonomy on their households' health and their level of education revealed a significant relationship ($\chi^2 = 46.5772$, $p < 0.05$). The proportion of women who made self-decisions about their households' health issues slightly increased with level of education such that the proportion of women with post-secondary education who made self-decision on their households' health issues was 20 percent point greater than the proportion of women in other level of education categories. Also, the study revealed that more than one-fifth of the women with no education (23.5%), primary (33.3) and secondary education (32.1%) have their husbands making decisions on households' health while only about one-tenth of women with post-secondary education (11.1%) have their husbands making sole decisions. In the same vain, Asiyanbola, (2006) examined women's involvement in residential location/relocation decision-making among tenants in Ibadan, Nigeria found out that there is a significant relationships between the level of women involvement in residential location/relocation decision-making and their educational level, occupation, and marital status.

However, on the overall, the findings revealed no significant relationship between women's health seeking behaviour and their level of education ($\chi^2 = 110.9514$, $p > 0.05$). The proportion of women that did not go to hospital (18.5% for primary; 25.9% for secondary) or take their children to hospital (17.1% for primary; 31.4% for secondary) among those who were educated did not significantly differ from their counterparts without any formal education (24.1% or 20.0%). Additionally, the proportion of non-educated women that did not go to the hospital when pregnant or proportion of those who preferred going to the prayer houses during pregnancy (22.2% & 24.4%) did not significantly differ from that of their educated counterparts who did not go to the hospital or preferred prayer houses during pregnancy: 17.8% & 15.4% for primary; 24.4% & 24.3% for secondary education.

The trend noticed above is a dangerous one due to the fact that husbands' decision about health issues most times prevailed over their wives own. Also is the fact that there is no significant relationship between women's health seeking behaviour between their levels of education. This shows the effect of culture and ways of life on the health seeking behaviour of the women whether they are educated or not.

Implication for the Study

1. Unfortunately about two-third of the women still had their husbands as sole decision maker on their personal health related issue. This implies that most women are not in control of their health. Considering the high poverty rate in Nigeria, women who do not have control over their health may surfer as fund could rather be used for things the men considered profitable.
2. On the positive side, majority of the women said they went to the hospital with their children. The implication is a reduced mortality rate.
3. Husband's decision prevailing over the women's decision on household's health as stated in the findings is dangerous especially in a patriarchal society as Nigeria where the male sex is seen as superior to that of their male counterpart.
4. The inability of some of the women to understand health related issues like reading of appointment slips, administering drugs, etc. implies that these women will have difficulty in caring for themselves and children.
5. Fortunately, the proportion of women who have never allowed their husband's decision to prevail over theirs increased with level of education. This implies that education has a lot of influence on women's decision making on health.

Suggestions for Further Studies

1. In future, other researchers may look at the effect of literacy education and women's decision making on mother and children's mortality rate in Nigeria.
2. Also, the types of decisions women make about household health can be investigated.
3. This study can also be duplicated in other parts of Nigeria using a qualitative method.

REFERENCES

Asiyanbola, R. A. (2006). Residential location decision making and gender in Nigeria. *Geoforum, 37*(6), 1059–1065. doi:10.1016/j.geoforum.2006.01.006

Bhola, H. S., & Gomez, S. V. (2006). *Signposts to literacy for sustainable development.* Germany: UNESCO: Institute for Lifelong Learning.

Cohen, L., Maniom, L., & Morrison, K. (2011). *Research methods in education.* New York, NY: Routledge.

Huebler, F. (2008). Adult literacy in Nigeria. Retrieved from http://huebler.blogspot.com

Ibrahim, J., & Salihu, A. (2004). *Women marginalisation and politics in Nigeria.* Nigeria; OSIWA: Global Rights, CDD.

Kagitcibasi, C., Goksen, F., & Gulgoz, S. (2005). Functional adult literacy and empowerment of women: Impact of a functional literacy program in Turkey'. *Journal of Adolescent & Adult Literacy, 48*(6), 472–489. doi:10.1598/JAAL.48.6.3

Kwapong, O. A T. F. (2006). In their own way at their own level: Empowerment among rural women, the case of the Mo communities of Ghana. *Jenda: A Journal of Culture and African Women Studies, 8.* Retrieved from http://www.jendajournal.com/issue8/Kwaponh.html

Mejiuni, O. (2012). *Women and power: Education, religion and identity*. Ibadan, Nigeria: University press.

Nworgu, B. G. (2006). *Educational research: Basic issues and methods*. Ibadan, Nigeria: Wisdom Publisher Limited.

Odufuwa, B. O. (2007). Women participation in household automobile decision making in a developing economy-Nigeria. *Pakistan Journal of Social Sciences, 4*, 739–745.

Robinson-Pant. A. (n. d.). The Social Benefits of Literacy. Retrieved from http://portal.unesco.org/education/en/files/43483/11315414221

UNDP. (2006). Taking Gender Equality Seriously: Making Progress, Meeting New Challenges Taking Gender Equality Seriously. Retrieved from http://www.undp.org/gender

UNESCO. (2006). *EFA global monitoring report 2006. Literacy for life*. Paris, France: UNESCO.

UNESCO. (2008). *EFA global monitoring report*. Paris, France: Oxford University Press.

Wagner, D. A. (2000). *Literacy and adult education*. Darka, Georgia: UNESCO.

KEY TERMS AND DEFINITIONS

Decision Making: This is the act of choosing between two or more courses of action.

Health Issues: This can be defined as different aspects of health of women and children, e.g. children upkeep, physical, well-being and drug use.

Literacy: Here, literacy is defined as the ability to read, write and understand.

Maternal Knowledge: Maternal knowledge enables women to know more about their health issues and to take appropriate steps towards enhancing their health status. For example, ability to understand appointment slips, medical forms, medication labels, patients' educational materials and hospital clinics signs easily will afford women the opportunity to take appropriate care of their health and that of their children.

Patriarchal Society: This is a society where the male sex is seen as superior to the female counterpart.

Women's Autonomy: This is the ability of the women to make self-decisions about their households' health issues.

This work was previously published in the Handbook of Research on Advancing Health Education through Technology edited by Victor C.X. Wang, pages 191-212, copyright year 2016 by Medical Information Science Reference (an imprint of IGI Global).

Chapter 24
The Power of Collaborative Inquiry and Metaphor in Meeting the Health Literacy Needs of Rural Immigrant Women:
A Case of Parent Education

Al Lauzon
University of Guelph, Canada

Rachel Farabakhsh
University of Guelph, Canada

ABSTRACT

Rural communities often face the need to reach out to immigrant groups to help sustain their populations. However, rural communities often lack the necessary support and resources required to meet the needs of immigrant communities. This chapter reports on the role of a participatory education project in meeting the needs of immigrant Old Colony Mennonite women. Building on an existing ESL program in a rural community in Southwestern Ontario, a participatory health literacy pilot project was developed employing an action research format. With the participants, the authors explored the participant identified topic of dealing with the stress of parenting, using metaphors (presentational knowing) and collaborative inquiry. Post-project, in-depth, semi-structured interviews were completed with participants and program staff. Interview data was analyzed using a constant comparison method and five themes are identified and discussed: (1) reconsidering the nature of their children; (2) the power of language to transform; (3) modeling with language; (4) changing parental behaviours; and (5) normalizing what happens at home. The authors then discuss the efficacy of utilizing presentational knowing and collaborative inquiry as a pedagogical strategy for meeting the learning needs of rural immigrants.

DOI: 10.4018/978-1-5225-1928-7.ch024

INTRODUCTION

Canadian adult education has a long and proud history of working with marginalized people who have been socially excluded from educational opportunities and have developed innovative programs in the early days of Canadian adult education to address this exclusion: Frontier College, Farm Radio Forum, and the Antigonish Movement/Coady Institute to name just three. There is a long proud history in adult education of reaching out to those who live in margins of society. In a contemporary context, Canadian adult educators have reached out to the increasing immigrant population in an attempt to ease their way into becoming full participants in Canadian society. And while this is often addressed in the context of metropolitan and urban environments where most immigrants have settled, there are increasing numbers of immigrants settling in rural areas of Canada, areas that do not always have the resources to meet the learning needs of the immigrant population.

This chapter describes a unique rural based pilot project that attempts to meet the needs of immigrant women living in a southwestern rural Ontario community, and in this case it is a population of Old Colony Mennonite Women and the focus of the educational intervention can be broadly construed as health literacy. Specifically it is a participatory educational intervention that focused on the women's articulated need of being more effective parents.

We begin the chapter by providing an overview of the context for this pilot project.

SETTING THE CONTEXT

While Canadians generally have a high level and standard of health, it is not shared equitably across the population, and for those populations who do not have adequate literacy skills it can have a profound impact upon social and economic outcomes—key determinants of health (Health Canada, 2004). Rural communities have differed significantly demographically than larger urban centres on these key determinants of health, including levels of literacy, with rural communities being characterized by poorer overall health (DesMeules & Pong, 2006). In fact, DesMeules and Pong state, rurality in the Canadian context is now classified as a determinant of health. It has also been noted that rural women often face greater physical and mental health challenges than their urban counterparts (Leipert, 2005; McCallum & Lauzon, 2006). This is even further compounded for rural women immigrants who are faced with the responsibility of overseeing the healthcare of their families in a context where they lack culturally appropriate quality health information, access to services in their own language and the skills or confidence to question or validate their own health practices within a new culture (Jennisen, 1992). For rural communities who seek to attract immigrants to shore up their declining populations, being able to have the capacity to develop culturally sensitive and appropriate programs becomes a very important component of a rural development strategy.

Increasingly, there has been an emphasis on participatory approaches to adult education, including health literacy programming as this fosters participants' ability to think critically, construct knowledge and affect change in their lives (Auerbach, 2001). In other words, health literacy provides the skills, confidence and knowledge to make sound health choices, particularly among those who may feel disempowered to make such decisions. Thus health literacy is a form of nonformal education whereby its purpose is to help people be in control of their lives through making informed choices and decisions, and to take appropriate actions with regard to their individual health, health of their family and health of their community. And like the idea of differential health gradients for differing socioeconomic populations, health literacy programming needs to take into consideration variations in differing populations when giving consideration to program development. For example, Sparks (2002) highlights these differences, noting literate women in the context of parenting education rely upon experts and printed materials whereas poor and functionally illiterate women prefer oral traditions as a means of transmitting parenting information.

The project reported in this chapter is focused on rural immigrant women and their involvement in a participatory health literacy pilot program. The participants were Old Colony Mennonite women who have recently immigrated to Canada from Mexico, and who were living in rural Southwestern Ontario. We begin by providing an overview of the Old Colony Mennonites, their culture and history.

OLD COLONY MENNONITES

The Old Colony Mennonites have a long and geographically transitory history as they have faced periodic persecution since their inception in the sixteenth century and have made their home in Russia, the Ukraine, and the Netherlands and in the mid 1800s immigrated to Manitoba, Canada all in an attempt to "preserve a distinctive lifestyle" (Bowen, 2001, p. 462). Having always sought control of their own educational system—which allowed a grade 7 education for boys and a grade 6 education for girls—they immigrated to Mexico in the 1920s in response to Manitoba's *School Attendance Act of 1916* which prevented the Old Colony Mennonites from running their own schools. As Quiring (2003) notes, in Mexico Old Colony Mennonites were allowed to be landowners, were exempted from military service, were granted freedom in matters of religion, internal property and economic administration, and were allowed to establish and run their own educational system. Despite being very devout, the Old Colony Mennonites did not engage in proselytization strategies to convert others, but believed that the best way to influence others was through exemplary living. Rigid rules for 'living' were established by a church patriarchy and violation of these rules could lead to excommunication whereby the offending individual would be banned from "attending church, community functions, and from entrance to heaven (Quiring, 2003, p. 32)". In this sense the Old Colony Community had been rigid in its norms and values with very little tolerance for community members who did not subscribe to those norms and values.

As Redekop (1986) notes, the family has always been of central concern to the Mennonites, however there has been neither historical nor contemporary detailed documentation of Mennonite family life with most writings simply noting its importance, the size of family and their interactions with extended kin.

While Mennonites have a diversity of beliefs and practices with regard to family life, there has been a core set of beliefs that have endured over time. The marital relationship is considered to be a sacred relationship, a union of "heart and mind" premised on shared loyalty to God (Redekop, 1986). However, the marital relationship is embedded within a patriarchal social system whereby women were understood as "the weak sex and their role was to bear children and work silently beside their husbands" (Kulig et al., 2009, p. 326); women were primarily responsible for the domestic sphere of family life and Kulig et al. maintain this is accomplished through limiting their access to information to prevent them from questioning decisions. In many ways women's voices are quiet if not silent.

While children were viewed as innocent, they were also seen as having a capacity for evil (Redekop, 1986). Parents were responsible for being "vigilant and strict toward their children and not let their 'natural' love for their own offspring interfere with their Christian duty as parents" (p. 86). The old adage children should be seen and not heard, in many ways applies here. Parents expected and required obedience from their children, required them to complete assigned chores, and did not involve them in family decision-making. In order to keep children obedient, Mennonite parents are more prone than their Ontario neighbours to use marshal punishments such as spanking and strapping of their children (Redekop, 1986).

While education is often seen as a means of offering new and widened opportunities for youth that go beyond that of their parents, education in the context of the Old Colony Mennonite community was essential in protecting the community and maintaining its cultural isolation; its job was to prepare students for life in their community, a community that was isolated from the wider cultural world in which it was embedded. The school was run in conjunction with the rhythm of agrarian life, with schools running for six months of the year. The language of the texts in school is High German, distinct from their oral language of Low German, technically a West Prussian dialect, but one which incorporates some Dutch, Russian and some English words that the Mennonite community has encountered over the course of its history. High German is taught primarily through religious materials: the Bible, catechism, and song books as well as a primary reader, the *Fibel;* consequently some students are not truly literate upon graduation.

Over the past 80 years many Mennonites who have inherited farms in northern Mexico have undertaken secondary migration in search for new sources of land in southern Mexico, Belize, Bolivia, Paraguay and Argentina. Those who have not moved have found themselves on smaller and smaller parcels of land as it is further divided, resulting in the majority of Old Colony Mennonite families in northern Mexico owning only a minimal amount of land. This is no surprise given that the 6,000 migrants who left Manitoba in the 1920s numbered over 150,000 by 1997 (Quiring, 2003). As a result, many of the Old Colony Mennonites have traveled from Mexico to Canada and the United States, and especially to Ontario, to work as migrant farm workers to earn additional income. Repeated droughts in Mexico during the 1990s coupled with NAFTA and a low Mexican currency, and few forms of government sponsored social support have made life difficult for this population. In contrast, in Canada they experienced higher wages, provincial and federal social programs as well as support through the Mennonite Central Committee, offering an attractive alternative to life in Mexico. Subsequently, many Old Colony Mennonites have decided to emigrate from Mexico back to Canada and have been settling in Southwestern Ontario. And while many first worked in agriculture, after a number of years many take up other occupations such as construction, house renovations, trucking and in some cases developing small businesses (Janzen, 2004).

Berger (2004, p. 12) proposes that while immigrants may experience difficulty and conflict as they settle in their new cultural home, they enter into a three phase process that leads, he argues, to eventually reflect upon these two cultures, eventually developing "ways to function in their new reality by reinventing themselves and developing a new sense of identity". In this case, the Old Colony Mennonites have had to surrender some of their cultural autonomy and isolation as they are integrated into the host culture. Most men are not farming, nor can they afford farm land, so they have taken various jobs as have some of the women. Children attend a local school, and while there are Old Colony Mennonite schools within Ontario, for many families either the school is too far away or else they cannot afford it (Janzen, 2004). Furthermore, and unprecedented, many of the Old Colony Mennonite children are now attending a public high school. All of this points to a changing culture, a culture that seemingly can no longer isolate itself. This, from our perspective, creates a learning opportunity as adults and children grapple with new ways-of-being in the world as they adjust to a new culture, for many a new language, and a new reality.

A HEALTH LITERACY INTERVENTION

Adult education has a rich history and tradition of working for and with those on what we often call the margins of society, or those who Sauve (2001) describes as non-mainstream learners. This tradition is rooted in a core set of values that prizes the ideas of meaningful learner participation, inclusiveness, and ownership; adult learners, if respected, should not be the mere recipients or beneficiaries of the pedagogical efforts of adult educators, but should be actively involved in the decision-making. As Toso et al. (2009) note, adult education programs "should be a program of and by learners" (p. 151). This approach to adult education we call participatory education, an approach Campbell (2001[a]) describes as bottom up. Its purpose is to enhance critical thinking, active citizenship, autonomy and collaborative capacity (Toso et al., 2009; Sauve, 2001). Sauve (1987, quoted in Campbell, 2001[b], p.4) describes it as a

Learning/teaching process wherein all participants are involved in and committed to defining their own learning needs and wants, working out an approach …all within a context of making life better for themselves and those around them (p. 19).

Sauve (2001), in examining participatory education from the perspective of the educator, argues it is the "enabling of a group of people to name their world, recognize their potential to create experience, and begin working to fulfill that potential as individuals and communities" (p. 17). She further adds that it provides learners with new opportunities to identify "life-giving choices and developing the confidence and skills to act on them" (p. 17). This is accomplished through their participation in developing curriculum that arises out of the daily needs of their everyday life. It is, as Torso et al. (2009) describe, a life contextualized and dialogic education rather than the mainstream decontextualized and monologic education, approaches that Freire (1973) called banking education and Lave (1996) refers to as the acquisition theory of learning. A contextualized and dialogic approach to education allows learners to address real lifeworld needs while allowing participants to exercise their agency within the classroom decision making processes; this exercise of agency may then have consequences beyond the classroom. For example, Toso et al. (2009) report that in a participatory family literacy program learners were better parents, which one would expect in a family literacy program, but they were also better able to pursue their own personal aspirations; exercising agency in class appears to have transferred beyond the classroom and this may be a function, as Toso *et al.* suggest, of enhanced self confidence and self esteem. Prins (2008) affirms this in her literacy study conducted in rural El Salvador, reporting that active participation in a literacy program resulted in numerous psycho-social benefits (i.e. enhanced self esteem) and planted the seeds of agency.

As stated previously, this intervention is a participatory education pilot project that utilized collaborative inquiry, which is described as a powerful means of facilitating adult learning by supporting the critical subjectivity of learners that fosters meaning-making from their experience (Yorks & Kasl, 2002). In characterizing collaborative inquiry, Yorks and Kasl describe it as:

- Democratic
- Honours multiple ways of knowing
- Meets conditions for free and open discourse

- Links learning to lived experience
- Values action
- And is often emancipatory in its intent (p. 93).

Yorks and Kasl also argue that presentational knowing may play a pivotal role in collaborative inquiry. Davis-Manigaulte et al. (2006) have defined presentational knowing as what "happens when conceptual processes interact with imagination and intuition so as to enable learners to perceive patterns" (p. 27). They further write that:

Imaginal and intuitive knowing manifested in expressive forms is an important bridge between precognitive, prelinguistic experiential knowing and conceptual knowing, which is often referred to as rational or analytical knowing (p. 30).

They also maintain that metaphors are powerful forms of presentational knowing that provide a foundation for developing codified knowledge from experience. Cook-Sather (2003) has argued that metaphors are a means for learners to free their minds while Garner (2005) argues that metaphor is the basis for everyday cognition, making it well suited for programs that focus on the marginalized, such as literacy programs where the focus of learning is on everyday activities. He further argues, however, that the use of metaphor must be based upon something that learners are intimately familiar with in order to transfer their understanding onto the other concept which is unknown, or in some cases learners are trying to reframe their current understanding of a concept through metaphor. Morgan (1998) describes metaphors as the "primal force through which humans create meaning by using one element of experience to understand another" (p. 4). He further adds that "metaphors extend insight and suggest action that may have not been possible before" (p. 6).

Prins et al. (2009) have maintained that marginalized women—such as those in health literacy programs— benefit from the social interaction with peers and teachers in nonformal educational programs and play a "vital role in enhancing poor women's access to social support and in turn their psychological well-being" (p. 336). In reviewing the pertinent literature, they also note that these interactions are often associated with "decreased anxiety and depression and greater self-esteem, sense of control, and ability to survive with scarce material resources" (pp. 336-337). They also noted that it reduces the stress of parenting and of day-to-day family life. Collaborative inquiry, with its emphasis on women constructing their own meaning from their own experience, would certainly seem to be an effective means for fostering the psychological well-being of women participants.

Given the above, we developed a participatory education pilot project that was premised on collaborative inquiry with a focus on forms of presentational knowing, focusing on metaphors as a means for the women participants to construct their own knowledge, both individually and collectively.

This pilot project was piggybacked upon a Mennonite ESL program in a rural community in Southwestern Ontario that has been running for ten years. The ESL program is intended as a newcomers' program and responds to the needs of newly immigrated Old Colony Mennonite women to learn English and to have access to health professionals who speak Low German. The program offered is conventional in that both an introductory and intermediate ESL class is offered in the morning followed by a short presentation on various health/family issues by invited outside speakers which are translated as needed into Low German by either the public health nurse or the social worker that oversee the program. The program coordinators are also available throughout the morning to discuss confidential health issues with any of the participants in Low German.

In discussion with professional staff we proposed that we might provide some supplementary programming premised on the principles of participatory education; we had hoped through this pilot project to develop the capacities of the women themselves so that they could develop culturally sensitive learning materials and become engaged in educating other members of their community. The staff members were supportive and gave us an opportunity to present our proposal to the intermediate ESL class. We presented our ideas to the intermediate ESL class which proposed that the class work with us on a meaningful issue of their choice with a goal of developing a resource book that would then be presented back to the community for future use with and by other learners. We also hoped that in the future the use of this learning resource would be facilitated by the participants of this study. The entire class of 12 agreed to participate, however, four women dropped out of the program as a result of employment conflict, leaving us with eight participants.

The first class was spent brainstorming with the women and discussing possible issues that they might investigate and selecting one issue they would like to explore; they decided upon dealing with the stress of motherhood and ways of bringing the best out in children. The class met eight times over a period of five months and engaged the women in discussion of various metaphors as they relate to understanding children and parenting, and in sharing and discussing parenting scenarios (stories) from their experience followed by the collective generation of possible responses to those scenarios. The course culminated with the collective authoring and development of the booklet *Bringing Out the Best in Our Children* by the participants which was then presented to program staff and the community and has since become a community learning resource for parent education.

RESEARCH METHODOLOGY

William Torbert (2001) wrote:

Action inquiry is a research practice inspired by the primitive sense that all our actions, including those we are most certain about and are most committed to, are in fact also inquiries. Conversely, action inquiry is also inspired by the primitive sense that all our inquiries, including those we most painstakingly construct to detach ourselves as researchers, in as far as possible from biasing interests, are in fact also actions. (p. 250)

As practitioners and academics that operate out of a capacity development framework, the above quote is quite fitting. The pilot project described here is both action and research. The pilot project as described above was our action. What we describe here is our process of inquiry. However, it is important to note that while the intervention was participatory, the research component was not: the researchers set the research agenda and developed interview schedules independent of the participants from the pilot project.

From the beginning, we knew we were interested in what difference, if any, participating in the pilot project made to the participants, and how it affected them with an emphasis on how their understanding of children and parenting may have changed. To this end, we aligned ourselves with the interpretivist perspective for the inquiry component of the project. This seemed to best align with what we hoped to accomplish, given that it operates on the principle of individuals subjectively constructing their understanding of their reality while engaging in their social context (Merriam & Associates, 2002). Providing opportunities to explore the evolution of their perspectives allows participants to critically reflect upon the genesis of their current knowledge and their process of reconstructing and negotiating new meaning. The participants describe what is significant and meaningful to them from their personal perspective as new understandings and ways of knowing emerge.

In-depth, semi-structured interviews were conducted with the eight women who were members of the Old Colony community and had completed the program, as well as with the four staff members. The learner interviews took place in their homes over a period of three months; however, one participant opted to be interviewed over the phone, as she was not comfortable in having the interviewer in her home. All interviews were conducted in English, ranged in length from approximately 30 to 60 minutes, and were recorded and transcribed immediately following the interview. In addition to recording and transcribing the interviews, the interviewer made notes throughout the interviews. A translator was present during three of the interviews to provide clarifications as necessary.

Interviews were structured to flow as a conversation, taking the participants from their upbringing in Mexico through to their emigration to Canada, with a specific focus on parenting. Participants were also asked about participating in the project, and their thoughts and experiences related to producing the booklet. The interviews concluded by asking the women if they thought they had changed over the course of the pilot project, and if so, how they had changed. None of the participants were employed outside the home during the period of the study.

The four staff members (the nurse, social worker, and two ESL instructors) were also interviewed utilizing a semi-structured interview format. These interviews focused on their perceptions of the women and how the women had responded to, and changed, as a result of their participation in the pilot project.

Data analysis utilized a constant comparison method (Miles & Huberman, 1994), whereby interview transcripts were reviewed and themes identified. Participants and staff interviews were analyzed independently of one another. First, participant interviews were reviewed by reading through the interview transcripts to familiarize us with the dialogues. Then the first interview was reviewed to identify pertinent themes. Subsequent interviews were then read, using the codes identified in previous transcripts, and where data did not fit previous codes a new code was developed. Once all interviews had been coded, the codes were reviewed and, where appropriate, collapsed. The same process was then used to analyze the staff interviews. Once both sets of interviews were coded, a comparison was drawn between the women's self reports and staff's observation of changing behaviours.

FINDINGS

While the larger project did include examining the impact of developing and publicly presenting the booklet back to staff and the community on the participants, the findings for the purposes of this chapter will report only on the project and its impact upon the participants' perspectives and behaviour in terms of parenting, and the role of others in their learning. Given this, and our desire to let the women participants' voices speak for themselves, we have used staff voices sparingly while quoting the learners extensively. The themes that emerged from the data analysis are: re-considering the nature of children, the power of language to transform, modeling with language, changing parental behaviours, and normalizing what happens at home. We begin, however, by providing a brief overview of the women participants and staff.

Participants

The women participants in this project ranged in age from 21-38 and all have immigrated to Ontario, Canada from Mexico within the last two to ten years. All of them have achieved the maximum education allowed for women in Old Colony Mennonite communities—grade 6— and all have at least one child with one woman having 10 children. Six of the women are able to read simple English text fluently and five of them spoke simple English fluently. All of the women participants were enrolled in the intermediate ESL program.

The staff interviewed included the public health nurse and social worker, both of who come from a Mennonite background, speak Low German and have worked with this community for thirteen and five years respectively, and the two ESL teachers, one who has some Mennonite heritage but neither speak Low German. They have worked with this community for three and two years.

Re-Considering the Nature of Their Children

In the context of child rearing practices, nothing much had changed over the history of the Old Colony community. Simply stated, parenting was not reflected upon and hence for the participants of this program to reflect on their parenting was unprecedented. This process of reflecting, or looking at their children in a new way, was invaluably assisted with the use of metaphor. Many of the women reported that their approach to understanding the nature of their children and their way of interacting with them changed dramatically over the five month program. The use of metaphors triggered for many a transformation in their perception of their children, and children in general. As one participant told us,

I never thought that a child could be so beautiful and important until we looked at the rock with the shiny gems, I never thought about that.

Many of the women had been raised in large families which didn't acknowledge the uniqueness of each child. Children traditionally were viewed, even at an early age, as income earners on the farm or for the girls as caregivers for babies and housekeepers in the home. With many mouths to feed in an economically strained setting, the luxury of appreciating each child for their own gifts was not common, and when they began to parent their own children, the participants of this study approached parenting the same way as they had been parented. As one participant explained to us,

I never realized that there was a difference in children; that one could learn so differently from another and be so different from one another. We were always taught that we were the same... We would be punished for doing something different.

The use of the metaphor to assist with the process of reflection made little sense to the women at first. In fact, when we began to discuss the nature of children and brought out objects such as the rocks and plants to explore the concept of children, many of the women said such things as, 'Yes, children like rocks'. After exploring the metaphorical parallels between children and the various objects, the women's perception of their children began to change.

When we first talked about the seeds and the plants, it didn't make sense because most Mennonites in Mexico don't look at plants and then see children. Once I got it though, I started to look at my children differently. My parents in Mexico saw all children as the same. They all thought the same way.

For some participants, the use of the metaphor startled them into re-thinking their understanding of their children.

What really made my head turn was the rock with the gems and to think about it as a child and to bring out the best in them. I didn't know what a rock would have to do with that, I didn't get it, but now I do. I found that really interesting. I didn't think a rock had anything to do with a child, but I see that children have all this hidden in them.

The metaphors gave the women a chance to play with the analogy themselves and develop it as they thought more deeply about the nature of their children.

I liked those shiny gems in that ugly rock. Sometimes the children don't act that nicely on the outside, but are still beautiful on the inside; I liked that!

For others, the metaphor translated quickly into reconsidering the way they interact with their children.

I liked using the plants and the rocks and the seeds to talk about the children. At first it seemed strange because a plant is not alive like a human, but then I liked it. It helped me think about what to say to my children when they were being bad. It helped me not to get so angry with them, to think about what to say...I thought about how children are all so different and need patience; it made me think about how we have to take care of our children.

The Power of Language to Transform

Most of the women had been raised in large families with parents who didn't analyze the art of parenting, but instead simply coped with the stress of poverty with the noodles to make, the clothes to sew, the challenge of farming in drought condition all within the context of the cultural religious norms that guided their uniform approach to child rearing. As the women told us, there was not an emphasis upon softening one's language; often only the most essential things were said. This was how the use of language was modeled while discipline was used to shape children's behaviour uniformly without room for verbal affection, encouragement or appreciation of an individual child's unique gifts, needs, challenges and potential.

Many of the women recounted that in their family of origin experience, there was little verbal interaction between parents and children at all. Most often parents would be silent and walk away rather than praise a child; encouragement was not a part of the culture. For some of the women, encouragement became perceived to be like a nutrient to help a child grow.

When my parents saw something I did that was good, they didn't say anything. I think it is important to thank my children, to help them grow.

Many of the women lamented that they had not thought about the power of language earlier, however they seemed inspired now to infuse a spirit of encouragement through language with their children.

I never thought about how to learn to raise kids and bring out the best in them, though I wish I had earlier. I never learned that from my parents....I never thought about the way to speak to children, I had never learned it. I had never thought about how important it is to tell them how good they are.

When discussing the power of language to transform situations, many of the women expressed how much more carefully they now select words and choose phrases when they interact with their children.

I never thought so carefully about what I say to my children. I now think about what I say, more carefully than I did before. I am more patient with them. I want to do more of this.

Acquiring language within a context of exploring its role in relationship to something meaningful to them—their children—seemed to inspire the learners to re-evaluate their use and understanding of language.

Modeling with Language

Besides lacking a tradition of encouragement in their communication, many of the women expressed that that they never learned to be courteous within their families because it had never been modeled for them.

I was never taught about being polite; I never thought about how my manners will teach my kids. We never did that in Mexico.

Another participant told us,

If someone did say thank you, we wouldn't have even known what to say, because we were shy and we hadn't learned that, and that is horrible!

Now becoming more aware of their role as parents to model behaviour, they became aware that their own actions and use of language deeply affected the actions and language of their children.

Using language to bring out virtues was not something I ever heard or learned growing up. I never thought that language had anything to do with that. Sometimes I will say something and think that is not so bad, and then when I hear the children say it, I'll ask where they heard it and they will say, I heard it from you. I want the children to see good things from me; I don't want them to do bad things, so now I am more careful with how I speak.

Many of the women began to see parenting as a progressive learning process, one in which their children should eventually surpass them—especially in the use of language and in their knowledge and skills of parenting.

I love it when the small children speak kindly, so now I do it to show them. If we read about it, we can think about it and do it. I hope my children will be better parents than me.

While rethinking the role of parents as role models, the mothers still recognized that simply knowing what one wanted to do did not always translate easily into doing it.

Even if you know it, it is hard sometimes to talk to the kids the way we should. I want to be a good model for my kids, then my kids will be even better.

To become more conscious of the impact of modeling language challenged many of the women to re-think their patterns of communication with their children.

Changing Parental Behaviors

The lack of encouragement did not only extend to verbal communication; among the Old Colony Mennonites, demonstrating physical affection to children was also uncommon. When we discussed the importance of expressing love to our children, the women began to re-examine this practice in the context of nurturing their young "tender plants".

I think my mother gave me four hugs [A day? she was asked.] No, all my life. Hugging was for people in love.

Showing affection was considered only appropriate for courtship. Many women described how they now make a conscious effort to hug their children, because as they explained, until they observed Canadian parents demonstrating affection to their children and then discussed it in class, they never thought about its importance. When we initially discussed the importance of a minimum of four hugs a day as being important for a child's health, many of the women looked shocked.

I never thought that a child could be so beautiful and important. ... I hug my children so much now ... I never thought about how important it is to hug them many times a day. I think my parents would think they should have learned it too.

The participants also described changes they perceived within themselves and these changes took two forms: in terms of their actual interactions with their children, and their own self-perception. For the former, many of the women described specific changes in their behavior after the pilot program; changes in their level of patience, self reflection or strategies that they had never considered before. Many of the women began thinking about how they spend time with their children, how they communicate with them and encourage them to reflect:

Change, ya the group changed me. After, I started reading more to my kids before they went to bed, I tell them stories, and I think a lot more about how I can be a better mom. Before they wouldn't pick up their toys but now I talk with them and they are more helpful. I give them a choice and they do it. They are happier now and thank me a lot more too.

Many of the women utilized strategies such as giving their children choices as a means to help their children develop a sense of responsibility. This indicated a change in the way they interacted; they were becoming less frustrated and clearer about their role as parents.

The thing that really helped me was talking about giving choices; this was new and it is important for them. If I asked my boys to clean up, and they wouldn't I would just clean up for them, but now I give them choices so that they can be more responsible.

Many of the women described a change in themselves in terms of becoming more loving and patient; it seemed to be related to the different perception of their role as parents:

I think I am more loving with my children now when I am home with them; I look at them differently. After talking about it in our group, I find I don't yell at my kids, and I find we listen to each other better when I am calm. I try and model what I want to see in them. I think I am calmer when things get difficult. I am thinking about ways and words to calm down. I think I am a better person in that way.

The majority of the women described the changes in the interactions with their children as positive; none of the women described a frightening aspect of that shift, however as described by the senior staff member, this culture has traditionally resisted change.

They all changed in some way, but you know change is also very frightening. So much of their culture is about not needing to change—this is the way it has always been done and this is the way you are going to keep on doing it and some of these women are ready to move on beyond that and evaluate their approach to child rearing… That type of reflection is not encouraged in their community and especially for the women, for the women to do a lot of thinking—that is not the norm.

Despite cultural traditions, the women were indicating signs of re-evaluating their interactions with their children and changing the parent/child relationship.

Normalizing What Happens at Home

The collaborative dimension of this project offered these women a unique opportunity to share their perceptions of both the nature of their children and their role as parents. This was the first time they had to share the challenges of parenting as groups that offered support and new approaches to parenting did not exist in the Old Colony community in Mexico. In fact, the women were historically isolated from one another, having very little contact with other women beyond their immediate family when living in Mexico. And as we have seen in the previous findings, reflection on parenting was not the norm.

Normalizing what happens at home became a very key event for "freeing" the women to explore the nature of children and parenting. Much of this can be attributed to the frankness and courage of one woman to share the difficulties she experienced with her children that created the freedom for other women in the group to honestly acknowledge the parenting challenges they faced. As one participant told us,

I was surprised when Anna told us what happens when her son doesn't clean up his mess; I thought that just doesn't happen in my house. The other women know everybody has that problem and we talked about ideas. Now I don't get that much angry.

Many of the women described their impatience with their children related to feeling they were facing unique family situations and a sense of personal shame that their children acted in a certain way.

I often feel that other women are always doing a better job than me, but when we talked about examples at home and how to bring out a virtue, we could all relate to the same things. ...I liked how we made up examples together because it showed we all had the same at home.

The sharing of situations helped generate creativity together to develop strategies based upon their emerging understanding of the nature of their children. As one staff member observed,

I have seen many of them more eager to share, more willing to talk since then. It is important for them to be talking together about raising children and getting new ideas.

This also constituted the first time these women having shared stories and generated possible solutions to some of their parenting challenges, actively tried out the ideas of others. As one participant told us,

I liked the idea of getting more ideas from moms. If it is a good idea and it fits, I will try and use it.

Clearly the collaborative nature of this pilot project provided a wide variety of new resources—other moms— while at the same time removed the sense of isolation, frustration and feeling of being ineffective as a mother.

DISCUSSION

For the women who participated in the pilot project, the use of metaphors was essential to their learning. It was by looking at their children through metaphors that they came to see them differently. The capacity to view their children differently allowed the women to call into question the behaviours they used in response to their children, and redefining their understanding of children calls into question the underlying assumptions they have with regard to parenting. Hence the metaphors also helped them to reflect on what they had learned from their culture about raising children, which was learned mostly through the role modelling provided by their parents and other parents in their community. As Lakoff and Johnson (1980) and Morgan (1998) have reminded us, metaphors are pervasive in our lives and are the very heart of our thought, knowledge and action, particularly as it relates to everyday life (Cook-Sather, 2003). Clearly this is the case for the participants in this study. While it was not cognitively easy for the women to explore children through the use of metaphor, it did open up a whole new way for them to look at their own children, and children in general, leading them to recognize the importance of actively nurturing and encouraging their children, challenging their assumptions about effective parenting and a recognition of the transformative role that language plays in the parenting process. As a result, the participants of this project became very aware of the role of language in parenting and consequently learned to choose their words carefully when speaking to their children. The women learned and acknowledged that they needed to model communication patterns they wished their children to emulate; they needed to be a positive role model for their children.

The women, through learning to reflect on how they had "learned" to be parents, then brought this capacity to reflect on their parenting on an ongoing basis. This, coupled with opportunities to explore various parenting scenarios generated out of their collective experience and alternative ways of responding to each, provided them with an opportunity to develop a wider repertoire of behaviours to deal with situations with their children as they arose; within the context of parenting the women had learned something very valuable—that they had choices and choices requires reflection to differentiate between circumstances or situations. Hence the women were developing a capacity for reflection, a requisite capacity to having choice.

While the metaphors opened up a space for reflecting on children, and exploring scenarios allowed them to explore multiple responses to various situations, which ultimately led to changes in how the women spoke to and with their children; it also manifest in changed behaviours as women learned to question other aspects of what they had learned about parenting through being parented. One issue that emerged that we believe is significant, at least from our perspective, is the physical expression of affection. This clearly was not part of the parental repertoire of Old Colony culture, yet through metaphorically exploring the nature of children and their needs, the women came to understand the importance of expressing physical affection to their children. It also led to other changing behavioural patterns, including reading and telling their children stories, and giving children opportunities to make choices and decisions.

Over all, the participants expressed that through participating in this pilot project they were more patient and loving with their children than they had been before they participated in the project. This was also bore out in the observations of staff who communicated that they had noticed changes in the women's interactions with their children. The women who participated in this project have become, we believe, more effective mothers.

But the changes outlined above would not have been possible, we believe, in the absence of a supportive environment. Clearly a pivotal moment in the pilot project was when one member courageously shared what happened in her home with her children, opening up not only the discussion but giving other women permission to share what happened in their homes. This then allowed them to directly look at specific issues, to collectively identify strategies to deal with the common challenges of parenting and then try them out at home. As Prins et al. (2009) noted, the social interaction within a collaborative environment benefits marginalized women, enhancing their social support and their well-being. Certainly the women speak about how the sharing of these stories from home normalized what happens at home, allowing them to set aside their feelings of shame and erroneous beliefs about their efficacy as mothers, enhancing their psychological well-being. With enhanced well-being they were able to develop new understanding of both children and parenting, and consequently to change their parenting to be more nurturing, tending to their "young seedlings". And while the metaphors were powerful vehicles for the learning of individual participants, a supportive social environment that permits free and open discussion and sharing of experiences is also essential. While individuals were constructing their own emerging perspectives on parenting, collectively they were articulating a new discourse on parenting for their community that was embodied in their booklet *Bringing Out the Best in Our Children*. As a community resource and a resource that was intended to be used with other Old Colony Mennonite women in the community, it was an active attempt to transform the parenting discourse in the Old Colony Mennonite community in this rural Southern Ontario community.

CONCLUSION

This study sought to assess the efficacy of using collaborative inquiry and metaphors as pedagogical strategies within the context of participatory health education. First, using collaborative inquiry as part of the pedagogical strategy allowed the participants in the study to focus on something important to them from their daily life—parenting. In Toso et al. (2009) words, it was a "program of and by the learner" (p. 151)".

Second, metaphors were a powerful tool for making explicit assumptions as the participants in this study did with regard to parenting. It is also valuable for seeing specific phenomenon from new perspectives (i.e., children and parenting). In this study we have seen how these women were able to see their children differently and in doing so were able to examine and change their approach to parenting. And while metaphors can be a powerful means of learning and constructing knowledge, their effectiveness was enhanced by not simply being an individual exploration, but in this study it was a social exploration; the collaborative inquiry provided a forum for dialogue whereby the women collectively explored the meanings of the metaphors. It also provided a forum for them to share their parenting experiences and challenges, and collectively look for different ways of handling these situations. The results of this pilot project are that the women participants viewed children differently, they viewed parenting differently, they actively experimented with new parenting behaviours and subsequently changed the nature of the relationship they had with their children. And we can see as Davis-Manigualte et al. (2006) suggested, metaphors are a means of bridging presentational knowledge with codified knowledge and in this case the women were able to codify their understanding of parenting in the context that children's growth needs to be nurtured. And while this may sound somewhat obvious, this was not a consideration nor was it a part of the parental repertoire of behaviours these women report exhibiting prior to their participating in this pilot project. Furthermore, once codified it become a guiding principle by which they can assess their parenting activities.

Third, the women in this study developed a capacity for reflection; a capacity we would argue is a prerequisite to exercising in meaningful ways one's agency. Even in the context of the pilot project itself these women demonstrated a new found sense of agency that was not present at the beginning of the pilot project.

In conclusion, collaborative inquiry and presentational knowing through the use of metaphors are congruent with the goals of participatory education and in this case have been deemed efficacious strategies for bringing about significant learning and change for non-mainstream learners, and in particular may be appropriate for rural immigrant women as they struggle to make a new life for their families in a foreign culture. As rural communities seek to attract immigrants they must develop effective means for supporting their integration into a new community as they negotiate between their culture of origin and their new host culture (Berger, 2004).

As one staff member told us,

Their voice (as an Old Colony Mennonite community) has been a quiet one, and among the women it is even quieter...They are not used to being asked what they are thinking and sometimes they don't know. It hasn't been cultivated. They are not used to articulating it.

It is apparent to us that through this short participatory health literacy project these eight Old Colony Mennonite women have begun to find their voice and have begun to exercise their agency. As the staff member who made the above quote later told us, when the experts come in to speak to them the women are no longer sitting silently listening but are actively engaged with the expert, asking for clarification, questions and on occasion challenging them. This, we believe, speaks to the efficacy of this pilot project and participatory approaches to working with rural immigrants. While Canadian rural communities increasingly look to emigrating populations as a source to sustain communities, they also need active, involved and engaged citizens. This participatory approach to rural programming assists in developing the foundations for new citizens so they may play an active and vital role in sustaining rural Canada.

REFERENCES

Auerbach, E. (2001). Yes, but… problematizing ESL pedagogy. In P. Campbell & B. Burnaby (Eds.), *Participatory practice in adult education* (pp. 267–306). Mahwah, NJ: Lawrence Erlbaum Associates.

Berger, R. (2004). *Women immigrants tell their story*. New York, NY: Haworth Press.

Bowen, D. S. (2001). Die Auswanderung: Religion, culture and migration among old colony mennonites. *The Canadian Geographer*, *45*(4), 461–473. doi:10.1111/j.1541-0064.2001.tb01496.x

Campbell, P. (2001a). Participatory literacy practices: Exploring pedagogy. In P. Campbell & B. Burnaby (Eds.), *Participatory practices in adult education* (pp. 55–76). Mahwah, NJ: Lawrence Erlbaum Associated Ltd.

Campbell, P. (2001b). Introduction. In P. Campbell & B. Burnaby (Eds.), *Participatory practices in adult education* (pp. 1–14). Mahwah, NJ: Lawrence Erlbaum Associated Ltd.

Cook-Sather, A. (2003). Movements of the mind: Matrix, metaphors and re-imagining education. *Teachers College Record*, *105*(6), 946–977. doi:10.1111/1467-9620.00274

Davis-Manigaulte, J., Yorks, L., & Kasl, E. (2006). Expressive ways of knowing and transformative learning. *New Directions for Adult and Continuing Education*, *109*(109), 27–35. doi:10.1002/ace.205

DesMeules, M., & Pong, R. (2006). *How healthy are rural Canadians? An assessment of their health status and health determinants*. Ottawa, Canada: CIHI.

Freire, P. (1973). *Pedagogy of the oppressed*. New York, NY: The Seabury Press.

Garner, R. (2005). Humor, analogy, and metaphor: H.A.M. it up in teaching. *Radical Pedagogy*, *6*(2), 1.

Health Canada. (2004). *What determinants of health?* Retrieved from http://phac-aspc.g.ca/ph-sp/phhd/determinants/determinants.htm

Janzen, W. (2004). Welcoming the returning 'Kanadier' Mennonites from Mexico. *Journal of Mennonite Studies*, *22*, 11–24.

Jennisen, T. (1992). *Health issues in rural Canada*. Ottawa, Canada: Health Canada.

Kulig, J. C., Babcock, R., Wall, M., & Hall, S. (2009). Being a woman: Perspectives of low-German speaking mennonite women. *Health Care for Women International*, *30*(4), 324–338. doi:10.1080/07399330802694989 PMID:19255886

Lakoff, G., & Johnson, M. (1980). *The metaphors we live by*. Chicago, IL: University of Chicago Press.

Lave, J. (1996). Teaching, as learning. In practice. *Mind, Culture, and Activity*, *3*(3), 149–164. doi:10.1207/s15327884mca0303_2

Leipert, B. (2005). Rural women's health issues in Canada: An overview and implications for policy and research. *Canadian Women's Studies*, *24*(4), 109–116.

McCallum, M., & Lauzon, A. C. (2006). If there is no mark, there is no crime: Help seeking behaviours of psychologically abused rural women. *Canadian Women's Studies*, *24*(4), 130–135.

Merriam, S. B. et al. (2002). *Qualitative research in practice*. San Francisco, CA: Jossey Bass.

Miles, M. B., & Huberman, M. (1994). *Qualitative analysis: A sourcebook of new methods*. London, UK: Sage Publications.

Morgan, G. (1998). Images of organization (the executive Ed.). Thousand Oaks, CA: Sage Publications.

Prins, E. (2008). Adult literacy education, gender equity and empowerment: Insights from a Freirean-inspired literacy programme. *Studies in the Education of Adults*, *40*(1), 24–39.

Prins, E., Toso, B. W., & Schafft, K. A. (2009). It feels like a little family: Social interaction and support among women in adult education and literacy programs. *Adult Education Quarterly*, *59*(4), 335–352. doi:10.1177/0741713609331705

Quiring, D. M. (2003). *Mennonite Old Colony vision: Under siege in Mexico and the Canadian connection*. Steinbach, Canada: Crossway Publications.

Redekop, P. (1986). The Mennonite family in transition. *Journal of Mennonite Studies*, *4*, 77–93.

Sauve, V. L. (1987). *From one educator to another: A window on participatory education*. Edmonton, Canada: Grant MacEwan Community College.

Sauve, V. L. (2001). A personal journey into participatory education. In P. Campbell & B. Burnaby (Eds.), *Participatory practices in adult education* (pp. 15–30). Mahwah, NJ: Lawrence Erlbaum Associated Ltd.

Sparks, B. (2002). Adult literacy as cultural practice. *New Directions for Adult and Continuing Education*, *96*(96), 59–68. doi:10.1002/ace.79

Torbert, W. R. (2001). The practice of action inquiry. In P. Reason & H. Bradbury (Eds.), *Handbook of action research* (pp. 250–260). London, UK: Sage Publications.

Toso, B. W., Prins, E., Drayton, B., Gnanadass, E., & Gungor, R. (2009). Finding voice: Shared decision-making and student leadership in a family literacy program. *Adult Basic Education and Literacy*, *3*(3), 151–160.

Yorks, L., & Kasl, E. (2002). Learning from inquiries: Lessons for using collaborative inquiry as an adult learning strategy. *New Directions for Adult and Continuing Education*, *94*(94), 93–104. doi:10.1002/ace.63

KEY TERMS AND DEFINITIONS

Capacity Development: A participatory process that utilizes experience to collectively construct tacit and intimate knowledge.

Collaborative Inquiry: Inquiry 'with' rather than 'on' people, emphasizing the active engagement of participants as fully engaged collaborators who participate in determining the goal, direction and process of the inquiry.

Health Literacy: The ability to utilize health information and knowledge to inform health related decisions.

Metaphor: A word or object that describes a subject by asserting that it is, on some point of comparison, the same as the otherwise unrelated object whose delineation leads to insights and understanding.

Nonformal Education: Organized educational activity that does not take place in the formal system and is intended to achieve learning objectives for a particular audience.

Participatory Adult Education: Adult education characterized by learner control and ownership over the learning objectives, learning processes, and learning outcomes which are usually facilitated by someone outside the learner group.

Presentational Knowing: An intuitive grasp of patterns and wholes.

This work was previously published in the Handbook of Research on Adult and Community Health Education edited by Victor C. X. Wang, pages 51-67, copyright year 2014 by Medical Information Science Reference (an imprint of IGI Global).

Index

M

N

O

P

Q

R

S

T

U

W

CPSIA information can be obtained
at www.ICGtesting.com
Printed in the USA
BVOW07*0022210417
481343BV00007B/78/P

9 781522 519